Infective Endocarditis
A Multidisciplinary Approach

感染性心内膜炎多学科诊疗

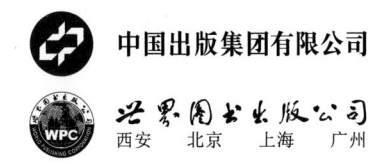

主　编　[美]阿尔曼·科里克（Arman Kilic）

简旭华　译

中国出版集团有限公司

世界图书出版公司
西安　北京　上海　广州

图书在版编目（CIP）数据

感染性心内膜炎多学科诊疗 /（美）阿尔曼·科里克（Arman Kilic）主编；简旭华译 . -- 西安：世界图书出版西安有限公司，2025.4. -- ISBN 978-7-5232-2003-0

Ⅰ . R542.4

中国国家版本馆 CIP 数据核字第 2025F5Q729 号

Infective Endocarditis: A Multidisciplinary Approach
Arman Kilic
ISBN: 9780128206577
Copyright © 2022 Elsevier Inc. All rights reserved.
Authorized Chinese translation published by World Publishing Xi'an Corporation Limited.

《感染性心内膜炎多学科诊疗》（简旭华 译）
ISBN: 9787523220030
Copyright © Elsevier Inc. and World Publishing Xi'an Corporation Limited. All rights reserved.
No part of this publication may be reproduced or transmitted in any form or by any means, electronic or mechanical, including photocopying, recording, or any information storage and retrieval system, without permission in writing from Elsevier Inc. Details on how to seek permission, further information about the Elsevier's permissions policies and arrangements with organizations such as the Copyright Clearance Center and the Copyright Licensing Agency, can be found at our website: www.elsevier.com/permissions.
This book and the individual contributions contained in it are protected under copyright by Elsevier Inc. and World Publishing Xi'an Corporation Limited (other than as may be noted herein).

This edition of Infective Endocarditis: A Multidisciplinary Approach is published by World Publishing Xi'an Corporation Limited under arrangement with ELSEVIER INC.
This edition is authorized for sale in Mainland of China only, excluding Hong Kong, Macau and Taiwan. Unauthorized export of this edition is a violation of the Copyright Act. Violation of this Law is subject to Civil and Criminal Penalties.

本版由 ELSEVIER INC. 授权世界图书出版西安有限公司在中国大陆地区（不包括香港、澳门以及台湾地区）出版发行。
本版仅限在中国大陆地区（不包括香港、澳门以及台湾地区）出版及标价销售。未经许可之出口，视为违反著作权法，将受民事及刑事法律之制裁。
本书封底贴有 Elsevier 防伪标签，无标签者不得销售。

注　意

本书涉及领域的知识和实践标准在不断变化。新的研究和经验拓展我们的理解，因此须对研究方法、专业实践或医疗方法作出调整。从业者和研究人员必须始终依靠自身经验和知识来评估和使用本书中提到的所有信息、方法、化合物或本书中描述的实验。在使用这些信息或方法时，他们应注意自身和他人的安全，包括注意他们负有专业责任的当事人的安全。在法律允许的最大范围内，爱思唯尔、译文的原文作者、原文编辑及原文内容提供者均不对因产品责任、疏忽或其他人身或财产伤害及（或）损失承担责任，亦不对由于使用或操作文中提到的方法、产品、说明或思想而导致的人身或财产伤害及（或）损失承担责任。

书　　名	感染性心内膜炎多学科诊疗
	GANRANXING XINNEIMOYAN DUOXUEKE ZHENLIAO
主　　编	[美]阿尔曼·科里克（Arman Kilic）
译　　者	简旭华
责任编辑	马可为
装帧设计	新纪元文化传播
出版发行	世界图书出版西安有限公司
地　　址	西安市雁塔区曲江新区汇新路 355 号
邮　　编	710061
电　　话	029-87214941　029-87233647（市场营销部）
	029-87234767（总编室）
网　　址	http://www.wpcxa.com
邮　　箱	xast@wpcxa.com
经　　销	新华书店
印　　刷	西安雁展印务有限公司
开　　本	787mm×1092mm　1/16
印　　张	20.75
字　　数	390 千字
版次印次	2025 年 4 月第 1 版　2025 年 4 月第 1 次印刷
版权登记	25-2025-030
国际书号	ISBN 978-7-5232-2003-0
定　　价	218.00 元

医学投稿　xastyx@163.com　‖　029-87279745　029-87285296
☆如有印装错误，请寄回本公司更换☆

主编简介 Editor

阿尔曼·科里克
ARMAN KILIC
John M. Kratz Endowed Chair in Cardiac Surgery
Associate Professor of Surgery
Surgical Director, Heart Failure and Heart Transplant Program
Director, Harvey and Marcia Schiller Surgical Innovation Center
Division of Cardiothoracic Surgery
Department of Surgery
Medical University of South Carolina
Charleston, SC, United States

原著作者 Contributors

Abdul Rahman Akkawi Heart and Vascular Institute, University of Pittsburgh Medical Center, Pittsburgh, PA, United States

M. Almela Microbiology Service, Hospital Clinic-IDIBAPS, University of Barcelona, Barcelona, Spain

Andrea Amabile Division of Cardiac Surgery, Yale School of Medicine, New Haven, CT, United States

J. Ambrosioni Infectious Diseases Service, Hospital Clinic-IDIBAPS, University of Barcelona, Barcelona, Spain

George J. Arnaoutakis Division of Thoracic and Cardiovascular Surgery, University of Florida, Gainesville, FL, United States

Hamza Aziz The Johns Hopkins Hospital, Baltimore, MD, United States

Cayley Bowles Department of Cardiothoracic Surgery, Stanford University School of Medicine, Stanford, CA, United States

Paul Brocklebank Division of Cardiothoracic Surgery, Medical University of South Carolina, Charleston, SC, United States

N.E. Bruun Department of Cardiology, Zealand University Hospital, Roskilde, Denmark

Edwin Chen Department of Internal Medicine, Division of Infectious Disease, University of Pittsburgh Medical Center, Pittsburgh, PA, Unites States

Abby L. Chiappelli University of Pittsburgh Medical Center, Pittsburgh, PA, United States

Sung-Min Cho Division of Neurocritical Care, Departments of Neurology, Neurosurgery, Anesthesiology and Critical Care Medicine, Johns Hopkins University School of Medicine, Baltimore, MD, United States; Neuroscience Critical Care Division, Departments of Anesthesiology and Critical Care Medicine, Neurology, and Neurosurgery, Johns Hopkins School of Medicine Baltimore, MD, United States

Chun Woo Choi Division of Cardiac Surgery, Cardiovascular Surgical Intensive Care, Department of Surgery, Heart and Vascular Institute, Johns Hopkins University School of Medicine, Baltimore, MD, United States

A. Dahl Infectious Diseases Service, Hospital Clinic-IDIBAPS, University of Barcelona, Barcelona, Spain; Department of Cardiology, Herlev Gentofte University Hospital, Herlev, Denmark

Laurent de Kerchove Division of Cardiothoracic and Vascular Surgery, Cliniques Universitaires Saint-Luc, Brussels, Belgium; Pôle de Recherche Cardiovasculaire, Institut de Recherche Expérimentale et Clinique (IREC), Université Catholique de Louvain, Brussels, Belgium

Sami El-Dalati Division of Infectious Diseases, University of Pittsburgh Medical Center, Pittsburgh, PA, United States

Cetin Erol Ankara University School of Medicine, Cardiology Department, Samanpazari, Ankara, Turkey

N. A. Mark Estes, III Heart and Vascular Institute, University of Pittsburgh Medical Center, Pittsburgh, PA, United States

Eric W. Etchill Division of Cardiac Surgery, Department of Surgery, Johns Hopkins Hospital, Baltimore, MD, United States

C. Falces Cardiovascular Institute, Hospital Clinic-IDIBAPS, University of Barcelona, Barcelona, Spain

Lloyd M. Felmly Medical University of South Carolina, Charleston, SC, United States; Division of Cardiothoracic Surgery, Department of Surgery, Medical University of South Carolina, Charleston, SC, United States

Carolyn R. Fernandes Division of Infectious Diseases, Department of Medicine, University of Pittsburgh School of Medicine, Pittsburgh, PA, United States; University of Pittsburgh Medical Center, Pittsburgh, PA, United States

Shinichi Fukuhara University of Michigan Health Systems, Ann Arbor, MI, United States

D. Fuster Nuclear Medicine Service, Hospital Clinic-IDIBAPS, University of Barcelona, Barcelona, Spain

D. García-Pares Infectious Diseases Service, Hospital Clinic-IDIBAPS, University of Barcelona, Barcelona, Spain; Internal Medicine Service, Clinica Sagrada Familia, Barcelona, Spain

C. García de la Maria Infectious Diseases Service, Hospital Clinic-IDIBAPS, University of Barcelona, Barcelona, Spain

Arnar Geirsson Division of Cardiac Surgery, Yale School of Medicine, New Haven, CT, United States

Katherine A. Giuliano Division of Cardiac Surgery, Department of Surgery, Johns Hopkins Hospital, Baltimore, MD, United States

Corbin E. Goerlich The Johns Hopkins Hospital, Baltimore, MD, United States

Priya Gopalan University of Pittsburgh Medical Center, Pittsburgh, PA, United States

Thomas Gossios Department of Cardiology, St Thomas' Hospital, London, United Kingdom

M. Hernandez-Meneses Infectious Diseases Service, Hospital Clinic-IDIBAPS, University of Barcelona, Barcelona, Spain

William Hiesinger Department of Cardiothoracic Surgery, Stanford University School of Medicine, Stanford, CA, United States

Edward T. Horn University of Pittsburgh School of Pharmacy, Pittsburgh, PA, United States

Elizabeth Hovis University of Pittsburgh Medical Center, Pittsburgh, PA, United States

Lauren V. Huckaby University of Pittsburgh Medical Center, Pittsburgh, PA, United States

Alex Israel University of Pittsburgh Medical Center, Pittsburgh, PA, United States

Cansin Tulunay Kaya Ankara University School of Medicine, Cardiology Department, Samanpazari, Ankara, Turkey

Maxwell Kilcoyne Division of Cardiothoracic Surgery, Medical University of South Carolina, Charleston, SC, United States

Arman Kilic John M. Kratz Endowed Chair in Cardiac Surgery, Medical University of South Carolina and Surgical Director of the Heart Failure and Heart Transplant Program, Charleston, SA, United States; Division of Cardiothoracic Surgery, Medical University of South Carolina, Charleston, SC, United States

Ahmet Kilic The Johns Hopkins Hospital, Baltimore, MD, United States

Sui Kwong Li Division of Infectious Diseases, Department of Medicine, University of Pittsburgh School of Medicine, Pittsburgh, PA, United States; University of Pittsburgh Medical Center, Pittsburgh, PA, United States

Nicholas Marschalk Department of Internal Medicine, Division of Infectious Disease, University of Pittsburgh Medical Center, Pittsburgh, PA, Unites States

Shayna McEnteggart Heart and Vascular Institute, University of Pittsburgh Medical Center, Pittsburgh, PA, United States

Lauren B. McKibben University of Pittsburgh Medical Center, Pittsburgh, PA, United States

J.M. Miro Infectious Diseases Service, Hospital Clinic-IDIBAPS, University of Barcelona, Barcelona, Spain

A. Moreno Infectious Diseases Service, Hospital Clinic-IDIBAPS, University of Barcelona, Barcelona, Spain

Makoto Mori Division of Cardiac Surgery, Yale School of Medicine, New Haven, CT, United States

Sowmya Nanjappa Division of Infectious Diseases, Department of Medicine, University of Pittsburgh School of Medicine, Pittsburgh, PA, United States; University of Pittsburgh Medical Center, Pittsburgh, PA, United States

Chukudi Onyeukwu Heart and Vascular Institute, University of Pittsburgh Medical Center, Pittsburgh, PA, United States

Christian O. Perez Division of Infectious Diseases, Department of Medicine, University of Pittsburgh School of Medicine, Pittsburgh, PA, United States; University of Pittsburgh Medical Center, Pittsburgh, PA, United States

J.M. Pericàs Infectious Diseases Service, Hospital Clinic-IDIBAPS, University of Barcelona, Barcelona, Spain

A. Perissinotti Nuclear Medicine Service, Hospital Clinic-IDIBAPS, University of Barcelona, Barcelona, Spain

Bernard Prendergast Department of Cardiology, St Thomas' Hospital, London, United Kingdom

E. Quintana Cardiovascular Institute, Hospital Clinic-IDIBAPS, University of Barcelona, Barcelona, Spain

Ronak Rajani Department of Cardiology, St Thomas' Hospital, London, United Kingdom

Hariharan Regunath University of Missouri, Columbia, MO, United States

Ryan M. Rivosecchi University of Pittsburgh Medical Center, Pittsburgh, PA, United States

Robert M. Sade Medical University of South Carolina, Charleston, SC, United States; Division of Cardiothoracic Surgery, Department of Surgery, Medical University of South Carolina, Charleston, SC, United States

E. Sandoval Cardiovascular Institute, Hospital Clinic-IDIBAPS, University of Barcelona, Barcelona, Spain

Neel Shah Department of Internal Medicine, Division of Infectious Disease, University of Pittsburgh Medical Center, Pittsburgh, PA, Unites States

Alaa Shalaby Heart and Vascular Institute, University of Pittsburgh Medical Center, Pittsburgh, PA, United States

Neeta Shenai University of Pittsburgh Medical Center, Pittsburgh, PA, United States

Brandon J. Smith Department of Internal Medicine, Division of Infectious Disease, University of Pittsburgh Medical Center, Pittsburgh, PA, Unites States; University of Pittsburgh Medical Center, Pittsburgh, PA, United States

Jessica Snawerdt AdventHealth Celebration, Kissimmee, FL, United States

Silvia Solari Division of Cardiothoracic and Vascular Surgery, Cliniques Universitaires Saint-Luc, Brussels, Belgium

Matthew Suffoletto Department of Medicine, University of Pittsburgh, Pittsburgh, PA, United States

Lise Tchouta Columbia University Medical Center, New York City, NY, United States

J.M. Tolosana Cardiovascular Institute, Hospital Clinic-IDIBAPS, University of Barcelona, Barcelona, Spain

Tamara L. Trienski Allegheny General Hospital, Pittsburgh, PA, United States

Ken Uchino Cerebrovascular Center, Neurological Institute, Cleveland Clinic, Cleveland, OH, United States

B. Vidal Cardiovascular Institute, Hospital Clinic-IDIBAPS, University of Barcelona, Barcelona, Spain

J. Alexander Viehman Division of Infectious Diseases, Department of Medicine, University of Pittsburgh School of Medicine, Pittsburgh, PA, United States; University of Pittsburgh

Medical Center, Pittsburgh, PA, United States

Tyler J. Wallen   Division of Thoracic and Cardiac Surgery, Geisinger Health System, Wilkes-Barre, PA, United States

Gabe Weininger   Division of Cardiac Surgery, Yale School of Medicine, New Haven, CT, United States

Glenn J.R. Whitman   Division of Cardiac Surgery, Department of Surgery, Johns Hopkins Hospital, Baltimore, MD, United States

Stevan P. Whitt   University of Missouri, Columbia, MO, United States

Lucy Q. Zhang   Division of Neurocritical Care, Departments of Neurology, Neurosurgery, Anesthesiology and Critical Care Medicine, Johns Hopkins University School of Medicine, Baltimore, MD, United States

译序一 Foreword

感染性心内膜炎是一种致死率极高的感染性疾病，常累及多个器官，临床表现复杂多样，诊断和治疗面临诸多挑战。由于其病情复杂且严重，多学科协作在感染性心内膜炎的诊治中就显得尤为重要。

《感染性心内膜炎多学科诊疗》一书基于当前医学研究和临床诊疗的需求，凝聚了多国学者的心血，是他们长期临床实践的结晶。本书从流行病学、病因、诊断、内外科治疗、伦理学及多学科协作等方面，全面阐述了感染性心内膜炎的历史、演变及现状。

在流行病学方面，本书探讨了社会因素对感染性心内膜炎流行病学的影响，特别是葡萄球菌成为主要致病菌的社会原因。在诊断方面，以 Duke 标准为基础，详细分析了临床表现、血培养、超声检查及现代影像技术的应用，阐述了提高诊断准确性的路径。在内科治疗方面，本书对抗生素的使用进行了细化和规范，并为围手术期的管理提供了方案。外科治疗则分左、右心感染进行阐述，讨论了手术适应证、时机及不同病理改变下的手术方式。此外，本书还强调了多学科协作的重要性，并提供了多器官受累时的外科诊疗策略及流程。最后，从伦理学角度探讨了感染性心内膜炎治疗中的社会问题。

在当前感染性心内膜炎治疗面临挑战、国内相关研究论著较为缺乏的情况下，本书中文版的出版无疑具有重要的学术价值，它将为国内临床医生和研究人员提供宝贵的学习资源。

我诚挚推荐《感染性心内膜炎多学科诊疗》一书，希望它能为临床医生和相关研究者提供有益的指导。

广东省心血管病研究所 所长

陈寄梅

2025 年 3 月

译序二 Foreword

《感染性心内膜炎多学科诊疗》是一部由多国临床从业者合力编著，旨在为感染性心内膜炎的诊疗提供全面、前沿指导的著作。作为一种表征多变的疾病，感染性心内膜炎由病原微生物侵袭心内膜或心瓣膜引起，其严重性及复杂性常使临床处理陷于两难的境地，死亡率至今居高不下。

译者在行医期间，深刻感受到广东地区这类疾病发病率较高，即使已完成千例相关病例的手术，积累了一定的临床经验，仍不时会感到这类疾病的复杂、处理的棘手、相关指导资料的缺乏与不足，部分相关文献与临床实际还存有差距，经常要面临诸如"出血与抗凝的矛盾""体外循环禁忌与不手术心力衰竭无法纠正的矛盾""冠状动脉的评估与造影禁忌的矛盾"等现实困境。*Infective Endocarditis: A Multidisciplinary Approach* 一书的问世有针对性地对以上问题做了回应，并从多学科角度阐述了感染性心内膜炎的流行病学、病因、诊断、治疗等多方面的问题。书中整合了欧洲心脏病学会（ESC）心内膜炎管理指南、美国胸外科协会（AATS）专家共识等最新循证证据，更将临床的处理难题通过结构化框架、多学科协作方式转化为可操作的临床路径，为感染性心内膜炎，尤其是那些疑难病例提供了全面、系统的指导。

在本书翻译过程中，译者根据自己对感染性心内膜炎的认知和理解，尽可能使用通俗的语言，使表达更为清晰；在术语标准化方面，则严格参照全国科学技术名词审定委员会的规范，最大限度保留原著的学术严谨性。本书数据的引用主要基于欧美相关数据、文献及指南，其患者人群特点及构成可能与我国患者人群存在差异，所以参照本书进行实践时，一定要结合患者的实际情况。此外，医学翻译是一门高深的学问，我们的工作一定存在不足之处，恳请读者予以批评指正。

本书的翻译出版得到了王维腾、甘礼溪、叶兰心、庄乐泉、陈欧迪、刘洋和孙涛涛等众多同道的指导和帮助，在此表示诚挚感谢。希望这部译著能成为我们应对感染性心内膜炎复杂战局的"战术手册"，协助临床医生解决一些临床难题。

简旭华
2025 年 3 月

目 录 Contents

第1章	感染性心内膜炎的流行病学与病理生理学	/ 1
第2章	感染性心内膜炎临床诊断的基本方法	/ 22
第3章	感染性心内膜炎的微生物学	/ 39
第4章	感染性心内膜炎的超声心动图评估	/ 56
第5章	感染性心内膜炎的其他影像学检查	/ 68
第6章	感染性心内膜炎的预防	/ 91
第7章	感染性心内膜炎的抗菌治疗	/ 103
第8章	危重感染性心内膜炎患者的术前准备	/ 124
第9章	危重感染性心内膜炎患者的术后处理	/ 134
第10章	感染性心内膜炎的神经系统并发症	/ 142
第11章	静脉吸毒并发感染性心内膜炎的精神问题	/ 158
第12章	心脏植入式设备相关心内膜炎	/ 176
第13章	感染性心内膜炎患者的门诊随访与处理	/ 195
第14章	手术时机与手术指征	/ 211
第15章	右心感染性心内膜炎的外科治疗	/ 221

第 16 章	自体二尖瓣心内膜炎的外科治疗	/ 233
第 17 章	自体主动脉瓣心内膜炎的外科治疗	/ 239
第 18 章	主动脉根部脓肿的外科治疗	/ 248
第 19 章	感染性心内膜炎的复杂多瓣膜手术	/ 258
第 20 章	感染性心内膜炎并发急性卒中的手术时机	/ 264
第 21 章	静脉吸毒者心内膜炎的医疗伦理	/ 272
第 22 章	感染性心内膜炎的多学科服务	/ 291
第 23 章	感染性心内膜炎的未来研究方向	/ 309

第 1 章
感染性心内膜炎的流行病学与病理生理学

Edwin Chen, Brandon J. Smith, Nicholas Marschalk, Neel Shah

Department of Internal Medicine, Division of Infectious Disease, University of Pittsburgh Medical Center, Pittsburgh, PA, Unites States

流行病学

引 言

早在 16 世纪，法国医生 Jean François Fernel 首先对感染性心内膜炎（IE）的临床特征进行了描述，也成为将"生理学"一词引入生物体功能研究的第一人[1]。接下来的几个世纪，多位杰出医学家通过对人体生理学和病理生理学的细心研究，阐述了 IE 的微生物学发病机制、瓣膜病变与感染相关性以及栓塞临床后遗症等，从而奠定了对该病的认知基础[2]。1885 年，因"Osler 结节"而闻名的 William Osler 爵士发表了一系列具有里程碑意义的演讲，在这些讲座中，他通过对前期大量相关知识的总结，构建出 IE 的系统性概念框架，并引发了医学界对心内膜炎的关注[3-5]。

20 世纪初，尽管临床医生对心内膜炎的认识不断深入，但由于缺乏有效的治疗方法，IE 的发病率和死亡率一直居高不下。早期的治疗方案包括使用磺胺类药物、汞和砷等毒性物质以及热疗，治愈率几乎为零[1-2]。幸运的是，20 世纪微生物学和生物化学领域同时取得了长足的进步。1928 年，Alexander Fleming 爵士发现青霉素，20 世纪 40 年代该药首次临床试验成功。其后，Howard Florey、Ernst Chain 和 Norman Heatley 对青霉素大规模生产工艺进行了改进，为 IE 的治愈铺平了道路。

青霉素的出现彻底改变了 IE 的自然进程，其对抗生素出现之前尚未经历人工选择压力的野生型葡萄球菌和链球菌菌株非常有效。伴随青霉素在心内膜炎之外的临床广泛使用，这一医学奇迹也使 Alexander Fleming 爵士实至名归地获得了 1945 年诺贝尔生理学或医学奖。当然，青霉素的耐药性也不可避免地出现了[6]。事实上，在青霉素广泛使用后的短短几年内，耐药金黄色葡萄球菌就出现在临床多药耐药微生物中。由此，一场旷日持久的人类与致病微生物的攻防之战拉开了序幕，并延续至今[7]。

青霉素还标志着不断变化的 IE 临床治疗模式的开端。20 世纪末 21 世纪初，医学取得了长足发展，伴随新型抗生素的开发，心脏植入式电子设备（CIED）、人工瓣膜、长期留置的静脉导管的普遍使用，以及血液透析人数的增长，临床诊疗也发生了明显变化[8-14]。此外，在美国，日益流行的阿片类药物应用已影响右侧心内膜炎的患病率和发病率，一些罕见微生物成为导致 IE 的致病微生物[15-16]，所有这些变化均显著影响了心内膜炎的流行病学。

概　述

　　IE 仍然是一种罕见的疾病，发病率为（2～10）/10 万，在世界不同区域、不同国家，甚至同一国家的不同地区其发病率都存在差异[17-22]。不同国家的报道情况基本一致，即 IE 总体发病率稳定，偶有轻微增加[23-24]。虽然统计数据没有大的变化，但随着时间的推移，其流行病学还是发生了显著改变。在抗生素出现前，IE 发病主要集中在 30～40 岁人群，通常以风湿性瓣膜病患者为主，链球菌为主要病原体[21,25-27]。而从 20 世纪开始，随着世界各国在工业化和富裕程度上的差异，低收入和高收入国家 IE 的特征也出现了变化。低收入国家仍保留抗生素出现前的疾病特征，风湿性疾病仍然是关键的风险因素，占比高达 2/3[28]。相反，在高收入国家，生活条件改善，链球菌性咽炎治疗便捷，风湿性疾病已不再是 IE 的主要易感因素[23,29]，取而代之的是老龄，且风险因素和微生物学特征与之前相比也有较大差异[30]。

　　21 世纪初，高收入国家 IE 的平均患病年龄已上升至 60～70 岁，两性发病率分布相对平均[21,26,31-32]。这种年龄的变化直接反映了发达国家人均寿命的延长，同时伴随着与年龄相关的共病，以及治疗中必须实施的一些操作[8,33-34]。与年龄相关的风险因素通常包括高血压、糖尿病、冠状动脉疾病以及肝肾疾病[35-36]。由于终末期肾病（ESRD）人群的增加，血液透析现已成为 IE 的最大风险因素之一，占 IE 病例的 25% 以上[37-38]。瓣膜病也是感染的风险因素，常见病变包括先天性二叶主动脉瓣，以及与年龄相关的退行性瓣膜反流和脱垂[38-40]。左侧瓣膜受累为主，最常见的是主动脉瓣，而右侧 IE 相对罕见，占 5%～10%[17,41]。此外，目前用于各种瓣膜置换的假体材料也成为可能带来感染的因素，此类人工瓣膜感染占到总病例的 20% 以上[35-36,42-43]。同样，随着 CIED 使用的增多，与之相关的感染所引发的 IE 也在增加[9,44]。

　　作为医学进步的直接结果，高收入国家 IE 的微生物学也发生了变化。在二十世纪六七十年代之前，草绿色链球菌感染占大多数[23]。然而，在过去几十年中，葡萄球菌已取代草绿色链球菌，占比达 40%，其中，金黄色葡萄球菌已成为主要致病菌[23,30,45-46]。这一变化主要是由于免疫功能低下人群的增加，源于长期服用类固醇或其他免疫抑制药物，以及实体器官或骨髓移植病例的增加[47]。此外，还包括长期留置导管的应用和经导管主动脉瓣置换术（TAVR）等侵入性手术的增加，以及人工瓣膜和 CIED 的广泛使用等[30,34,43,48]。由于同样的原因，肠球菌、β-溶血性链球菌和营养变异链球菌的致病也在增加[43,49-51]。而以往少见的病原菌如革兰氏阴性菌、真菌和非典型细菌目前占比仍然较低[17,23,50-51]。

静脉吸毒者的 IE

静脉吸毒（IVDU）者 IE 是一个独特的流行病学群体。该人群较为年轻，中位年龄40岁，男性(55%~58%)的发病率高于女性[32,52-53]。年发病率为1.5‰~20‰，高出普通人群20倍[54-55]。发病率与阿片类药物的使用增多相关，在某些三级医疗中心因阿片滥用导致的 IE 占总 IE 病例的1/3[56-60]。与非吸毒者相比，IVDU 者的 IE 主要发生在右心（76%~79%），影响左侧瓣膜的比例较低（16%~30%），累及双侧瓣膜者更少（5%~10%）[61-64]。在受累的右侧瓣膜中，三尖瓣受累最常见（高达69%）[65-66]。这种右侧瓣膜的受累倾向可能与毒品的静脉注射和随之进入的致病微生物有关，化学物质的注射可对瓣膜组织造成化学性和物理性损伤，继而引起瓣膜感染[52,54]。有数据显示，某些毒品具有血管活性作用，特别是可卡因，可能引起瓣膜内膜的血管痉挛，导致瓣膜局部损伤和血栓形成，成为感染病灶[54]。这一机制可以解释为什么非注射类毒品使用者 IE 的发病率较高的现象[61]。

与非吸毒感染者类似，金黄色葡萄球菌也是吸毒患者最常见的致病微生物，但在后者中致病率更高。一项比较研究显示：IVDU 者 IE 中有68%为金黄色葡萄球菌感染，而非吸毒 IE 者中的比例仅为28%[17,63]。这种明显的差异推测是由于该人群较高的金黄色葡萄球菌定植率造成的[67-68]。继葡萄球菌之后，其他常见的病原体有链球菌和肠球菌[52]。一些在非吸毒者中较罕见的致病菌，如革兰氏阴性菌（假单胞菌）、真菌（尤其是念珠菌）以及多种致病菌的混合感染，在吸毒患者中都较为常见[52,69-70]。另外，由 IVDU 者的注射习惯及注射用具（如用嘴部舔舐针头和注射部位）造成的 HACEK（包括嗜血杆菌属、凝聚杆菌属、心杆菌属、艾肯菌属、金氏杆菌属）及其他口腔菌群感染，在吸毒者 IE 中并不少见[70]。

并发症发生率和死亡率

IE 具有很高的并发症发生率和死亡率，其总体预后受多因素影响，包括病原体种类、栓塞和感染并发症严重程度、感染前的共病、瓣膜受累程度以及手术干预的必要性[71]。根据临床症状轻重不同，院内早期死亡率差异很大，可低至个位数或高达45%[17,19,72-77]。不良预后因素包括左侧感染或瓣周受累、人工瓣膜心内膜炎（PVE）、多共病、中枢神经系统受累、高龄和葡萄球菌或真菌感染[26,77-80]。即使拥有现代医学多种治疗手段，预后仍然很差，1年死亡率高达40%[17,71,73,81]。在一项使用数学模型进行的研究中，将 IE 患者与普通人群比较，其1年、3年及5年生存率均较低（分别为90% vs. 92%、81% vs. 86%、70% vs. 82%），表明 IE 在初诊后数年内，可持续导致较高的并发症发生率和死亡率[73]。

与非 IVDU IE 患者相比，IVDU 感染者具有更高的并发症发生率和死亡率。一项比较研究显示：两者住院死亡率和1年全因死亡率无明显差异（IVDU 与非 IVDU 分别为：6% vs. 9%，$P>0.05$；16% vs. 13%，$P>0.05$）[72]。另一项比较研究表明，尽管 IVDU 者的首次住院死亡率和 30 d 再入院死亡率更低（IVDU 与非 IVDU 分别为：6.8% vs. 9.6%，P<0.001；3.4% vs. 7.9%，P<0.001），但 30~180 d 的再入院死亡率无差异（IVDU 与非 IVDU：4% vs. 3.8%，P>0.05）[59]。IVDU 者的长期预后很差，纵向研究显示总体死亡率高达 30%~40%[82-83]。尽管 IVDU 者有高风险行为，但生存率并无显著下降，可能与他们多为年轻人，临床共病较少有关[72]。另一种可能就是他们多为右侧瓣膜受累，而右侧 IE 的预后更佳[84-86]。与这一情形相反，如果他们出现左侧感染，相比非吸毒患者，IVDU 者的预后则较差[87]。

由于 IE 预后不良，临床有必要找到根源以改善临床结局。众所周知，及时诊断、适当使用抗生素和早期评估手术适应证对于提高生存率至关重要[88-89]。但实际工作中常常会发生诊断延误、抗生素使用不当、手术延误，或者根本不遵循或偏离指南等情况[80,90-92]。鉴于疾病的复杂性，多个专家组提议应建立多学科团队开展急性疾病的管理[36,71,93]。这些"心内膜炎团队"已被证明可降低住院死亡率和长期死亡率，减少感染栓塞并发症，缩短等待手术的时间，降低手术死亡率[71,94-96]。事实上，已证明"心内膜炎团队"是 1 年生存率的独立阳性预测因子[81]。

感染的病理生理学

概　述

血管内皮层发挥多种重要功能，包括血管张力的调节、血液和组织间隙之间的分子交换、免疫系统调节和内稳态[97]，而这些功能中缺少促进细菌和真菌黏附这一功能，这不是物种进化的遗漏，而是一种保护机制。血液被认为是无菌的环境[98]，当微生物进入血液时，内皮层可以起到屏障隔离保护的作用（图 1.1）。

通常，IE 的发生发展必须依次经历 4 个步骤，即内皮的损伤、病原体侵入血管、病原体黏附于内皮、病原体增殖[99]。

多种因素可导致内皮损伤，包括机械力、自身抗体、炎症损伤以及病原体对内膜的直接伤害[100]。这些因素中最重要的是病原菌的毒力，后文将对此进行更详细的讨论。一旦瓣膜的内皮层受到损害，下一步就是病原体进入血液。无论是通过破损的黏膜、来自其他处受感染组织的血行传播，还是经 IVDU 或留置导管的直接血流接种，一旦病原体进入血流，它就有可能黏附在受损的瓣膜上并启动发病机制。

病原体可以直接黏附在受损的内膜上，也可以黏附在无菌的血小板 - 纤维蛋白血栓上，成为感染灶[101]。不同的病原体对内皮层的黏附力不同，例如金黄色葡萄球菌具有非常高的黏附亲和力，而大多数肠杆菌的黏附力就要低得多。金黄色葡萄球菌的另一个独特之处在于它具有直接感染完整内皮的能力，这也造成了其总体的高感染率[101]。

随着病原体附着在瓣膜上，持续的复制会导致赘生物形成以及感染团块的不

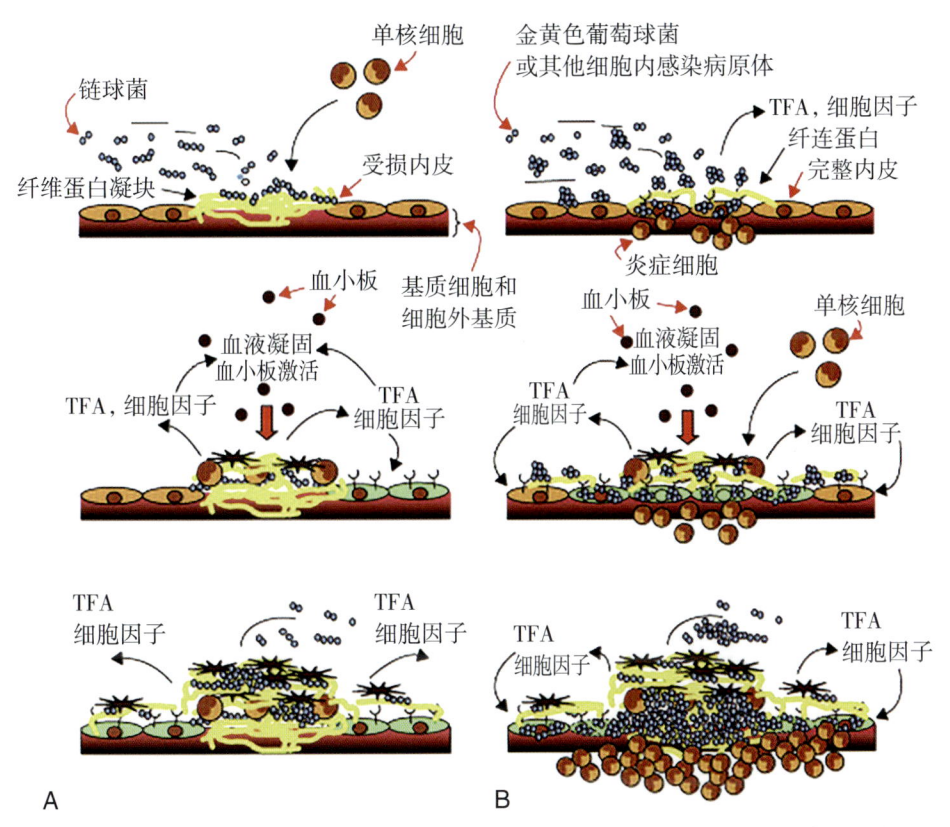

图 1.1 细菌在瓣膜定植的早期步骤。A. 在受损上皮的定植过程：暴露的基质细胞和细胞外基质蛋白促进纤维蛋白-血小板凝块形成，成为链球菌黏附位点（左上）；纤维蛋白上已黏附的链球菌吸引单核细胞并诱导它们产生组织因子活性（TFA）和细胞因子（左中）；这些介质激活凝血级联反应，吸引和激活血小板，并诱导邻近内皮细胞产生细胞因子、整合素和 TFA（左下），促进赘生物生长。B. 在炎性瓣膜组织的定植过程：对于瓣膜局部炎症的反应，内皮细胞表达整合素以结合血浆纤连蛋白，微生物通过已附壁的纤连蛋白结合蛋白黏附内皮，借此侵入内皮（右上）；作为应对，内皮细胞产生 TFA 和细胞因子，引发血液凝固和炎症扩大，激发赘生物的形成（右中）；侵入细胞的细菌通过分泌活性蛋白，如溶血素最终裂解内皮细胞（绿色细胞）（右下）。改编自：Moreillon P., Que Y.-A. Infective endocarditis. Lancet, 2004, 363: 139–149. https://doi.org/10.1016/S0140-6736（03）15266-X. Moreillon P., Que, Y.-A, Bayer A.S. Pathogenesis of streptococcal and staphylococcal endocarditis. Infect Dis Clin North Am, 2002, 16: 297–318. 经 Elsevier 许可使用

断增大。在这一过程中，病原体的毒力因素和宿主免疫系统起到了至关重要的作用，两方面的作用决定了病原体能否在体内持续繁殖并得以生存[101]。

病原体

对患者病情的深入了解可以帮助临床医生相对准确地预判致病微生物。一般而言，患者的既往接触史与感染的微生物病原体之间存在直接相关性，这种关联在 IE 中显得尤其密切。革兰氏阳性球菌包括葡萄球菌属（皮肤）、链球菌属（皮肤、口腔、胃肠道）和肠球菌（胃肠道和泌尿生殖道），构成了独特的人体正常菌群。皮肤和（或）黏膜的破损促进了它们的血源性接种，一旦进入血流，病原体表现

出不同程度对受损心血管组织的黏附，以增进其对心脏组织的感染能力。相反，革兰氏阴性杆菌主要定植于呼吸道、胃肠道和泌尿生殖道，所表现的对心血管组织的黏附能力相对较低。但消化道和泌尿生殖道破损时，也可出现革兰氏阴性杆菌的血行传播，伴随着不同程度的 IE 风险，这取决于潜在的患者因素和病原体特异性因素。第三种重要的病原体是酵母菌，特别是念珠菌属。这些真菌通常定植在胃肠道，在院内感染和 PVE 中发挥重要作用。相关病原体的细节将在后续章节中进一步讨论。

微生物在赘生物形成中的作用

随着赘生物的成熟，它成为一个由纤维蛋白、血小板、红细胞、白细胞以及分布在其中的菌团共同构成的网状结构，形成一个用以保护细菌或真菌免于人体固有免疫系统和抗生素攻击的复杂生态系统。外层的纤维蛋白可防御吞噬细胞的侵入，细菌藏于结构深层以减少免疫系统的攻击，同时还通过降低自身代谢以降低抗生素的效能，因为抗生素（如 β-内酰胺类）主要针对快速分裂和代谢活跃的细菌[102]。纤维蛋白/细胞基质这一结构可以在赘生物的感染成分被消除后长期存在，如果不通过手术清除赘生物，免疫系统可能需要数月甚至数年才能清除赘生物中的死细菌和微生物碎片[103]。

瓣膜完整性在 IE 发展中的作用

IE 的发生通常必须依次经过上述 4 个步骤。如果宿主的免疫系统能够在此过程完成之前有效干预，感染则不会发生。然而，需要指出的是，心脏瓣膜的潜在完整性在感染的发生机制中也起着关键作用，它们的损伤会显著增加感染的风险。短暂性菌血症是一种常见现象，可在对未消毒的身体部位进行操作后发生[104]，这一现象的代表性事例是刷牙。在一项对 290 名受试者比较刷牙和单次拔牙（使用或不使用阿莫西林预防感染）的研究中，发现 3 种情况都出现了短暂性菌血症。作者得出结论：虽然刷牙组的短暂性菌血症总体发生率最低，但患者每天都要刷牙，这种频率可能使心内膜炎的总体发生风险最高[105]。那么，设想如果为了保持口腔卫生而较高频率去刷牙，为什么我们并没有更高频地患上心内膜炎呢？答案似乎在于瓣膜的完整性，只要保持这种完整性，总体上感染的风险就会很低；而心脏瓣膜完整性损害引起的结构性改变可增加 IE 的发生风险。与瓣膜完整性受损相关的最常见情况包括二尖瓣脱垂（MVP）、风湿性心脏病（RHD）、先天性心脏畸形和人工心脏瓣膜植入。

·二尖瓣脱垂（MVP）

美国人群的 MVP 发病率为 2%~3%。20 世纪 80 年代的一项描述性分析首次提出 MVP 与草绿色链球菌心内膜炎之间存在关联[104]。2007 年之前，美国心脏协会（AHA）的指南将 MVP 作为术前预防性使用抗生素的指征。然而，由于缺乏证据表明在已有 MVP 的情况下发生术后菌血症的风险高到足以超过抗生素治疗带来的相关不良事件的风险，因此后来又将 MVP 排除在风险因素之外[105]。为了进一步量化其感染风险，一项研究根据是否存在心脏杂音比较了 MVP 患者发生心内膜炎的风险，发现有杂音患者的年化感染风险为 1/1400，虽然风险似乎很低，但它比未听见杂音的 MVP 患者高了 35 倍[106]。

- **风湿性心脏病（RHD）**

RHD 是急性风湿热的后遗症，由 A 型链球菌（化脓性链球菌）性咽炎诱发自身免疫反应引起。其发生基于该型链球菌的 M 蛋白中含有一段心肌肌球蛋白样序列结构，从而引起免疫交叉反应导致瓣膜损伤，二尖瓣和主动脉瓣最常受累。此外，免疫反应引起的相关慢性炎症可导致瓣膜狭窄、前向流量减少，或瓣膜关闭不全出现反流增加[107]。RHD 可以是一次急性风湿热严重反应或多次反复作用的结果[108]。除了损害心脏瓣膜外，广泛的炎症反应还会损害多种其他组织，包括皮肤、关节和神经系统。1940 年前，80%～90% 诊断为心内膜炎的患者存在 RHD[109]。

20 世纪下半叶，RHD 的发病率显著下降，特别是在发达国家。20 世纪 80 年代，在英国的两个样本人群中，这一比例已降至 23%～35%[110-112]。卫生条件的改善、人口密度的降低和医疗服务的可及性都被认为是贡献因素。然而，广泛使用青霉素治疗急性链球菌性咽炎是唯一被证明可以降低急性风湿热发病率的有效干预措施[113]。

- **先天性心脏病（CHD）**

CHD 以多种先天性解剖异常为特征，包括瓣膜或大血管的结构和功能异常以及间隔缺损[114]。CHD 是发生心内膜炎的重要风险因素，特别是在儿科人群中，其发病率是普通人群的 2～7 倍[42,115]。

发绀型 CHD、左侧心脏病变和心内膜垫缺损与儿童时期心内膜炎风险增加有关。随着医学的进步，许多 CHD 儿童得以接受矫治性手术或瓣膜置换术。然而，在术后 6 个月内，这类患者发生 IE 的风险将进一步升高[43]。与自体瓣膜先天异常需要接受手术的患者相比，因其他 CHD 而接受瓣膜置换术的患者发生院内 IE 的比率显著升高（61% vs.14%）[116]。

- **人工瓣膜 IE（PVE）**

包括人工瓣膜在内的人工材料可成为感染发生的原发灶。PVE 约占所有心内膜炎病例的 20%[117]，患者的年发病率为 0.3%～1.2%[80,117-118]。所有人工瓣膜都存在风险，但这种风险根据瓣膜手术后的时间长短和瓣膜类型而有所不同。PVE 传统上分为早期（术后 ≤ 12 个月）和晚期（术后 > 12 个月）[119]。临床上认识这种区别很重要，因为早期和晚期感染在流行病学和微生物学上均存在差异。

早 期

人工瓣膜放置后早期存在较高的感染风险。PVE 早期，病原体可经手术过程直接侵入，或术后通过血行传播。在此期间，人工瓣膜内皮化尚未完成，病原体可以直接进入黏附于假体瓣环及周边尚未愈合的组织，也可沿着缝合线侵入瓣膜及瓣周组织。缝合线可以作为病原体黏附的额外病灶。在愈合的关键时期，直接接触这些暴露的组织可增加瓣周脓肿的发生风险[120]。

根据病原体不同，可将术后早期进一步细分为术后<2个月和2~12个月。近期（<2个月）PVE，最可能的病原体是金黄色葡萄球菌和凝固酶阴性葡萄球菌（CoNS），其次是革兰氏阴性杆菌和念珠菌。鉴于院内感染率很高，这种病原学特征并不令人意外；此外，在这一人群中出现抗生素耐药也更加普遍。术后2~12个月的PVE，CoNS最常见，其次是金黄色葡萄球菌、链球菌和肠球菌[43,48,118]。其间，PVE病原体多兼具医院和社区获得性二重性，常有不同程度的耐药性。

晚 期

术后12个月以上发生的PVE表现与自体瓣膜心内膜炎（NVE）相似，在瓣膜完整性的破坏上与RHD和CHD近似。此时的瓣周组织虽已内皮化，但心脏结构的变化改变了瓣膜表面及血流特征。无论是生物瓣还是机械瓣，换瓣后瓣膜形态及组织的这一改变都很容易引起血小板-纤维蛋白微栓的沉积。最终，内皮化作为一种保护机制可降低毒力较弱的病原体（如CoNS）在人工瓣膜上定植并形成赘生物的能力。另外，内皮化还对防止迟发性瓣周脓肿具有一定作用[120]。

晚期PVE的病原体构成类似传统的NVE。链球菌和金黄色葡萄球菌是非IVDU患者最常见的病原体，其次是CoNS和肠球菌；而在IVDU或中心静脉导管留置的病例中，还可见到革兰氏阴性杆菌和念珠菌等病原体[121-122]。

人工瓣膜类型

与机械瓣置换相比，以往认为生物瓣置换发生PVE的风险较高。但目前文献显示，瓣膜类型带来的感染风险差异很小。瑞典国家患者登记处1997—2012年主动脉瓣置换术（患者为50~69岁）的数据表明：接受生物瓣置换术的患者平均随访时间为5.0年，PVE发生率为8.6%；机械瓣置换患者平均随访8.8年，PVE发生率为7.3%[123]。另外3项随机试验纳入了1400多名患者，随访时间为8~20年，结果显示：与机械瓣相比，生物瓣PVE发生率有增加的倾向，但没有统计学意义[124-126]。还有一项研究纳入了超过3.8万名≥65岁的患者，随访12年，生物瓣PVE的发生率为2.2%，机械瓣PVE的发生率为1.4%，校正后的风险比（HR）为1.65（95%CI=1.31~1.95）[127]。

同样受到关注的是TAVR术后发生PVE的风险。TAVR于2002年首次在美国使用[128]，与开胸主动脉瓣置换术（SAVR）类似，TAVR手术放置的外源材料为病原体生长提供了基础。来自斯堪的纳维亚国家登记处和临床试验的数据表明，SAVR和TAVR相关PVE的发生率相似，且术后第1年的风险较高[129-130]。

TAVR 相关 PVE 的微生物学病因与 SAVR 相似，但肠球菌感染率较高，推测可能与 TAVR 腹股沟操作位置接近泌尿生殖道和胃肠道有关，确切机制目前尚不清楚。

临床表现

概　述

IE 的影响可仅限于心脏，也可累及身体几乎每个器官系统。感染对心脏瓣膜及心肌组织的侵犯可引起瓣膜关闭不全，甚至瓣叶-瓣环分离，乳头肌、室间隔和心室壁、心包穿孔，心肌脓肿和完全性房室传导阻滞。无菌及带菌栓子可导致肺、脾、血管、皮肤、肾、眼和大脑栓塞等灾难性事件。免疫现象并不罕见，同样可累及眼、肾和大脑。这一可对全身造成如此广泛损害的病症，对临床而言是一个重大挑战，同时也预示着高并发症发生率和致死率（图 1.2 至图 1.7）。

心血管

IE 最可怕的后果之一是感染从心脏瓣膜局部向心肌蔓延导致瓣周脓肿，引起致命并发症，包括瓣膜功能不全、心室破裂、瘘管形成和心脏传导阻滞[131]。因此，诊断脓肿的存在预示高死亡率[132]。心肌脓肿的发生风险及随之可能的心脏传导阻滞，因感染病原体的毒力和感染严重程度的不同而异[77]。与亚急性感染相比，葡萄球菌多引起急性感染，更容易出现脓肿[133]。其他风险因素包括主动脉瓣心内膜炎、PVE 和 IVDU[134-135]。与身体其他位置脓肿的形成方式相似，心内脓肿的形成也是由病原体直接侵入心脏组织，继发组织坏死，随后免疫细胞裂解，形成脓液[136]。脓肿最常见的部位是纤维瓣环，它是维持瓣膜稳定性的重要结构[137]。

如果感染累及传导系统，可出现房室传导阻滞和快速型心律失常。由于希氏

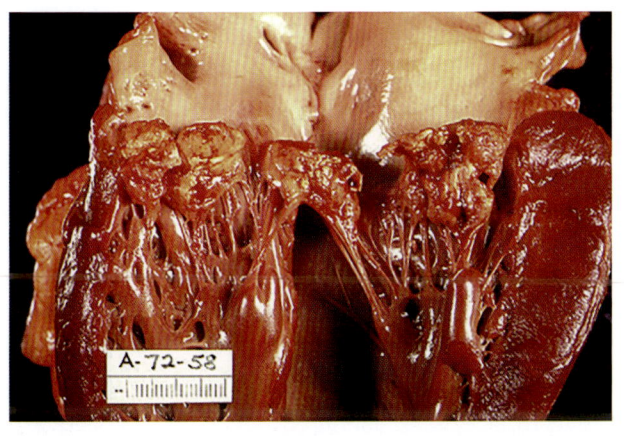

图 1.2 感染性心内膜炎（IE）赘生物大体病理样本。图片是人类心脏的一个切面，取自尸检。显示一例亚急性细菌性心内膜炎的大体病理改变，病原菌是副流感嗜血杆菌。在左心室内部的视图中，可见二尖瓣瓣叶上附着的巨大赘生物或细菌团块

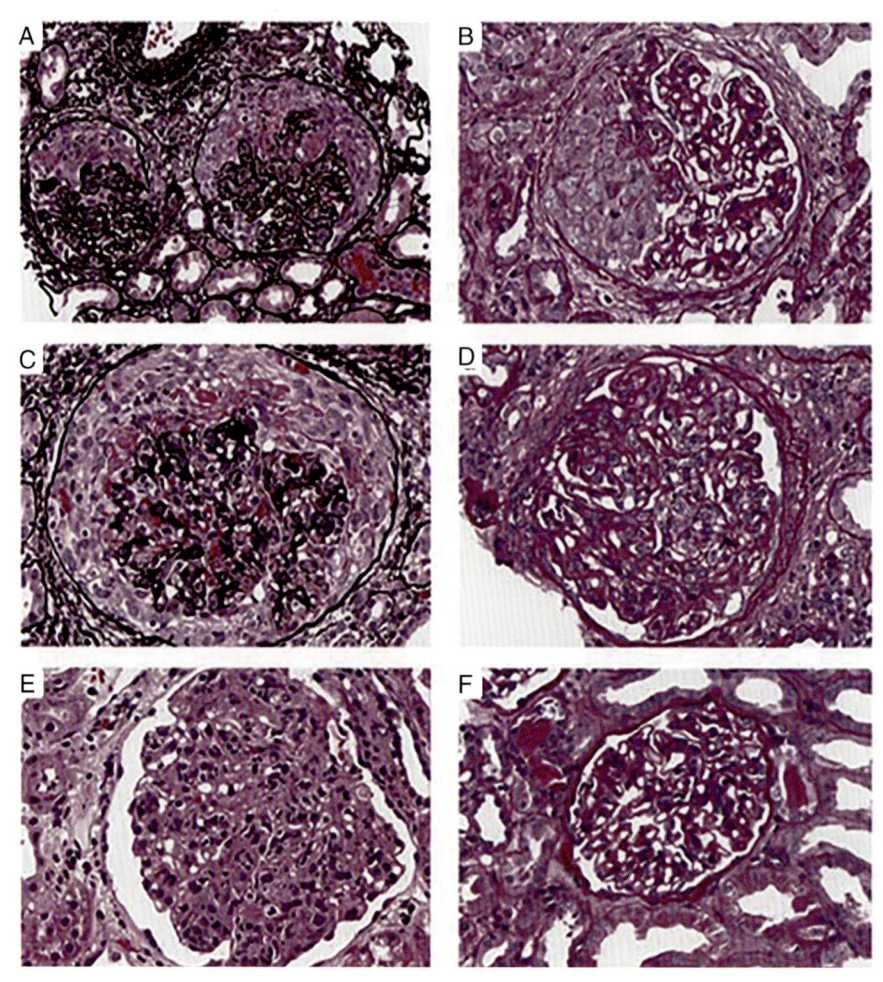

图 1.3　心内膜炎患者的组织病理学结果显示免疫复合物肾小球肾炎

束邻近主动脉瓣，因此心脏传导阻滞在主动脉瓣 IE 时较为常见；而房室结靠近二尖瓣，累及二尖瓣和主动脉瓣的瓣周脓肿均可出现相应的传导问题[138]。心脏传导阻滞可表现为束支或Ⅰ度、Ⅱ度或完全性房室传导阻滞，这一过程可表现为进行性加重，提示感染对传导系统的侵蚀在不断进展[139]。也可以发生无心肌脓肿的传导异常，这种情况起因不明，推测与局部感染炎症浸润相关，而非脓肿形成[140]。根据传导系统损伤的严重程度，这类病例多需要手术治疗并安装永久起搏器。最后，冠状动脉的栓塞可导致急性心肌梗死、心功能损害、心力衰竭，也可以引起心律失常[141]。

神经系统

中枢神经系统是 IE 栓塞最常见的部位[142]。心源性缺血性卒中可发生在不同的血管区域，严重的可危及生命，轻微的可无临床症状，仅通过影像学检查才得以明确[143-144]。脑血管事件的发生风险与赘生物增大密切相关[145]。出血性卒中不

感染性心内膜炎的流行病学与病理生理学 第 1 章

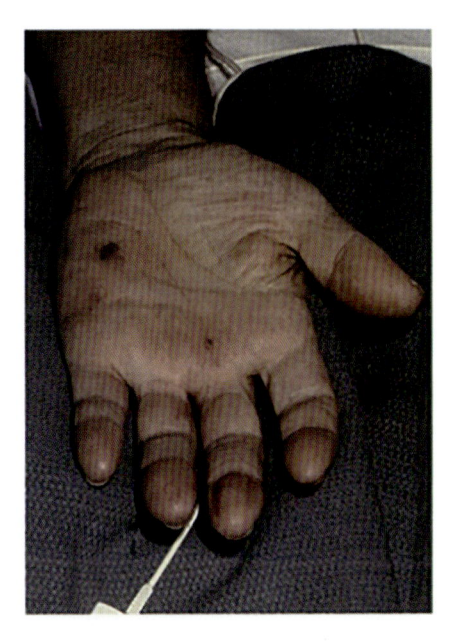

图 1.4 心内膜炎患者的 Janeway 病变

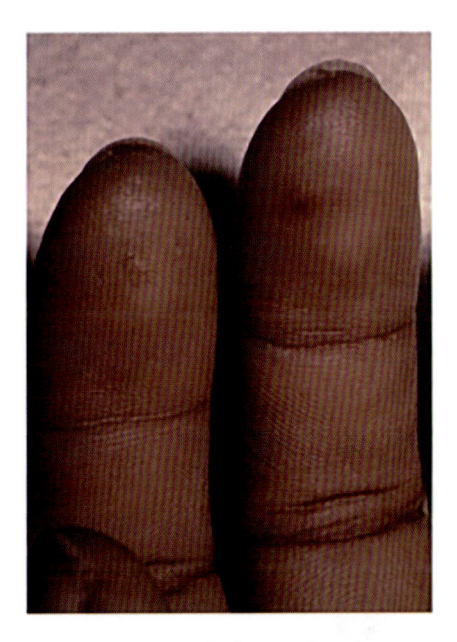

图 1.5 心内膜炎患者的血管内表现——Osler 结节

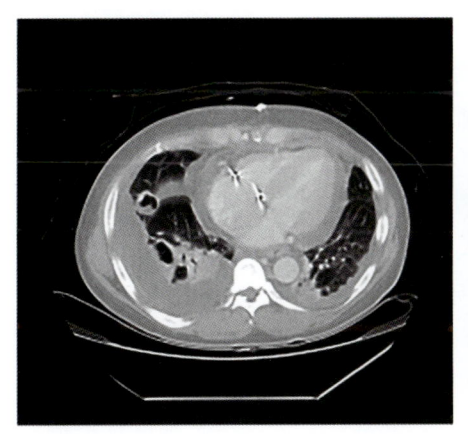

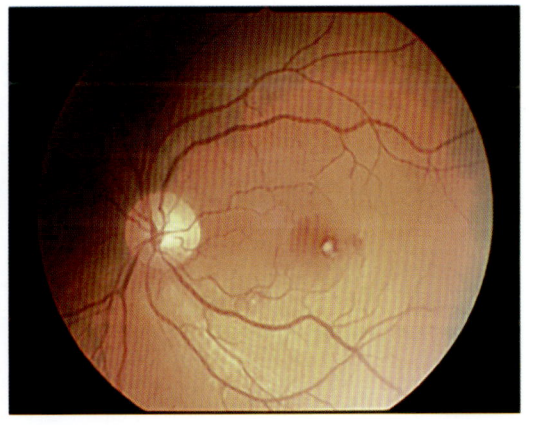

图 1.6 脓毒性肺栓塞，常见于累及三尖瓣和肺动脉瓣的心内膜炎

图 1.7 心内膜炎患者的眼部表现——眼底镜检查中的 Roth 斑

太常见，但往往是致命的，常见于梗死病灶的出血转化；其次是栓子中的病原菌侵入血管壁，导致管壁受损破裂所致[146-147]。真菌性动脉瘤由 William Osler 爵士首次命名，主要是根据尸检血管大体标本类似真菌感染引起的动脉瘤形态，而事实是大多数真菌性动脉瘤是由细菌引起的。真菌性动脉瘤最常见于大脑，也可以出现在全身其他部位相对较大的动脉[148]。局部脑脓肿的发生也可源于脓毒性栓塞，当带有病原菌的栓子通过循环抵达脑组织时，就有可能形成局部脓肿。同理，脑炎和脑膜炎也可源于同一侵入性病原体的致病过程。

肺

脓毒性肺栓塞通常由累及三尖瓣或肺动脉瓣的心内膜炎引起（右侧心内膜炎），因为这些结构将血液直接泵入肺。与中枢神经系统的栓塞性疾病类似，并发症可由血管栓塞引起，也可由感染的局部扩散导致。广泛的栓塞还可引起肺动脉高压，与慢性血栓栓塞性疾病类似，使用肺动脉内膜剥脱术已成功治疗这类病例[149]。细菌还可通过栓塞和感染性播散侵入局部肺组织导致肺空洞、肺脓肿和脓胸，这些病理改变可单独或合并存在[150-151]。

皮肤和指甲

受心内膜炎的影响，皮肤和指甲的异常因其位置浅表在视诊时最易发现，瘀点、Janeway病变、Osler结节和碎片状出血是典型表现。虽然这些均非心内膜炎的特异性表现，但其存在提示有较高的并发症发生风险[152]。其中最常见的是瘀点，它是真皮出血引起的针状红色和棕色非褪色斑点；Janeway病变是手掌和脚底出现的无痛性红色出血斑疹、丘疹或结节；而Osler结节则是疼痛性的紫色或红色结节，通常出现在指尖和脚趾。一般认为，Janeway病变是微脓肿，由脓毒性栓子引起，活检时病变组织培养呈阳性支持这一观点[153]；与之不同，Osler结节则推测是血管炎所致，早期活检显示血管周围存在炎症反应，而组织培养结果呈阴性。当然也存在一些争议，因为从Osler结节中同样也培养出了病原体。从组织学角度来看，两者病理结构也相似[154-155]，因此有学者推测可能只是同一病理过程发生在不同解剖部位的表现而已，而疼痛性Osler结节可能是血管球体炎症所致[156-158]。这两种表现都很罕见，尤其是在抗生素时代。碎片状出血源于甲床血管出血，表现为手指甲和脚趾甲下方垂直的红色或棕色条纹[159]，其本质是脓毒性栓子累及甲床脉管系统引起的甲床瘀斑[160]。然而，健康成年人中孤立性的碎片状出血并不罕见，因此要做出心内膜炎的诊断必须进行全面的临床评判[161]。

肾

IE相关的肾脏损害主要源于脓毒性栓塞及免疫反应[162]，其中急性肾损伤和肾病综合征并不少见。IE相关肾病综合征的临床表现轻重不一，从寡免疫复合物型新月体肾小球肾炎到伴有广泛补体和免疫球蛋白沉积的弥漫性增殖性肾小球肾炎[163-164]。新月体肾小球肾炎最常见，特征是C3补体沉积，而无免疫球蛋白沉积[165]。实验室检查可发现血清补体水平下降和自身抗体血清学检测阳性，包括抗核抗体、类风湿因子、抗核细胞质抗体和抗磷脂抗体。以上结果必须结合临床病情慎重判断，以排除免疫性疾病的可能；因为非感染性肾小球肾炎的主要治疗方法是免疫抑制，而感染相关的肾小球肾炎需要积极治疗潜在的感染[163]。当伴有IE时，积极的抗生素治疗可改善肾小球疾病，因为细菌负荷的减轻会减少循环免疫复合物[166]。与其他器官一样，脓毒性栓子进入肾脏还可导致肾梗死及肾脓肿[167]。梗死有时无症状,脓肿对抗生素治疗多有效,很少有脓肿大到需要外科干预。

眼

心内膜炎的眼部病变具有广泛的临床表现,从良性结膜出血、棉絮斑、Roth 斑,到危及视力的脉络膜视网膜炎和眼内炎[168]。与心内膜炎的其他外周表现类似,这些表现并非血管内感染所特有,也可由各种其他传染性和非传染性疾病引起。眼内炎是由感染播散进入玻璃体和(或)房水引起,也可由菌血症或真菌血症血行播散至眼所致。然而,与单纯的菌血症相比,这一病症只有在 IE 相关的菌血症中才较为常见[169-170]。眼内炎的进展速度与严重程度与致病微生物的毒力和数量相关[171],细菌和真菌可以从血管丰富的脉络丛播散,导致眼的破坏并危及视力。而心内膜炎引起的结膜出血与瘀斑及碎片状出血的起因相同。

Roth 斑通常被描述为白色的中心性视网膜出血,同样是因栓塞所致。组织学检查通常看不到细菌,所见多为局部毛细血管破裂以及出血性病变中央纤维蛋白栓形成[172]。这些改变推测可能是获得性血小板减少和弥漫性血管内凝血等因素所致,而非感染的直接蔓延[173],这一观点因在血液系统恶性疾病及创伤中存在同样病变而得到了进一步证实[172]。

需指出,用"Roth 斑"一词定义上述病变不够准确。其实 Moritz Roth 博士原来所描述的特征性的绒毛状白色斑点,有明显且独立的红色出血点,是我们现在所说的棉绒斑[174]。首先描述这一以白色为中心周围有出血的特征性病变的是 Litten 博士,但基于 Roth 的前期工作,业内误将这一病变发现归于 Roth。因此,我们今天所说的 Roth 斑,更恰当地说应该是"Litten 征"[174]。

肌肉和骨骼

心内膜炎的感染可累及肌肉、骨骼和关节,这与持续性菌血症有关,而非心源性栓塞或免疫反应。肌痛和关节痛很常见,考虑与增强的炎症反应有关[175]。骨髓炎和化脓性关节炎因感染的血行播散导致,与微生物的毒力相关[176]。金黄色葡萄球菌是最有可能引起这些感染的病原体,如上所述,它也常常引起心内膜炎。

血液

IE 还可引起脾脏、骨髓和血液的一些病症。脾脏是脓毒性栓塞的另一个常见累及器官,多导致梗死和脓肿[177-178]。在亚急性心内膜炎病例中,还可出现脾大,考虑与免疫系统活性增加、脾组织增生以及可能的免疫复合物沉积有关[179],在 ^{18}F-FDG PET 上常常表现为心内膜炎患者的脾脏、骨髓代谢亢进[180],这提示高炎症状态,但更深入的机制尚未阐明。赘生物本身,尤其是附着于人工瓣膜时,可因剪切应力引起红细胞溶血,导致溶血性贫血[181]。清除赘生物以及进行人工瓣膜置换可解决这一问题。

参考文献

[1] Grinberg M, Solimene MC. Historical aspects of infective endocarditis. Rev Assoc Med Bras, 2011, 57: 228–233.

[2] Millar BC, Moore JE. Emerging issues in infective endocarditis. Emerg Infect Dis, 2004, 10: 1110–1116.

[3] Osler W. The Gulstonian lectures, on malignant endocarditis, lecture I. Br Med J, 1885, 1: 467–470.

[4] Osler W. The Gulstonian lectures, on malignant endocarditis, lecture II. Br Med J, 1885, 1: 522–526.

[5] Osler W. The Gulstonian lectures, on malignant endocarditis, lecture III. Br Med J, 1885, 1: 577–579.

[6] Rosenblatt-Farrell N. The landscape of antibiotic resistance. Environ Health Perspect, 2009, 117: A244–A250.

[7] Lobanovska M, Pilla G. Penicillin's discovery and antibiotic resistance: lessons for the future? Yale J Biol Med, 2017, 90: 135–145.

[8] Slipczuk L, et al. Infective endocarditis epidemiology over five decades: a systematic review. PloS One, 2013, 8: e82665.

[9] Cabell CH, et al. Increasing rates of cardiac device infections among medicare beneficiaries: 1990—1999. Am Heart J, 2004, 147: 582–586.

[10] Darouiche RO. Treatment of infections associated with surgical implants. N Engl J Med, 2004, 350: 1422–1429.

[11] McCarthy JT, Steckelberg JM. Infective endocarditis in patients receiving long-term hemodialysis. Mayo Clin Proc, 2000, 75: 1008–1014.

[12] Martin GS, Mannino DM, Eaton S, et al. The epidemiology of sepsis in the United States from 1979 through2000. N Engl J Med, 2003, 348: 1546–1554.

[13] Wisplinghoff H, et al. Nosocomial bloodstream infections in US hospitals: analysis of 24 179 cases from a prospective nationwide surveillance study. Clin Infect Dis, 2004, 39: 309–317.

[14] Fluit AC, et al. Antimicrobial susceptibility and frequency of occurrence of clinical blood isolates in Europe from the SENTRY antimicrobial surveillance program, 1997 and 1998. Clin Infect Dis, 2000, 30: 454–460.

[15] Meisner JA, Anesi J, Chen X, et al. Changes in infective endocarditis admissions in Pennsylvania during the opioid epidemic. Clin Infect Dis, 2019. https://doi.org/10.1093/cid/ciz1038.

[16] Wallen TJ, et al. Tricuspid valve endocarditis in the era of the opioid epidemic. J Card Surg, 2018, 33: 260–264.

[17] Murdoch DR, et al. Clinical presentation, etiology, and outcome of infective endocarditis in the 21st century: the International Collaboration on Endocarditis-Prospective Cohort Study. Arch Intern Med, 2009, 169: 463–473.

[18] Duval X, et al. Temporal trends in infective endocarditis in the context of prophylaxis guideline modifications:three successive population-based surveys. J Am Coll Cardiol, 2012, 59: 1968–1976.

[19] Hoen B, et al. Changing profile of infective endocarditis: results of a 1-year survey in France. J Am Med Assoc, 2002, 288: 75–81.

[20] Berlin JA, et al. Incidence of infective endocarditis in the Delaware Valley, 1988—1990. Am J Cardiol, 1995, 76: 933–936.

[21] Hogevik H, Olaison L, Andersson R, et al. Epidemiologic aspects of infective endocarditis in an urban population. A 5-year prospective study. Medicine, 1995, 74: 324–339.

[22] Bin Abdulhak AA, et al. Global and regional burden of infective endocarditis, 1990—2010: a systematic review of the literature. Glob Heart, 2014, 9: 131–143.

[23] Ambrosioni J, et al. The changing epidemiology of infective endocarditis in the twenty-first century. Curr Infect Dis Rep, 2017, 19: 21.

[24] Pant S, et al. Trends in infective endocarditis incidence, microbiology, and valve replacement in the United States from 2000 to 2011. J Am Coll Cardiol, 2015, 65: 2070-2076.

[25] Yew HS, Murdoch DR. Global trends in infective endocarditis epidemiology. Curr Infect Dis Rep,

2012, 14: 367-372.
[26] Watanakunakorn C, Burkert T. Infective endocarditis at a large community teaching hospital, 1980—1990. A review of 210 episodes. Medicine, 1993, 72: 90-102.
[27] Letaief A, et al. Epidemiology of infective endocarditis in Tunisia: a 10-year multicenter retrospective study. Int J Infect Dis, 2007, 11: 430-433.
[28] Carapetis JR, Steer AC, Mulholland EK, et al. The global burden of group A streptococcal diseases. Lancet Infect Dis, 2005, 5: 685-694.
[29] Seckeler MD, Hoke TR. The worldwide epidemiology of acute rheumatic fever and rheumatic heart disease.Clin Epidemiol, 2011, 3: 67-84.
[30] Fowler VG, et al. Staphylococcus aureus endocarditis: a consequence of medical progress. J Am Med Assoc, 2005, 293: 3012-3021.
[31] Correa de Sa DD, et al. Epidemiological trends of infective endocarditis: a population-based study in Olmsted County, Minnesota. Mayo Clin Proc, 2010, 85: 422-426.
[32] Kadri AN, et al. Geographic trends, patient characteristics, and outcomes of infective endocarditis associated with drug abuse in the United States from 2002 to 2016. J Am Heart Assoc, 2019, 8: e012969.
[33] Forestier E, Fraisse T, Roubaud-Baudron C, et al. Managing infective endocarditis in the elderly: new issues for an old disease. Clin Interv Aging, 2016, 11: 1199-1206.
[34] Prendergast BD. The changing face of infective endocarditis. Heart, 2006, 92: 879-885.
[35] Toyoda N, et al. Trends in infective endocarditis in California and New York State, 1998—2013. J Am Med Assoc, 2017, 317: 1652-1660.
[36] Habib G, et al. ESC guidelines for the management of infective endocarditis: the task force for the management of infective endocarditis of the European Society of Cardiology (ESC). Endorsed by: European Association for Cardio-Thoracic Surgery (EACTS), theEuropean Association of Nuclear Medicine (EANM). Eur Heart J, 2015, 36: 3075-3128.
[37] Saran R, et al. US renal data system 2019 annual data report: epidemiology of kidney disease in the United States. Am J Kidney Dis, 2019. https://doi.org/10.1053/j.ajkd.2019.09.002.
[38] Mostaghim AS, Lo HYA, Khardori N. A retrospective epidemiologic study to define risk factors, microbiology,and clinical outcomes of infective endocarditis in a large tertiary-care teaching hospital. SAGE Open Med, 2017, 5. 2050312117741772.
[39] Hill EE, et al. Infective endocarditis: changing epidemiology and predictors of 6-month mortality: a prospective cohort study. Eur Heart J, 2007, 28: 196-203.
[40] Cahill TJ, Prendergast BD. Infective endocarditis. Lancet, 2016, 387: 882-893.
[41] Chan P, Ogilby JD, Segal B. Tricuspid valve endocarditis. Am Heart J, 1989, 117: 1140-1146.
[42] Mylonakis E, Calderwood SB. Infective endocarditis in adults. N Engl J Med, 2001, 345: 1318-1330.
[43] Regueiro A, et al. Association between transcatheter aortic valve replacement and subsequent infective endocarditis and in-hospital death. J Am Med Assoc, 2016, 316: 1083-1092.
[44] Carrasco F, et al. Clinical features and changes in epidemiology of infective endocarditis on pacemaker devices over a 27-year period (1987—2013). Europace, 2016, 18: 836-841.
[45] Vogkou CT, Vlachogiannis NI, Palaiodimos L, et al. The causative agents in infective endocarditis: a systematic review comprising 33 214 cases. Eur J Clin Microbiol Infect Dis, 2016, 35: 1227-1245.
[46] Liesman RM, Pritt BS, Maleszewski JJ, et al. Laboratory diagnosis of infective endocarditis. J Clin Microbiol, 2017, 55: 2599-2608.
[47] Cabell CH, et al. Changing patient characteristics and the effect on mortality in endocarditis. Arch Intern Med, 2002, 162: 90-94.
[48] Amat-Santos IJ, et al. Infective endocarditis after transcatheter aortic valve implantation: results from a large multicenter registry. Circulation, 2015, 131: 1566-1574.
[49] Benito N, et al. Health care-associated native valve endocarditis: importance of non-nosocomial acquisition. Ann Intern Med, 2009, 150: 586-594.

[50] Fernández-Hidalgo N, et al. Contemporary epidemiology and prognosis of health care-associated infective endocarditis. Clin Infect Dis, 2008, 47: 1287–1297.

[51] Muñoz P, et al. Current epidemiology and outcome of infective endocarditis: a multicenter, prospective, cohort study. Medicine, 2015, 94: e1816.

[52] Colville T, Sharma V, Albouaini K. Infective endocarditis in intravenous drug users: a review article. Postgrad Med, 2016, 92: 105–111.

[53] Hilbig A, Cheng A. Infective endocarditis in the intravenous drug use population at a tertiary hospital in Melbourne, Australia. Heart Lung Circ, 2020, 29: 246–253.

[54] Sanaiha Y, Lyons R, Benharash P. Infective endocarditis in intravenous drug users. Trends Cardiovasc Med, 2019. https://doi.org/10.1016/j.tcm.2019.11.007.

[55] Levine DP, Crane LR, Zervos MJ. Bacteremia in narcotic addicts at the detroit medical center. II. Infectious endocarditis: a prospective comparative study. Clin Infect Dis, 1986, 8: 374–396.

[56] Cooper HLF, et al. Nationwide increase in the number of hospitalizations for illicit injection drug use-related infective endocarditis. Clin Infect Dis, 2007, 45: 1200–1203.

[57] Shrestha NK, et al. Injection drug use and outcomes after surgical intervention for infective endocarditis. Ann Thorac Surg, 2015, 100: 875–882.

[58] Wang A, Gaca JG, Chu VH. Management considerations in infective endocarditis: a review. J Am Med Assoc, 2018, 320: 72–83.

[59] Rudasill SE, et al. Clinical outcomes of infective endocarditis in injection drug users. J Am Coll Cardiol, 2019, 73: 559–570.

[60] Wurcel AG, et al. Increasing infectious endocarditis admissions among young people who inject drugs. Open Forum Infect Dis, 2016, 3: ofw157.

[61] Chambers HF, Morris DL, Täuber MG, et al. Cocaine use and the risk for endocarditis in intravenous drug users. Ann Intern Med, 1987, 106: 833–836.

[62] Chambers HF, Korzeniowski OM, Sande MA. Staphylococcus aureus endocarditis: clinical manifestations in addicts and nonaddicts. Medicine, 1983, 62: 170–177.

[63] Frontera JA, Gradon JD. Right-side endocarditis in injection drug users: review of proposed mechanisms of pathogenesis. Clin Infect Dis, 2000, 30: 374–379.

[64] Miró JM, Moreno A, Mestres CA. Infective endocarditis in intravenous drug abusers. Curr Infect Dis Rep, 2003, 5: 307–316.

[65] Robbins MJ, Soeiro R, Frishman WH, et al. Right-sided valvular endocarditis: etiology, diagnosis, and an approach to therapy. Am Heart J, 1986, 111: 128–135.

[66] Roberts R, Slovis CM. Endocarditis in intravenous drug abusers. Emerg Med Clin, 1990, 8: 665–681.

[67] Tuazon CU, Sheagren JN. Increased rate of carriage of Staphylococcus aureus among narcotic addicts. J Infect Dis, 1974, 129: 725–727.

[68] Gordon RJ, Lowy FD. Bacterial infections in drug users. N Engl J Med, 2005, 353: 1945–1954.

[69] Ellis ME, Al-Abdely H, Sandridge A, et al. Fungal endocarditis: evidence in the world literature, 1965—1995. Clin Infect Dis, 2001, 32: 50–62.

[70] Sousa C, Botelho C, Rodrigues D, et al. Infective endocarditis in intravenous drug abusers: an update. Eur J Clin Microbiol Infect Dis, 2012, 31: 2905–2910.

[71] Botelho-Nevers E, et al. Dramatic reduction in infective endocarditis-related mortality with a management-based approach. Arch Intern Med, 2009, 169: 1290–1298.

[72] Leahey PA, LaSalvia MT, Rosenthal ES, et al. High morbidity and mortality among patients with Sentinel admission for injection drug use-related infective endocarditis. Open Forum Infect Dis, 2019, 6: ofz089.

[73] Thuny F, et al. Excess mortality and morbidity in patients surviving infective endocarditis. Am Heart J, 2012, 164: 94–101.

[74] Fernández Guerrero ML, González López JJ, Goyenechea A, et al. Endocarditis caused by Staphylococcus aureus: a reappraisal of the epidemiologic, clinical, and pathologic manifestations with analysis of factors determining outcome. Medicine, 2009, 88: 1–22.

[75] Moreillon P, Que Y-A. Infective endocarditis. Lancet, 2004, 363: 139–149.
[76] Fefer P, Raveh D, Rudensky B, et al. Changing epidemiology of infective endocarditis: a retrospective survey of 108 cases, 1990—1999. Eur J Clin Microbiol Infect Dis, 2002, 21: 432–437.
[77] Miro JM, et al. Staphylococcus aureus native valve infective endocarditis: report of 566 episodes from the International Collaboration on Endocarditis Merged Database. Clin Infect Dis, 2005, 41: 507–514.
[78] Julander I. Unfavourable prognostic factors in Staphylococcus aureus septicemia and endocarditis. Scand J Infect Dis, 1985, 17: 179–187.
[79] Mylotte JM, TayaraA. Staphylococcus aureus bacteremia: predictors of 30-day mortality in a large cohort. Clin Infect Dis, 2000, 31: 1170–1174.
[80] Kiefer T, et al. Association between valvular surgery and mortality among patients with infective endocarditis complicated by heart failure. J Am Med Assoc, 2011, 306: 2239–2247.
[81] Kaura A, et al. Inception of the "endocarditis team" is associated with improved survival in patients with infective endocarditis who are managed medically: findings from a before-and-after study. Open Heart, 2017, 4: e000699.
[82] Goodman-Meza D, et al. Long term surgical outcomes for infective endocarditis in people who inject drugs: a systematic review and meta-analysis. BMC Infect Dis, 2019, 19: 918.
[83] Rodger L, et al. Clinical characteristics and factors associated with mortality in first-episode infective endocarditis among persons who inject drugs. JAMA Netw Open, 2018, 1: e185220.
[84] Kamaledeen A, Young C, Attia RQ. What are the differences in outcomes between right-sided active infective endocarditis with and without left-sided infection? Interact Cardiovasc Thorac Surg, 2012, 14: 205–208.
[85] Moss R, Munt B. Injection drug use and right sided endocarditis. Heart, 2003, 89: 577–581.
[86] Musci M, et al. Surgical treatment of right-sided active infective endocarditis with or without involvement of the left heart: 20-year single center experience. Eur J Cardiothorac Surg, 2007, 32: 118–125.
[87] Thalme A, Westling K, Julander I. In-hospital and long-term mortality in infective endocarditis in injecting drug users compared to non-drug users: a retrospective study of 192 episodes. Scand J Infect Dis, 2007, 39: 197–204.
[88] Thuny F, et al. The timing of surgery influences mortality and morbidity in adults with severe complicated infective endocarditis: a propensity analysis. Eur Heart J, 2011, 32: 2027–2033.
[89] Kang D-H, et al. Early surgery versus conventional treatment for infective endocarditis. N Engl J Med, 2012, 366: 2466–2473.
[90] González De Molina M, Fernández-Guerrero JC, Azpitarte J. Infectious endocarditis: degree of discordance between clinical guidelines recommendations and clinical practice. Rev Esp Cardiol, 2002, 55: 793–800.
[91] Muhlestein JB. Infective endocarditis: how well are we managing our patients? J Am Coll Cardiol, 1999, 33: 794–795.
[92] Delahaye F, Rial MO, de Gevigney G, et al. A critical appraisal of the quality of the management of infective endocarditis. J Am Coll Cardiol, 1999, 33: 788–793.
[93] Baddour LM, et al. Infective endocarditis in adults: diagnosis, antimicrobial therapy, and management of complications: a scientific statement for healthcare professionals from the american heart association. Circulation, 2015, 132: 1435–1486.
[94] Lancellotti P, et al. ESC Working Group on Valvular Heart Disease position paper–heart valve clinics: organization, structure, and experiences. Eur Heart J, 2013, 34: 1597–1606.
[95] Baumgartner H, et al. ESC/EACTS Guidelines for the management of valvular heart disease. Eur Heart J, 2017, 38: 2739–2791.
[96] Chirillo F, et al. Management strategies and outcome for prosthetic valve endocarditis. Am J Cardiol, 2013, 112: 1177–1181.
[97] Nguyen D, Coull BM. Primer on cerebrovascular diseases. Elsevier, 2017: 108–113.

[98] Minnesota Department of Health. Normally sterile sites: invasive bacterial diseases, 2019. at: https://www.health.state.mn.us/diseases/invbacterial/sterile.html.
[99] Sullam PM, Drake TA, Sande MA. Pathogenesis of endocarditis. Am J Med, 1985, 78: 110–115.
[100] Leask RL, Jain N, Butany J. Endothelium and valvular diseases of the heart. Microsc Res Tech, 2003, 60: 129–137.
[101] Vilcant V, Hai O. StatPearls. StatPearls Publishing, 2020.
[102] McDonald JR. Acute infective endocarditis. Infect Dis Clin, 2009, 23: 643–664.
[103] Lang S, Watkin RW, Lambert PA, et al. Detection of bacterial DNA in cardiac vegetations by PCR after the completion of antimicrobial treatment for endocarditis. Clin Microbiol Infect, 2004, 10: 579–581.
[104] DeSimone DC, et al. Association of mitral valve prolapse with infective endocarditis due to viridans group streptococci. Clin Infect Dis, 2015, 61: 623–625.
[105] Daly CG. Antibiotic prophylaxis for dental procedures. Aust Prescr, 2017, 40: 184–188.
[106] MacMahon SW, et al. Risk of infective endocarditis in mitral valve prolapse with and without precordial systolic murmurs. Am J Cardiol, 1987, 59: 105–108.
[107] Harris C, Croce B, Cao C. Rheumatic heart disease. Ann Cardiothorac Surg, 2015, 4: 492.
[108] Sika-Paotonu D, Beaton A, Raghu A, et al. Acute Rheumatic Fever and Rheumatic Heart Disease // Ferretti JJ, Stevens DL, Fischetti VA. Streptococcus pyogenes: basic biology to clinical manifestations. University of Oklahoma Health Sciences Center, 2016.
[109] Weinstein L, Rubin RH. Infective endocarditis–1973. Prog Cardiovasc Dis, 1973, 16: 239–274.
[110] Ormiston JA, Neutze JM, Agnew TM, et al. Infective endocarditis: a lethal disease. Aust N Z J Med, 1981, 11: 620–629.
[111] Bayliss R, et al. The microbiology and pathogenesis of infective endocarditis. Br Heart J, 1983, 50: 513–519.
[112] Neutze JM, WHO Study Group on Rheumatic Fever/Rheumatic Heart Disease. Infective endocarditis and rheumatic heart disease. 1987.
[113] Carapetis JR. Rheumatic heart disease in developing countries. N Engl J Med, 2007, 357: 439–441.
[114] What are congenital heart defects?: CDC; n.d. at: https://www.cdc.gov/ncbddd/heartdefects/facts.html.
[115] Verheugt CL, et al. Turning 18 with congenital heart disease: prediction of infective endocarditis based on a large population. Eur Heart J, 2011, 32: 1926–1934.
[116] Fortún J, et al. Infective endocarditis in congenital heart disease: a frequent community-acquired complication. Infection, 2013, 41: 167–174.
[117] Vongpatanasin W, Hillis LD, Lange RA. Prosthetic heart valves. N Engl J Med, 1996, 335: 407–416.
[118] Wang A, et al. Contemporary clinical profile and outcome of prosthetic valve endocarditis. J Am Med Assoc, 2007, 297: 1354–1361.
[119] Agnihotri AK, McGiffin DC, Galbraith AJ, et al. The prevalence of infective endocarditis after aortic valve replacement. J Thorac Cardiovasc Surg, 1995, 110: 1708–1720. Discussion 1720.
[120] Carpenter JL. Perivalvular extension of infection in patients with infectious endocarditis. Rev Infect Dis, 1991, 13: 127–138.
[121] Rivas P, et al. The impact of hospital-acquired infections on the microbial etiology and prognosis of late-onset prosthetic valve endocarditis. Chest, 2005, 128: 764–771.
[122] Lee JH, et al. Prosthetic valve endocarditis: clinicopathological correlates in 122 surgical specimens from 116 patients (1985—2004). Cardiovasc Pathol, 2011, 20: 26–35.
[123] Bjursten H, et al. Infective endocarditis after transcatheter aortic valve implantation: a nationwide study. Eur Heart J, 2019, 40: 3263–3269.
[124] Hammermeister K, et al. Outcomes 15 years after valve replacement with a mechanical versus a bioprosthetic valve: final report of the Veterans Affairs randomized trial. J Am Coll Cardiol, 2000, 36: 1152–1158.
[125] Oxenham H, et al. Twenty year comparison of a Bjork-Shiley mechanical heart valve with

porcine bioprostheses. Heart, 2003, 89: 715–721.
[126] Stassano P, et al. Aortic valve replacement: a prospective randomized evaluation of mechanical versus biological valves in patients ages 55 to 70 years. J Am Coll Cardiol, 2009, 54: 1862–1868.
[127] Brennan JM, et al. Long-term safety and effectiveness of mechanical versus biologic aortic valve prostheses in older patients: results from the Society of Thoracic Surgeons Adult Cardiac Surgery National Database. Circulation, 2013, 127: 1647–1655.
[128] Cribier A. The development of transcatheter aortic valve replacement (TAVR). Glob Cardiol Sci Pract, 2016, 2016: e201632.
[129] Butt JH, et al. Long-term risk of infective endocarditis after transcatheter aortic valve replacement. J Am Coll Cardiol, 2019, 73: 1646–1655.
[130] Moriyama N, et al. Prosthetic valve endocarditis after transcatheter or surgical aortic valve replacement with a bioprosthesis: results from the FinnValve Registry. EuroIntervention, 2019, 15: e500–e507.
[131] d'Udekem Y, David TE, Feindel CM, et al. Long-term results of surgery for active infective endocarditis. Eur J Cardiothorac Surg, 1997, 11: 46–52.
[132] Choussat R, et al. Perivalvular abscesses associated with endocarditis; clinical features and prognostic factors of overall survival in a series of 233 cases. Perivalvular Abscesses French Multicentre Study. Eur Heart J, 1999, 20: 232–241.
[133] Arnett EN, Roberts WC. Valve ring abscess in active infective endocarditis. Frequency, location, and clues to clinical diagnosis from the study of 95 necropsy patients. Circulation, 1976, 54: 140–145.
[134] Graupner C, et al. Periannular extension of infective endocarditis. J Am Coll Cardiol, 2002, 39: 1204–1211.
[135] Omari B, et al. Predictive risk factors for periannular extension of native valve endocarditis. Clinical and echocardiographic analyses. Chest, 1989, 96: 1273–1279.
[136] Singer AJ, Talan DA. Management of skin abscesses in the era of methicillin-resistant Staphylococcus aureus. N Engl J Med, 2014, 370: 1039–1047.
[137] Rouzé S, et al. Infective endocarditis with paravalvular extension: 35-year experience. Ann Thorac Surg, 2016, 102: 549–555.
[138] Roberts NK, Child JS, Cabeen WR. Infective endocarditis and the cardiac conducting system. West J Med, 1978, 129: 254–256.
[139] Mehta NJ, Nehra A. A 66-year-old man with fever, hypotension, and complete heart block. Chest, 2001, 120: 2053–2056.
[140] Weisse AB, Khan MY. The relationship between new cardiac conduction defects and extension of valve infection in native valve endocarditis. Clin Cardiol, 1990, 13: 337–345.
[141] Glazier JJ. Interventional treatment of septic coronary embolism: sailing into uncharted and dangerous waters. J Intervent Cardiol, 2002, 15: 305–307.
[142] Snygg-Martin U, et al. Cerebrovascular complications in patients with left-sided infective endocarditis are common: a prospective study using magnetic resonance imaging and neurochemical brain damage markers. Clin Infect Dis, 2008, 47: 23–30.
[143] Johnson MD, Johnson CD. Neurologic presentations of infective endocarditis. Neurol Clin, 2010, 28: 311–321.
[144] Hess A, et al. Brain MRI findings in neurologically asymptomatic patients with infective endocarditis. AJNR Am J Neuroradiol, 2013, 34: 1579–1584.
[145] Mohananey D, et al. Association of vegetation size with embolic risk in patients with infective endocarditis: a systematic review and meta-analysis. JAMA Intern Med, 2018, 178: 502–510.
[146] Goldschmidt E, Faraji AH, Salvetti D, et al. Intracranial vessel occlusion preceding the development of mycotic aneurysms in patients with endocarditis. BMJ Case Rep, 2019, 12.
[147] Morris NA, Matiello M, Lyons JL, et al. Neurologic complications in infective endocarditis: identification, management, and impact on cardiac surgery. Neurohospitalist, 2014, 4: 213–222.

[148] González I, et al. Symptomatic peripheral mycotic aneurysms due to infective endocarditis: a contemporary profile. Medicine, 2014, 93: 42–52.

[149] Crosland W, et al. Pulmonary endarterectomy for pulmonary hypertension from septic emboli. Ann Thorac Surg, 2015, 99: 1814–1816.

[150] Cheng Y-F, Hsieh Y-K, Wang B-Y, et al. Tricuspid valve infective endocarditis complicated with multiple lung abscesses and thoracic empyema as different pathogens: a case report. J Cardiothorac Surg, 2019, 14: 41.

[151] Chahoud J, Sharif Yakan A, Saad H, et al. Right-sided infective endocarditis and pulmonary infiltrates. Cardiol Rev, 2016, 24: 230–237.

[152] Servy A, et al. Prognostic value of skin manifestations of infective endocarditis. JAMA Dermatol, 2014, 150:494–500.

[153] Kerr A, Tan JS. Biopsies of the Janeway lesion of infective endocarditis. J Cutan Pathol, 1979, 6: 124–129.

[154] Alpert JS, Krous HF, Dalen JE, et al. Pathogenesis of Osler's nodes. Ann Intern Med, 1976, 85: 471–473.

[155] Farrior JB, Silverman ME. A consideration of the differences between a Janeway's lesion and an Osler's node in infectious endocarditis. Chest, 1976, 70: 239–243.

[156] Alpert JS. Osler's nodes and Janeway lesions are not the result of small-vessel vasculitis. Am J Med, 2013, 126: 843–844.

[157] Von Gemmingen GR. Osler's node of subacute bacterial endocarditis. Arch Dermatol, 1967, 95: 91.

[158] Gunson TH, Oliver GF. Osler's nodes and Janeway lesions. Australas J Dermatol, 2007, 48: 251–255.

[159] Fawcett RS, Linford S, Stulberg DL. Nail abnormalities: clues to systemic disease. Am Fam Physician, 2004, 69: 1417–1424.

[160] Young JB, Will EJ, Mulley GP. Splinter haemorrhages: facts and fiction. J R Coll Physicians Lond, 1988, 22: 240–243.

[161] Robertson JC, Braune ML. Splinter haemorrhages, pitting, and other findings in fingerrnails of healthy adults. Br Med J, 1974, 4: 279–281.

[162] Mittal BV. Renal lesions in infective endocarditis (an autopsy study of 55 cases). J Postgrad Med, 1987, 33: 193–197.

[163] Satoskar AA, Parikh SV, Nadasdy T. Epidemiology, pathogenesis, treatment and outcomes of infection-associated glomerulonephritis. Nat Rev Nephrol, 2020, 16: 32–50.

[164] Lee LC, et al. "Full house" proliferative glomerulonephritis: an unreported presentation of subacute infective endocarditis. J Nephrol, 2007, 20: 745–749.

[165] Boils CL, Nasr SH, Walker PD, et al. Update on endocarditis-associated glomerulonephritis. Kidney Int, 2015, 87: 1241–1249.

[166] McKenzie PE, et al. Serum and tissue immune complexes in infective endocarditis. J Clin Lab Immunol, 1980, 4: 125–132.

[167] Majumdar A, et al. Renal pathological findings in infective endocarditis. Nephrol Dial Transplant, 2000, 15: 1782–1787.

[168] Jung J, et al. Incidence and risk factors of ocular infection caused by Staphylococcus aureus bacteremia. Antimicrob Agents Chemother, 2016, 60: 2012–2017.

[169] Vaziri K, Pershing S, Albini TA, et al. Risk factors predictive of endogenous endophthalmitis among hospitalized patients with hematogenous infections in the United States. Am J Ophthalmol, 2015, 159: 498–504.

[170] Durand ML. Endophthalmitis. Clin Microbiol Infect, 2013, 19: 227–234.

[171] Vallejo-Garcia JL, Asencio-Duran M, Pastora-Salvador N, et al. Role of inflammation in endophthalmitis. MediatInflamm, 2012, 2012: 196094.

[172] Ling R, James B. White-centred retinal haemorrhages (Roth spots). Postgrad Med, 1998, 74: 581–582.

[173] Fred HL. Little black bags, ophthalmoscopy, and the Roth spot. Tex Heart Inst J 2013, 40: 115–116.

[174] Khawly JA, Pollock SC. Litten's sign (Roth's spots) in bacterial endocarditis. Arch Ophthalmol, 1994, 112: 683–684.

[175] González-Juanatey C, et al. Rheumatic manifestations of infective endocarditis in non-addicts. A 12-year study. Medicine, 2001, 80: 9–19.

[176] Murillo O, et al. Endocarditis associated with vertebral osteomyelitis and septic arthritis of the axial skeleton. Infection, 2018, 46: 245–251.

[177] Aalaei-Andabili SH, et al. Management of septic emboli in patients with infectious endocarditis. J Card Surg, 2017, 32: 274–280.

[178] Dvoretsky LI, Yakovlev SV, Sergeeva EV, et al. Abscess of the spleen in a patient with infectious endocarditis. Ter Arkh, 2018, 90: 98–101.

[179] Nast CC, Colodro IH, Cohen AH. Splenic immune deposits in bacterial endocarditis. Clin Immunol Immunopathol, 1986, 40: 209–213.

[180] Boursier C, et al. Hypermetabolism of the spleen or bone marrow is an additional albeit indirect sign of infective endocarditis at FDG-PET. J NuclCardiol, 2020. https://doi.org/10.1007/s12350-020-02050-2.

[181] Gradon JD, Hirschbein M, Milligan J. Fragmentation hemolysis: an unusual indication for valve replacement in native valve infective endocarditis. South Med J, 1996, 89: 818–820.

第2章
感染性心内膜炎临床诊断的基本方法

Sami El-Dalati

Division of Infectious Diseases, University of Pittsburgh Medical Center, Pittsburgh, PA, United States

引 言

感染性心内膜炎（IE）的诊断通常很复杂，可能是当今医疗人员面临的最具挑战性的疾病诊断之一。患者临床表现多样，而现有诊断检查及标准并不完善。尽管早期诊断和及时治疗可以明显改善临床结局，但仍有近25%的病例是在发病后1个月才得以确诊[1-4]。虽说改良Duke标准、经食管超声心动图（TEE）和正电子发射断层扫描（PET）等多种手段已被广泛用于诊断，但IE的诊断仍侧重临床，需综合考虑多种因素才能确诊，包括患者罹患感染的风险因素、临床症状和体征、微生物学证据、超声心动图和放射学检查结果，以及临床病程。

心内膜炎以往被分为急性（具有暴发性）或亚急性（过程较为平缓）两大类。目前，临床表现上的急缓已不作为诊断标准的一部分，也不被纳入治疗决策时的考量。但两大分类临床表现的差异在临床观察并做出IE可能性诊断时至关重要：因为这类患者症状和体征多样化，可表现为急危重症，也可能有几个月的漫长病史，且涉及多学科。此外，伴随接受人工瓣膜、心脏植入式电子设备（CIED）和左心室辅助装置（LVAD）人数的增多，带来感染风险人群数量的增加，而新的对感染诊断更为灵敏的检查方式的出现（例如心脏PET），为早期诊断带来便利。综合以上因素，临床须保持高度警觉，使用敏感仪器在患者出现明显的临床表现之前积极寻找心内膜炎的证据，这也是临床对IE诊断模式的重要转变。换言之，以往医生对于该病的诊断严重依赖感染的检查结果，而未积极查找感染源头（部分由于Duke诊断标准的缘故）。

本章我们将重点讲述IE的临床特征、回顾现有的诊断流程和检查方法，并总结出一套适用性强的诊断方案。这里要强调的一个理念是：没有任何一种体征、症状或检查对于诊断IE是绝对灵敏或特异的。有了这种认知，在临床上我们就要对每个患者进行个体化的全面的了解和分析，而不是过分强调某些表现或检查结果。从这一角度而言，由包括心外科、心内科、感染科及神经科医护人员组成的多学科团队一定会有助于IE的准确诊断。

临床表现

一般体征和症状

IE 的初始症状，无论其严重程度如何，通常都是非特异性的，包括发热、畏寒、不适、厌食、盗汗、呼吸困难、头痛和体重减轻[5]。发热是最常见的症状，可出现在 90% 的患者中[6-7]，程度差异很大，不能用于确诊或排除诊断。需注意的是：60 岁以上的患者可以没有发热，而所有病例中一半以上年龄超过了 60 岁[8-10]。发热的持续时间，特别是在开始适当的抗菌治疗后的发热时间，已被证明与死亡率增加相关。对 26 名发热超过 2 周的患者研究发现，有 27% 合并心内脓肿[11]。呼吸困难和咳嗽是常见的症状，可能与充血性心力衰竭或（和）右侧心内膜炎中的脓毒性肺栓塞有关。

肌肉骨骼症状与心内膜炎也密切相关，包括关节痛（17% 的患者）和腰痛（1/3 的患者）等，且在许多情况下可能先于其他症状出现[8,12]。有报道显示，有 14% 的患者可合并滑膜炎（伴或不伴化脓性关节炎）[12]。此外，还有报道显示自发性椎体骨髓炎和 IE 的重叠发生率高达 30.8%[13]；因此，椎体骨髓炎在没有其他病因可解释的情况下，需慎重考虑是否还合并 IE。

心血管体征和症状

该类患者多原有瓣膜病变，心脏杂音成为其最常见的体检异常，可见于 85% 的病例[6]，仅 8%~15% 是新发或加重了的杂音[8]。此外，心力衰竭发生率差异很大：1986 年的一组 40 例患者中，78% 存在心力衰竭[14]；而最近对 234 731 名诊断为心内膜炎的病例的回顾性数据调查显示，仅有 28.9% 并发心力衰竭[15]。造成这种差异的原因有多种因素，包括心力衰竭定义的标准化和大型电子数据库的推出，这些数据库可对海量病例进行数据提取，而未进行病历审查。

神经系统体征和症状

除心脏表现外，10%~35% 的左侧心内膜炎患者因并发栓塞性卒中而出现神经系统异常[16-17]。鉴于所有卒中病例中 15%~70% 是栓塞性的，而未确诊的 IE 具有很高的栓塞发生率，两者存在很强的关联性，为此，美国超声心动图学会指南推荐：对所有缺血性卒中的患者应进行经胸超声心动图（TTE）或 TEE 排查[18]。对于是否需要在卒中评估中常规加入血培养以便于 IE 的更早诊断，尚待进一步的研究。此外，约 75% 的患者可出现临床不明显的神经系统并发症，包括无症状栓塞、微出血、真菌性动脉瘤或脑脓肿等，可在进一步的影像学检查中得以明确[19]。后文将对此进行讨论。

1%~20% 的心内膜炎患者可出现脑膜炎或脑膜反应（脑脊液白细胞计数升高但培养阴性）。这通常不作为心内膜炎的表现[18,20]，较常见于金黄色葡萄球菌感染菌血症[21-22]。对于脑膜炎症状和体征，应进行腰椎穿刺。如果脑脊液培养阳性，依结果选择抗生素。在所有细菌性脑膜炎患者中，心内膜炎占比约为2%[21]，但很多IE病例可出现脑病症候，这或许是先前描述的神经系统并发症的结果，如卒中、颅内出血、真菌性动脉瘤和脑脓肿，也可能是继发于其他多种因素，包括疾病严重程度和（或）尿毒症[20]。

眼部体征和症状

心内膜炎很少出现原发性的眼部症状，但有不到1%的心内膜炎患者可因视网膜中央动脉栓塞导致视力丧失而就诊[23]。内源性眼内炎，主要表现为视力下降，虽仅占所有眼内炎病例的2%~8%，但近40%的患者是由IE引起，在某些情况下，眼内炎成为部分心脏感染病例的主要临床表现[24]。约3%的无眼部症状的心内膜炎患者在随后散瞳检查时可发现有Roth斑或眼底小白斑，伴视网膜出血[25]。

皮肤体征和症状

IE的皮肤异常表现随抗生素的应用而减少。典型的表现包括碎片状出血或与指甲平行的瘀斑，约19%的病例具有这种表现，但这些表现是非特异性的，还可见于手部反复受伤、二尖瓣狭窄和肾衰竭腹膜透析的患者[8]。2.2%的患者可因微栓塞在手掌和足底表面出现Janeway病变或无痛性斑块。Osler结节是出现在手掌、手指或脚趾上的疼痛性红斑结节，推测可能是继发于免疫反应或栓塞。一项对139例心内膜炎患者的回顾性研究显示：Osler结节的发生率已从抗生素使用前的40%~90%下降到1995年的6.7%[25-26]。尽管皮肤表现越来越少，但它们仍具有重要的临床意义，已被纳入改良Duke标准[7]。

实验室检查

血培养和微生物学检查

目前缺乏一种对IE既灵敏又特异的血清学诊断方法，实验室检查的主要方法仍然是在使用抗生素前进行血培养。目前的美国心脏协会（AHA）指南建议，在评估心内膜炎时抽取3组血培养[27]。血培养的检出率随着抽血样本数量的增加而提高，文献显示血培养频次由1次增加到3次可将检出率由73%提高到98%[28]。不同医疗机构血培养阴性率差异很大：有的报道只有2%，也有的报道接近70%[29]，2015年AHA指南估计这一数值约为20%[27]。培养阴性最常见的原因是抽血培养时间点在使用抗生素后。在2项共计204例血培养阴性心内膜炎患者的研究中，有46%的病例在血培养采样前接受了抗菌治疗[30-31]。其实在这些病例中，部分病例的病情已清晰提示血培养的必要性；然而，多数情况下，即便患者存在心内膜炎风险因素，但由于临床表现仅仅是一些模棱两可的非特异性症状，常常导致临床医生根据个人经验使用口服或静脉注射抗生素。为此，我们认为，在这类人群中，有必要大幅降低血培养的门槛。这样做虽然存在 1%～5% 的假阳性率，但与心内膜炎诊断延迟所带来的并发症乃至死亡相比，这一假阳性率对临床影响相对较小[4,32]。另外，虽然降低培养门槛可能带来培养污染假阳性问题，但相比因乱用抗生素导致培养阴性而没有针对性地使用广谱抗生素所带来的副作用及药物毒性，根据培养结果有针对性地使用窄谱抗生素，可以抵消上述假阳性的负面作用。

革兰氏阳性菌是心内膜炎的主要致病菌，多项大样本研究显示，其占比在 80% 以上，以金黄色葡萄球菌最常见[33]。而以往链球菌更为常见，出现这一流行病学变化的原因可能与静脉吸毒的增多以及高危患者普遍给予预防性抗感染治疗有关[34]。还有研究显示，培养短于 10 h 即出现血培养阳性的金黄色葡萄球菌菌血症病例已被证实与随后诊断为金黄色葡萄球菌 IE 存在关联，而培养短于 13.7 h 即出现阳性与高死亡率相关[35]。

除金黄色葡萄球菌外，草绿色链球菌，其他类型链球菌如 A 族和 B 族链球菌、营养变异链球菌和解没食子酸链球菌，以及肠球菌和凝固酶阴性葡萄球菌，是其他常见的革兰氏阳性致病菌。2011 年一项对 115 名革兰氏阳性菌血症患者进行的研究显示：与医生依据经验判断决定是否进行超声心动图检查相比，对该类患者常规行超声心动图检查，可使心内膜炎的诊出率增加近 3 倍[36]。

革兰氏阴性菌在 IE 中相对少见，估计占比为 1.3%～10%[33-34,36-37]，半数病例由 HACEK 病原体（嗜沫嗜血杆菌、凝聚杆菌、人心杆菌、侵蚀艾肯菌和金氏金氏菌）引起，另一半则是临床较常见的革兰氏阴性致病菌引起，其中铜绿假单胞菌、大肠杆菌、肺炎克雷伯菌和黏质沙雷菌所导致的感染约占非 HACEK 病例的 2/3。据报道，HACEK 菌血症对随后诊断为心内膜炎有 60% 的阳性预测率，这提示临床应尽早评估 IE 存在的可能性。此前，静脉吸毒被认为是非 HACEK 革兰氏阴性菌心内膜炎的主要风险因素；但最近的文献表明，这一人群仅占此类病例的 4%，而半数以上病例以医疗暴露为主要风险因素[38]，其中包括心血管装置的植入（如人工瓣膜和 CIED）。

真菌是心内膜炎的少见致病菌，占比 2%～4%，约半数病例由念珠菌引起[39-40]；但随着一些治疗手段使用的增多，估计发病率还可能升高。虽然真菌还不作为心内膜炎的"典型"致病菌，但 2016 年对 187 名念珠菌菌血症患者进行的研究发现，接受超声心动图检查的病例中有 5.9% 检出了赘生物[41]。

其他实验室检查

· 全血细胞计数

除血培养外，血常规虽然是非特异性的，但可提示心内膜炎的存在。典型的正常色素性和正常细胞性贫血可见于 80% 的心内膜炎病例[8]。溶血性贫血可见于人工瓣膜 IE，与血液流经病损瓣膜后形成湍流导致红细胞发生机械破坏有关。此外，超过半数病例可出现白细胞增多（>10×10⁹/L），而白细胞减少也可见于 5%～15% 的病例[42]。还有报道显示，5%～15% 的患者可出现血小板减少[8]。

- **血清生化检测和尿液分析**

常规生化检测可发现心内膜炎的常见并发症，即急性肾损伤。一项对 185 例心内膜炎病例的研究发现，1/3 的患者合并急性肾衰竭 [血肌酐>2.0 mg/dL（176.8 μmol/L）][43]。另一项对 112 名患者的研究显示，急性肾损伤发生率为 68.8%[44]。心内膜炎相关肾衰竭是多因素导致的，包括急性肾小管坏死、脓毒性栓塞、伴或不伴间质性肾炎的药物肾毒性，以及肾小球肾炎，其在 IE 中的发生率高达 22%[45]。金黄色葡萄球菌性心内膜炎是导致急性肾损伤和肾小球肾炎的风险因素[43,46]。在心内膜炎相关肾小球肾炎中：97% 的患者有血尿，6% 有肾性蛋白尿[46]；低补体血症也很常见，37% 的患者补体 C3 偏低，16% 补体 C3 和 C4 偏低；此外，28% 的患者抗中性粒细胞胞质抗体（ANCA）阳性[46]。如果尿常规提示存在尿路感染的可能性，尿培养则有助于确定心内膜炎的来源。然而，对没有可靠感染病史、无临床症状的尿培养阳性结果的解读必须非常谨慎，因为阳性结果可能是严重的菌血症的结果而非原因，也可能仅仅是无症状菌尿。

IE 的免疫检测结果也可异常，但用于诊断缺乏特异性。法国一项包含 56 名确诊病例的研究显示：56% 的患者红细胞沉降率（ESR）增高，84% 的患者 C- 反应蛋白（CRP）升高，36% 的患者类风湿因子升高[47]。在另一组 85 例的患者中：CRP>40 mg/L 被确定为死亡及主要不良事件的预测因子，不良事件包括急性肾损伤、脓毒性脑栓塞和非脑部栓塞事件以及心脏并发症[48]。

- **血培养阴性 IE 的检测**

如前所述，血培养阴性在 IE 中占有可观的比例。原因部分归于过早使用抗生素，另外，有些病原菌常规血培养不能生长，如巴尔通体（包括汉赛巴尔通体和五日热巴尔通体）及贝纳柯克斯体，由它们引起的心内膜炎约占 0.8%，可靠的诊断方法就是血清学或聚合酶链反应（PCR）检测[33]。布鲁氏菌、军团菌和肺炎支原体也无法通过常规血培养进行可靠鉴定，需要对外科切除的瓣膜标本进行血清学或 PCR 检测确定。此外，非结核分枝杆菌（NTM）是一种罕见的引起 IE 的细菌，需要特殊抗酸血液培养基才能生长。尽管 NTM 心内膜炎的总体发病率很低，但自 2011 年以来，奇美拉分枝杆菌（*Mycobacterium chimaera*）导致的人工瓣膜心内膜炎在全球有增加的趋势，可能与心脏直视手术使用了受污染的加热 - 冷却消毒设备有关[49]。为此，2011 年后有过心脏手术史、血培养阴性的患者，临床应高度怀疑这一诊断的可能性。最后，还有一些培养阴性也可能是非细菌性血栓性心内膜炎，以心脏瓣膜赘生物为特征。赘生物由纤维蛋白和血小板聚集物组成，没有炎症反应或细菌存在，最常见于风湿性疾病，如系统性红斑狼疮、抗中性粒细胞胞质抗体血管炎，也可见于转移性恶性肿瘤。

虽然目前已知血培养阴性心内膜炎发生的原因多种多样，但临床要制定一套针对这一患者人群的评估体系还存在一定困难。为此，2017年马赛一家三级医疗中心发布了他们的一套标准化评估程序[29]，即利用血清学检测柯克斯体、巴尔通体、布鲁氏菌、军团菌和支原体，同时还可补充使用血清广谱检测和特异性PCR检测以及瓣膜广谱16S核糖体RNA PCR检测等手段。通过这些方法，他们在177例血培养阴性病例中明确了138例（78%）的病原体。

作为疑似心内膜炎常规评估的一部分，血液及血清学检测具有合理性，内容包括全血细胞计数、肌酐、ESR、CRP、补体水平检测以及尿液分析。对于血培养阴性心内膜炎患者，血清检测巴尔通体、布鲁氏菌、柯克斯体、军团菌和支原体可能有助于明确诊断。血培养阴性的人工瓣膜心内膜炎，如果是2011年以后接受过心脏直视手术，应使用抗酸血培养以排除奇美拉分枝杆菌感染。针对培养阴性的心内膜炎确诊手术病例，使用广谱16S核糖体RNA PCR检测切除的瓣膜组织，灵敏度约为80%，假阳性率为3%[50]；但这一检查对血清标本的检测在心内膜炎诊断中的作用尚不明确。

超声心动图

经胸超声心动图（TTE）和经食管超声心动图（TEE）在心内膜炎的诊断中发挥着重要作用，是检查瓣膜赘生物这一IE标志性特征的最佳影像学方式。其他与心内膜炎相关的超声心动图表现包括：瓣周脓肿、人工瓣膜与自体瓣环分离或新出现的瓣膜反流[7]。虽然TEE是公认的影像诊断"金标准"，但其尚存不足之处[6]：首先，对人工瓣膜病变诊断不够灵敏；其次是其侵入性，且需镇静处理，这就可能因患者需要相关准备或存在相关禁忌导致检查延迟，部分甚至完全不能接受这类检查。

经胸超声心动图（TTE）

经体表超声心动图是AHA和欧洲心脏病学会（ESC）指南推荐的针对心内膜炎的一线影像检查方法[6,27]。ESC报道TTE对诊断自体瓣膜和人工瓣膜IE的灵敏度分别为70%和50%，这一数字主要基于1989年的一项研究结果。该研究招募了80名患者，共涉及91个病变瓣膜[51]。在这个特定队列中，使用TTE在69个自体瓣膜感染中的47个瓣膜上发现了赘生物，超声诊断灵敏度为68.1%；而在22个人工瓣膜感染中的6个瓣膜上发现了赘生物，灵敏度为27.3%。同期其他研究也都提示TTE的灵敏度较低（28%～63%）[52-55]。最近的一次回顾性研究是在2017年，29名金黄色葡萄球菌心内膜炎确诊病例接受了TTE和TTE检查，TTE的灵敏度仅为21%[56]，原因是很多瓣周脓肿位置都靠后，TTE对这一位置病变的灵敏度非常低，只有4%～28%[57-58]。因此，所有TTE诊断为左侧心内膜炎的病例都应接受 TEE 来评估心内膜炎的瓣环并发症，例如脓肿、假性动脉瘤、心脏内瘘等。同理，对于人工瓣膜 TTE 阴性而临床高度怀疑心内膜炎的病例也应该进行 TEE 检查。有报道提及 TTE 诊断的高特异性可能存在一些误导性，超声心动图诊断 IE 的重要指标主要是发现瓣膜赘生物（本章后续部分将讨论）[7]，而忽视了感染并发的其他病理改变。准确意义上讲，只有将 TTE 与手术切除瓣膜或尸检的病理结果进行比较得出的结果，TTE 的特异性才能真正确定。TTE 的主要优点是已被广泛使用、检查快捷方便且无创。此外，在右侧心内膜炎患者中，TTE 已被证实与 TEE 具有相似的灵敏度[59]。然而，如果临床高度怀疑 IE，明智的做法是立即进行 TEE 检查，而不是等待 TTE 阳性结果的出现，以致延误治疗时机[27]。

经食管超声心动图（TEE）

如前所述，TEE 公认是诊断 IE 的最佳影像手段；但患者检查前要禁食准备，检查时需要镇静处理，为此可能很大一部分患者需要延迟检查。此外，不同医院实施 TEE 的具体情况不同，有些医疗机构周末不提供这类检查，对于这些因素带来的影响尚未得到充分研究。

据 ESC 报道，目前 TEE 诊断自体瓣膜和人工瓣膜心内膜炎的灵敏度分别为 96% 和 92%[6]。但当对这些数据进行更详尽的分析时，有证据显示这一数值可能被高估，因为这一结论是基于 1989—1994 年间的 4 项研究得出的[51-54]。这些研究都是在改良 Duke 诊断标准引入之前进行的，而且在 Shapiro、Erdel 和 Shively 的 3 项研究中，仅少量患者接受了手术或尸检，这就导致了这些高灵敏度数据的获得是基于超声心动图检测的赘生物而非病理检查。Shively 等报道的 TEE 灵敏度为 94%，而其队列中仅有 16 名患者。Mugge 等的研究是 4 项研究中唯一一项所有患者都接受了手术或尸检，他们报道 TEE 对自体瓣膜和人工瓣膜心内膜炎的灵敏度分别为 94% 和 77%。值得注意的是，该研究仅有 22 例人工瓣膜心内膜炎患者。后续的文献报道显示，在所有心内膜炎病例中，13%~44% 可无超声心动图异常[33,60-61]。此外，TEE 在 IE 早期可呈假阴性，如果临床高度怀疑 IE，欧美共识指南均建议间隔 5~7 d 复查一次 TEE[6,27]。综上所述，虽然文献报道 TEE 的灵敏度很高，临床医生还是应该意识到现有数据的缺陷，不过分依赖 TEE 检查结果，保持临床警觉性，进行综合判断。近来心脏 PET 作为辅助性影像手段引入临床，特别是用于人工瓣膜心内膜炎的诊断，具有较大作用。

其他影像学检查与心电图

正电子发射断层扫描（PET/CT）

心脏 ^{18}F- 氟脱氧葡萄糖（^{18}F-FDG）PET/CT 是一种相对较新的核成像工具，可以协助诊断 IE。它利用了 PET 的双重成像功能：①可以检测炎症区域，通过识别炎症白细胞（表达大量葡萄糖转运蛋白、代谢异常活跃）进行确认；②可以判断结构异常，心脏 CT 可以发现与心内膜炎相关的结构异常。多项研究表明，将 ^{18}F–FDG PET/CT 引入 Duke 标准可将其对人工瓣膜心内膜炎诊断的灵敏度提高到约 90%[62-63]。回顾性研究还表明，对临床病史提示存在心内膜炎的病例，^{18}F–FDG PET/CT 检查结果与术中的感染发现具有良好相关性[64]。

^{18}F–FDG PET/CT 很少用于诊断自体瓣膜心内膜炎。2020 年一项针对 115 名自体瓣膜心内膜炎的研究显示灵敏度仅有 22%。当将 PET/CT 与 Duke 标准结合用于诊断自体瓣膜心内膜炎时，灵敏度也仅为 65%[65]。作者推测，PET/CT 之所以对自体瓣膜感染诊断的灵敏度低，是因为自体瓣膜标本中纤维化组织占主导，而人工瓣膜感染病理上以多形核细胞浸润为主。心脏 PET/CT 还有一个不足之处，即在瓣膜置换术后 1 年内进行该检查，存在人工瓣膜引起的生理性中低程度 FDG 摄取增加的现象[66]。有文献认为，术后的这种摄取增加与外科黏合剂的使用有关，非人工瓣膜所致，且这是瓣膜置换术后出现的非感染性摄取增加的典型模式[67-68]。这一现象的存在可能不利于对该类病例核医学影像的解读，但如果由经验丰富的核医学医生进行分析，即便患者近期做过瓣膜置换，存在摄取异常，^{18}F–FDG PET/CT 在鉴定是否存在心内膜炎时仍有价值。目前 ESC 将心脏 ^{18}F–FDG PET/CT 包含在人工瓣膜心内膜炎诊断标准中，前提是瓣膜置换术后 ≥ 3 个月[6]。

尽管具有诸多优点，但心脏 ^{18}F–FDG PET/CT 在北美医疗机构尚未广泛使用。部分原因是设备昂贵，另外就是能熟练解读这些结果的专业人员数量较少。此外，标准化的 PET 检查需要限制碳水化合物 24～36 h，检查前还需禁食[69-70]，这些准备可能导致诊疗延误，并可能出现不良临床结果。基于以上原因，^{18}F–FDG PET/CT 目前仍局限于部分患者人群；但伴随其临床研究应用的深入与拓展，相信将有更多的患者从中获益。

计算机断层扫描（CT）

以往，CT 不作为 IE 的常规诊断手段，但目前多层门控心脏 CT 在识别瓣膜赘生物方面已被证明与 TEE 具有相似效果[71-72]，在检测瓣周脓肿和假性动脉瘤方面，甚至优于后者[6,71]。然而，CT 在临床主要用于诊断 IE 的栓塞并发症，如中枢神经系统、肺、肾、脾等的栓塞事件。CT 血管造影（CTA）还可用于脓毒性栓塞引起的周围血管闭塞和肠系膜缺血。因此，当临床出现栓塞相关体征和症状时，专业上的一致意见就是使用 CT 进行评估，而对无症状者经验性地使用 CT 评估头部、胸部、腹部和（或）骨盆的栓塞情况，目前尚存争议。2015 年埃及的一项研究显示：对 81 例左侧心内膜炎确诊病例常规进行 CTA 检查，63% 的病例发现有中枢神经系统栓塞的证据[73]，其中 1/3 无临床症状，CTA 结果导致 25.6% 的入组病例改变了治疗计划。但临床具体有多少无症状患者因为 CTA 影像结果而改变治疗计划，急性肾损伤发生率又是多少等数据未予报道。理论上讲，栓塞一旦被 CT 或 CTA 检查证实，可以帮助一部分按 Duke 标准被认为是疑似的病例，升级为确诊病例。

而在以上所有作用当中，CT检查最重要的作用可能就是检测颅内出血和（或）真菌性动脉瘤。如果证实存在这些并发症，则很大程度上需要调整手术治疗方案。临床需要注意，单纯CT平扫即可检测到颅内出血，无须使用碘造影剂，可避免使用造影剂诱发肾病的风险。目前，CT检查对于胸部、腹部和（或）盆腔栓塞等病变的使用多为经验性，且数据有限。常规使用这类检查前，必须权衡检查可能的获益与造成肾损伤和辐射风险等方面的弊端。

磁共振成像（MRI）

相比CT，MRI对心内膜炎脑血管并发症更灵敏[6]。近2/3接受常规脑部MRI的患者发现有栓塞病变[74]，其中约30%的病例没有临床症状。与CT相似，MRI发现脑部栓塞并发症同样可以升级心内膜炎的诊断。在对53名疑似心内膜炎患者的研究中，常规脑部MRI使32%的病例得以明确诊断，还有18%的患者因MRI结果而改变治疗计划[75]。中枢神经系统栓塞的风险因素包括赘生物>10mm、金黄色葡萄球菌菌血症、高龄、糖尿病和心房颤动[76]。

研究显示，腹部MRI可以检出约34%的临床无症状系统性栓塞，不过检出率明显低于脑部[77]。2012年法国的一项研究评估了常规脑部和腹部MRI在58例疑似心内膜炎患者中的作用，腹部MRI检查结果仅使1名患者升级为确诊，没有患者因此而需修正治疗方案。虽然资料有限，但证据表明脑部MRI可能有助于临床医生对疑似心内膜炎的诊断升级，以明确诊断，并调整治疗计划；而常规腹部MRI似乎没有这些益处。目前，AHA和ESC指南推荐所有疑似心内膜炎合并头痛、神经功能缺损或脑膜症状的病例均需接受脑血管影像学检查[6,27]。

血管造影（CTA/MRA）

对于疑似或确诊心内膜炎的患者，CT或MRI上蛛网膜下腔出血的证据可提示真菌性动脉瘤的存在。传统的血管造影公认是诊断真菌性动脉瘤的"金标准"，但在操作上存在引起卒中、颅内出血、动脉夹层和穿刺部位血肿等风险[78]，而CTA和MR血管造影（MRA）没有上述风险。对此，2018年对10项研究（包括868个病例）进行的meta分析发现：与MRA相比，CTA具有更高的诊断灵敏度和准确性[79]，且更为简单易行，使用更广泛；而MRA的优点则是使用造影剂较少、肾毒性低。

心电图（ECG）

ECG检查对心内膜炎的灵敏度较低，但对疑似病例的诊断可提供重要信息。冠状动脉栓塞导致的心肌梗死占所有心内膜炎病例的2.9%~10.6%，ECG可以通过ST段变化进行判断[80]。ECG对心包炎也可以通过ST段抬高进行鉴别。高达30%的心内膜炎病例可能出现心内膜脓肿，这种情况最常见于主动脉瓣感染[81]，脓肿可侵犯心脏传导系统，导致约25%的病例出现房室传导阻滞。据报道，ECG

对疑似心内膜炎脓肿的阳性预测值为88%，但灵敏度仅有45%[58]。

诊断标准

改良 Duke 标准

第一套常用的心内膜炎诊断标准是 Von Reyn 标准，首次发表于1981年。Von Reyn 标准主要依赖于微生物学和其他相关检查结果，该标准的使用早于超声心动图的应用，存在诸多不足。为此，1994年推出了 Duke 标准，并于2000年进一步更新[7,82]。虽然制定这些改良标准的初衷是为流行病学研究及临床试验提供更好的准入标准，但改良的 Duke 标准一经推出即被临床用作心内膜炎的主要诊断标准（表2.1）。该诊断标准结合微生物学和超声心动图检查的主要标准和临床及微生物学检查的次要标准对患者进行分层，分为确诊、疑似或排除心内膜炎三大类。主要标准包括：①心内膜炎典型致病微生物血培养持续呈阳性或多次呈阳性，或②超声心动图发现心内膜受累的证据或新的瓣膜反流。次要标准包括：①发热；②心内膜炎风险因素；③免疫并发症；④血管并发症；⑤不符合主要标准的血培养阳性。患者满足2项主要标准，或1项主要标准和3~4项次要标准，或5项次要标准，均可确诊 IE。符合1项主要标准和1~2项次要标准，或符合3~4项次要标准的被归类为疑似 IE。所有其他病例均可排除 IE。

尽管改良 Duke 标准在临床上得到了广泛和长期的应用，报道显示，其灵敏度也仅有70%~79%[83]。为此，对心内膜炎的诊断不能仅凭这几项指标，而是要全盘考虑临床各种因素来判断。Duke 标准灵敏度的不尽如人意可归因于心内膜炎病例中很大一部分血培养或超声心动图阴性[29,33,60-61]。此外值得注意的是，除了静脉吸毒，Duke 标准没有具体说明其他哪些因素会增加 IE 的风险。因此，临床上应该对相关风险因素有清晰的认识，具体包括：既往心内膜炎病史，年龄>60岁，男性，人工瓣膜置换术后，先天性心脏病，安装有植入式心脏装置，留置中心静脉导管，心脏瓣膜病（特别是二叶主动脉瓣畸形和二尖瓣脱垂伴中重度反流），血液透析[6]。

为能更准确地诊断心内膜炎，2015年 ESC 对心内膜炎指南做了补充：^{18}F-FDG PET/CT 检测到人工瓣膜植入部位周围存在异常炎症活动（但瓣膜植入须>3个月）和心脏 CT 检测到明确的瓣周病变。这两点被加入 Duke 标准的主要标准[6]。为提高人工瓣膜心内膜炎的诊断灵敏度，一些研究机构主张进一步修正 Duke 标准的条款，将新出现的杵状指、脾大、指/趾端裂片状出血、皮下瘀点、ESR 和 CRP 升高、镜下血尿以及中心静脉或外周静脉置管的存在纳入诊断标准[84]。

表 2.1 感染性心内膜炎（IE）的改良 Duke 诊断标准

确诊心内膜炎	疑似心内膜炎	排除心内膜炎
·2 项主要标准	·1 项主要标准和 1~2 项次要标准	·0 项主要标准和 1~2 项次要标准
·1 项主要标准和 ≥ 3 项次要标准	·3~4 项次要标准	·1 项主要标准和 0 项次要标准
·5 项次要标准		

主要标准

A. 实验室证据：
- 2 次独立的血培养结果均提示为 IE 的典型微生物：草绿色链球菌、金黄色葡萄球菌、牛链球菌、HACEK（嗜血杆菌、凝聚杆菌、人心杆菌、侵蚀艾肯菌和金氏金氏菌）或社区获得性肠球菌（缺乏原发病灶）
- 贝纳柯克斯体单次血培养阳性或 I 期抗体效价 > 1∶800

B. 心内膜受累的证据：
- 超声心动图支持 IE
  阳性结果的定义：瓣膜或瓣膜支撑结构上振荡的心内团块，或在反流束路径上，或在植入材料上，没有其他解剖学结构可以解释；或心肌脓肿，或新出现的人工瓣膜与自体瓣环部分分离
- 新的瓣膜反流（先前杂音强度增加，或杂音性质改变而强度改变不多）

次要标准

A. 心脏感染易患因素或静脉吸毒者
B. 发热 ≥ 38℃
C. 血管表现：主要动脉栓塞、脓毒性肺梗死、真菌性动脉瘤、脑出血、结膜出血、Janeway 病变
D. 免疫表现：肾小球肾炎、Osler 结节、Roth 斑、类风湿因子阳性
E. 血培养阳性但不符合之前提到的主要标准（不包括单次凝固酶阴性葡萄球菌血培养阳性，不引起心内膜炎的微生物）或缺乏与 IE 相符的微生物活动性感染的血清学证据

总体方案

本章概述了 IE 的临床体征和症状、最常见的病原体、多种影像方式在诊断中的作用，并讨论了主要的诊断标准。掌握这些内容除了对于快速准确诊断心内膜炎非常重要外，还有助于制定疾病的总体评估方案。各医疗机构可根据自身现有的影像设备及相关的专业经验，制定出自身对 IE 的诊治方案，以降低该患者人群的院内死亡率（图 2.1）[85-87]。

在评估新患者时，考虑患者是否有 IE 的风险因素可能会对诊断有所帮助。例如，如果患者为二叶主动脉瓣，或进行过人工瓣膜置换，或植入有心内装置，或为静脉吸毒者，或在接受血液透析，那么接诊人员应考虑心内膜炎的可能性，尤其是当这种患者出现一些非特异性表现时（例如不明原因的发热、卒中或新诊断的肾小球肾炎）。还有数据支持对所有表现为典型病原体菌血症的患者采用 TTE 检查，初步评估心内膜炎存在的可能性，可使患者获益[36]。多达 30% 的金黄色葡萄球菌菌血症患者在随后的诊疗过程中发现患有心内膜炎[88]，在此基础上，针

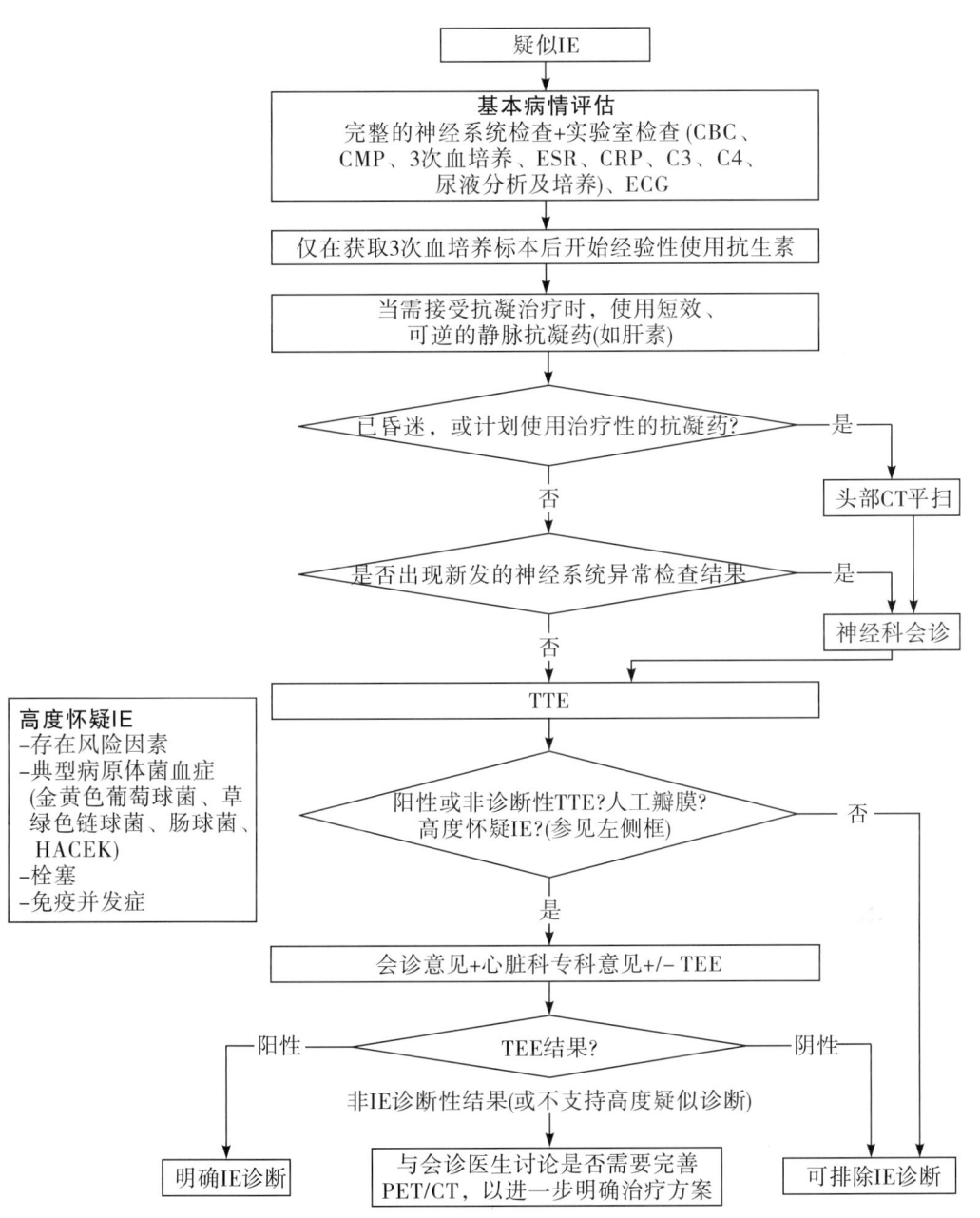

```
                        ┌─────────┐
                        │ 疑似IE  │
                        └────┬────┘
                             ↓
            ┌──────────────────────────────────┐
            │          基本病情评估              │
            │ 完整的神经系统检查+实验室检查(CBC、│
            │ CMP、3次血培养、ESR、CRP、C3、C4、  │
            │  尿液分析及培养)、ECG              │
            └──────────────┬───────────────────┘
                           ↓
            ┌──────────────────────────────────┐
            │ 仅在获取3次血培养标本后开始经验性使用抗生素 │
            └──────────────┬───────────────────┘
                           ↓
            ┌──────────────────────────────────┐
            │ 当需接受抗凝治疗时，使用短效、       │
            │ 可逆的静脉抗凝药(如肝素)            │
            └──────────────┬───────────────────┘
                           ↓
                  ┌────────────────────┐    是    ┌──────────┐
                  │已昏迷，或计划使用治疗│────────→│头部CT平扫│
                  │性的抗凝药?          │         └──────────┘
                  └─────────┬──────────┘
                         否 ↓
                  ┌────────────────────┐    是    ┌──────────┐
                  │是否出现新发的神经系统│────────→│神经科会诊│
                  │异常检查结果         │         └──────────┘
                  └─────────┬──────────┘
                         否 ↓
                      ┌────────┐
                      │  TTE   │
                      └────┬───┘
                           ↓
┌──────────────┐   ┌────────────────────┐                ┌──────────────┐
│高度怀疑IE     │   │阳性或非诊断性TTE?人工│    否          │              │
│-存在风险因素  │   │瓣膜?高度怀疑IE?(参见 │──────────────→│              │
│-典型病原体菌血症│  │左侧框)              │                │              │
│(金黄色葡萄球菌、│  └─────────┬──────────┘                │              │
│草绿色链球菌、肠│         是 ↓                            │              │
│球菌、HACEK)   │   ┌────────────────────┐                │              │
│-栓塞          │   │会诊意见+心脏科专科意见│                │              │
│-免疫并发症    │   │+/- TEE              │                │              │
└──────────────┘   └─────────┬──────────┘                │              │
                              ↓                           │              │
                   阳性 ┌──────────┐ 阴性                  │              │
              ┌───────│ TEE结果?  │──────┐                │              │
              ↓        └──────────┘      ↓                │              │
                  非IE诊断性结果(或不支持高度疑似诊断)
         ┌──────────┐  ┌──────────────────┐   ┌──────────┐
         │明确IE诊断│  │与会诊医生讨论是否需要│   │可排除IE诊断│
         └──────────┘  │完善PET/CT，以进一步│   └──────────┘
                       │明确治疗方案        │
                       └──────────────────┘
```

图2.1 感染性心内膜炎（IE）诊疗流程，由密歇根大学心内膜炎多学科医疗团队制定。CBC：全血细胞计数；CMP：综合代谢检测；ESR：红细胞沉降率；CRP：C-反应蛋白；ECG：心电图；TTE：经胸超声心电图；TEE：经食管超声心电图；HACEK：参见表2.1

对何时进行TEE检查设计了有效评分系统，包括VIRSTA评分（针对金黄色葡萄球菌菌血症）和NOVA评分（针对肠球菌菌血症）[89-90]。即使通过TTE已确诊的心内膜炎患者，仍有必要进行TEE检查，以评估是否存在侵袭性瓣环并发症，例如心内脓肿。当临床高度怀疑人工瓣膜心内膜炎而超声心动图阴性时，^{18}F-FDG PET/CT是一种有用的辅助工具，可以实现准确的诊断。神经系统CT和MRI均可用于检测心内膜炎的栓塞并发症,从而协助疾病的诊断和随后的治疗。鉴于 IE 相关的高并发症发生率和致死率,以及延迟诊断及误诊可能带来的灾难性后果,对于具有相应的症状、风险因素、典型病原体以及(或)实验室检查或放射学结果符合心内膜炎诊断的患者,有必要制定一套排查程序。

总　结

IE 仍然是一种复杂的疾病,临床表现多种多样。尽管心血管影像检查和治疗方法取得了长足进步,但目前的诊断标准和检测手段仍不完善,导致该病的院内死亡率居高不下。鉴于此,同时考虑到医疗实践中不同机构间存在广泛差异,利用现有文献、当前的检查手段和诊断标准,加上合理的临床判断(最重要),制定一套针对疑似心内膜炎的系统性评估方案,对于解决这一致命性疾病至关重要。

参考文献

[1] Bishara J, Leibovici L, Gartman-Israel D, et al. Long-term outcome of infective endocarditis: the impact of early surgical intervention. Clin Infect Dis, 2001, 33: 1636.

[2] Nadji G, Goissen T, Brahim A, et al. Impact of early surgery on 6-month outcome in acute infective endocarditis. Int J Cardiol, 2008, 129: 227.

[3] Kang D, Kim Y, Kim S, et al. Early surgery versus conventional treatment for infective endocarditis. N Engl J Med, 2012, 366(26): 2466–2473.

[4] N'Guyen Y, Duval X, Revest M, et al. Time interval between infective endocarditis first symptoms and diagnosis: relationship to infective endocarditis characteristics, microorganisms and prognosis. Ann Med, 2016, 49(2): 117–125.

[5] Cahill TJ, Prendergast BD. Infective endocarditis. Lancet, 2016, 387(10021): 882–893.

[6] Habib G, Lancellotti P, Antunes M, et al. ESC guidelines for the management of infective endocarditis: the task force for the management of infective endocarditis of the European Society of Cardiology (ESC). Eur Heart J, 2015, 36(44): 3075–3128.

[7] Li J, Sexton D, Mick N, et al. Proposed modifications to the Duke criteria for the diagnosis of infective endocarditis. Clin Infect Dis, 2000, 30(4): 633–638.

[8] Armstong W, Shea M. Clinical diagnosis of infective endocarditis//Vlessia AA, Bolling SF, editors. Endocarditis: a multidisciplinary approach to modern treatment. NY. Futura: Armonk, 1999: 107–133.

[9] Terpenning MS, Buggy BP, Kauffman CA. Infective endocarditis: clinical features in you and elderly patients. Am J Med, 1987, 83: 626–634.

[10] Hill EE, Herijgers P, Claus P, et al. Infective endocarditis: changing epidemiology and predictors of 6-month mortality: a prospective cohort study. Eur Heart J, 2007, 28(2): 196–203.

[11] Blumberg EA, Robbin N, Adimora A, et al. Persistent fever in association with infective endocarditis. Clin Infect Dis, 1992, 15: 983–990.

[12] Churchill MA, Geraci JE, Hunder GG. Musculoskeletal manifestations of bacterial endocarditis. Ann Intern Med, 1966, 87: 754–759.

[13] Pigrau C, Almirante B, Flores X, et al. Spontaneous pyogenic vertebral osteomyelitis and endocarditis: incidence, risk factors, and outcome. Am J Med, 2005, 118(11): 1287–1294.

[14] Varma MP, McCluskey DR, Khan MM, et al. Heart failure associated with infective endocarditis. A review of 40 cases. Br Heart J, 1986, 55(2): 191–197.

[15] Pati P, Khalif A, Shanmugam B, et al. Trends in infective endocarditis complicated by congestive

heart failure: data from the national inpatient sample from 1999—2014. Chest, 2017, 3692(17): 3692.
[16] Hart R, Foster J, Luther M, et al. Stroke in infective endocarditis. Stroke, 1990, 21: 695–700.
[17] Grecu N, Tiu C, Terecoasa E, et al. Endocarditis and stroke. Maedica, 2014, 9(4): 375–381.
[18] Saric M, Armour A, Arnaout S, et al. Guidelines for the use of echocardiography in the evaluation of a cardiac source of embolism. J Am Soc Echocardiogr, 2016, 29: 1–42.
[19] Singhal AB, Topcuoglu MA, Buonanno FS. Acute ischemic stroke patterns in infective and nonbacterial thrombotic endocarditis: a diffusion-weighted magnetic resonance imaging study. Stroke, 2002, 33(5): 1267–1273.
[20] Morris NA, Matiello M, Lyons JL, et al. Neurologic complications in infective endocarditis: identification, management, and impact on cardiac surgery. Neurohospitalist, 2014, 4(4): 213–222.
[21] Lucas MJ, Brouwer MC, van der Ende A, et al. Endocarditis in adults with bacterial meningitis. Circulation, 2013, 127(20): 2056–2062.
[22] Pedersen M, Benfield TL, Skinhoej P, et al. Haematogenous Staphylococcus aureus meningitis. A 10-year nationwide study of 96 consecutive cases. BMC Infect Dis, 2006, 6(49).
[23] Piqueras FJ, Esquinas BG, Pinilla Rivas M, et al. Central retinal artery occlusion and infective endocarditis: rigor does matter. Arch Soc Esp Oftalmol, 2015, 90(11): 546–548.
[24] Carmelli G, Surles T, Brown A. Endophthalmitis and mycotic aneurysm: the only clues to underlying endocarditis. Clin Pract & Cases Emerg Med, 2018, 2(1): 16–20.
[25] Yee J, McAllister CK. Osler's nodes and the recognition of infective endocarditis: a lesson diagnostic importance. South Med J, 1987, 80: 753–757.
[26] Sandre RM, Shafran SD. Infective endocarditis: review of 135 cases over 9 years. Clin Infect Dis, 1996, 22(2): 276–286.
[27] Baddour L, Wilson W, Bayer A, et al. Infective endocarditis in adults: diagnosis, antimicrobial therapy, and management of complications a scientific statement for healthcare professionals from the American Heart Association. Circulation, 2015, 132: 1–53.
[28] Lee A, Mirrett S, Reiler LB, et al. Detection of bloodstream infection in adults: how many blood cultures are needed? J Clin Microbiol, 2007, 45(11): 3546–3548.
[29] Fournier PE, Gouriet F, Casalta JP, et al. Blood culture-negative endocarditis: improving the diagnostic yield using new diagnostic tools. Medicine, 2017, 96(47).
[30] Werner M, Andersson R, Olaison L, et al. A clinical study of culture-negative endocarditis. Medicine, 2003, 82(4): 263–273.
[31] Hoen B, Selton-Suty C, Lacassin F, et al. Infective endocarditis in patients with negative blood cultures: analysis of 88 cases from a one-year nationwide survey in France. Clin Infect Dis, 1995, 20: 501–506.
[32] Hall KK, Lyman JA. Updated review of blood culture contamination. Clin Microbiol Rev, 2006, 19(4): 788–802.
[33] Murdoch DR, Corey GR, Hoen B, et al. Clinical presentation, etiology, and outcome of infective endocarditis in the 21st century: the International Collaboration on Endocarditis-Prospective Cohort Study. Arch Intern Med, 2009, 169(5): 463–473.
[34] Vlessis AA, Hovaguimian H, Jeggers J, et al. Infective Endocarditis: ten-year review of medical and surgical therapy. Ann Thorac Surg, 1996, 61: 1217–1222.
[35] Siméon S, Le Moing V, Tubiana S, et al. Time to blood culture positivity: an independent predictor of infective endocarditis and mortality in patients with Staphylococcus aureus bacteraemia. Clin Microbiol Infect, 2019, 25(4): 481–488.
[36] Vos FJ, Bleeker-Rovers CP, Sturm PD, et al. Endocarditis: effects of routine echocardiography during Gram-positive bacteraemia. Neth J Med, 2011, 69(7): 335–340.
[37] Raza SS, Sultan OW, Sohail MR. Gram-negative bacterial endocarditis in adults: state-of-the-heart. Expert Rev Anti Infect Ther, 2010, 8(8): 879–885.
[38] Morpeth S, Murdoch D, Cabell CH, et al. Non-HACEK Gram-negative bacillus endocarditis. Ann Intern Med, 2007, 147(12): 829–835.

[39] Dignani MC, Solomkin JS, Anaissie EJ. Candida//Anaissie EJ, McGinnis MR, Pfaller MA. Clinical mycology. New York, NY: Churchill Livingstone, 2009: 197–229.
[40] Ellis ME, Al-Abdely H, Sandridge A, et al. Fungal endocarditis: evidence in the world literature, 1965—1995. Clin Infect Dis, 2001, 32(1): 50–62.
[41] Fernández-Cruz A, Cruz Menárguez M, Muñoz P, et al. The search for endocarditis in patients with candidemia: a systematic recommendation for echocardiography? A prospective cohort. Eur J Clin Microbiol Infect Dis, 2015, 34(8): 1543–1549.
[42] Garvey GJ, Neu HC. Infective endocarditis: an evolving disease: a review of endocarditis at the Columbia Presbyterian Medical Center, 1968—1973. Medicine, 1975, 57: 105–127.
[43] Conlon PJ, Jefferies F, Krigman HR, et al. Predictors of prognosis and risk of acute renal failure in bacterial endocarditis. Clin Nephrol, 1998, 49(2): 96–101.
[44] Gagneux-Brunon A, Pouvaret A, Maillard N, et al. Acute kidney injury in infective endocarditis: a retrospective analysis. Medicine et Maladies Infecieuses, 2019, 49(7): 527–533.
[45] Neugarten J, Gallo GR, Baldwin DS. Glomerulonephritis in bacterial endocarditis. Am J Kidney Dis, 1984, 3(5): 371–379.
[46] Boils CL, Nasr SH, Walker PD, et al. Update on endocarditis-associated glomerulonephritis. Kidney Int, 2015, 87(6): 1241–1249.
[47] Raoult D, Casalta JP, Richet H, et al. Contribution of systematic serological testing in diagnosis of infective endocarditis. J Clin Microbiol, 2005, 43(10): 5238–5242.
[48] Mohanan S, Gopalan NR, Vellani H, et al. Baseline C-reactive protein levels and prognosis in patients with infective endocarditis: a prospective cohort study. Indian Heart J, 2018, 70(Suppl. 3): S43–S49.
[49] Inojosa WO, Gioббia M, Muffato G, et al. Mycobacterium chimaera infections following cardiac surgery in Treviso Hospital, Italy, from 2016 to 2019: cases report. World J Clin Cases, 2019, 7(18): 2776–2786.
[50] Shrestha NK, Ledtke CS, Wang H, et al. Heart valve culture and sequencing to identify the infective endocarditis pathogen in surgically treated patients. Ann Thorac Surg, 2015, 99(1): 33–37.
[51] Mugge A, Daniel WG, Frank G, et al. Echocardiography in infective endocarditis: reassessment of prognostic implications of vegetation size determined by the transthoracic and the transesophageal approach. J Am Coll Cardiol, 1989, 14: 631–638.
[52] Shapiro SM, Young E, De Guzman S, et al. Transesophageal echocardiography in diagnosis of infective endocarditis. Chest, 1994, 105: 377–382.
[53] Erbel R, Rohmann S, Drexler M, et al. Improved diagnostic value of echocardiography in patients with infective endocarditis by transoesophageal approach. A prospective study. Eur Heart J, 1988, 9: 43–53.
[54] Shively BK, Gurule FT, Roldan CA, et al. Diagnostic value of transesophageal compared with transthoracic echocardiography in infective endocarditis. J Am Coll Cardiol, 1991, 18: 391–397.
[55] Drexler M, Erbel R, Rohmann S, et al. Diagnostic value of two-dimensional transoesophageal versus transthoracic echocardiography in patients with infective endocarditis. Eur Heart J, 1987, 8: 303–306.
[56] Sekar P, Johnson JR, Thurn JR, et al. Comparative sensitivity of transthoracic and transesophageal echocardiography in diagnosis of infective endocarditis among veterans with Staphylococcus aureus bacteremia. Open Forum Infect Dis, 2017, 4(2): ofx035.
[57] Ellis SG, Goldstein J, Popp RL. Detection of endocarditis-associated perivalvular abscesses by two-dimensional echocardiography. J Am Coll Cardiol, 1985, 5(3): 647–653.
[58] Blumberg EA, Karalis DA, Chandrasekaran K, et al. Endocarditis-associated paravalvular abscesses. Do clinical parameters predict the presence of abscess? Chest, 1995, 107(4): 898–903.
[59] San Román JA, Vilacosta I, Zamorano J, et al. Transesophageal echocardiography in right-sided endocarditis. J Am Coll Cardiol, 1993, 21(5): 1226–1230.

[60] Habib G, Badano L, Tribouilloy C, et al. Recommendations for the practice of echocardiography in infective endocarditis. Eur J Echocardiogr, 2010, 11: 202–219.
[61] Hershman-Sarafov M, Paz A, Potasman I, et al. Echo-negative endocarditis: analysis of 538 consecutive transesophageal echocardiographies. Open Forum Infect Dis, 2016, 3(1): 1105.
[62] Pizzi M, Roque A, Fernandez-Hidalgo N, et al. Improving the diagnosis of infective endocarditis in prosthetic valves and intracardiac devices with ^{18}F-fluorodeoxyglucose positron emission tomography/compute tomography angiography: initial results at an infective endocarditis referral center. Circulation, 2015, 132(12): 1113–1126.
[63] Saby L, Laas O, Habib G, et al. Positron emission tomography/computed tomography for diagnosis of prosthetic valve endocarditis: increased valvular ^{18}F-fluorodeoxyglucose uptake as a novel major criterion. J Am Coll Cardiol, 2013, 61(23): 2374–2382.
[64] El-Dalati S, Murthy VL, Owczarczyk AB, et al. Correlating cardiac F-18 FDG PET/CT results with intra-operative findings in infectious endocarditis. J Nucl Cardiol, 2019, 28: 289–294.
[65] de Camargo RA, Sommer Bitencourt M, Meneghetti JC, et al. The role of ^{18}F-fluorodeoxyglucose positron emission tomography/computed tomography in the diagnosis of left-sided endocarditis: native vs prosthetic valves endocarditis. Clin Infect Dis, 2020, 70(4): 583–594.
[66] Wahadat AR, Tanis W, Scholtens AM, et al. Normal imaging findings after aortic valve implantation on ^{18}F-Fluorodeoxyglucose positron emission tomography with computed tomography. J Nucl Cardiol, 2020.
[67] Roque A, Pizzi MN, Fernández-Hidalgo N, et al. Morpho-metabolic post-surgical patterns of non-infected prosthetic heart valves by [18F]FDG PET/CTA:"normality"is a possible diagnosis. Eur Heart J Cardiovasc Imaging, 2020, 21(1): 24–33.
[68] Swart LE, Gomes A, Scholtens AM, et al. Improving the diagnostic performance of ^{18}F-fluorodeoxyglucose positron-emission tomography/computed tomography in prosthetic heart valve endocarditis. Circulation, 2018, 138(14): 1412–1427.
[69] Scholtens AM, Swart LE, Kolste HJT, et al. Standardized uptake values in FDG PET/CT for prosthetic heart valve endocarditis: a call for standardization. J Nucl Cardiol, 2018, 25(6): 2084–2091.
[70] Larson SR, Pieper JA, Hulten EA, et al. Characterization of a highly effective preparation for suppression of myocardial glucose utilization. J Nucl Cardiol, 2020, 27(3): 849–861.
[71] Feuchtner GM, Stolzmann P, Dichtl W, et al. Multislice computed tomography in infective endocarditis: comparison with transesophageal echocardiography and intraoperative findings. J Am Coll Cardiol, 2009, 53(5): 436–444.
[72] Fagman E, Perrotta S, Bech-Hanssen O, et al. ECG-gated computed tomography: a new role for patients with suspected aortic prosthetic valve endocarditis. Eur Radiol, 2012, 22(11): 2407–2414.
[73] Meshaal MS, Kassem HH, Samir A, et al. Impact of routine cerebral CT angiography on treatment decisions in infective endocarditis. PloS One, 2015, 10(3): e0118616.
[74] Snygg-Martin U, Gustafsson L, Rosengren L, et al. Cerebrovascular complications in patients with left-sided infective endocarditis are common: a prospective study using magnetic resonance imaging and neurochemical brain damage markers. Clin Infect Dis, 2008, 47(1): 23–30.
[75] Duval X, Iung B, Klein I, et al. Effect of early cerebral magnetic resonance imaging on clinical decisions in infective endocarditis: a prospective study. Ann Intern Med, 2010, 152: 497–504.
[76] Hubert S, Thuny F, Resseguier N, et al. Prediction of symptomatic embolism in infective endocarditis: construction and validation of a risk calculator in a multicenter cohort. J Am Coll Cardiol, 2013, 62(15): 1384–1392.
[77] Iung B, Klein I, Mourvillier B, et al. Respective effects of early cerebral and abdominal magnetic resonance imaging on clinical decisions in infective endocarditis. Eur Heart J Cardiovasc Imaging, 2012, 13(8): 703–710.
[78] Lin A, Rawal S, Agid R, et al. Cerebrovascular imaging: which test is best? Neurosurgery, 2018, 83(1): 5–18.

[79] Chen X, Liu Y, Tong H, et al. Meta-analysis of computed tomography angiography versus magnetic resonance angiography for intracranial aneurysm. Medicine (Baltim), 2018, 97(20): e10771.

[80] Murtaza G, Rahman ZU, Sitwala P, et al. Case of acute ST segment elevation myocardial infarction in infective endocarditis-management with intra coronary stenting. Clin Pract, 2017, 7(3): 950.

[81] Choussat R, Thomas D, Isnard R, et al. Perivalvular abscesses associated with endocarditis; clinical features and prognostic factors of overall survival in a series of 233 cases. Perivalvular Abscesses French Multicentre Study. Eur Heart J, 1999, 20(3): 232–241.

[82] Durack DT, Lukes AS, Bright DK, et al. Evaluation of new clinical criteria for the diagnosis of infective endocarditis. Am J Med, 1994, 96: 211–219.

[83] Shrestha N, Shakya S, Hussain S, et al. Sensitivity and specificity of Duke criteria for diagnosis of definite infective endocarditis: a cohort study. Open Forum Infect Dis, 2017, 4(1): S550–S551.

[84] Lamas CC, Eykyn SJ. Suggested modifications to the Duke criteria for the clinical diagnosis of native valve and prosthetic valve endocarditis: analysis of 118 pathologically proven cases. Clin Infect Dis, 1997, 25: 713–719.

[85] Botelho-Nevers E, Thuny F, Casalta JP, et al. Dramatic reduction in infective endocarditis—related mortality with a management-based approach. Arch Intern Med, 2009, 169(14): 1290–1298.

[86] Carrasco-Chinchilla F, Sanchez-Espin G, Ruiz-Morales J, et al. Influence of a multidisciplinary alert strategy on mortality due to left-sided infective endocarditis. Spanish Soc Cardiol, 2014, 67(5): 380–386.

[87] Chirillo F, Scotton P, Rocco F, et al. Management of patients with infective endocarditis by a multidisciplinary team approach: an operative protocol. J Cardiovasc Med, 2013, 14(9): 659–668.

[88] Rasmussen RV, Høst U, Arpi M, et al. Prevalence of infective endocarditis in patients with Staphylococcus aureus bacteraemia: the value of screening with echocardiography. Eur J Echocardiogr, 2011, 12(6): 414–420.

[89] Tubiana S, Duval X, Alla F, et al. The VIRSTA score, a prediction score to estimate risk of infective endocarditis and determine priority for echocardiography in patients with Staphylococcus aureus bacteremia. J Infect, 2016, 72(5): 544–553.

[90] Bouza E, Kestler M, Beca T, et al. The NOVA score: a proposal to reduce the need for transesophageal echocardiography in patients with enterococcal bacteremia. Clin Infect Dis, 2015, 60(4): 528–535.

第 3 章
感染性心内膜炎的微生物学

J. Alexander Viehman [1,2], *Brandon J. Smith* [2], *Sowmya Nanjappa* [1,2], *Sui Kwong Li* [1,2], *Christian O. Perez* [1,2], *Carolyn R. Fernandes* [1,2]

[1]Division of Infectious Diseases, Department of Medicine, University of Pittsburgh School of Medicine, Pittsburgh, PA, United States; [2]University of Pittsburgh Medical Center, Pittsburgh, PA, United States

引 言

近年来，随着感染性心内膜炎（IE）流行病学的显著变化，明确哪些病原体是其主要致病因素显得非常重要。在美国，金黄色葡萄球菌已取代链球菌成为 IE 最常见的致病菌，约占所有病例的 30%。这一转变是多因素的，包括人工瓣膜、起搏器等心脏植入装置的广泛应用，以及静脉吸毒人群的不断扩大[1]。主要的革兰氏阳性菌感染趋势参见图 3.1[2]。要了解心内感染时宿主–病原体的相互作用，首先要从病原体分类、起源、毒力因子和抗生素耐药性等方面进行探讨。

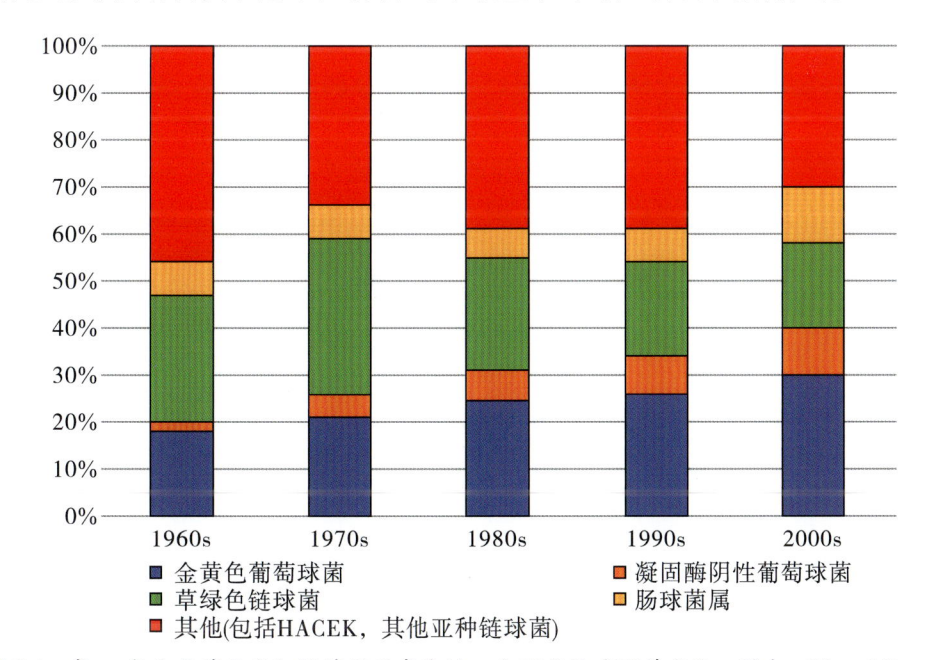

图 3.1 每 10 年主要革兰氏阳性菌所致感染性心内膜炎的病因学变化。引自：Slipczuk L, et al. Infective endocarditis epidemiology over five decades: a systematic review. PloS One, 2013, 8(12): e82665

自体瓣膜 IE 相关病原体

金黄色葡萄球菌

金黄色葡萄球菌（S.aureus）是一种普遍存在的革兰氏阳性球菌，在革兰氏染色中呈现典型的"葡萄样"形态。其命名来自拉丁语单词 aureus，意为"金色"，这源于培养基上菌落呈现金黄色。金黄色葡萄球菌为需氧生长，但也是兼性厌氧。所有葡萄球菌均为过氧化氢酶试验阳性，这一点可将其与链球菌区别开。凝固酶试验用于鉴别金黄色葡萄球菌（凝固酶阳性）与其他大多数临床相关并统称为凝固酶阴性的葡萄球菌（CoNS）[3]。包括金黄色葡萄球菌在内的葡萄球菌，一般共生于人类的皮肤和黏膜。人类是葡萄球菌的主要宿主，约 30% 的人群体内有金黄色葡萄球菌定植，金黄色葡萄球菌广泛存在的状态及其多种毒力因子使之成为 IE 的常见病因[4]，这也决定了为什么出现金黄色葡萄球菌血培养呈阳性是严重的医疗事件。除非在极其罕见的情况下，否则，金黄色葡萄球菌培养阳性绝不应该被视为采样过程中的污染；即便患者已从金黄色葡萄球菌菌血症中逐渐恢复，但只要血培养阳性，临床就应考虑 IE 的可能性。

·毒力因子

金黄色葡萄球菌可产生多种毒力因子（本文涵盖了其中最相关的因子），它们的作用包括促进自身生长和定植、入侵宿主、逃避免疫系统和组织破坏等。

广义上讲，鼻腔携带的金黄色葡萄球菌代表了该菌毒力因子的集合。虽然鼻腔携带已被证明会增加金黄色葡萄球菌感染的风险，但有限的证据表明，定植个体的病情可能比未定植个体的病情更轻[5]。进一步的证据表明，这种定植会产生适应性免疫，这可以解释定植者病情较轻的原因[6]。一旦进入体内，金黄色葡萄球菌既可以在细胞外也可以在细胞内生存。在细胞外，细菌更容易受到免疫系统的作用，包括补体级联反应的调理作用、白细胞吞噬作用和被抗体结合。为应对这些免疫过程，金黄色葡萄球菌可表达多种表面蛋白，包括聚集因子 A、蛋白 A 和多种补体抑制因子[7-8]。

金黄色葡萄球菌可产生多种毒力因子，可直接破坏宿主细胞和组织。研究最深入的是 Pantone-Valentine 白细胞毒素（PVL）。PVL 毒素于 1932 年首次被描述，其作用是引起宿主防御细胞（包括白细胞）的膜破裂，最终导致细胞死亡[9]。这种毒素通常与社区获得性耐甲氧西林金黄色葡萄球菌（MRSA）感染有关[10]，但其在鼻腔定植中的作用尚不清楚。然而，它与严重坏死性皮肤和软组织感染以及肺炎有着某种关联[11]。

·流行病学

鉴于耐药模式存在广泛的地理差异，因此在临床诊治中，当地流行病学是一个重要的考虑因素。例如，在美国，南部和东北部 MRSA 感染率历年来是较高的，而西部各州的耐药病例则有所下降[12-14]。在同一时期（1999—2003年），欧洲也出现了类似的差异性：冰岛的MRSA感染率为0.5%，而希腊则高达44%[13]。即便同一地区，不同人群的耐药率也存在差异：儿童与成人、住院患者与门诊患者、同一医院内的不同病房、静脉吸毒者与非静脉吸毒者等都存在差异。

甲氧西林敏感金黄色葡萄球菌（MSSA）

在发现并广泛使用青霉素治疗金黄色葡萄球菌感染之前，其导致的菌血症死亡率超过80%[15]。青霉素问世后，死亡率急剧下降，但不久之后耐药株接踵而至。1942年，科研人员首次阐明了相关耐药机制[16]。金黄色葡萄球菌由 blaZ 基因编码产生β-内酰胺酶，该酶可水解青霉素的β-内酰胺环，使其永久失活[17]。青霉素、氨基青霉素（阿莫西林、氨苄西林）和脲青霉素（哌拉西林）均可被这些细胞外β-内酰胺酶水解。

为解决青霉素耐药的问题，甲氧西林问世并于1961年用于临床[18]。甲氧西林属于青霉素的一个亚类，称为抗葡萄球菌青霉素，可对抗 blaZ 编码的β-内酰胺酶的水解作用。由于药物毒性问题，特别是间质性肾炎的出现，甲氧西林已退出临床。然而，苯唑西林和萘夫西林（也是抗葡萄球菌青霉素）仍在广泛使用。

现有文献进一步表明，在MSSA菌血症和心内膜炎的治疗中，与万古霉素作为终极治疗相比，使用β-内酰胺类药物可获得更好的临床结局[19]。但并非所有β-内酰胺类均具有同样好的疗效。第一代头孢菌素，如头孢唑林，就被发现疗效不亚于抗葡萄球菌青霉素。有证据表明，与萘夫西林相比，头孢唑林对β-内酰胺酶具有相对较好的耐受性[20]，但业界对于是否选择β-内酰胺类治疗MSSA仍存争议。值得注意的是，回顾性证据表明，与苯唑西林、萘夫西林和头孢唑林相比，β-内酰胺与β-内酰胺酶抑制剂的组合治疗方案（氨苄西林-舒巴坦和哌拉西林-他唑巴坦）的死亡率可能较高[21]。

耐甲氧西林金黄色葡萄球菌（MRSA）

1961年，英国首次报道了耐甲氧西林现象，当时刚引入抗葡萄球菌青霉素[22]。如上所述，金黄色葡萄球菌由于产生β-内酰胺酶而对青霉素产生耐药性；而它对抗葡萄球菌青霉素和头孢菌素的耐药性，主要是通过改变靶向青霉素结合蛋白（PBP）上的结合位点结构产生的。PBP是细菌细胞壁合成所必需的酶，在细胞壁合成的交联阶段发挥特殊作用。金黄色葡萄球菌产生4种PBP——PBP1~4，由 mecA 基因编码的变异PBP2蛋白名为PBP2a，这种改变可引起该蛋白质对大多数β-内酰胺的亲和力降低，导致细菌的强耐药性[23]。万古霉素仍然是治疗严重MRSA感染的主要手段，但鉴于其肾毒性和不断需要进行剂量调整所带来的挑战，人们一直在研发利用更新、更安全的替代药品。

万古霉素中敏和耐药金黄色葡萄球菌

自20世纪50年代以来,万古霉素一直是治疗MRSA的主要药物。耐万古霉素金黄色葡萄球菌(VRSA)于2002年在美国首次被发现,但相当罕见,报道的病例不足20例[24]。耐药性是由从肠球菌质粒获得的 vanA 操纵子在不同的接合作用(译者注:细菌通过菌毛相互接触时,质粒DNA从一个细菌转移至另一个细菌,这种类型的DNA转移称为接合作用)中产生的。万古霉素与D-Ala-D-Ala肽聚糖前体结合,最终干扰细胞壁的合成。vanA通过编码不易受万古霉素结合影响的D-Ala-D-Lac来改变细胞壁的合成,从而产生耐药性[24]。

比VRSA更常见的分离株是万古霉素中敏金黄色葡萄球菌(VISA),它们对万古霉素的敏感性降低,但没有完全耐药。这种表型出现之前,通常存在的是万古霉素敏感和万古霉素中敏分离株的混合菌群,称为杂合VISA(hVISA)[25]。至于VISA出现和向hVISA过渡背后的机制本文不赘述,这仍是一个有待研究的领域。重要的是:hVISA菌群暴露于糖肽(万古霉素)时间过长与其转化为VISA相关[26]。因此,当怀疑hVISA存在时,通常会采用达托霉素、头孢洛林或利奈唑胺等替代治疗。

α-溶血性链球菌

α-溶血性链球菌具有所有链球菌共同拥有的普遍特征:兼性厌氧,成对或成链的革兰氏阳性球菌,不产生过氧化氢酶或凝固酶[27]。α-溶血是指当将微生物在血琼脂上培养时,由于红细胞破坏而出现的绿色变色。

草绿色链球菌(*Viridans Streptococci*)包括多种α-溶血和非溶血性链球菌,通常定植于口咽部和上呼吸道。"Viridans"一词在拉丁语中意为"绿色",指的是α-溶血。该组包括缓症链球菌(*Str. mitis*)、血液链球菌(*Str. sanguinis*)、变异链球菌(*Str. mutans*)和唾液链球菌(*Str. salivarius*)等亚种[28]。实验室分子诊断技术极大改变了对单个链球菌亚种的识别,但一些传统诊断技术仍在不同医疗机构的临床中使用(不被胆汁溶解和对奥普托欣抵抗是鉴别出草绿色链球菌的主要特征)。尽管该菌全球各地的估测发病率各不相同,但推测它约占自体瓣膜IE病例的20%[29]。毒力因子包括产生细胞外葡聚糖[30],与不产生葡聚糖的链球菌相比,区别在于它具有黏附心脏瓣膜的能力,并具有不同程度的青霉素耐药性,导致的IE临床类型多为亚急性。

咽峡炎链球菌(*Streptococcus anginosus*)由3个亚群组成:咽峡炎链球菌(*Str. anginosus*)、星座链球菌(*Str. constellatus*)和中间型链球菌(*Str. intermedius*)[31]。它们是口咽部和胃肠道的共生菌群,可以通过在常规琼脂培养基上形成相对较小的菌落来与其他Lancefield链球菌区分开来。咽峡炎链球菌仅占自体瓣膜IE病例的5%,但它容易引发脓肿[32]。毒力因子包括纤连蛋白结合增强、血小板聚集和通过水解酶产生的凝血酶样活性[33]。咽峡炎链球菌通常对青霉素敏感,但之前也有过其对青霉素敏感性降低和耐药的报道。

肺炎链球菌（Streptococcus pneumoniae）是引起细菌性肺炎、中耳炎、鼻窦炎和脑膜炎的常见病原体，而引起 IE 等血管内感染则较为罕见[34]。鼻咽定植率在出生后的第 2 年和第 3 年达到峰值，而后下降至成人的 10% 左右。侵袭性肺炎链球菌疾病往往更高比例地发生在年龄 > 65 岁、有潜在器官功能障碍（心、肺、肾、肝和脾）以及存在各种免疫缺陷（例如补体缺乏、抗体缺陷、中性粒细胞减少等）的人群。肺炎链球菌可以通过 α-溶血、对奥普托欣的敏感性以及在胆汁盐中的溶解度进行微生物学鉴定。毒力因子主要包括多糖荚膜，它具有抵抗调理作用、抗吞噬作用和细胞内杀伤的能力[35]。临床绝大多数疾病是由血清型 23 引起，肺炎链球菌多糖疫苗（PPSV-23）专门针对这一类型[36]，但在儿童人群 PCV-7 和 PCV-13 的全面疫苗接种将有助于降低这一成人侵袭性肺炎链球菌疾病的发病率。目前，β-内酰胺类抗生素仍然是该类疾病的标准治疗方案，但肺炎链球菌对青霉素敏感性降低和耐药现象越来越常见。

肠球菌

肠球菌（Enterococcus）以前被归类为 D 组链球菌，后来独立命名。最常见的致病亚种是粪肠球菌（E. faecalis）和屎肠球菌（E. faecium），通常构成胃肠道、肝胆道和泌尿生殖道菌群。其所导致的 IE 占自体瓣膜病例的 10%，其中粪肠球菌是最常见的病因。它们产生光滑、灰色的菌落，这些菌落可以是 α-溶血的，也可以是非溶血性的，能够在 10~45℃ 含有 6.5%NaCl 的培养基中生长[37]。毒力因子包括聚集物质蛋白和细胞外表面蛋白：在动物模型中，前者可促进肠球菌黏附在心脏赘生物上[38]，后者可参与生物膜形成[39]。由于青霉素和头孢菌素的最低抑菌浓度（MIC）相对较高，因此与其他链球菌相比，肠球菌的抗菌治疗更为复杂。其根源在于肠球菌细胞壁 PBP 的亲和力降低，以及新出现的耐万古霉素肠球菌（主要是屎肠球菌）。耐药机制是由于 *vanA* 和 *vanB* 突变（最常见），导致 D-Ala-D-Lac 取代了细胞壁肽聚糖末端的 D-Ala-D-Ala，从而阻止万古霉素抑制细胞壁交联的作用。治疗肠球菌通常为二联用药，一般是氨苄西林与氨基糖苷类药物联合，而近年来氨苄西林与头孢曲松联合使用更普遍。

营养变异链球菌

营养变异链球菌（NVS）于 1961 年首次从心内膜炎患者中分离出来，因其特征而被认为是缓症链球菌的亚种[40]。随着时间的推移，基于对 16S 核糖体 RNA 序列的分析，它们被重新分类为引起人类感染的 2 个属、4 个种：缺陷乏养菌（Abiotrophia defectiva）、毗邻颗粒链球菌（Granulicatella adiacens）、苛养颗粒链球菌（Granulicatella elegans）和副毗邻颗粒链球菌（Granulicatella paraadiacens）[41]。它们是人类上呼吸道和胃肠道正常菌群的一部分。所有 NVS 都很"挑剔"，需要有吡哆醛或 L-半胱氨酸才能在次代培养基中生长。它们可以通过不同的革兰氏染色呈现多形性，并在血琼脂上形成非溶血性或 α-溶血小菌落[42]。

NVS 感染只占 IE 病例的一小部分，通常表现为在原有瓣膜疾病基础上出现的惰性感染。除分离和鉴别困难之外，对于大多数常规临床实验室来说，NVS 的体外抗菌药物敏感性测试都很具挑战性。多项体外研究显示，所有 NVS 分离株均对万古霉素敏感，对氨基糖苷类耐药性也不强，但对青霉素、头孢菌素、克林霉素和达托霉素的敏感性差异很大[43-45]。另一项对美国各地 599 株 NVS 临床分离株的大型研究显示：所有 NVS 对万古霉素敏感，90% 以上对左氧氟沙星敏感，但对青霉素和头孢曲松的敏感性存在显著的菌株和地域差异，缺陷乏养菌对青霉素最不敏感[46]。体外试验和实验动物模型已显示出青霉素或万古霉素与氨基糖苷类药物之间的协同作用。

与其他链球菌引起的 IE 相比，NVS 引起的 IE 往往具有更高的并发症发生率和死亡率。一项研究对比了 NVS 与其他链球菌引起的 IE，结果显示：死亡率分别为 14% 和 5%，栓塞事件发生率分别为 33% 和 11%，心力衰竭发生率为 33% 和 18%[47]。另一项针对 33 例患者的研究指出：50% 的患者需要手术，2/3 的患者在术后 10 年时仍然存活[48]。即使是对青霉素敏感的菌株也可能出现复发。因此当药敏试验无法进行时，细菌种类的鉴定有助于临床治疗方法的选择。目前主张联合用药时间为 4~6 周。

- **解没食子酸链球菌**（*Str. gallolyticus*）

这类革兰氏阳性球菌通常表达 Lancefield D 群抗原，是 IE 的重要病因。值得注意的是，由它们引起的菌血症或 IE 与成人结肠恶性肿瘤或其他结肠疾病存在密切关联[49]。此外，解没食子酸链球菌菌血症和肝病之间也存在关联，据此认为是网状内皮系统功能受损导致门静脉或体循环细菌清除率降低所致[50]。该类细菌以前被称为牛链球菌，最近重新分类，这给临床医生造成了困扰，因为新的名称忽略了它们分离来源的重要性，而仅仅注重了其培养特征。Ⅰ型牛链球菌（引起 IE 和菌血症最常见的一种），现在被命名为解没食子酸链球菌解没食子酸亚种；Ⅱ/1 型牛链球菌被命名为婴儿链球菌大肠亚种，而 Ⅱ/2 型牛链球菌被称为解没食子酸链球菌巴氏亚种[51]。该类细菌菌落通常很小，在血琼脂上不溶血，可在 40% 胆汁中生长并水解七叶苷[42,52]。种系之间的区分很具挑战性，多数实验室使用自动化系统、基因测序或其他方法进行亚种鉴定。

该菌引起的 IE 症状通常是亚急性表现，也可以是非特异性的发热、盗汗、厌食和体重减轻。与其他链球菌和非链球菌病原体引起的 IE 相比，解没食子酸链球菌 IE 所形成的赘生物可能很大（通常>10 mm）（20% *vs.* 34% *vs.*50%）[53]。对于所有病例，如果存在菌血症，应尽快进行超声心动图和结肠镜检查，特别是病原菌为解没食子酸链球菌解没食子酸亚种时，还要进行肝功能评估。青霉素、头孢曲松、碳青霉烯类、万古霉素、达托霉素和利奈唑胺疗效可靠[54-55]。美国心脏协会（AHA）推荐使用 β-内酰胺类（青霉素 G 或头孢曲松）或万古霉素，或与氨基糖苷类药物联用，疗程 2~6 周，具体取决于分离株的青霉素 MIC，以及治疗的是自体瓣膜 IE 还是人工瓣膜 IE[56]。

- **单核细胞增生李斯特菌（*Listeria monocytogenes*）**

李斯特菌是兼性厌氧、非分枝、短杆状革兰氏阳性细菌，在光学显微镜下具有特征性的翻滚运动[57]。只有单核细胞增生李斯特菌可引起人类感染，通常与零星的食源性接触有关，可感染新生儿、老年人、孕妇和细胞介导免疫缺陷的人群[42]。它通常引起胃肠道疾病，对中枢神经系统致病有趋向性，常引起脑膜脑炎和脑脓肿，也可引起菌血症且没有明确病灶，罕见情况下也会引起 IE，可累及自体瓣膜和人工瓣膜[58]。对文献报道的 68 例病例的回顾发现，单用青霉素或氨苄西林治疗，或前两者之一与庆大霉素联合治疗对大多数病例有效，万古霉素加庆大霉素是合理的替代方案。这类病例并不一定需要手术治疗[59]。

β-溶血性链球菌

β-溶血性链球菌是革兰氏阳性球菌，过氧化氢酶试验呈阴性，在革兰氏染色中以成对或链状出现。它们是兼性厌氧的，可以在人体皮肤、口咽和胃肠道及泌尿生殖道定植。与 α-溶血性链球菌不同，β-溶血性链球菌在血琼脂平板上呈现完全性溶血，二者可以此进行鉴别。这些链球菌的特异性细胞壁碳水化合物抗原决定了它们的 Lancefield 分组，其中 A 组（化脓性链球菌）和 B 组（无乳链球菌）可引起 IE，但很少见（约占所有 IE 病例的 1%~2%）。很少观察到化脓性链球菌、无乳链球菌对青霉素耐药，因此 β-溶血性链球菌 IE 的治疗通常采用青霉素和氨基糖苷类联合用药[60-61]。

化脓性链球菌虽为人类常见致病菌，但很少引起 IE。它更常引起咽炎和皮肤感染（丹毒）以及坏死性感染。一个重要的毒力因子是 M 蛋白，它是细胞壁上的一种纤维蛋白，可防止吞噬作用，并有助于细菌黏附细胞，同时阻止补体的结合[62]；透明质酸荚膜是阻止吞噬作用的另一个关键毒力因子；链球菌溶血素 O 则可通过在细胞膜上成孔而导致红细胞和中性粒细胞破坏，这一分泌物还有降低吞噬作用的用途[63]。

无乳链球菌已知可引起新生儿脓毒症、尿路感染和皮肤感染。其引起 IE 的风险因素包括人类免疫缺陷病毒（HIV）感染、糖尿病、恶性肿瘤和肝硬化。约 1/3 的人在胃肠道和会阴存在该菌定植。类似化脓性链球菌，无乳链球菌具有多糖荚膜，有助于防止吞噬作用；它还分泌一种 β-溶血素/溶细胞素，通过成孔作用破坏宿主细胞；另外，还可产生 C5a 肽酶，干扰补体的结合[64]。

HACEK 细菌

HACEK 细菌由来自 5 个属的革兰氏阴性菌组成，所引起的 IE 占美国总 IE 的比例不到 1%[65]，主要侵犯已有心脏病或（和）牙病基础的人群，多累及自体左侧瓣膜。HACEK 引起的 IE 通常表现为亚急性病程，就诊时已有数周的症状。在过去的几十年里，这类微生物通常被认为是"培养阴性"心内膜炎的病原体，需要长时间培养才能识别，但最近开始的在常规培养加入血培养的技术提升了培养的阳性率[66]。HACEK IE 患者的中位年龄比非 HACEK 患者更年轻，总体死亡率也更低[67]。

副流感嗜血杆菌（*Haemophilus parainfluenzae*）仍然是 HACEK IE 最常见的病因。它是一种多形性不动革兰氏阴性杆菌，是正常呼吸道菌群的一部分，可引起上呼吸道和下呼吸道感染。与副流感嗜血杆菌相关的典型感染是慢性阻塞性肺疾病的急性加重。鉴于其引起非 IE 感染的能力，血液中副流感嗜血杆菌的存在对 IE 的阳性预测值仅为 55%[68]。虽然 1/3 的分离株为青霉素耐药，但氨基青霉素、头孢曲松、左氧氟沙星、四环素和碳青霉烯类药物在体外对该菌药效可靠（95%～100%）[67,69]。

凝聚杆菌（*Aggregatibacter*）以前被分类为放线杆菌或嗜血杆菌属，是 HACEK IE 的第二类常见病原菌。凝聚杆菌（伴放线凝聚杆菌、嗜沫凝聚杆菌和惰性凝聚杆菌）是人类口腔中的定植菌群，与牙周炎和牙菌斑有关[67]。这些细菌是不动兼性厌氧菌。伴放线凝聚杆菌（最常见）常与放线菌种混合感染，多见于侵袭性感染，这类细菌引起的菌血症可高度预警心内膜炎的存在[68]。据报道，1/5 的分离株为青霉素耐药[69]。

心杆菌（*Cardiobacterium*）包括人心杆菌和瓣膜心杆菌，是多形性不动兼性厌氧菌。它们属于正常的口腔菌群，也是呼吸道菌群，还可以定植于女性生殖道[67]。心杆菌引起的非 IE 感染十分罕见，因此其菌血症的出现对心内膜炎的阳性预测值 >90%[68]。某些分离株具有 β-内酰胺酶，可灭活青霉素[70]。

侵蚀艾肯菌（*Eikenella corrodens*）引起的 IE 是 HACEK 中最少见的，典型的情况是被受感染的人咬伤导致的 IE。这些兼性厌氧菌是人类的口腔菌群，与牙齿感染有关，可以通过舔或咬传播到伤口，导致皮肤感染。其菌血症并不是 IE 的强预测因素，因为其他类型的感染更常见[67]。已有青霉素耐药的报道，但耐药发生率较低[69]。

金氏金氏菌（*Kingella kingae*）和反硝化金氏菌（*Kingella denitrificans*）是人类口咽和泌尿生殖道的正常菌群，兼性不动厌氧菌。虽然在 HACEK 中金氏金氏菌引起心内膜炎并不常见，但它可导致幼儿化脓性关节炎，并与该人群的脑膜炎有关[67]。其菌血症对心内膜炎的阳性预测值不足 50%[68]。约 1/4 的分离株被发现对青霉素和氨基青霉素具有耐药性，对头孢菌素的敏感性为 100%[71]。

静脉吸毒相关病原体

流行病学

随着时间的推移，引起静脉吸毒者 IE 的病原体分布也发生了变化。20 世纪

80年代之前，金黄色葡萄球菌引起的IE（40%）数倍于铜绿假单胞菌和念珠菌感染，后两者分别各占15%[72]。最近的研究表明，金黄色葡萄球菌目前占到了静脉吸毒者IE病例的绝大多数（近60%）[73-74]。然而，大多数假单胞菌IE病例还是与静脉吸毒有关，而黏质沙雷菌和念珠菌IE与注射毒品关系密切[75]。虽然黏质沙雷菌属于肠杆菌家族，但它很少成为内源性菌群的一部分，而更多被看作一种环境病原体，其发病多与水污染有关[76]。铜绿假单胞菌和黏质沙雷菌引起IE可能是注射前使用未煮沸灭菌的自来水或淡香水溶解药物所致[77]。静脉吸毒者一些常见的做法包括舔针、用嘴咬碎药物，而所接触到的唾液含有口咽微生物群（包括草绿色链球菌和口腔革兰氏阴性菌）。其他因素，如皮肤破裂、用唾液涂拭注射部位等，则会因皮肤菌群的存在而增加感染、菌血症和IE的风险。与非静脉吸毒的人相比，静脉吸毒人群的皮肤葡萄球菌定植率更高[78]，罕见情况下，他们会因感染不常见的细菌而出现IE，包括棒状杆菌属、梭状杆菌属、梭状芽胞杆菌属和奈瑟菌属。多种微生物混合感染的IE常见于静脉吸毒者中，曾从单个病例的血培养中培养出了多达8种不同的病原体[79-80]。由于该人群右侧瓣膜IE的发生率高，故其IE的症状与其他人群IE的表现有所不同，杂音、全身栓塞以及血管和免疫问题的发生率较低。

- **铜绿假单胞菌**（*Pseudomonas aeruginosa*）

机会致病菌铜绿假单胞菌是一种专性需氧革兰氏阴性杆菌。它是一种环境微生物，可在土壤和水中找到。菌落上常因产生绿脓菌素和荧光嗜铁素而呈现绿色或蓝绿色。其并非健康人类微生物组的一部分，但可以在呼吸道、泌尿道和皮肤（例如烧伤）中定植，通过多种毒力因子在这些部位和其他部位引起感染[81]。

铜绿假单胞菌关键的毒力因子包括极鞭毛和多个菌毛。鞭毛有助于杆菌定向并提供急性感染所需的运动能力。菌毛可以黏附细胞并促进细菌在细胞表面聚集。聚集作用还可以为铜绿假单胞菌提供另一个关键毒力因子——生物膜。生物膜是一种细胞外多糖基质，还包括蛋白质和脂质。生物膜可以充当屏障，保护细菌免受免疫细胞和抗菌剂的攻击；也可以充当锚，起到固定的作用。在生物膜内，铜绿假单胞菌维持低生长，这会导致抗菌剂活性的下降。此外，绿脓菌素会增加宿主吞噬细胞的氧化应激，降低其吞噬能力[82]。

耐药性是铜绿假单胞菌感染的一个标志性特征，其发生机制多样。外排泵和外膜通透性降低是铜绿假单胞菌对多类抗生素产生耐药的内在机制。多染色体β-内酰胺酶包括AmpC和OXA-50也能水解β-内酰胺类抗生素。获得性耐药机制包括DNA旋转酶突变、氨基糖苷类修饰酶的产生以及β-内酰胺酶的过量产生或修饰[76,82]。

假单胞菌IE通常采用联合药物治疗，一般是一种抗假单胞菌β-内酰胺类药物联合一种氨基糖苷类药物，治疗6周。氟喹诺酮类药物可作为二线用药。如果不进行瓣膜置换术，左侧IE的死亡率非常高，因此需请外科会诊[83-84]。

- 念珠菌属（*Candida*）

念珠菌属是大小为 1~8 μm 的芽生酵母。致病性念珠菌属也可以是正常人类菌群的一部分，主要存在于黏膜、皮肤和胃肠道，是引起真菌性心内膜炎最常见的原因[85]。念珠菌心内膜炎于 1940 年首次报道，患者为静脉吸毒者，致病菌为近平滑念珠菌（*Candida parapsilosis*）[86]。过去 10 年，美国静脉吸毒人群的增加导致了更多的念珠菌菌血症[87]。念珠菌 IE 的其他风险因素主要与医疗相关，包括中心静脉插管、人工瓣膜植入、植入式心脏装置的使用、免疫抑制剂和抗生素的临床使用以及血液透析[88]。

IE 中最常见的真菌感染种类是白色念珠菌（44%），其次是近平滑念珠菌（27%）、热带念珠菌（10%）和光滑念珠菌（6%）[88]。风险因素也因菌种不同有些差异：近平滑念珠菌可能与静脉插管和肠外营养有关，热带念珠菌与恶性肿瘤和化疗有关。值得注意的是，光滑念珠菌为单倍体，对氟康唑的耐药率高于白色念珠菌[89]。

念珠菌 IE 的死亡率高于细菌性 IE，需要积极检查和治疗。其菌血症并发眼内炎的比例高于细菌性心内膜炎，因此对于疑似念珠菌 IE 的患者需要进行眼科评估[88,90-91]。鉴于死亡风险较高，需要进行手术评估，建议起始治疗采用脂质制剂两性霉素 B 或高剂量棘白菌素[56,92]。

IE 相关的人畜共患病原体

布鲁氏菌属（*Brucella species*）

布鲁氏菌是一种小型、不动的革兰氏阴性球杆菌，可通过接触受感染的动物组织、吸入受感染的雾化颗粒或食用受感染的动物产品（如肉类或奶制品）引起人畜共患传播，从而导致人类感染。3 种较为常见的引起人畜共患感染的病原体为羊布鲁氏菌（*Brucella melitensis*）、流产布鲁氏菌（*Brucella abortus*）和猪布鲁氏菌（*Brucella suis*）[93]。在布鲁氏菌病中，心血管并发症是造成死亡的主要原因[94]。虽然该病可发生在普通人群，且具有世界范围的广泛性，但多与职业暴露有关，例如肉类包装、乳业、畜牧业、兽医。在西方国家，则多见于微生物实验室技术人员。临床上，急性感染可出现持续数天或数周的全身症状，如发热、寒战、盗汗、体重减轻和关节痛。心血管感染被归类为慢性感染，通常表现为符合心内膜炎表现的终末期器官损伤，而常规检查多为阴性[95]。

采用培养这一公认的金标准技术确诊布鲁氏菌心内膜炎非常困难，因为该菌对培养的条件十分苛刻，尤其是在慢性感染中。送检时应告知微生物学实验室存在布鲁氏菌鉴别诊断的问题，以采取适当的预防措施。将培养时间延长到 6 周可提高阳性培养检出，适当临床情况下可使用血清学方法进行诊断。血清凝集试验（SAT）滴度增加 4 倍、持续 2 周，即可确诊感染[96]。一般 SAT 滴度＞1∶160 时即可做出诊断，但应注意，流行地区与非流行地区诊断要求的滴度有所不同，流行地区要求SAT滴度达到1:160,而非流行区域为1:80[95]。PCR技术可以帮助诊断，但不是所有单位均具备PCR检测条件，且这一检测尚未标准化。

目前没有正式的治疗指南，通常使用三联疗法，包括多西环素、利福平至少12周，前4周联合使用氨基糖苷类。与单独药物治疗相比，瓣膜置换与抗菌治疗相结合被证明可以降低总体死亡率，尽管目前手术指征尚不明确[97]。

巴尔通体属（*Bartonella species*）

血培养阴性心内膜炎最常见的原因之一为巴尔通体感染，它是一种较难培养的革兰氏阴性菌，大部分病例为汉赛巴尔通体（*Bartonella henselae*）和五日热巴尔通体（*Bartonella quintana*）感染[98]。涉及五日热的病例通常与环境卫生条件差有关，例如存在大量虱子（主要的传播媒介）。汉赛巴尔通体感染是由于接触带菌的猫（猫因跳蚤叮咬或接触其他猫的体液而带有汉赛巴尔通体菌血症）而引起。除去以上病原菌来源外，人类自身存在的瓣膜病和人工瓣膜置换成为导致IE风险因素[99]。另外，在这类病例中，由免疫复合物介导的肾小球肾炎的发病率有增加趋势，临床表现为坏死性抗中性粒细胞胞质抗体（ANCA）阳性肾小球肾炎[100]。

鉴于巴尔通体在培养时很难生长，因此诊断具有挑战性。通常是采用血清学方法来完成，包括酶联免疫吸附试验和间接荧光抗体检测，其缺点是与衣原体、贝纳柯克斯体之间存在交叉反应[101]。此外，急性感染时IgM可能较低，因此可能导致假阴性[101]。使用Warthin-Starry染色对瓣膜进行组织病理学检查也有助于诊断。分子学方法诊断，特别是DNA扩增和16S rRNA测序，即使先前使用过抗生素治疗也有助于提高检测的灵敏度和特异性，但这些技术尚未被广泛应用[100]。目前尚无针对性的治疗指南，专家一般推荐6周的多西环素治疗，前2周联合使用氨基糖苷类药物[102]。

Q热（*Q fever*）

慢性Q热继发于贝纳柯克斯体（*C. burnetii*）感染，该微生物是一种小的、专性细胞内生长的革兰氏阴性杆菌。其最常见的表现是亚急性心内膜炎，通常可在初次感染后12个月内发病[103]。Q热心内膜炎是血培养阴性心内膜炎的第二常见原因，仅次于巴尔通体。这种细菌的感染是通过吸入雾化的受感染动物体液（例如出生时带出的体液、尿液、粪便）或摄入受污染的未经巴氏消毒的乳制品而发生的。贝纳柯克斯体分布于世界大部分地区。发生心内膜炎的主要风险因素是原有瓣膜疾病，其他风险因素包括怀孕和免疫功能低下[104]。

由于经胸和经食管超声心动图（TTE和TEE）很少能观察到赘生物病变，因此这类感染诊断起来很困难。即便发现赘生物，多半是在主动脉瓣和二尖瓣上，常常很小[105]。因此，当患者符合Duke标准并具有符合慢性感染的血清学结果（例如Ⅰ期IgG滴度＞1∶800）时，即可确诊。当Ⅰ期IgG滴度范围在1∶128～1∶800时，血清学数据可以提供支持，但不能确诊[105]。此外，培养阳性、16S rRNA PCR或心脏瓣膜免疫组织化学检测也可支持诊断。血液16S rRNA PCR阳性可提供进一步的支持证据[105]。

Q热心内膜炎的治疗包括口服多西环素（每次100mg，每天2次）和羟氯喹（每次200 mg，每天3次），治疗持续时间至少为18个月或直到Ⅰ期IgG＜1∶200[106]。临床上，这类病例应请外科会诊考虑瓣膜置换手术，多数患者存在血流动力学问题[107]。

人工瓣膜IE相关病原体

人工瓣膜心内膜炎（PVE）通常分为早、晚两期，以瓣膜置换后1年为界。早期PVE，金黄色葡萄球菌感染占主导地位，凝固酶阴性葡萄球菌（CoNS）感染居第二位。需提到的是，CoNS是自体瓣膜IE的一个非常罕见的病因[108]。在PVE晚期，一些自体瓣膜IE的常见致病菌，如链球菌和肠球菌，在这一时期则更常见，而在此期CoNS的风险仍然存在。另外，PVE中念珠菌及其他细菌（包括棒状杆菌属）的感染风险增加[109-110]。

凝固酶阴性葡萄球菌（CoNS）

所有CoNS均为革兰氏阳性球菌，过氧化氢酶试验呈阳性。表皮葡萄球菌群（CoNS的一种），包括表皮葡萄球菌、人葡萄球菌、溶血葡萄球菌和头状葡萄球菌，还有其他一些菌种，它们具有相似的微生物学和临床特征。它们与路邓葡萄球菌（*S. lugdunensis*）的区别有3点：路邓葡萄球菌可以独特地产生导致过氧化氢酶试验假阳性的聚集因子；表皮葡萄球菌几乎总是导致PVE，而路邓葡萄球菌在80%的情况下导致自体瓣膜IE；大多数情况下，表皮葡萄球菌对β-内酰胺类抗生素耐药，而路邓葡萄球菌通常对苯唑西林敏感。临床上，血培养过程中对路邓葡萄球菌的处理与金黄色葡萄球菌类似[111]。

表皮葡萄球菌是分布在整个身体表面的皮肤菌群，不同部位的细菌存在一些差异。它们的主要毒力因子包括对异物表面的黏附和生物膜的产生。这类细菌的二次侵袭能力有限，但它们可以首先黏附到血管内导管、心脏装置或假体关节上，然后再黏附到一些细胞外蛋白质上，例如纤维蛋白原和胶原蛋白，它们产生生物膜使其免受宿主免疫系统和抗菌剂的攻击[112]。

表皮葡萄球菌中经常含有允许表达PBP2a的基因，这赋予了该菌对β-内酰胺类药物的耐药性。在大多数情况下，这些蛋白质由*mecA*基因编码[112]。表皮葡萄球菌感染常规使用万古霉素进行治疗，但对葡萄球菌引起的PVE采用联合用药也是合理的选择[56]。

参考文献

[1] Murdoch DR, et al. Clinical presentation, etiology, and outcome of infective endocarditis in the 21st century: the International Collaboration on Endocarditis-Prospective Cohort Study. Arch Intern Med, 2009, 169(5): 463–473.

[2] Slipczuk L, et al. Infective endocarditis epidemiology over five decades: a systematic review. PloS One, 2013, 8(12): e82665.

[3] Taylor TA, Unakal CG. Staphylococcus aureus. Treasure Island (FL): StatPearls, 2020.

[4] Wertheim HF, et al. The role of nasal carriage in Staphylococcus aureus infections. Lancet Infect Dis, 2005, 5(12): 751–762.

[5] Wertheim HF, et al. Risk and outcome of nosocomial Staphylococcus aureus bacteraemia in nasal carriers versus non-carriers. Lancet, 2004, 364(9435): 703–705.

[6] Ritz HL, et al. Association of high levels of serum antibody to staphylococcal toxic shock antigen with nasal carriage of toxic shock antigen-producing strains of Staphylococcus aureus. Infect Immun, 1984, 43(3): 954–958.

[7] Foster TJ. Immune evasion by staphylococci. Nat Rev Microbiol, 2005, 3(12): 948–958.

[8] Rooijakkers SH, van Kessel KP, van Strijp JA. Staphylococcal innate immune evasion. Trends Microbiol, 2005, 13(12): 596–601.

[9] Prevost G, et al. Panton-Valentine leucocidin and gamma-hemolysin from Staphylococcus aureus ATCC 49775 are encoded by distinct genetic loci and have different biological activities. Infect Immun, 1995, 63(10): 4121–4129.

[10] Miller LG, et al. Necrotizing fasciitis caused by community-associated methicillin-resistant Staphylococcus aureus in Los Angeles. N Engl J Med, 2005, 352(14): 1445–1453.

[11] Gillet Y, et al. Association between Staphylococcus aureus strains carrying gene for Panton-Valentine leukocidin and highly lethal necrotising pneumonia in young immunocompetent patients. Lancet, 2002, 359(9308): 753–759.

[12] Kuehnert MJ, et al. Methicillin-resistant-Staphylococcus aureus hospitalizations, United States. Emerg Infect Dis, 2005, 11(6): 868–872.

[13] Tiemersma EW, et al. Methicillin-resistant Staphylococcus aureus in Europe, 1999—2002. Emerg Infect Dis, 2004, 10(9): 1627–1634.

[14] Fukunaga BT, et al. Hospital-acquired methicillin-resistant Staphylococcus aureus bacteremia related to medicare antibiotic prescriptions: a state-level analysis. Hawaii J Med Public Health, 2016, 75(10): 303–309.

[15] Skinner D, Keefer CS. Significance of bacteremia caused by Staphylococcus aureus: a study of one hundred and twenty-two cases and a review of the literature concerned with experimental infection in animals. Arch Intern Med, 1941, 68(5): 851–875.

[16] Rammelkamp CH, Maxon T. Resistance of Staphylococcus aureus to the action of penicillin. PSEBM (Proc Soc Exp Biol Med), 1942, 51(3): 386–389.

[17] Kernodle DS. Mechanisms of resistance//Fischetti VA, et al. Gram-positive pathogens. American Society of Microbiology, 2019.

[18] Lowy FD. Antimicrobial resistance: the example of Staphylococcus aureus. J Clin Invest, 2003, 111(9): 1265–1273.

[19] McDanel JS, et al. Comparative effectiveness of beta-lactams versus vancomycin for treatment of methicillin susceptible Staphylococcus aureus bloodstream infections among 122 hospitals. Clin Infect Dis, 2015, 61(3): 361–367.

[20] Burrelli CC, et al. Does the beta-lactam matter? Nafcillin versus cefazolin for methicillin-susceptible Staphylococcus aureus bloodstream infections. Chemotherapy, 2018, 63(6): 345–351.

[21] Beganovic M, et al. Comparative effectiveness of exclusive exposure to nafcillin or oxacillin, cefazolin, piperacillin/tazobactam, and fluoroquinolones among a national cohort of veterans with methicillin-susceptible Staphylococcus aureus bloodstream infection. Open Forum Infect Dis,

2019, 6(7): ofz270.

[22] Jevons MP, Coe AW, Parker MT. Methicillin resistance in staphylococci. Lancet, 1963, 1(7287): 904–907.

[23] Fishovitz J, et al. Penicillin-binding protein 2a of methicillin-resistant Staphylococcus aureus. IUBMB Life, 2014, 66(8): 572–577.

[24] Walters MS, et al. Vancomycin-resistant Staphylococcus aureus- Delaware, 2015. MMWR Morb Mortal Wkly Rep, 2015, 64(37): 1056.

[25] Howden BP, et al. Isolates with low-level vancomycin resistance associated with persistent methicillin-resistant Staphylococcus aureus bacteremia. Antimicrob Agents Chemother, 2006, 50(9): 3039–3047.

[26] McGuinness WA, Malachowa N, DeLeo FR. Vancomycin resistance in Staphylococcus aureus. Yale J Biol Med, 2017, 90(2): 269–281.

[27] Sinner SWTAR. Manndell, Douglas, and Bennett's principles and practice of infectious diseases. 8th. Philadelphia: Elsevier, 2015.

[28] Procop GW, et al. Koneman's color atlas and textbook of diagnostic microbiology. 7th. Philadelphia: Wolters Kluwer, 2017.

[29] Fowler Jr VG, et al. Staphylococcus aureus endocarditis: a consequence of medical progress. J Am Med Assoc, 2005, 293(24): 3012–3021.

[30] Scheld WM, Valone JA, Sande MA. Bacterial adherence in the pathogenesis of endocarditis. Interaction of bacterial dextran, platelets, and fibrin. J Clin Invest, 1978, 61(5): 1394–1404.

[31] Petti CAS, C W. Mandell, Douglas, and Bennett's principles and practice of infectious diseases. 8th. Philadelphia: Elsevier, 2015.

[32] Whiley RA, et al. Streptococcus intermedius, Streptococcus constellatus, and Streptococcus anginosus (the Streptococcus milleri group): association with different body sites and clinical infections. J Clin Microbiol, 1992, 30(1): 243–244.

[33] Willcox MD. Potential pathogenic properties of members of the "Streptococcus milleri"group in relation to the production of endocarditis and abscesses. J Med Microbiol, 1995, 43(6): 405–410.

[34] Janoff ENM, D M. Mandell, Douglas, and Bennett's principles and practice of infectious diseases. 8th. Philadelphia: Elsevier, 2015.

[35] Mitchell AM, Mitchell TJ. Streptococcus pneumoniae: virulence factors and variation. Clin Microbiol Infect, 2010, 16(5): 411–418.

[36] Shapiro ED, et al. The protective efficacy of polyvalent pneumococcal polysaccharide vaccine. N Engl J Med, 1991, 325(21): 1453–1460.

[37] Arias CAM, Bennett E. Mandell, Douglas, and Bennett's principles and practice of infectious diseases. 8th. Philadelphia: Elsevier, 2015.

[38] Schlievert PM, et al. Aggregation and binding substances enhance pathogenicity in rabbit models of Enterococcus faecalis endocarditis. Infect Immun, 1998, 66(1): 218–223.

[39] Heikens E, Bonten MJ, Willems RJ. Enterococcal surface protein Esp is important for biofilm formation of Enterococcus faecium E1162. J Bacteriol, 2007, 189(22): 8233–8240.

[40] Frenkel A, Hirsch W. Spontaneous development of L forms of streptococci requiring secretions of other bacteria or sulphydryl compounds for normal growth. Nature, 1961, 191: 728–730.

[41] Collins MD, Lawson PA. The genus Abiotrophia (Kawamura et al.) is not monophyletic: proposal of Granulicatella gen. nov., Granulicatella adiacens comb. nov., Granulicatella elegans comb. nov. and Granulicatella balaenopterae comb. nov. Int J Syst Evol Microbiol, 2000, 50(Pt 1): 365–369.

[42] Bennett JE, Dolin R, Blaser MJ. Mandell, Douglas, and Bennett's principles and practice of infectious diseases. 8th. Philadelphia: Elsevier, 2020. p. 1 [Online resource].

[43] Alberti MO, Hindler JA, Humphries RM. Antimicrobial susceptibilities of Abiotrophia defectiva, Granulicatella adiacens, and Granulicatella elegans. Antimicrob Agents Chemother, 2015, 60(3): 1411–1420.

[44] Zheng X, et al. Antimicrobial susceptibilities of invasive pediatric Abiotrophia and Granulicatella

isolates. J Clin Microbiol, 2004, 42(9): 4323–4326.
[45] Liao CH, et al. Nutritionally variant streptococcal infections at a University Hospital in Taiwan: disease emergence and high prevalence of beta-lactam and macrolide resistance. Clin Infect Dis, 2004, 38(3): 452–455.
[46] Prasidthrathsint K, Fisher MA. Antimicrobial susceptibility patterns among a large, nationwide cohort of Abiotrophia and Granulicatella clinical isolates. J Clin Microbiol, 2017, 55(4): 1025–1031.
[47] Roberts RB. Streptococcal endocarditis: the viridans and β-hemolytic streptococci//Kaye D. Infective endocarditis. New York: Raven Press, 1992.
[48] Fida M, et al. 1074. Management and outcomes of infective endocarditis due to nutritionally variant streptococci. Open Forum Infectious Diseases, 2018, 5(Suppl. 1_1): S321–S322.
[49] Klein RS, et al. Association of Streptococcus bovis with carcinoma of the colon. N Engl J Med, 1977, 297(15): 800–802.
[50] Tripodi MF, et al. Streptococcus bovis endocarditis and its association with chronic liver disease: an underestimated risk factor. Clin Infect Dis, 2004, 38(10): 1394–1400.
[51] Schlegel L, et al. Reappraisal of the taxonomy of the Streptococcus bovis/Streptococcus equinus complex and related species: description of Streptococcus gallolyticus subsp. gallolyticus subsp. nov., S. gallolyticus subsp. macedonicus subsp. nov. and S. gallolyticus subsp. pasteurianus subsp. nov. Int J Syst Evol Microbiol, 2003, 53(Pt 3): 631–645.
[52] Chuard C, Reller LB. Bile-esculin test for presumptive identification of enterococci and streptococci: effects of bile concentration, inoculation technique, and incubation time. J Clin Microbiol, 1998, 36(4): 1135–1136.
[53] Pergola V, et al. Comparison of clinical and echocardiographic characteristics of Streptococcus bovis endocarditis with that caused by other pathogens. Am J Cardiol, 2001, 88(8): 871–875.
[54] Beck M, Frodl R, Funke G. Comprehensive study of strains previously designated Streptococcus bovis consecutively isolated from human blood cultures and emended description of Streptococcus gallolyticus and Streptococcus infantarius subsp. coli. J Clin Microbiol, 2008, 46(9): 2966–2972.
[55] Streit JM, et al. Daptomycin tested against 915 bloodstream isolates of viridans group streptococci (eight species) and Streptococcus bovis. J Antimicrob Chemother, 2005, 55(4): 574–578.
[56] Baddour LM, et al. Infective endocarditis in adults: diagnosis, antimicrobial therapy, and management of complications: a scientific statement for healthcare professionals from the American Heart Association. Circulation, 2015, 132(15): 1435–1486.
[57] Billie J. Listeria and erysipelothrix//Murray PR, Baron EJ. Manual of clinical microbiology. Washington DC: ASM Press, 2007.
[58] Nieman RE, Lorber B. Listeriosis in adults: a changing pattern. Report of eight cases and review of the literature, 1968—1978. Rev Infect Dis, 1980, 2(2): 207–227.
[59] Fernandez Guerrero ML, et al. Prosthetic valve endocarditis due to Listeria monocytogenes. Report of two cases and reviews. Int J Infect Dis, 2004, 8(2): 97–102.
[60] Sambola A, et al. Streptococcus agalactiae infective endocarditis: analysis of 30 cases and review of the literature, 1962—1998. Clin Infect Dis, 2002, 34(12): 1576–1584.
[61] Oppegaard O, et al. Clinical and molecular characteristics of infective beta-hemolytic streptococcal endocarditis. Diagn Microbiol Infect Dis, 2017, 89(2): 135–142.
[62] Wong SS, Yuen KY. Streptococcus pyogenes and re-emergence of scarlet fever as a public health problem. Emerg Microb Infect, 2012, 1(7): e2.
[63] Zhu L, et al. Contribution of secreted NADase and streptolysin O to the pathogenesis of epidemic serotype M1 Streptococcus pyogenes infections. Am J Pathol, 2017, 187(3): 605–613.
[64] Liu GY, Nizet V. Extracellular virulence factors of group B Streptococci. Front Biosci, 2004, 9: 1794–1802.
[65] Holland TL, et al. Infective endocarditis. Nat Rev Dis Primers, 2016, 2: 16059.
[66] Baron EJ, Scott JD, Tompkins LS. Prolonged incubation and extensive subculturing do not increase recovery of clinically significant microorganisms from standard automated blood cultures.

Clin Infect Dis, 2005, 41(11): 1677–1680.
[67] Revest M, et al. HACEK endocarditis: state-of-the-art. Expert Rev Anti Infect Ther, 2016, 14(5): 523–530.
[68] Sen Yew H, et al. Association between HACEK bacteraemia and endocarditis. J Med Microbiol, 2014, 63(Pt 6): 892–895.
[69] Coburn B, et al. Antimicrobial susceptibilities of clinical isolates of HACEK organisms. Antimicrob Agents Chemother, 2013, 57(4): 1989–1991.
[70] Lu PL, et al. Infective endocarditis complicated with progressive heart failure due to beta-lactamase-producing Cardiobacterium hominis. J Clin Microbiol, 2000, 38(5): 2015–2017.
[71] Matuschek E, et al. Antimicrobial susceptibility testing of Kingella kingae with broth microdilution and disk diffusion using EUCAST recommended media. Clin Microbiol Infect, 2018, 24(4): 396–401.
[72] Watanakunakorn C. Changing epidemiology and newer aspects of infective endocarditis. Adv Intern Med, 1977, 22: 21–47.
[73] Jain V, et al. Infective endocarditis in an urban medical center: association of individual drugs with valvular involvement. J Infect, 2008, 57(2): 132–138.
[74] De Rosa FG, et al. Infective endocarditis in intravenous drug users from Italy: the increasing importance in HIV-infected patients. Infection, 2007, 35(3): 154–160.
[75] Cooper R, Mills J. Serratia endocarditis. A follow-up report. Arch Intern Med, 1980, 140(2): 199–202.
[76] Horcajada JP, et al. Acquisition of multidrug-resistant Serratia marcescens by critically ill patients who consumed tap water during receipt of oral medication. Infect Control Hosp Epidemiol, 2006, 27(7): 774–777.
[77] Wieland M, et al. Left-sided endocarditis due to Pseudomonas aeruginosa. A report of 10 cases and review of the literature. Medicine (Baltim), 1986, 65(3): 180–189.
[78] Tuazon CU, Sheagren JN. Increased rate of carriage of Staphylococcus aureus among narcotic addicts. J Infect Dis, 1974, 129(6): 725–727.
[79] Szabo S, Lieberman JP, Lue YA. Unusual pathogens in narcotic-associated endocarditis. Rev Infect Dis, 1990, 12(3): 412–415.
[80] Weber G, et al. Infective endocarditis due to Fusobacterium nucleatum in an intravenous drug abuser. Eur J Clin Microbiol Infect Dis, 1999, 18(9): 655–657.
[81] Araos R, D'Agata E. Pseudomonas aeruginosa and other Pseudomonas species//Bennett JE, Dolin R, Blaser MJ. Mandell, Douglas, and Bennett's principles and practice of infectious diseases. Philadelphia: Elsevier, 2019.
[82] Gellatly SL, Hancock RE. Pseudomonas aeruginosa: new insights into pathogenesis and host defenses. Pathog Dis, 2013, 67(3): 159–173.
[83] Baddour LM. Twelve-year review of recurrent native-valve infective endocarditis: a disease of the modern antibiotic era. Rev Infect Dis, 1988, 10(6): 1163–1170.
[84] Huang G, Barnes EW, Peacock Jr JE. Repeat infective endocarditis in persons who inject drugs:"take another little piece of my heart". Open Forum Infect Dis, 2018, 5(12): ofy304.
[85] Ellis ME, et al. Fungal endocarditis: evidence in the world literature, 1965—1995. Clin Infect Dis, 2001, 32(1): 50–62.
[86] Joachim H, Polayes SH. Subacute endocarditis and systemic mycosis (monilia). J Am Med Assoc, 1940, 115(3): 205–208.
[87] Poowanawittayakom N, et al. Reemergence of intravenous drug use as risk factor for Candidemia, Massachusetts, USA. Emerg Infect Dis, 2018, 24(4).
[88] Arnold CJ, et al. Candida infective endocarditis: an observational cohort study with a focus on therapy. Antimicrob Agents Chemother, 2015, 59(4): 2365–2373.
[89] Mamtani S, et al. Candida endocarditis: a review of the pathogenesis, morphology, risk factors, and management of an emerging and serious condition. Cureus, 2020, 12(1): e6695.
[90] Nguyen MH, et al. Candida prosthetic valve endocarditis: prospective study of six cases and review of the literature. Clin Infect Dis, 1996, 22(2): 262–267.

[91] Shin SU, et al. Clinical characteristics and risk factors for complications of candidaemia in adults: focus on endophthalmitis, endocarditis, and osteoarticular infections. Int J Infect Dis, 2020, 93: 126–132.

[92] Pappas PG, et al. Clinical practice guideline for the management of Candidiasis: 2016 update by the infectious diseases society of America. Clin Infect Dis, 2016, 62(4): e1–50.

[93] Pappas G, et al. The new global map of human brucellosis. Lancet Infect Dis, 2006, 6(2): 91–99.

[94] Jeroudi MO, et al. Brucella endocarditis. Br Heart J, 1987, 58(3): 279–383.

[95] Pappas G, et al. Brucellosis. N Engl J Med, 2005, 352(22): 2325–2336.

[96] Brucellosis reference guide. February, 2017 [cited 2020 July 15]; Available from: https://www.cdc.gov/brucellosis/pdf/brucellosi-reference-guide.pdf.

[97] Keshtkar-Jahromi M, et al. Medical versus medical and surgical treatment for Brucella endocarditis. Ann Thorac Surg, 2012, 94(6): 2141–2146.

[98] Fournier PE, et al. Comprehensive diagnostic strategy for blood culture-negative endocarditis: a prospective study of 819 new cases. Clin Infect Dis, 2010, 51(2): 131–140.

[99] Raoult D, et al. Diagnosis of 22 new cases of Bartonella endocarditis. Ann Intern Med, 1996, 125(8): 646–652.

[100] Babiker A, El Hag MI, Perez C. Bartonella infectious endocarditis associated with Cryoglobulinemia and multifocal proliferative glomerulonephritis. Open Forum Infect Dis, 2018, 5(8): ofy186.

[101] Fournier PE, Mainardi JL, Raoult D. Value of microimmunofluorescence for diagnosis and follow-up of Bartonella endocarditis. Clin Diagn Lab Immunol, 2002, 9(4): 795–801.

[102] Foucault C, Raoult D, Brouqui P. Randomized open trial of gentamicin and doxycycline for eradication of Bartonella quintana from blood in patients with chronic bacteremia. Antimicrob Agents Chemother, 2003, 47(7): 2204–2207.

[103] Stein A, Raoult D. Q fever endocarditis. Eur Heart J, 1995, 16(Suppl. B): 19–23.

[104] Fenollar F, et al. Risks factors and prevention of Q fever endocarditis. Clin Infect Dis, 2001, 33(3): 312e6.

[105] Anderson A, et al. Diagnosis and management of Q fever–United States, 2013: recommendations from CDC and the Q fever working group. MMWR Recomm Rep(Morb Mortal Wkly Rep), 2013, 62(RR-03): 1–30.

[106] Raoult D, et al. Treatment of Q fever endocarditis: comparison of 2 regimens containing doxycycline and ofloxacin or hydroxychloroquine. Arch Intern Med, 1999, 159(2): 167–173.

[107] Raoult D. Treatment of Q fever. Antimicrob Agents Chemother, 1993, 37(9): 1733–1736.

[108] Piper C, Korfer R, Horstkotte D. Prosthetic valve endocarditis. Heart, 2001, 85(5): 590–593.

[109] Nataloni M, et al. Prosthetic valve endocarditis. J Cardiovasc Med, 2010, 11(12): 869–883.

[110] Belmares J, et al. Corynebacterium endocarditis species-specific risk factors and outcomes. BMC Infect Dis, 2007, 7(1): 4.

[111] Sabe MA, et al. Staphylococcus lugdunensis: a rare but destructive cause of coagulase-negative staphylococcus infective endocarditis. Eur Heart J Acute Cardiovasc Care, 2014, 3(3): 275–280.

[112] Becker K, Heilmann C, Peters G. Coagulase-negative staphylococci. Clin Microbiol Rev, 2014, 27(4): 870–926.

第4章
感染性心内膜炎的超声心动图评估

Matthew Suffoletto

Department of Medicine, University of Pittsburgh, Pittsburgh, PA, United States

　　超声心动图是诊断和治疗感染性心内膜炎（IE）必不可少的影像方法。对可疑心内膜炎病例，超声心动图常常作为一线检查，而后续的一系列超声心动图复查可为病情追踪及临床决策提供信息。只要怀疑IE，就应尽早进行超声心动图检查，这已成为业内共识。IE的超声心动图表现是确诊这类疾病的基石。赘生物是改良Duke标准诊断IE的主要依据之一，许多已发表的文章和指南均以IE的超声心动图评估来确定诊断和指导治疗[1-3]。IE的并发症发生率和死亡率通常与感染并发症直接相关，这些并发症通过超声心动图一般较易被发现。例如，因感染破坏导致的瓣膜反流、基于赘生物大小和解剖位置可能引发的栓塞，以及瓣周的感染扩散。

　　2011年，美国超声心动图学会（ASE）合理使用指南指出，经胸超声心动图（TTE）适用于疑似IE、血培养呈阳性或出现新的心脏杂音的患者。此外，TTE或经食管超声心动图（TEE）也适用于评估栓子的心脏来源，这也是IE可能出现的临床问题[4]。而在某些情况下，TEE可能是更为恰当和临床首选的诊断检查（图4.1和图4.2），具体包括：根据患者特征考虑TTE不能诊断的可能性很高，或中高度预测为IE的病例（例如，有人工瓣膜置换或植入心内装置、葡萄球菌菌血症或真菌血症等）。TTE或TEE也适用于以下情况的再次评估：①已确诊IE，存在病情进展或并发症的高风险；②因临床病情或心脏相关检查发生变化而怀疑心内膜炎。然而，TTE不适用于评估与IE典型病原体无关的短暂性菌血症，或者比较明确的非血管内感染的病例[4]。

IE的超声心动图表现

　　心内膜炎的典型病变是赘生物。它由纤维蛋白基质和血小板、白细胞及细菌组成，是微观过程的肉眼大体表现，需要多种辅助因子参与形成。通常，首先是存在内皮破坏或损伤病灶，血小板和纤维蛋白得以黏附于此。引起内皮局部损伤的原因包括：①中心静脉导管或起搏器电极导线造成的机械性损伤，或通过反复静脉注射颗粒状毒品造成的内皮表面擦伤[5]；②获得性、自身免疫性疾病或既往IE相关的内皮炎性损伤；③室间隔缺损（VSD）或主动脉瓣关闭不全引起的高湍流。

　　血管内假体材料也可以成为纤维蛋白和血小板黏附的病灶，而后，血液中的

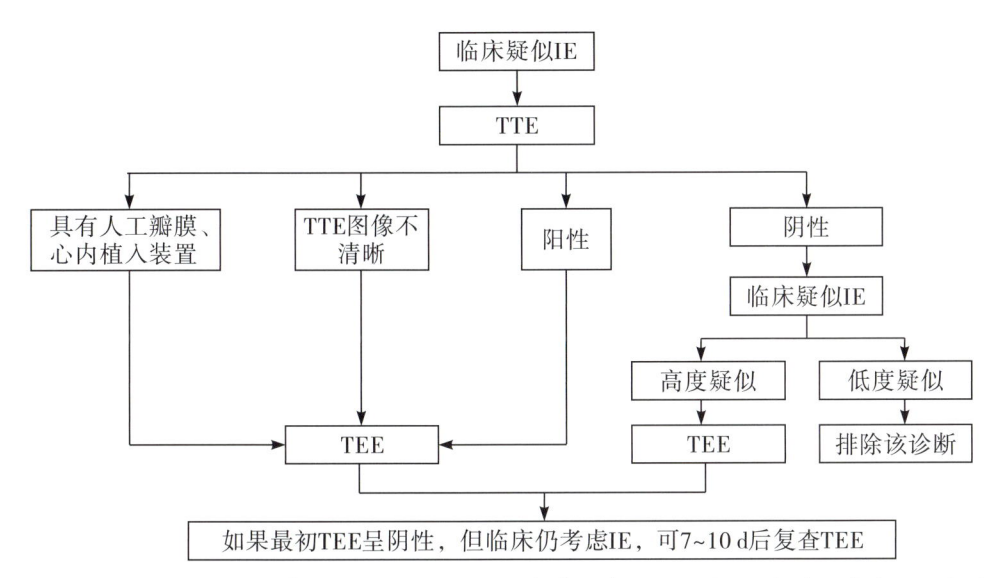

图 4.1　建议使用经胸超声心动图（TTE）和经食管超声心动图（TEE）诊断感染性心内膜炎（IE）的流程图。引自：Eur J Echocardiogr, 2010, 11(2): 201–219. https://doi.org/10.1093/ejechocard/jeg004. 本幻灯片的内容可能受版权保护：有关详细信息请参阅幻灯片注释

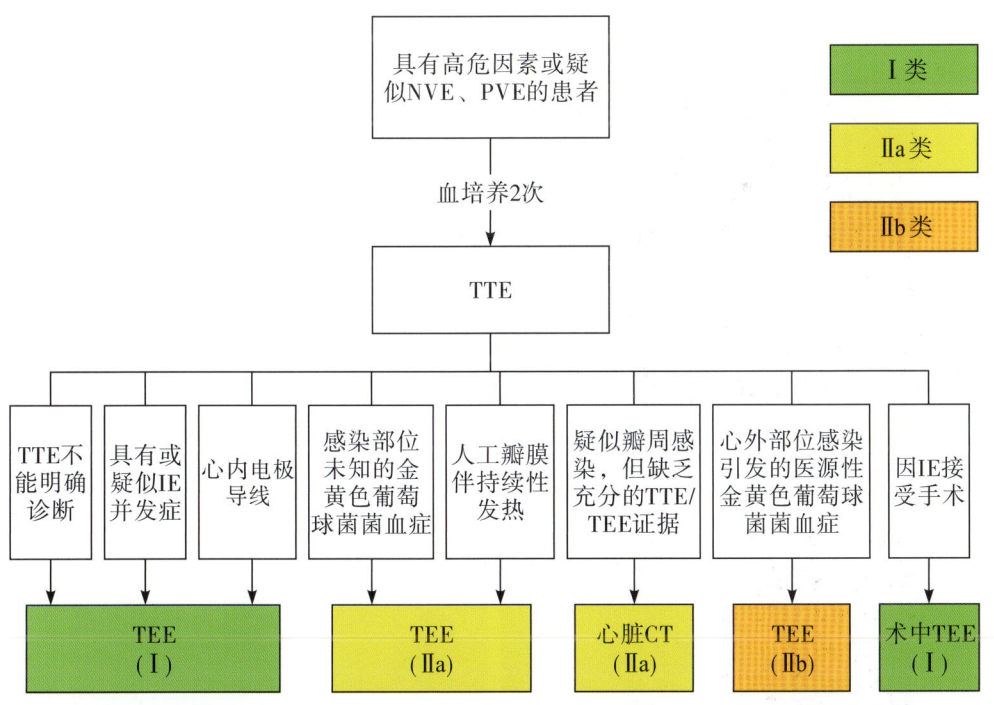

图 4.2　关于使用经胸超声心动图（TTE）和经食管超声心动图（TEE）诊断自体瓣膜心内膜炎（NVE）和人工瓣膜心内膜炎（PVE）的循证建议。引自：Nishimura RA, et al. JACC, 2014, 63: e57–e185.

病原微生物黏附在纤维蛋白－血小板基质上，为感染建立滩头阵地，通过病原体和血小板之间的相互作用使赘生物不断生长。以金黄色葡萄球菌为例，它有多种分子途径黏附血小板并与血小板相互作用，导致血小板活化和聚集，从而成为赘生物形成的关键机制[6-7]。

按超声心动图的定义，赘生物就是附着在瓣叶或心脏支撑结构、内皮组织或血管内假体材料上，独立振荡的回声团块[8]。图4.3显示了TEE检查中典型的二尖瓣赘生物。图4.4显示了TTE检查中的三尖瓣赘生物伴中度三尖瓣反流。

独立振荡是指独立于瓣叶运动或除瓣叶运动之外的运动，或者，特别是在人工瓣膜心内膜炎（PVE）或心脏装置感染的情况下，在心动周期中出现预期外的心内结构运动。与此不同，黏液样变的瓣叶可在超声下出现类似大的赘生物样改变，但它与瓣叶活动同步；还有来自起搏电极导线或人工瓣环的超声伪影可能看起来像肿块，但这些不会表现出独立于相关心脏结构之外的运动（图4.5）。

在自体瓣膜心内膜炎（NVE）中，赘生物通常见于瓣叶的"上游"表面，例如二尖瓣的左心房侧或左心室流出道侧或主动脉瓣，也可能附着在腱索、起搏电极导线、人工瓣膜或心内装置上[9-10]。由于瓣叶、反流束径路或心内假体材料上容易形成赘生物，因此超声心动图应对所有这类结构表面进行彻底评估。例如，主动脉瓣心内膜炎的主动脉瓣反流可导致二尖瓣瓣下结构和腱索的感染种植和

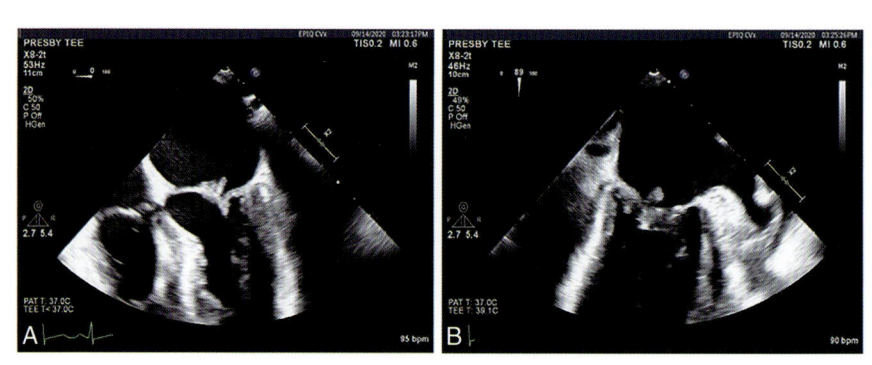

图4.3　TEE中的二尖瓣赘生物。A. 四腔心切面，显示赘生物主要累及前叶。B. 二腔心切面，显示后部P3段瓣叶异常增厚，提示更广泛的瓣膜感染

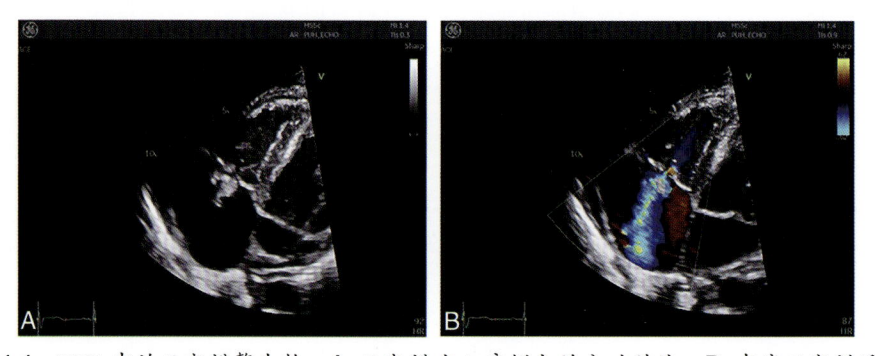

图4.4　TTE中的三尖瓣赘生物。A. 三尖瓣右心房侧大的分叶肿块。B. 中度三尖瓣反流

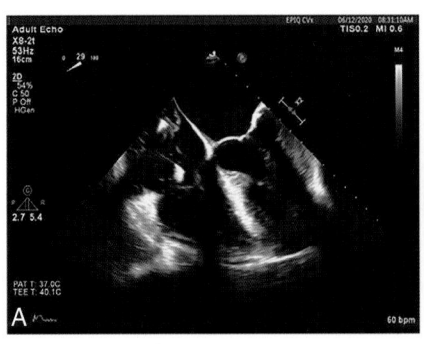

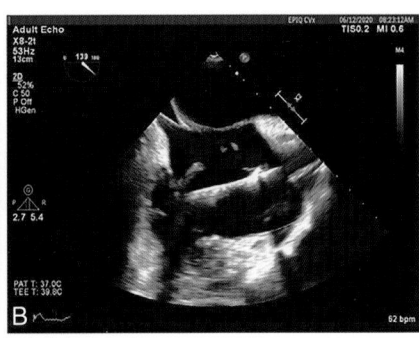

图 4.5　A. 未缩放的四腔心切面，起搏电极导线右心房部分可见相关的赘生物。多条起搏电极导线的存在会造成超声伪影，增加了赘生物的分辨难度。B. 适当放大调整的二腔心切面（140°）可以更好地区分起搏电极导线赘生物。注意：此视图中冠状窦和冠状窦电极导线清晰可见（左上）

播散，因此超声检查时应特别注意这些结构（尤其在术前超声检查时更应加倍注意）。

赘生物是 IE 肉眼可见的最基本病变，在感染的自然病程中还可能会出现侵袭性或其他复杂的病理改变和超声特征，下文将讨论相关内容。

Duke 标准中的超声心动图表现

改良 Duke 标准将以下超声心动图发现作为诊断 IE 的主要标准[2]：①赘生物；②心内或瓣周脓肿；③人工瓣膜与自体瓣环分离；④新出现瓣膜反流。

最后一项标准的判断最难，因为老年人群常见退行性瓣膜病，这一瓣膜病变可能是非感染性瓣膜异常和反流，判断不准就会出现假阳性诊断。

瓣叶上的赘生物或炎症引起的宿主防御反应可能导致瓣叶对合不良并出现反流（图 4.4B），IE 还可导致瓣叶穿孔、损毁，以致出现循环不稳的显著反流。根据 ASE 标准，可利用定量和半定量超声心动图技术来评估这些病例瓣膜反流的严重程度[3]。图 4.6 描绘了 TEE 发现的胸主动脉全舒张期逆向血流，这是自体主动脉瓣感染导致的严重主动脉瓣反流的征象。NVE 大的赘生物，尤其是 PVE 中的人工瓣膜赘生物，均可引起瓣口狭窄，导致瓣膜功能障碍。遇到这种情况时，应通过连续波多普勒超声测定跨瓣压差。图 4.7 显示了因二尖瓣赘生物阻塞而导致的二尖瓣流入道压差升高。

IE 的超声心动图评估

使用超声心动图评估 IE 时，须充分评估感染的程度，而不是简单地识别赘生物的存在与否，这包括对多瓣膜受累情况及侵袭性感染征象进行彻底评估。由于从开始感染到临床诊断，中间有较长的潜伏期，这段时间可能会有多个瓣膜受累，一方面可能是由于菌血症带来的种植播散，也可以是感染的直接蔓延。

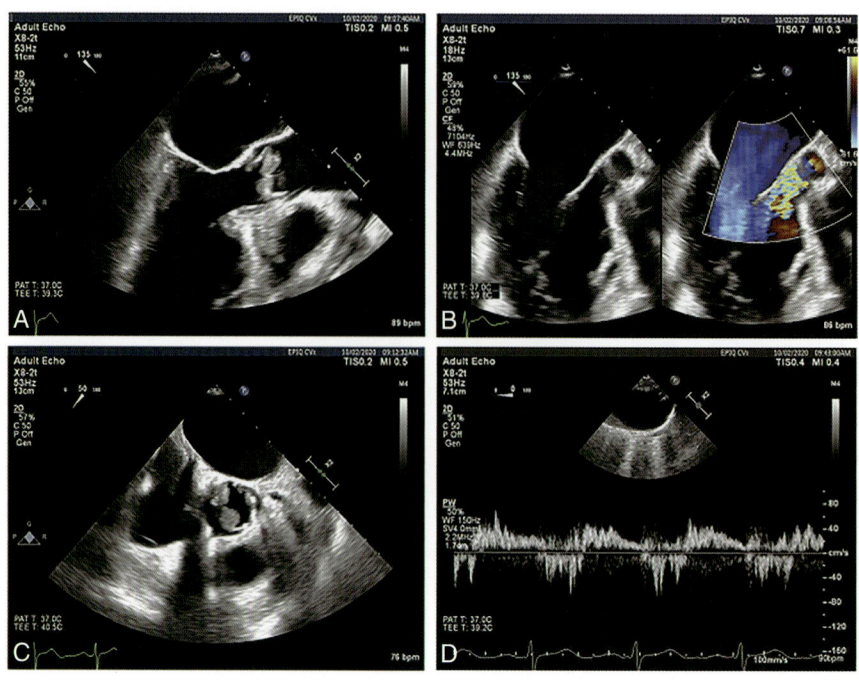

图4.6 二叶主动脉瓣IE和重度主动脉瓣反流。A.可见巨大赘生物伴瓣叶结构破坏。B.左心室流出道可见宽大的主动脉瓣反流束和左心室扩张。C. 0型二叶主动脉瓣开口呈椭圆形,右冠状动脉瓣叶上有大的赘生物。D.胸主动脉脉冲波多普勒可见全舒张期逆向血流

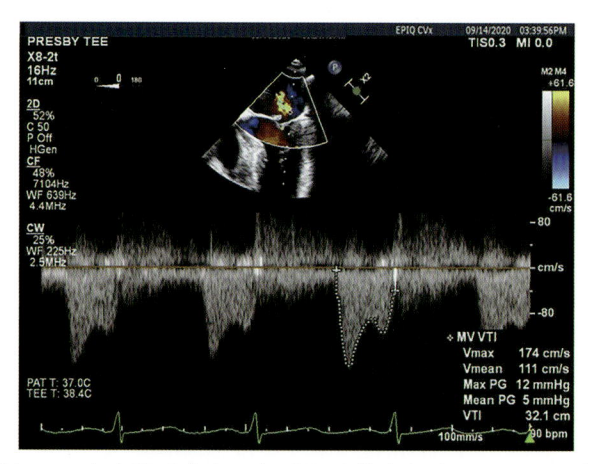

图4.7 自体瓣膜感染二尖瓣上的赘生物导致二尖瓣狭窄

超声心动图检查（TEE或TTE）应包括对瓣膜的完整二维（2D）和彩色多普勒评估，判定受累瓣膜的数量及心内结构的异常，测定赘生物的大小，适时结合瓣膜反流或狭窄的定量和半定量检测，判定瓣膜病变和瓣叶损害的临床意义。完整的超声心动图检查应包含对瓣膜病变的结构和血流动力学的评估，包括心腔扩大、心室功能和肺动脉高压等情况，如有可能，还应与之前的超声心动图检查进行比较。

通过同步显示彩色多普勒与二维灰阶图像，并进行"比较"，有助于更好地评价瓣膜结构异常，特别是在有瓣膜反流、穿孔或瓣周脓肿时。还有建议将瓣膜在多个心动周期的系列图像扫描也作为瓣膜评估的一部分。图 4.8 显示在发现大的三尖瓣赘生物后通过系列扫描检出了三尖瓣瓣叶穿孔，图 4.9 显示通过对图像的"颜色比较"来判断人工瓣膜感染流入和流出脓肿腔的血流。

对于有起搏电极导线和心内植入材料的患者必须充分评估赘生物或感染征象，使用 TEE 的精细探头进行操作，采集标准解剖切面可实现良好的评估（图 4.5B）。右心房的二腔心切面以及三尖瓣和右心室的经胃切面可以提供起搏电极导线最完整的图像，与标准的四腔心切面和 60° 三尖瓣切面相辅相成。二腔心切面通常可以在稍高位的全平面角度（100°～110°）下提供右心耳及相关右心房电极导线的良好影像。起搏电极导线的上腔静脉部分也可以从标准的二腔心切面上观察，一

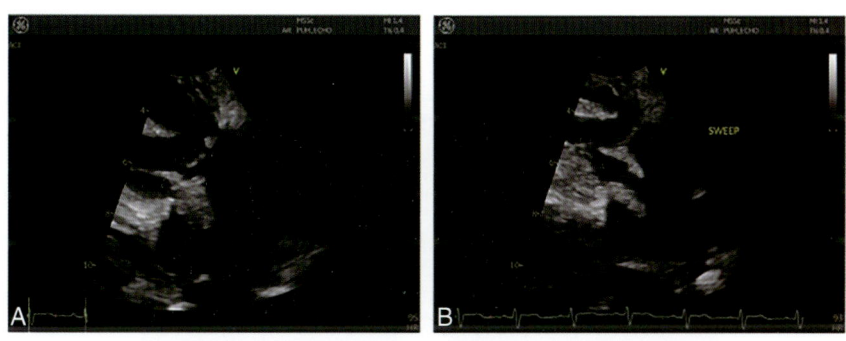

图 4.8 A. TTE 评估期间在右心室流入切面上发现大的三尖瓣赘生物。B. 从该成像位置进行多个心动周期的系列扫描，可判定三尖瓣瓣叶穿孔

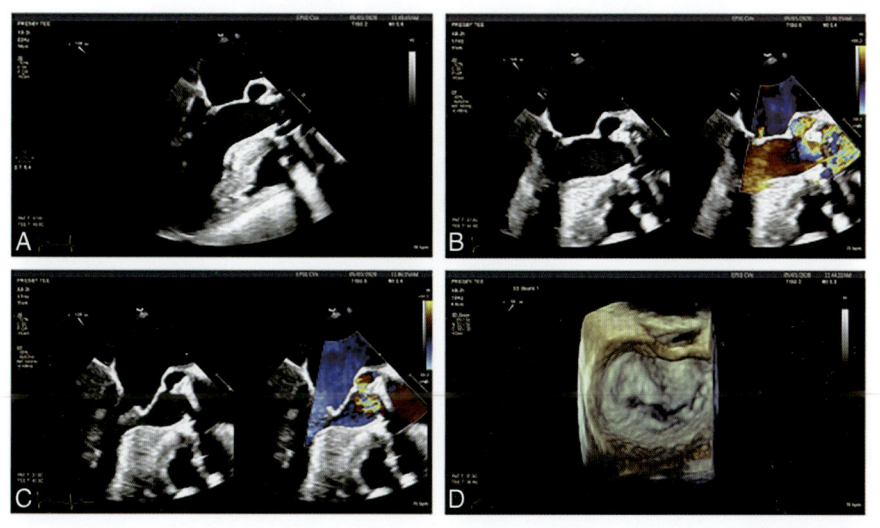

图 4.9 人工瓣膜心内膜炎（PVE）瓣周脓肿伴假性动脉瘤。A. 二维灰阶成像中人工主动脉瓣后部的无回声区可能与左心室流出道相交通（瘘）。B-C. 使用同步彩色多普勒比较成像显示收缩期血流进入假性动脉瘤或脓肿腔（B），舒张期血流经瘘管流出脓肿腔（C）。D. 与左心室流出道之间形成瘘管的假性动脉瘤的三维（3D）正面图像

般通过顺时针旋转 TEE 探头并向头侧后退完成。140°～150° 三尖瓣中心切面通常可提供三尖瓣瓣叶、瓣环、右心室起搏电极导线，以及双心室起搏或心脏再同步化治疗（CRT）起搏系统冠状窦电极导线的最佳影像。当超声设备具有同步双平面成像功能时，将可控光标调整到需要检查的电极导线段，便可获得清晰良好的图像（图 4.10）。

心内膜炎的侵袭性感染

感染侵犯到瓣叶外或心内膜表面外称为复杂性或侵袭性感染（图 4.11 和图 4.12），包括瓣周脓肿或心肌脓肿、假性动脉瘤或瘘，以及瓣膜瘤或穿孔。10%～20% 的 IE 患者可能存在瓣周感染，如果在适当的静脉抗生素治疗 5～7 d 后仍持续发热或血培养呈阳性，或者出现新的房室传导阻滞，或 12 导联心电图出现新的房室传导阻滞或传导异常，应怀疑存在瓣周感染。表 4.1 列出了侵袭性 IE 感染的各种病变类型。

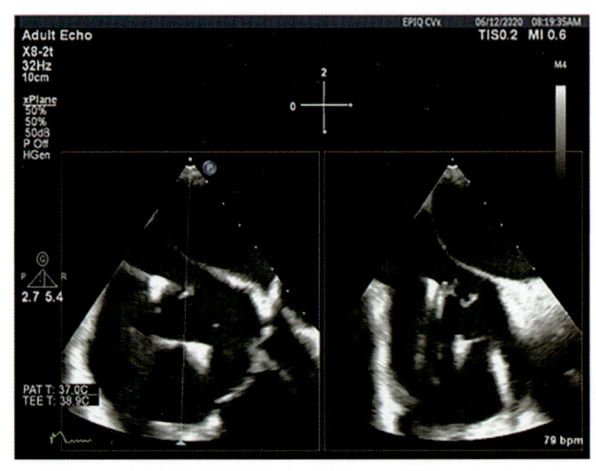

图 4.10　起搏电极导线右心房部分的同步可控双平面成像。将光标（细白线）放置在 0° 四腔心切面中起搏电极导线的需检查部分，右侧屏幕同时显示 90° 二腔心切面，确认起搏电极导线上存在赘生物

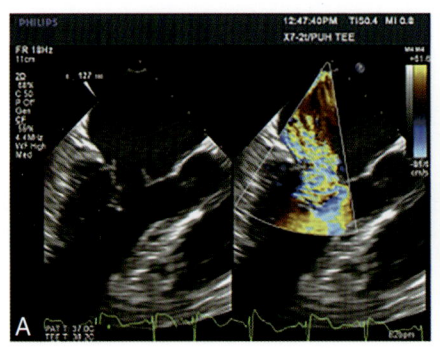

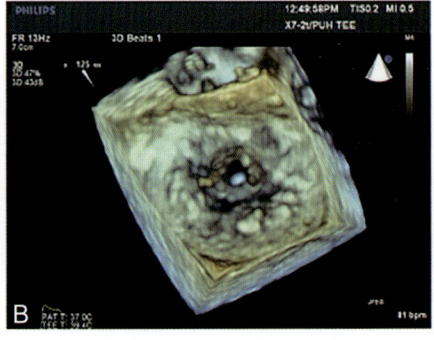

图 4.11　A. 二尖瓣前叶穿孔。B. 通过二尖瓣 3D 正面成像得到证实

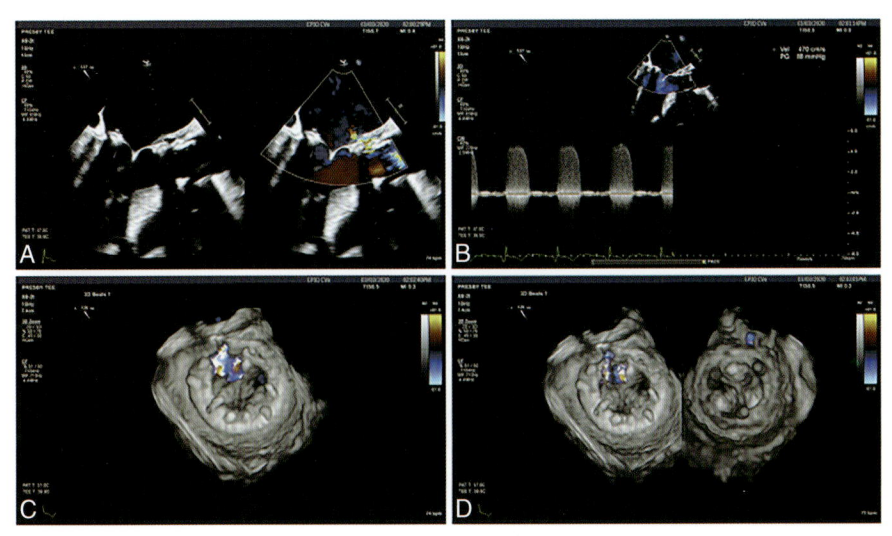

图 4.12 人工二尖瓣瓣周漏。A–B. 二尖瓣生物瓣和主动脉瓣生物瓣可见瓣周脓肿（人工二尖瓣、左心房壁和人工主动脉瓣之间的无回声区），彩色多普勒（A，右）和频谱多普勒（B）血流均符合人工二尖瓣前瓣瓣周漏。频谱多普勒信号可定义血流时相（本例为收缩期）和压差，二者均可帮助确定受累的心腔。C–D. 3D 彩色多普勒有助于确定瓣周漏的解剖位置和范围，特别是获取来自左心房和左心室的人工二尖瓣同步 3D 彩色多普勒成像时（D）

表 4.1　复杂性感染性心内膜炎（IE）的病理改变

- 脓肿：瓣周感染伴坏死或化脓性浸润，表现为增厚、不均匀的瓣周组织平面，外观可以是有回声或无回声的。当腔隙无回声时为脓肿腔。脓肿本身不与心腔或大血管腔直接连通，但在后期可出现与心腔或血管相通（参见瘘管或假性动脉瘤）。脓肿多见于主动脉瓣 IE 和人工瓣膜 IE（PVE）

- 假性动脉瘤：因感染形成的瓣周空腔，与心室或大血管相通，彩色多普勒显示血流可从中流入和（或）流出（图 4.9A）

- 瘘管：IE 导致两个相邻心腔或心腔与脓肿腔之间相通，最好通过彩色和频谱多普勒来确定（图 4.9B 和图 4.9C）

- 瓣叶穿孔：瓣叶在瓣口或瓣叶对合区位置之外出现不连续，允许心腔之间的血液流动。图 4.8B 和图 4.11 呈现了 IE 导致的瓣叶穿孔

- 瓣膜瘤：构成瓣叶的各组织层面出现分层改变，导致瓣膜变形和(或)功能障碍（图 4.13），可能与瓣叶穿孔有关或是瓣叶穿孔的先兆

- 腱索断裂：IE 导致腱索附着点破坏，是 IE 出现瓣膜反流的可能原因

- 瓣周漏：两个相邻心腔之间经瓣环裂隙出现的血液流动，通常限于 PVE（图 4.12）

- 人工瓣膜与自体瓣环分离：由于感染向瓣周扩散和瓣周漏扩大，人工瓣膜失去结构完整性，导致人工瓣膜出现异常摆动，通常伴有严重的瓣周漏

TTE 与 TEE

TTE 和 TEE 在 IE 的诊断和评估中都发挥着重要作用，一般根据临床情况来选择这两种检查方式。与 TEE 相比，TTE 的灵敏度较低（分别为 >90% 和 46%~75%）[8-14]，但 TTE 的优点是应用广泛、可及时使用、便携，且操作几乎无风险。因此，尽管灵敏度较低，但对疑似 IE 患者的初步评估通常还是选择 TTE（图 4.1 和图 4.2）。

对于 IE 可能性相对较低的患者，且 TTE 检查的影像质量较高，则仅需做 TTE 即可排除 IE 的诊断。2017 年的一项 meta 分析显示，对于没有进行人工瓣膜置换，TTE 谐波成像（目前超声心动图常用）完全排除了 IE 的患者，在 TEE 中检出赘生物的可能性非常低。

研究表明，TEE 在检测小赘生物、心内脓肿和人工瓣膜异常方面更为清晰。因此，美国心脏协会/美国心脏病学会（AHA/ACC）指南建议，对植入人工瓣膜或起搏器电极导线的病例，或尽管 TTE 呈阴性但仍高度怀疑 IE 的患者，应使用灵敏度和特异性更高的 TEE 进行检查（Ⅰ类，B 级证据）[8]。

对于 TTE 阳性病例，推荐进一步行 TEE 检查，用于评估瓣周病变范围、赘生物大小以及瓣膜反流程度，所有这些因素将影响临床决策和治疗方案。

对于疑似 IE，但 TEE 检查阴性，如果是自体瓣膜，已证明基本可排除 IE 的可能性；但对于植入了人工瓣膜的患者，TEE 检查阴性则有可能漏诊 IE[9-11]。因此，在高度怀疑 IE 而 TEE 阴性的情况下，特别是植入了人工瓣膜的患者，应考虑在 7~10 d 后复查 TEE。

假阳性结果

尽管在图像分辨率、放大倍率和三维（3D）成像技术上取得了长足进步，但 TTE 和 TEE 的特异性仍达不到 100%，很可能出现假阳性结果。以前传统超声无法看到的解剖结构变化现在可以通过超声成像技术发现，例如纤维蛋白链或退行性瓣膜变化，这些结构可能被误认为是赘生物。与 IE 无关的瓣叶脱垂、连枷腱索或乳头肌断裂在超声上可能有与赘生物相似的表现，加之伴有明显的瓣膜反流，而被误诊为 IE。脱垂的瓣叶一般不会表现出与赘生物一样的独立振荡运动，但冗余的腱索可以表现出独立于瓣叶的运动而被误认为是赘生物。保留腱索的二尖瓣置换后残留的腱索或二尖瓣瓣叶组织也很容易被误认为是人工瓣膜赘生物。二尖瓣环钙化，特别是干酪样二尖瓣环钙化，可表现为二尖瓣赘生物的超声特点。如果有可能（最好是在发生感染之前一段时间做过超声检查），将现行检查与之前的超声心动图进行比较，可为瓣膜异常的疑点问题提供宝贵信息。

心内血栓或肿瘤也可能会被误判为赘生物，因此诊断 IE 需要结合临床症状、血培养阳性或手术组织培养等结果。人工瓣膜血栓或起搏电极导线相关血栓可能与 PVE 或起搏电极导线相关感染难以区分，这就需要综合临床情况对 IE 做出诊断。当难以鉴别 PVE 与人工瓣膜血栓时，瓣周侵袭性感染的超声心动图表现，如瓣周漏或脓肿，有助于明确诊断。

成像伪影

正常的心脏结构也可能被误认为是赘生物。高度移动的三尖瓣环或右心房游离壁在成像平面可能被误认为是心内肿块或赘生物。三叶主动脉瓣的斜位成像可能会在左心室流出道中出现瓣下赘生物，这实际上是进入成像平面的第三个瓣叶。使用同步可控多平面成像有助于区分成像伪影和心内肿块或赘生物（图 4.13）。

3D 超声心动图

3D 超声心动图可作为 IE 诊断的辅助工具，是全面的 2D 成像和彩色多普勒评估的补充技术。虽然可能无法区分小赘生物，但大的赘生物通常可以通过 3D 成像技术轻松诊断。由于赘生物是三维结构，因此平面 2D 成像技术可能无法有效确定赘生物的大小及与其他解剖结构的关系。图 4.14 显示了二尖瓣赘生物，在各个切面图中均显示为中等大小；然而，当使用 3D 技术进行检查时，显示赘生物相当大，分布范围从二尖瓣环的 12 点钟到 4 点钟，可能同时累及二尖瓣前叶和后叶。图 4.15 很好地显示了累及 3 个主动脉瓣瓣叶的非细菌性血栓性心内膜炎（NBTE）。3D 超声心动图也可有效用于 PVE，以及观察瓣周病理变化（图 4.9D）。

非超声心动图影像学补充检查

在某些情况下，TTE 和 TEE 不足以提供充分的诊断证据，特别是对于 PVE。人工瓣膜的术后变化和声影可能会使 PVE 或侵袭性瓣周感染的诊断变得困难。在这些情况下，心脏 CT 和心脏 PET 成像可作为补充性影像学检查方式，具体取决于各机构对相关检查的熟悉程度[16-18]。由于时间分辨率较差，心脏 MRI 在这方面的作用十分有限。

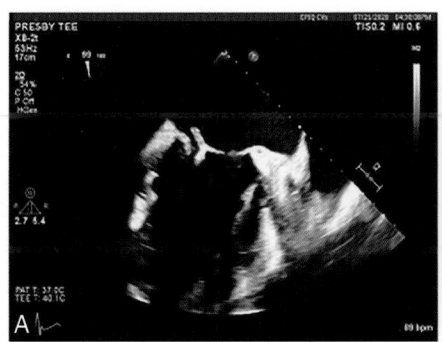

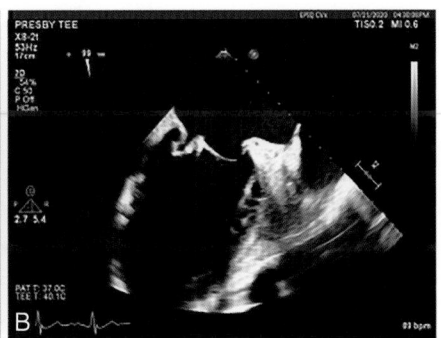

图 4.13 二尖瓣后叶瓣膜瘤。A. 收缩期。B. 舒张期

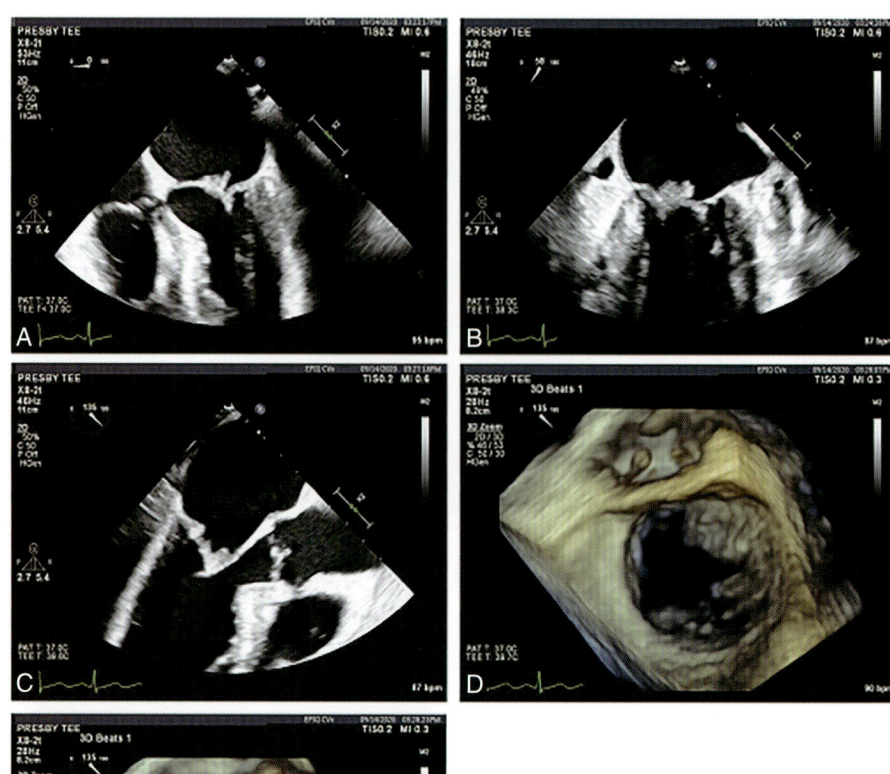

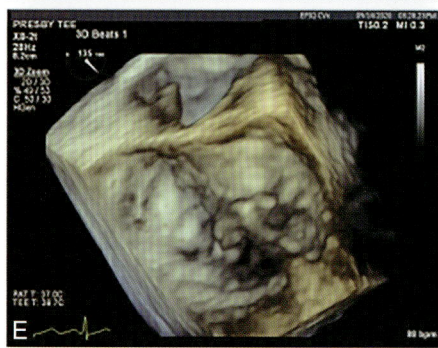

图 4.14　A-C. 2D 平面 TEE 成像显示 0°、60° 和 135° 标准解剖切面中的二尖瓣赘生物。D-E. 使用 3D 正面成像，从手术医生视角看到的同一赘生物舒张期（D）和收缩期（E）的表现。在标准解剖平面中最初看起来是中等大小的赘生物，在 3D 成像上显示为跨越二尖瓣环 1/3 的巨大多分叶赘生物

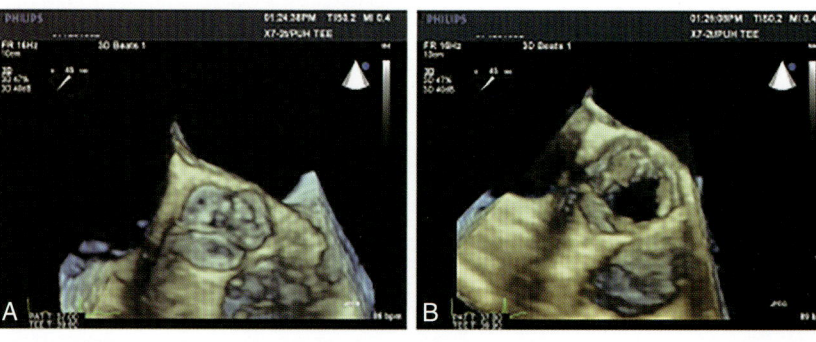

图 4.15　主动脉瓣非细菌性血栓性心内膜炎（NBTE）的 3D TEE 成像，显示 3 个瓣叶均受累。A. 舒张期。B. 收缩期。由于赘生物位于主动脉瓣叶的左心室侧，且 3D 成像是从瓣膜的主动脉侧"自上而下"进行的，因此在收缩期瓣膜打开期间，对赘生物的显示最佳。NBTE 最常涉及左侧瓣膜（在一项大型病例系列中显示：二尖瓣占 43%，主动脉瓣占 36%，三尖瓣占 4%，肺动脉瓣占 1%，主动脉瓣和二尖瓣交界处占 13%[15]）。虽然人们普遍认为 NBTE 的赘生物较小，但根据赘生物特征区分 NBTE 和 IE 是不可能的。然而，NBTE 中不会出现瓣周病变或其他侵入性感染的超声心动图征象。如果存在这些改变，则更符合 IE 的诊断

参考文献

[1] Durack DT, Lukes AS, Bright DK. New criteria for diagnosis of infective endocarditis: utilization of specific echocardiographic findings. Duke Endocarditis Service Am J Med. March, 1994, 96(3): 200–209.

[2] Li JS, Sexton DJ, Mick N, et al. Proposed modifications to the Duke criteria for the diagnosis of infective endocarditis. Clin Infect Dis, 2000, 30(4): 633.

[3] Nishimura RA, et al. AHA/ACC guideline for the management of patients with valvular heart disease, a report of the American College of Cardiology/American Heart Association task force on practice guidelines. JACC (J Am Coll Cardiol), 2014, 63: e57–e185.

[4] Douglas PS, et al. ACCF/ASE/AHA/ASNC/HFSA/HRS/SCAI/SCCM/SCCT/SCMR 2011 appropriate use criteria for echocardiography. J Am Soc Echocardiogr, 2011, 24: 229–267.

[5] Cahill TJ, Prendergast BD. Infective endocarditis. Lancet February 27, 2016, 387(10021): 882–893.

[6] Hannachi N, Habib G, Camoin-Jau L. Aspirin effect on Staphylococcus aureus-platelet interactions during infectious endocarditis. Front Med October, 15, 2019, 6: 217.

[7] Jung CJ, Yeh CY, Shun CT, et al. Platelets enhance biofilm formation and resistance of endocarditis-inducing streptococci on the injured heart valve. J Infect Dis April 01, 2012, 205(7): 1066–1075.

[8] Baddour LM, Wilson WR, Bayer AS, American Heart Association Committee on Rheumatic Fever, et al. Infective endocarditis in adults: diagnosis, antimicrobial therapy, and management of complications: a scientific statement for healthcare professionals from the American Heart Association. Circulation October 13, 2015, 132(15): 1435–1486.

[9] Bashore TM, Cabell C, Fowler VJ. Update on infective endocarditis. Curr Probl Cardiol, 2006, 4: 274–352.

[10] Krivokapich J, Child JS. Role of transthoracic and transesophageal echocardiography in diagnosis and management of infective endocarditis. Cardiol Clin, 1996, 14: 363–382.

[11] Roe MT, Abramson MA, Li J, et al. Clinical information determines the impact of transesophageal echocardiography on the diagnosis of infective endocarditis by the Duke criteria. Am Heart J, 2000, 139: 945–951.

[12] Lowry RW, Zoghbi WA, Baker WB, et al. Clinical impact of transesophageal echocardiography in the diagnosis and management of infective endocarditis. Am J Cardiol, 1994, 73: 1089–1091.

[13] Sochowski RA, Chan KL. Implication of negative results on a monoplane transesophageal echocardiographic study in patients with suspected infective endocarditis. J Am Coll Cardiol, 1993, 21: 216–221.

[14] Bai AD, et al. Diagnostic accuracy of transthoracic echocardiography for infective endocarditis findings using transesophageal echocardiography as the reference standard: a meta-analysis. J Am Soc Echocardiogr July, 2017, 30(7): 639–646.

[15] Bussani R, DE-Giorgio F, Pesel G, et al. Overview and comparison of infectious endocarditis and non-infectious endocarditis: a review of 814 Autoptic cases. In Vivo September-October, 2019, 33(5): 1565–1572.

[16] Feuchtner GM, Stolzmann P, Dichtl W, et al. Multislice computed tomography in infective endocarditis. J Am Coll Cardiol, 2009, 53: 436–444.

[17] Pizzi MN, et al. Improving the diagnosis of infective endocarditis in prosthetic valves and intracardiac devices with ^{18}F-fluordeoxyglucose positron emission tomography/computed tomography angiography. Circulation September 22, 2015, 132(12): 1113–1126.

[18] Zatorska K, Michalowska I, Abramczuk E, et al. The usefulness of cardiac computed tomography in the diagnosis of infective endocarditis and its perivalvular complications. Eur Heart J August 1, 2017, 38(Suppl. 1_1)

第 5 章
感染性心内膜炎的其他影像学检查

Thomas Gossios, Ronak Rajani, Bernard Prendergast
Department of Cardiology, St Thomas' Hospital, London, United Kingdom

引 言

目前，根据欧洲心脏病学会（ESC）和美国心脏病学会/美国心脏协会（ACC/AHA）的感染性心内膜炎（IE）诊断和治疗指南，要求将感染出现的一系列临床症状，结合心内膜受累相关证据，用于确定 IE 的诊断[1-2]。"标准化的改良 Duke 标准"是现今临床最常用的诊断标准，但对于人工心脏瓣膜、植入电子设备或超声心动图不能提供足够诊断依据时，仍存在诊断率较低的问题[3]。对此，2015 年 ESC 对标准进行了修改，纳入了其他的影像学方法，以提升上述情况的诊断准确性（表5.1）。具体包括：① 利用 CT 检测的瓣周病变（主要标准）；② ^{18}F-FDG PET/CT 检测到的人工心脏瓣膜置换术后 3 个月以上植入部位异常增高的放射摄取影（主要标准）；③ 影像学检测到近期栓塞事件（次要标准）。

这些补充并不是为了弱化超声心动图对于 IE 诊断的重要性，相反，这些措施可提高那些疑似 IE、超声心动图又无法提供足够证据的病例的诊断确定性。经胸超声心动图（TTE）作为 I 类指征依旧是临床首选的影像检查方式。经食管超声心动图（TEE）则在以下情况下作为 I 类推荐：所有临床怀疑 IE 且 TTE 呈阴性或 TTE 证据不足的患者，有人工心脏瓣膜和心内植入装置的患者 [这是基于 TTE 对检出赘生物的灵敏度低（人工瓣膜与自体瓣膜：50% *vs*.76%），而 TEE 的灵敏度则显著提高（人工瓣膜与自体瓣膜：96% *vs*.92%）][4-6]。

ESC 指南在改良 Duke 标准中引入了 CT 和 PET 影像结果作为诊断标准，而 ACC/AHA 指南则强调了这些成像方法在检出 IE 心脏以外并发症中的价值[7]。尽管存在上述细微差别，但两部指南均认为这些新的影像方法可在超声心动图的解剖和血流动力学发现之外提供具有辅助价值的诊断信息[8]。

CT 血管造影

心脏 CT 最初主要用于冠状动脉和血管成像，但其后多项研究显示，在疑似 IE 的诊断方面它已经得到了越来越广泛的应用。随着技术的进步，CT 扫描的空间分辨率已提高到 <0.5mm，这使得瓣膜形态（赘生物和穿孔）和瓣周并发症（脓肿

表 5.1 感染性心内膜炎（IE）的改良 Duke 诊断标准

主要标准

1）血培养
    a）2 次独立的血培养中培养出 IE 相关的典型微生物：
        · 草绿色链球菌、解没食子酸链球菌、HACEK[a]、金黄色葡萄球菌；或者
        · 社区获得性肠球菌，但未发现原发病灶；或者
    b）持续阳性血培养中培养出符合 IE 的微生物：
        · ≥2 次血培养呈阳性，抽血间隔>12 h；或者
        · 3 次血培养均阳性，或≥4 次血培养中的大部分呈阳性（第一个样本和最后一个样本间隔≥1 h）；或者
        · 单次血培养贝氏柯克斯体阳性或 IgG 抗体滴度>1：800

2）影像学
    a）超声心动图存在 IE 证据
        · 赘生物
        · 脓肿、假性动脉瘤、心内瘘
        · 瓣膜穿孔或瓣膜瘤
        · 人工瓣膜瓣周出现新的与自体瓣环的分离点——瓣周漏
    b）瓣膜置换术后 3 个月以上，通过 PET/CT 或放射性标记的白细胞 SPECT/CT 检测到人工瓣膜周围的异常代谢
    c）心脏 CT 发现明确的瓣周病变

次要标准

1）存在心脏易感因素或静脉吸毒
2）发热>38℃
3）血管表现（包括通过影像学检测到的）：动脉栓塞、脾梗死、真菌性动脉瘤、颅内出血、Janeway 病变
4）免疫表现：肾小球肾炎、Osler 结节、Roth 斑、类风湿因子
5）微生物学证据：血培养阳性但未达到主要标准，或具有符合 IE 的微生物感染的血清学证据

[a]HACEK：副流感嗜血杆菌、嗜沫嗜血杆菌、副嗜血杆菌、流感嗜血杆菌、凝聚杆菌，人心杆菌，侵蚀艾肯菌、金氏金氏菌、反硝化金氏菌。确诊 IE（2 个主要标准；1 个主要标准+3 个次要标准；5 个次要标准）。疑似 IE（1 个主要标准+1 个次要标准；3 个次要标准）

和假性动脉瘤）在 CT 影像上清晰可见[9-10]。

诊断性能

· 自体瓣膜 IE

鉴于 TEE 对自体瓣膜 IE 相关病变诊断的高准确性，因此其他影像方法在该领域诊断性能的相关数据很少。多排 CT 血管造影与作为 IE 成像金标准的 TEE 显示出相当的诊断效能，特别是在瓣膜和瓣周并发症的检测方面。一项针对 37 名临床疑似 IE 患者的研究表明：对比术中的解剖发现，心脏 CT 具有 96% 的诊断准确性（灵敏度 97%，特异性 88%），在诊断赘生物大小和活动性方面（不包括瓣叶穿孔）与 TEE 高度一致[11]。在对 19 名需要手术的主动脉瓣 IE 患者的进一步研究中，CT 对主动脉瓣假性动脉瘤（灵敏度 100%，特异性 87.5%）或瓣周病变（灵敏度

100%，特异性 100%）的诊断具有高度准确性。但 CT 检查也有其短板，尽管所有 >10 mm 的赘生物都能被准确检出，但 CT 无法识别更小的赘生物，因此，其对赘生物的总体诊断效能较差（灵敏度 71.4%，特异性 100%）[12]。在后来的一项对 71 个感染瓣膜（70% 是自体瓣膜）的研究中，CT 对检出瓣周脓肿和假性动脉瘤的灵敏度和特异性分别为 81% 和 90%。TEE 在检测赘生物和瓣叶穿孔方面优于 CT，因此，与单独使用超声心动图或 CT 相比，将两种方法结合可检测出所有（后经术中确认）的脓肿和假性动脉瘤[13]。

基于以上结果，在自体瓣膜 IE 怀疑出现瓣周并发症，而单纯超声心动图检查无法充分排除时，心脏 CT 作为一种辅助影像学检查对于明确诊断具有重要作用。

- **人工瓣膜 IE**

超声心动图对于检查人工心脏瓣膜有其局限性，主要是因为声影阻碍了对瓣叶和瓣周结构的有效观察。一项涉及 27 名（其中 16 人接受了手术）疑似人工瓣膜感染病例的研究显示：CT 在检出主动脉壁增厚方面与 TEE 的结果非常一致，但在脓肿或瓣裂方面 CT 与 TEE 结果则一致性略差（而在赘生物的检测方面仅为中等一致）[14]。在一项对 28 名疑似人工瓣膜 IE 的小样本研究中，作为 TTE 和 TEE 之外的补充检查，CT 的发现（主要是真菌性动脉瘤）使 21% 的患者接受了手术而非内科保守治疗[15]。在另一项对 67 名主动脉瓣人工瓣膜 IE 的进一步研究中，14% 的患者因 CT 检测到瓣周脓肿而得以手术治疗，但 TEE 未能检测到这一病变（图 5.1 和图 5.2）；相反，19% 的患者因 TEE 检测到具有手术指征的病变而推荐手术，但 CT 却没有相应发现（两种检查的完全一致率为 85%）[16]。正如后续多项研究所证实的，CT 对瓣周脓肿等并发症的诊断性能较好，而对赘生物、瓣膜穿孔和瓣周漏的诊断效能较差[17-22]。

以上研究表明，CT 可作为 TEE 的补充检查来评估疑似人工瓣膜 IE，两种影像检查方式相结合可提高 IE 相关病变的检出率，从而有效地对潜在并发症和其他相关诊断进行综合评估[23]。

CT 血管造影的其他应用及其主要局限性

心脏 CT 在再次心脏手术的手术准备中具有明确的作用（图 5.3），也是主动脉瓣 IE 患者冠状动脉及主动脉根部病变无创评估的首选方式，可避免导管操作引起的主动脉损伤和主动脉瓣赘生物医源性脱落导致全身性栓塞的风险[16,21,24-26]。在心脏影像正常时，CT 还可用于检测 IE 的栓塞并发症或排除其他隐匿性感染源（图 5.4A 和 B）[27-30]。

心脏 CT 的主要局限性是存在电离辐射、需要使用碘造影剂，以及与造影剂相关的急性肾损伤和过敏反应等风险。此外，冠状动脉和心脏瓣膜的成像需要缓慢且稳定的心率（受限于时间分辨率），控制心率可能需要静脉注射或口服 β 受体阻滞剂，但这对于存在充血性心力衰竭或严重瓣膜关闭不全的患者相对禁忌。

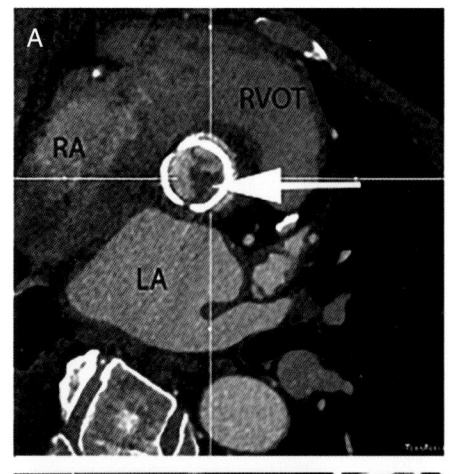

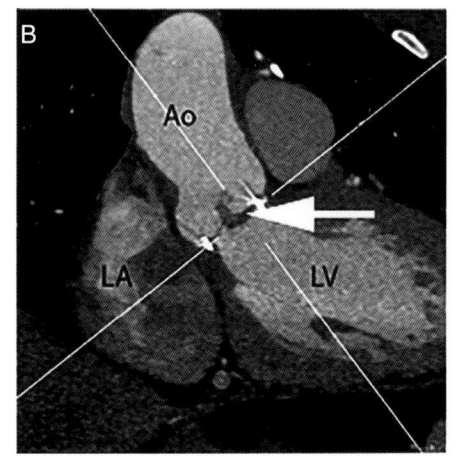

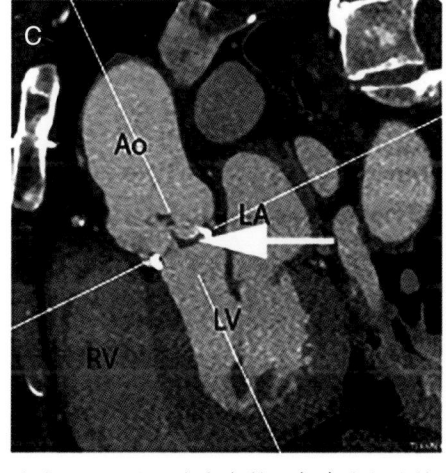

图 5.1 心脏 CT。A. 主动脉瓣水平的轴向切面。B. 左心室流出道水平的冠状切面。C. 三腔心切面。一名 70 岁男性患者因持续不适和寒战 1 周入院。既往史包括因复发性近平滑念珠菌主动脉瓣心内膜炎行再次主动脉瓣置换。血培养证实近平滑念珠菌菌血症复发。TEE 显示继发于主动脉瓣生物瓣赘生物（10 mm）的轻度瓣膜反流。CT 冠状动脉造影示先前的大隐静脉－右冠状动脉桥闭塞，其余血管桥通畅，自身冠状动脉多处狭窄，左冠瓣巨大赘生物及受累瓣叶增厚（箭头）。Ao：主动脉；LA：左心房；LV：左心室；RA：右心房；RV：右心室；RVOT：右心室流出道

人工心脏瓣膜和心脏植入式电子设备（CIED）也会产生大量硬束伪影，限制 CT 对某些关键结构的评估[31]。

分子影像学

对于自体心脏瓣膜，TTE 和 TEE 可提供良好的影像用于诊断。但在有人工心脏瓣膜和 CIED 时，却有其局限性，常规超声无法显示这些状态下的赘生物。此时，分子核医学技术可为定位潜在的感染源提供补充信息[32-33]。

分子影像的基本原理——优点和缺点

正电子发射断层扫描（PET）和单光子发射断层扫描（SPECT）的主要原理是使用放射性核素标记物定位炎症和感染病灶。临床上，^{111}In（铟）或 ^{99m}Tc（锝）标记的自体白细胞（WBC）和 ^{18}F-氟脱氧葡萄糖（^{18}F-FDG）已分别用于观察感染和

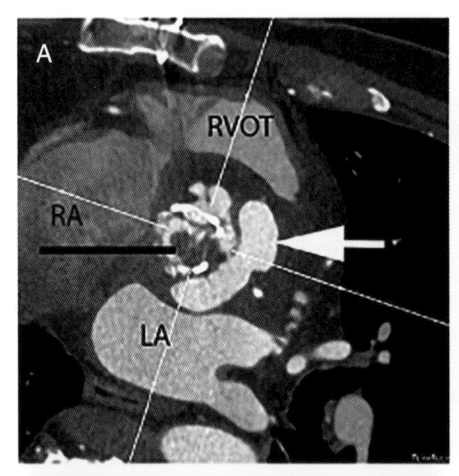

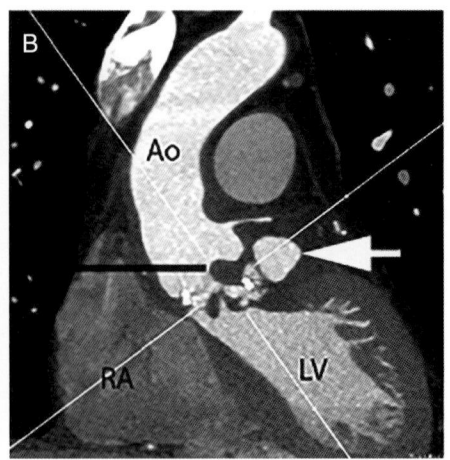

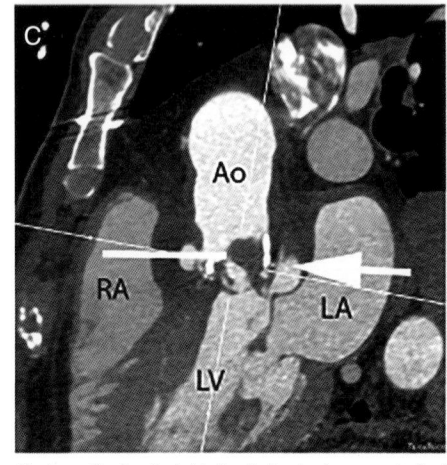

图 5.2 心脏 CT。A. 主动脉瓣水平的轴向切面。B. 左心室流出道水平的冠状切面。C. 三腔心切面。一名 78 岁男性患者，寒战、盗汗、厌食和背痛 3 周。既往曾行主动脉瓣生物瓣置换和冠状动脉旁路移植（LIMA-OM1）。血培养牛链球菌阳性。TEE 显示大的主动脉瓣赘生物和环绕主动脉根部的大脓肿，以及中度瓣周反流。CT 冠状动脉造影证实主动脉瓣损毁，伴赘生物和巨大瓣周脓肿，脓肿压迫左、右冠状动脉开口。Ao：主动脉；LA：左心房；LV：左心室；RA：右心房；RV：右心室；RVOT：右心室流出道

炎症病灶[34]。检查方式具有两方面功能——全身 γ 相机以评估放射性标记物的摄取（分子影像），CT 显像以进行解剖定位。将两种方法叠加使用，就能更好地获得病变与解剖的关系，用于临床诊治[35]。PET 辅以心电门控心脏 CT 血管造影已被推荐作为替代方法，它将分子成像与 CT 血管造影高时空分辨率的优点相结合，实现清晰、全面的解剖成像[36]。

与超声心动图相比，这两种方法都具有全身扫描采集信息的优点，可以准确检测 IE 的心外栓塞[34]。此外，两种方法都可识别潜在的感染源，既可用于判别 IE 的原发病灶，也可用于脓毒症患者的鉴别诊断（图 5.5）[37-39]。基于分子影像学原理，它们已被证明可用于评估炎症和感染的早期阶段，甚至在 IE 的一系列破坏导致出现可识别的解剖结构变化之前即可做出判断[40-41]。最后，这两种方法都能有效检测起搏器感染，范围包括从放置脉冲发生器的皮下囊袋到导线尖端可能存在的感染。同理，两种方法似乎都对诊断人工瓣膜 IE 较为敏感，并已用于评估疑似左心室辅助装置（LVAD）感染。

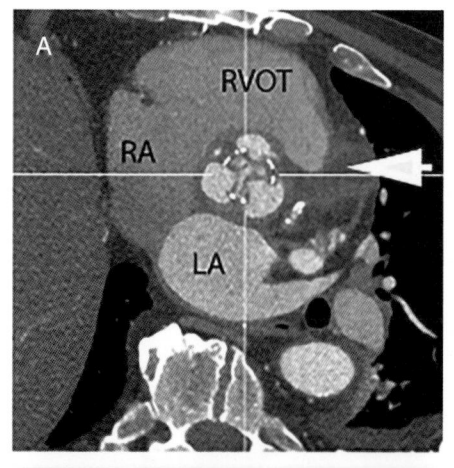

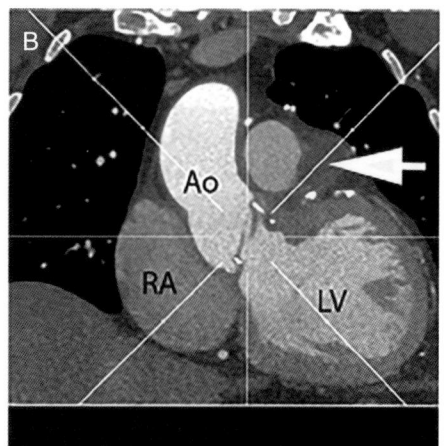

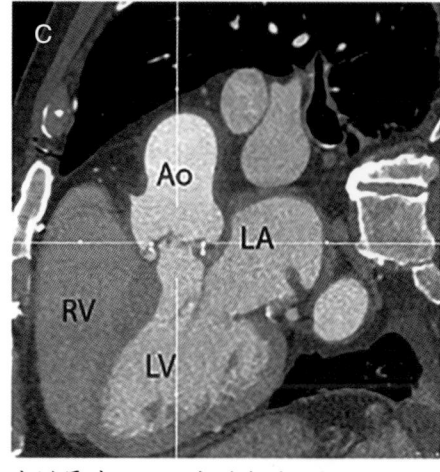

图5.3 心脏CT。A.主动脉瓣水平的轴向切面。B.左心室流出道水平的冠状切面。C.三腔心切面。一名87岁男性患者，因完全性房室传导阻滞和无乳链球菌血培养阳性而入院。既往有主动脉根部同种异体瓣膜植入和冠状动脉旁路移植手术史。超声心动图显示：除主动脉瓣轻度增厚外，无心内膜炎的证据。CT冠状动脉造影显示冠状动脉桥通畅，自身冠状动脉广泛钙化、狭窄；主动脉根部从左冠瓣向左延伸至主肺动脉根部的左侧可见一巨大低密度区域，其周围组织壁显著增强，提示主动脉根部脓肿（箭头）。手术证实主动脉根部瓣周脓肿导致左心室流出道与主动脉分离。Ao：主动脉；LA：左心房；LV：左心室；RA：右心房；RV：右心室；RVOT：右心室流出道

两种技术都需要电离辐射，示踪剂辐射剂量一般是3～8 mSv（毫西弗），CT扫描衰减校正所需的电离辐射约为5 mSv[42]。考虑到存在辐射，临床工作中需结合作为一线影像学方法的超声心动图，制定合理的检查方案。另外，虽然两种技术采集方式相似，但标记白细胞SPECT和 ^{18}F-FDG PET 成像在患者准备、放射标记和检查目的等方面存在根本不同，因此在评估疑似IE时可能会出现不同的结果。

放射性标记白细胞SPECT成像

·基本原理

在白细胞SPECT检查前，需要从血液样本（通常为40 mL）中采集患者的白细胞，并在体外进行放射性标记。放射性标记是一个复杂、耗时的过程，且花费

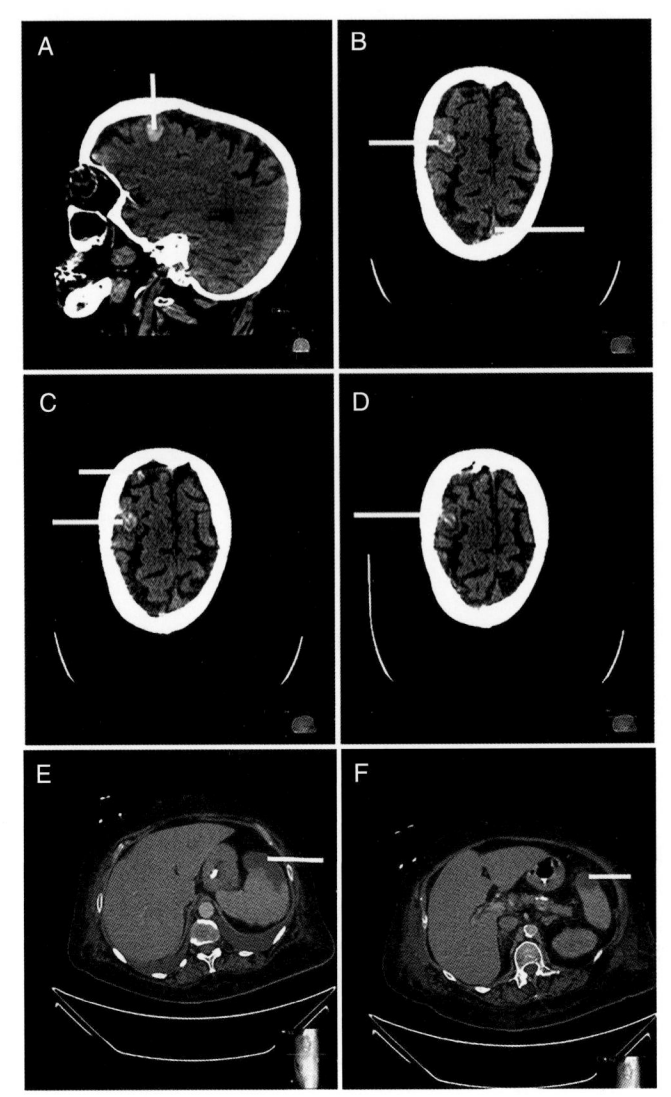

图 5.4　A. 脑部 CT 矢状切面。B-D. 脑部 CT 轴向切面。E-F. 腹部 CT 轴向切面。一名 54 岁女性患者，因突然意识丧失和金黄色葡萄球菌菌血症入院。既往有系统性红斑狼疮和抗磷脂综合征病史。超声心动图显示二尖瓣环后部脓肿。脑部 CT 显示创伤性额叶挫伤，右枕叶脑组织内出血，推测可能是脓毒性栓塞所致（实线）。腹部 CT 显示脾前极和下极多个低密度区域，提示脾梗死（实线）

不菲，还存在病原体污染的风险。最常用的标记试剂为 ^{99m}Tc-HMPAO（六亚甲基胺肟）。白细胞标记成功后，回输给患者，并在注射后 5 h 和 21 h 进行显像（结合低剂量 CT 扫描以获取与组织摄取相关的解剖关系），该检查对于患者的准备无特殊要求。

放射性标记物的摄取受许多因素的影响，例如放射标记的质量、前期的抗生素治疗效果（及持续时间）、感染组织的趋化特性以及微生物病原体的类型和数量[43]。与其他分子诊断技术相比，^{99m}Tc-HMPAO 标记的白细胞 SPECT/CT 的一

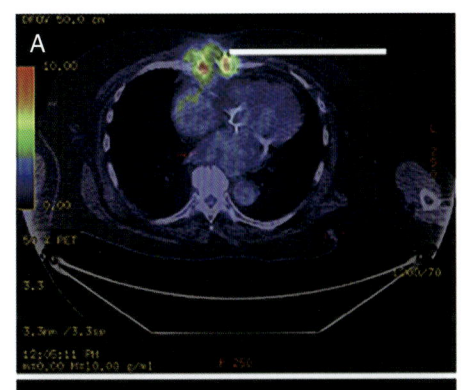

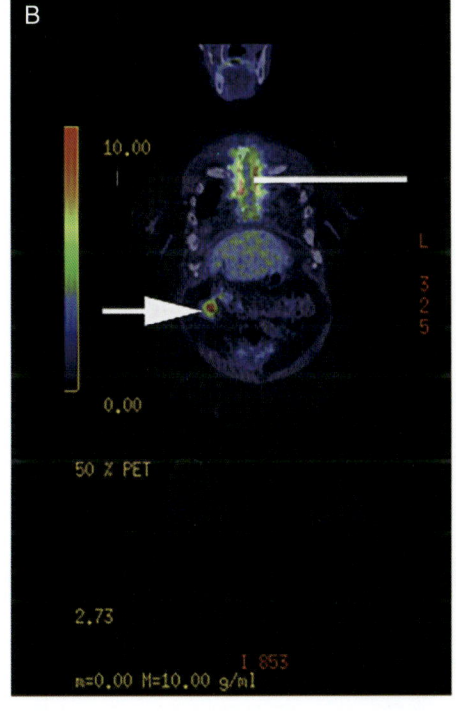

图5.5 ^{18}F-FDG PET/CT。A.轴向切面。B.冠状切面。一名80岁女性患者,因发热和近平滑念珠菌血培养呈阳性入院。1年前因牛链球菌心内膜炎而进行主动脉瓣置换。超声心动图显示瓣膜功能正常,无心内膜炎的证据。^{18}F-FDG PET/CT显示自体瓣膜或人工主动脉瓣周围无FDG摄取的异常增加。然而,胸骨正中切口局部显示存在弥漫性的FDG摄取显著增加,符合胸骨骨髓炎的表现(白色实线)。检查中偶然发现升结肠内有一FDG高摄取的(SUVmax=17.8)5 cm肿块(白色箭头),后证实为中分化腺癌

个突出优势是能够检测大脑中的感染病灶(而这是 ^{18}F-FDG 无法实现的,因为大脑组织存在对 ^{18}F-FDG 示踪剂固有的生理性摄取,与患者准备无关)。

- 诊断性能

在一组包括63例疑似 CIED 相关 IE 的研究中,^{99m}Tc-HMPAO- 白细胞 SPECT/CT 对 CIED 相关感染检测和定位的灵敏度为94%,12个月的随访显示,扫描呈阴性的患者均未出现 IE,估计的阴性预测值为95%[44]。

与 TTE 相比,^{99m}Tc-HMPAO- 白细胞 SPECT/CT 具有卓越的检测"真正"IE 的能力,即使在具有诊断意义病变的患者中表现同样出色。在40名疑似 IE 患者的研究中,14名患者得到临床确诊。放射性标记白细胞 SPECT 和 TTE 还可用于随访观察临床确诊 IE 的病理变化,两者具有相同的灵敏度(93%)。与 TTE 相比,

^{99m}Tc-HMPAO- 白细胞 SPECT/CT 诊断 IE 的假阳性率较低，这使得其特异性更高，两者分别为 42% 和 88%[45]。

根据改良 Duke 标准，将 ^{99m}Tc-HMPAO- 白细胞 SPECT/CT 纳入诊断程序，可能会使疑似 IE 患者被重新归类为确诊 IE。在对 131 名患者的进一步研究中，经 12 个月的随访，51 例确诊为 IE，其中 46 例患者经 ^{99m}Tc-HMPAO- 白细胞 SPECT/CT 检查确认为真阳性，无假阳性病例；依照改良 Duke 标准，11 名疑似 IE 患者因病理性外周摄取增加而重新调整为确诊 IE[46]。

^{99m}Tc-HMPAO- 白细胞 SPECT/CT 的阴性预测值超过 93%，这对于排除 CIED 相关感染特别有效[44,47]。一项包含 103 名患者的研究显示：根据改良 Duke 标准，49.5% 可能存在 CIED 感染的患者，经 ^{99m}Tc-HMPAO- 白细胞 SPECT/CT 检查排除了感染，使疑似 IE 的患者数量减少了 12.5%[47]。

以上研究表明了 ^{99m}Tc-HMPAO- 白细胞 SPECT/CT 在排除疑似 IE 方面的高度准确性，以及对相关 IE 病例确诊和正确分类的能力。但在某些情况下，使用这一检查时仍需谨慎。在非细菌性 IE（例如，无菌血栓性 IE 或真菌性 IE）中，因为 ^{99m}Tc-HMPAO- 白细胞 SPECT/CT 可能由于白细胞趋化作用降低而呈假阴性[46]。表皮葡萄球菌或肠球菌等则可能会通过形成生物膜来逃避宿主免疫系统的监视，从而导致感染灶内的白细胞聚集减少[35]。此外，前期的抗生素治疗也可能导致摄取减少，从而降低检查的灵敏度和特异性[48]。

^{18}F-FDG PET 成像

· 基本原理

^{18}F-FDG PET 成像的基本原理是：由于细菌和免疫细胞代谢需要，炎症区域局部会吸收大量葡萄糖，导致局部糖摄取增加。为消除所有背景代谢摄取的影响，检查前患者必须禁食 6~12 h 或低碳水化合物、高脂饮食至少 12~24 h，并在注射放射性示踪剂和图像采集前立即使用肝素[49-50]。这一处理过程主要是为抑制生理性心肌糖代谢，从而消除无炎症状态的心肌信号。生理性吸收还持续存在于脑组织（部分存在于肝脏和肠道），以及排泄示踪剂的泌尿道组织中。此外，肿瘤组织可表现出对葡萄糖的无抑制性摄取，这就造成了那些最初怀疑为 IE 的患者，最终确诊为恶性肿瘤[51]。

定性和半定量的影像学解读主要通过测量摄取区域的信号强度以计算出标准化摄取值（SUV）。测定的结果受多种因素影响，包括检查方案、图像采集时间、扫描仪性能、患者身体状况、血糖水平以及成像组织的解剖结构等[52-53]。已有学者提议将局部 SUV 达到肝实质测量值的 2 倍作为真正炎症的鉴别值，但目前缺乏大型前瞻性队列研究的支持[54]。

影像分析时必须考虑的一个关键因素是 ^{18}F-FDG PET 检测的是糖代谢本身，而并不等同于存在感染。在瓣膜术后早期没有感染的情况下，可能会观察到由于无菌性炎症而导致的摄取增加（图5.6）[55]。与感染相比，无菌性炎症的SUV测量值较小，但这一数值受患者准备情况、图像采集技术和扫描时间等多种因素影响。因此，区分感染和无菌性炎症的临界值变化较大[53]，这就限制了 ^{18}F-FDG PET 在诊断瓣膜术后早期 IE 中的作用。这种"生理性"摄取可能持续到术后 12 个月[56-57]，还有罕见的摄取长达 13 年的报道[58]。目前的指南推荐，对于 IE 可能性较高的患者，在人工瓣膜术后至少 3 个月可以进行 ^{18}F-FDG PET 检查[2]。但对于疑似早期 IE 的病例，也不应将患者排除在 ^{18}F-FDG PET 检查之外，因为根据摄取的形态分布有可能区分真正的感染和无菌性炎症（手术操作区域的摄取会更加均匀和局限）[59]。

非常重要的一点是，PET/CT 影像的解读需结合临床进行个体化处理。依据临床和血清学检测 IE 可能性较低的病例，在 PET 解读时出现假阳性的可能性较高。而前期经历过抗生素治疗的病例，则有出现假阴性检查的结果（当然不同证据之间存在矛盾）[60-63]。面对这些病例，可考虑使用放射性标记白细胞 SPECT 鉴别炎症和感染，以指导临床决策[64]。

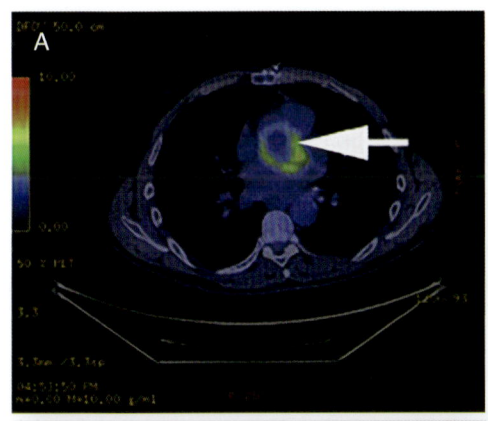

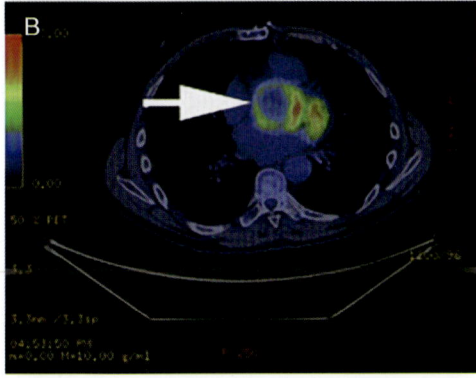

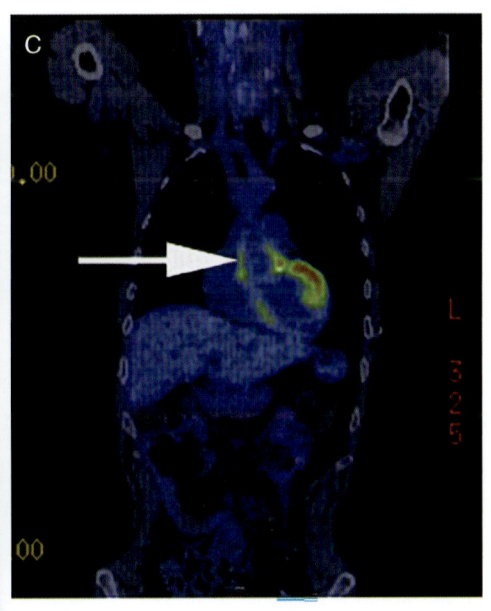

图5.6 ^{18}F-FDG PET/CT。A-B.轴向切面。C.冠状切面。一名 43 岁男性患者因中性粒细胞增多症入院，超声心动图检查怀疑心内膜炎。既往史包括因二叶主动脉瓣行主动脉瓣置换，后因反复出现人工瓣膜失功能而 4 次手术。^{18}F-FDG PET/CT 示主动脉根部周围的 FDG 摄取（SUVmax=9.1），主动脉周围软组织以及升主动脉近端的局灶摄取不高（SUVmax=2.8）。患者接受了急诊同种异体主动脉瓣移植，但血培养和血清学、切除的瓣膜组织革兰氏染色和培养未能确定病原体。组织学检查示广泛性坏死，不符合典型的 IE。有大量 IgG4 浆细胞浸润，符合自身免疫性血管炎

- **诊断性能**

^{18}F–FDG PET 无法独立对 IE 进行诊断，诊断需结合临床病情做出。欧洲心内膜炎登记处对这一检查方式的评价是：对人工瓣膜 IE 的诊断最为准确，对 CIED 相关感染的诊断则效果一般，而对自体瓣膜 IE 效果较差[65]。

自体瓣膜 IE

^{18}F–FDG PET/CT 在疑似自体瓣膜 IE 患者中的诊断作用仅做过小样本研究，结论是准确性较差。原因是赘生物内的代谢低，无法摄取足够的示踪剂。对 6 名已确诊自体瓣膜 IE 的患者的研究显示，尽管存在大的赘生物，但只有 1 例发现在自体瓣膜周围有示踪剂摄取[66]。在另一组对 10 例确诊自体瓣膜 IE 的研究中，只有 3 例存在瓣膜或瓣周摄取[67]。类似结果还出现在一个 88 例患者的队列中，20 例 IE 确诊患者仅 9 例表现出受感染的自体瓣膜周围存在异常摄取[67]。最后，一项针对 115 例患者采用 ^{18}F–FDG PET 诊断自体瓣膜 IE 的大型研究显示：其灵敏度为 22%，特异性为 100%，阳性预测值为 100%，阴性预测值为 66%，进一步显示了其对于自体瓣膜 IE 诊断的局限性[68]。因此在自体瓣膜 IE 的诊断过程中，^{18}F–FDG PET/CT 仅作为个别病例在其他影像检查无法确诊时的辅助诊断方式。

人工瓣膜 IE

由于人工瓣膜 IE 多并发瓣周脓肿（示踪剂摄取增加），^{18}F–FDG PET/CT 对这类患者具有较高的诊断价值[69]。一个纳入 8 项有关人工瓣膜患者研究的回顾性分析显示：^{18}F–FDG PET 检测人工瓣膜 IE 的灵敏度为 73%～100%，特异性为 71%～100%，阳性预测值为 67%～100%，阴性预测值为 50%～100%。这一研究的意义是，将 ^{18}F–FDG PET/CT 结果纳入改良 Duke 标准后，使该标准的诊断灵敏度从 52%～70% 大幅提高到 91%～97%[70-71]。据此，ESC 指南将瓣膜置换术 3 个月以后人工瓣膜周围存在病理性异常摄取（^{18}F–FDG PET/CT 或 ^{99m}Tc–HMPAO– 白细胞 SPECT/CT）纳入阳性影像发现的诊断标准，以提高改良 Duke 诊断标准的灵敏度[2]（尽管在这一时间点更早需要该影像诊断手段的仅为个别病例）[56]。

心脏植入式电子设备相关心内膜炎（CIED-IE）

^{18}F–FDG PET 在 CIED-IE 中的诊断作用因感染范围或程度（植入设备的脉冲发生器、皮下囊袋、起搏电极导线或右侧心脏瓣膜）的不同而异[72-74]。对于这类病例，准确的诊断至关重要。因为一旦确定是 CIED-IE，常常需要取出装置，而在这一过程中，^{18}F–FDG PET 是至关重要的判断手段[63,75]。一项对 21 名 CIED-IE 患者的研究显示，^{18}F–FDG PET/CT 对单纯囊袋部位感染的诊断灵敏度和特异性分别为 86.7% 和 100%，但对总体 CIED-IE（含各部位感染）的诊断灵敏度和特异性分别仅有 30.8% 和 62.5%（图 5.7）[76]，通过使用延迟钆显像观察人工装置材料中示踪剂的动态改变[77]，定量比较靶位 SUV 测量值与肝血池值、校正衰减伪影、减少金属伪影等措施可提高诊断准确性[78-79]。但对于设备植入早期影像学的结果需慎重解读，因为植入过程中的操作可能引起皮下囊袋和连接器周围组织的生理性摄

感染性心内膜炎的其他影像学检查 第 5 章

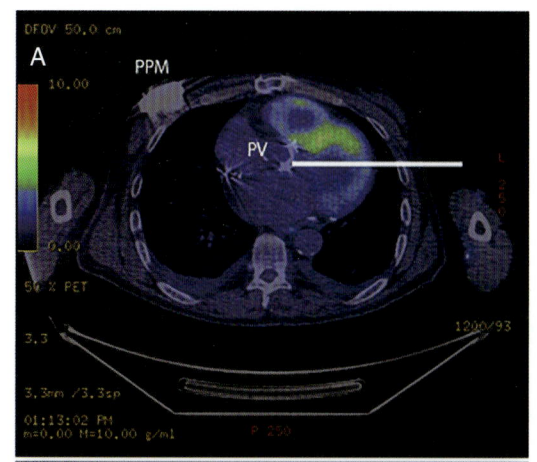

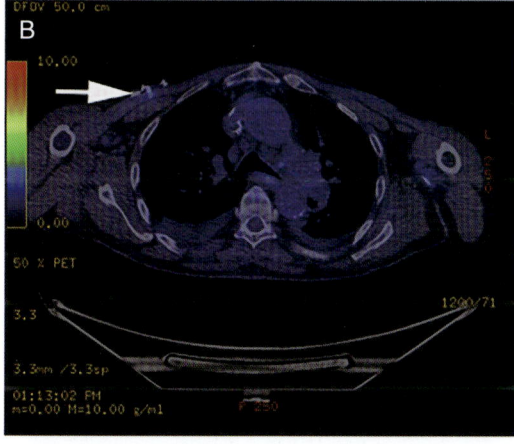

图 5.7 ^{18}F–FDG PET/CT。A–B. 轴向切面。一例 73 岁男性患者，既往有主动脉瓣机械瓣置换和心脏再同步治疗除颤器植入史，因近期身体不适就诊。血培养粪肠球菌阳性。超声心动图显示瓣膜位置、功能正常，没有心内膜炎证据。^{18}F–FDG PET/CT 成像显示邻近脉冲装置的电极导线近端部位的数个小灶性 FDG 摄取增加（箭头），而人工瓣膜、皮下囊袋及远端电极导线无摄取增加，证实电极导线连接部位存在 CIED-IE。伴随的心脏扩大和双侧少量胸腔积液符合充血性心力衰竭的表现。PPM：永久起搏器；PV：人工瓣膜（实线）

取[80]。另外，^{18}F–FDG PET/CT 还可用于诊断 CIED-IE 并发的隐匿性脓毒性栓塞[81]。

假体材料和其他装置相关的感染

　　对于人工血管相关感染的研究数据较少。一项包括 17 例疑似人工血管感染（非心脏原因）的研究显示：在最终诊断为 IE 的 9 例患者中（4 例为假阳性，其中 2 例最终确诊为主动脉炎），有 8 例 ^{18}F–FDG PET/CT 显示人工血管位置摄取不均匀，但主动脉瓣摄取均匀[82]。通常，对疑似血管移植物的感染，当传统 CT 无法诊断时，^{18}F–FDG PET/CT 具有辅助诊断价值[37,59,83]。同理，^{18}F–FDG PET/CT 对于先天性心脏病使用人工移植物、补片及心内装置的患者疑似发生 IE 同样具有辅助诊断价值（图 5.8A 和 B）[84-85]。

　　有数据显示，PET/CT 还可用于晚期心力衰竭和 LVAD 植入患者疑似 IE 的诊断[86-89]。由于心脏循环辅助设备很复杂，存在多个潜在感染部位（包括插管、经皮传动系统和皮肤植入点），因此，^{18}F–FDG PET/CT 具有超声心动图无法比拟的优势，可对所有可能感染部位进行全面评估。同时，与放射性标记白细胞闪烁扫描相比，它具有更高的灵敏度（但特异性较差）（放射性标记白细胞闪烁扫描因空间分辨率差而无法分辨软组织感染，也不能区分装置植入后的真正感染和炎症反应）[90]。

79

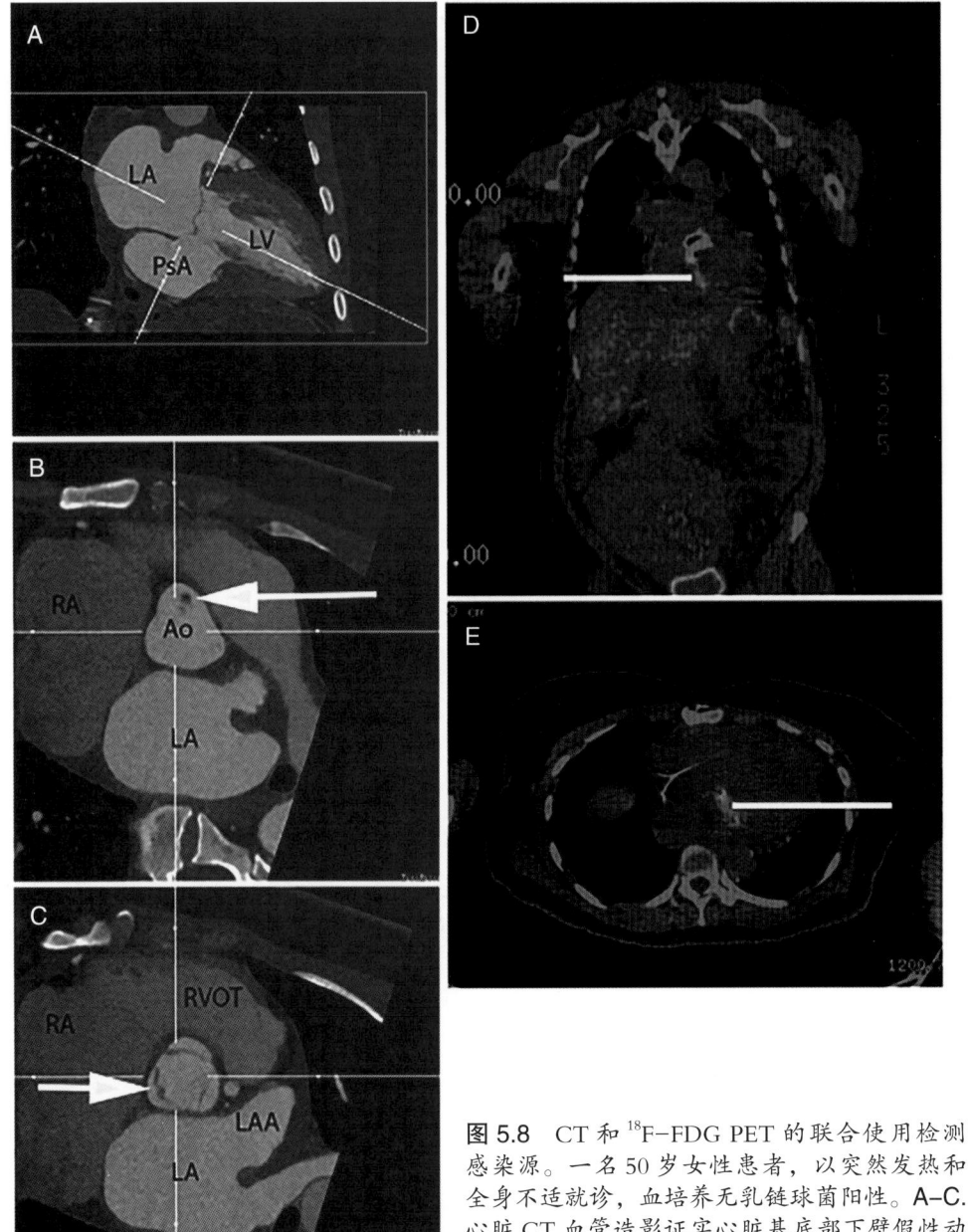

图 5.8 CT 和 ^{18}F-FDG PET 的联合使用检测感染源。一名 50 岁女性患者，以突然发热和全身不适就诊，血培养无乳链球菌阳性。A-C. 心脏 CT 血管造影证实心脏基底部下壁假性动脉瘤（A），以及右冠瓣（B，箭头）和无冠瓣（C，箭头）赘生物。患者接受了主动脉瓣-二尖瓣双机械瓣置换，以及先天性假性室壁瘤补片修复，术后 3 个月症状复发，血培养无乳链球菌呈阳性。Ao：主动脉；LA：左心房；LAA：左心耳；LV：左心室；PsA：假性动脉瘤；RA：右心房；RV：右心室；RVOT：右心室流出道。D-E. ^{18}F-FDG PET/CT 未显示人工瓣膜心内膜炎的证据，但在假性室壁瘤牛心包补片部位的摄取增加（实线，SUVmax=4.4）

磁共振成像

心脏磁共振成像

心脏磁共振（CMR）在 IE 的诊断及治疗中的作用有限，很大程度上是因为与超声心动图和 CT 相比，其空间分辨率较低。尽管对严重并发症，例如病损瓣膜的动脉瘤样改变，CMR 可轻易诊断[91-92]，但对于小赘生物则未必能发现[93-94]。而对于心脏内大肿块（尤其是出现在非典型位置）的组织特征，CMR 可用于鉴别赘生物、血栓或是其他性质的病变，同时还有助于手术方案的制定[95-96]。此外，CMR 还可提供有关心脏大小和功能的准确信息[97-99]，使用延迟钆增强成像和水肿特异性影像可早于超声心动图检查发现感染的瓣周扩散[93,100]。

CMR 还可用于 IE 伴心肌、心包受累，或自身免疫性炎症等其他组织特征的鉴别[100-101]。在 Libman-Sacks 心内膜炎，CMR 可以显示无菌性赘生物，并提供心肌浸润和心内血栓的相关信息[102-104]。在有自身免疫性疾病史的患者中，CMR 显示的心内膜下赘生物或斑片状延迟强化，可为非细菌性血栓性心内膜炎的诊断提供依据。

心外磁共振成像

磁共振成像（MRI）有助于识别多发的、无其他临床表现的栓塞病灶（这些病灶多半无临床症状）（图 5.9A 和 B）。

脑 MRI 可识别 70% 没有明显神经系统症状的中枢神经系统栓塞病变，其中急性缺血性卒中和颅内微出血最为常见[105]，目前已被归类为 Duke 诊断标准的次要标准[106-108]。大面积缺血性卒中或脑出血的手术预后较差，必须推迟外科瓣膜手术时间[109]。一项针对 130 名 IE 患者的研究显示：脑 MRI 检出了 68 名患者的栓塞和 10 名患者的动脉瘤，32% 的患者因此按改良 Duke 标准更新为确诊 IE，14% 的病例改变了手术计划[110]。

颅内微出血可通过 T2* 或磁敏感加权成像来检测。尽管它们对 IE 的手术结果没有影响，也未被纳入 Duke 标准[111]，但这是感染性脑内动脉瘤的前期表现，需使用数字减影血管造影（DSA）进一步明确病变程度[112-113]。这里需要提出的是，在检测真菌性动脉瘤方面，MR 血管造影的灵敏度显著低于 DSA（虽然阴性预测值较高），因此不应将其用作检测真菌性动脉瘤的一线检查手段[114]。

IE 常伴有背部疼痛，脊柱 MRI 在检测椎间盘炎症方面具有很高的灵敏度[114-115]。与脑内病变类似，脊髓栓塞已被纳入疑似 IE 患者的改良 Duke 诊断标准中。

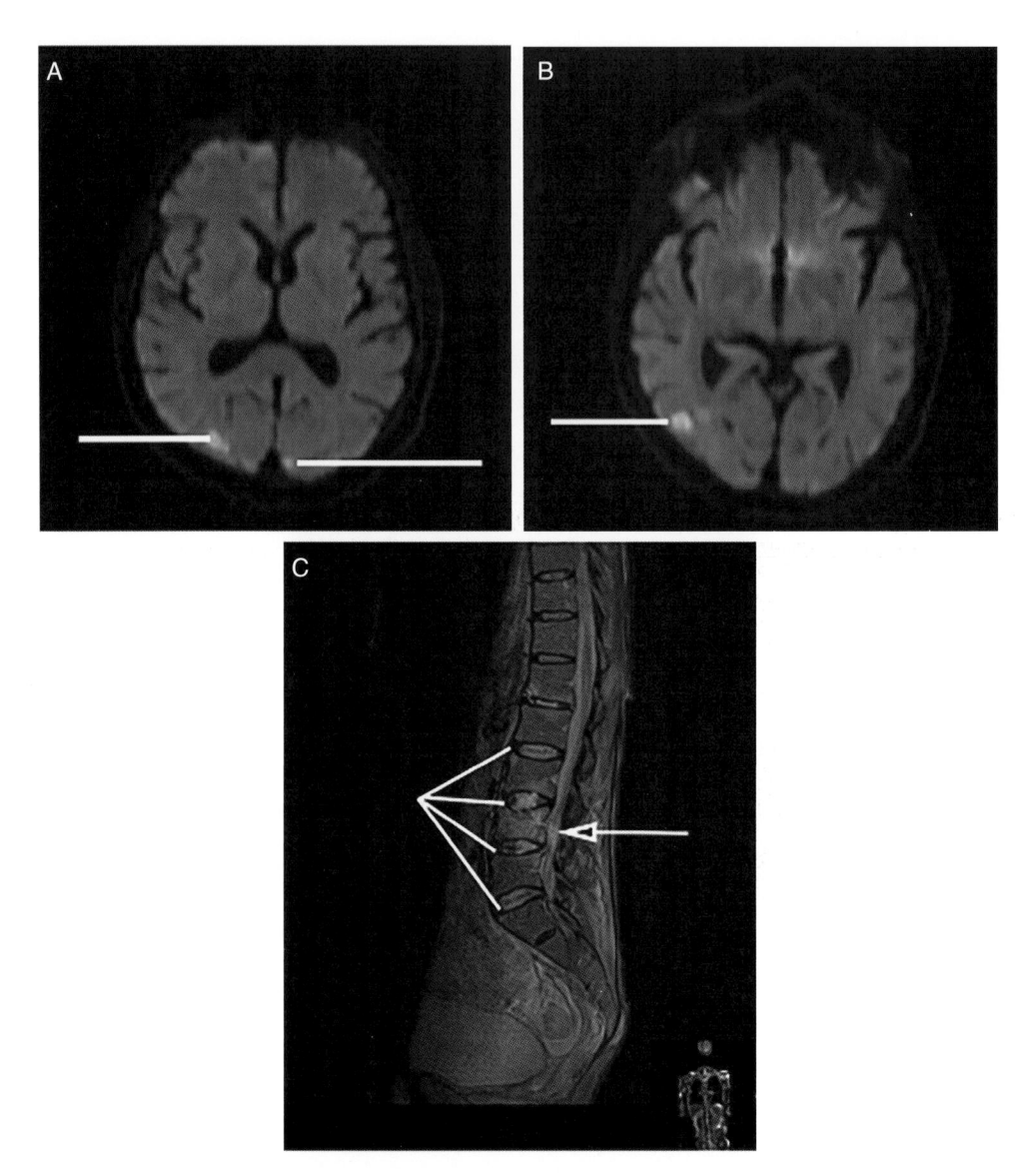

图 5.9 MRI 在 IE 栓塞并发症中的应用。一名 54 岁男性患者，既往有静脉吸毒史，以脓毒症和急性腹部及背部疼痛就诊，血培养金黄色葡萄球菌阳性。A-B. 脑部 MRI 扫描显示多个边缘模糊的皮质和皮质下信号异常病灶，涉及双侧枕顶叶和枕颞叶，伴有与脓毒性栓塞梗死和其他微脓肿病变相一致的组织水肿（实线）。C. 同一患者的脊柱 MRI，显示多节段化脓性腰椎间盘炎（实线）以及邻近椎旁和硬膜外的蜂窝织炎（箭头）

总 结

虽然超声心动图是 IE 诊治的主要影像手段，但其他一些影像学检查近些年在国际上也相继被纳入相关指南。CT 被推荐用于检测瓣周和主动脉根部并发症，提供无创的冠状动脉影像信息，辅助手术计划的制定。分子核医学成像则在人工瓣膜和 CIED 相关感染中表现出较高的诊断性能，还可提供有关转移病灶或其他感染源的信息。心脏 MRI 的作用相对有限，主要用于心肌受累的病例。但脑部和脊髓 MRI 对于外周栓塞的检测非常准确，检查结果常常会影响患者的诊断分类和手术时机。各种检查方式在 IE 的诊断和治疗中具有互补作用，充分了解各种检查方式的优劣及其适应证有助于临床医护人员更好地为患者提供优质的医疗服务（表 5.2 和图 5.10）。

表 5.2 感染性心内膜炎（IE）不同辅助影像学检查方法的优劣

	TEE	CMR/MRI	MDCTA	^{18}F-FDG PET	白细胞 SPECT
分辨率					
空间	高	中	高	低	低
时间	高	高	心率依赖	不适用	不适用
诊断性能					
NVIE	高	低	高	低	低
PVIE	中	低	高	高	高
瓣周并发症	中	低	高	高	高
外周栓塞	不适用	高	高	高	高
CIED	高	不适用	高	高	高
临床应用考量					
可获得性	广泛	中等	中等	较低	较低
检查前准备	要求镇静	造影要求 eGFR>30 mL/（min·kg）	造影要求 eGFR>30 mL/（min·kg）	24h 的 HFLC 饮食	白细胞体外标记
患者监护	可持续监护	监护受限	中等受限	中等受限	中等受限
放射剂量	无	无	约 24 mSv	16~24 mSv	16~24 mSv

TEE：经食管超声心动图；CMR：心脏磁共振；MRI：磁共振成像；MDCTA：多排计算机断层扫描血管造影；^{18}F-FDG PET：^{18}F-氟脱氧葡萄糖正电子发射断层扫描；白细胞 SPECT：放射性标记白细胞单光子发射断层扫描；NVIE：自体瓣膜感染性心内膜炎；PVIE：人工瓣膜感染性心内膜炎；CIED：心脏植入式电子设备；eGFR：估计的肾小球滤过率；HFLC：高脂低碳水化合物

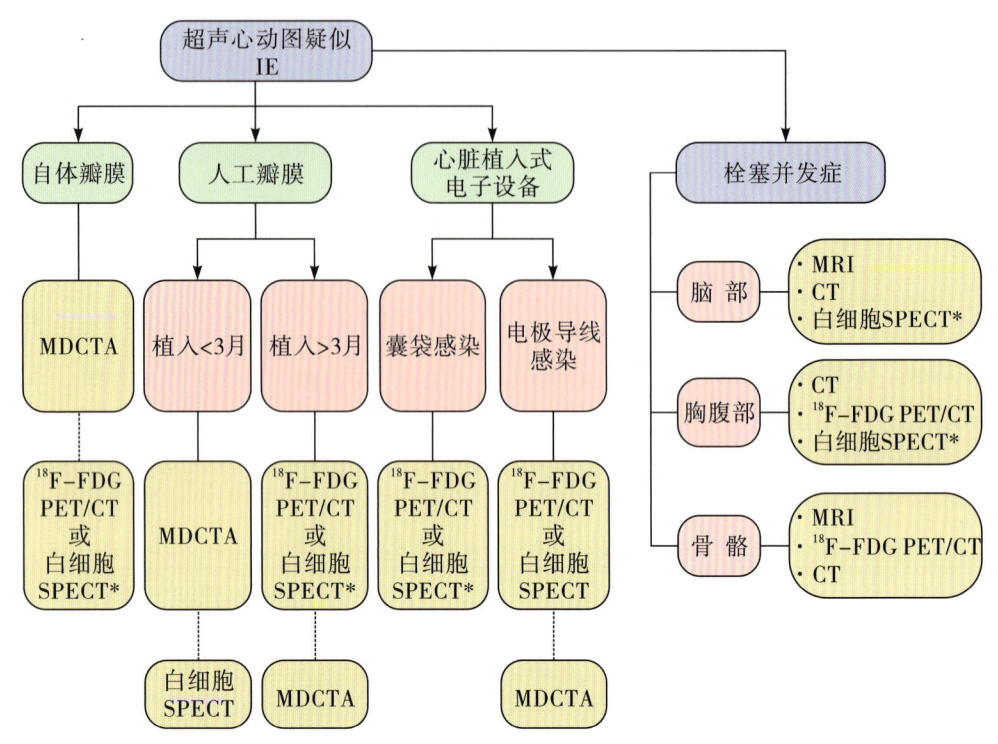

图 5.10 不同临床情况下影像学检查的选择流程。实线表示主要成像方式。虚线表示补充检查选项。*白细胞 SPECT 可能无法检测到表皮葡萄球菌和肠球菌属感染。^{18}F-FDG PET：^{18}F- 氟脱氧葡萄糖正电子发射断层扫描；IE：感染性心内膜炎；MDCTA：多排计算机断层扫描血管造影；白细胞 SPECT：放射性标记白细胞单光子发射断层扫描

参考文献

[1] Nishimura RA, Otto CM, Bonow RO, et al. AHA/ACC guideline for the management of patients with valvular heart disease: a report of the American College of Cardiology/American Heart Association Task Force on practice guidelines. Circulation, 2014, 129(23): e521–e643.

[2] Habib G, Lancellotti P, Antunes MJ, et al. ESC guidelines for the management of infective endocarditis: the task force for the management of infective endocarditis of the European Society of Cardiology (ESC). Endorsed by: European association for cardio-thoracic surgery (EACTS), the European association of nuclear medicine (EANM). Eur Heart J, 2015, 36(44): 3075–3128.

[3] Bruun NE, Habib G, Thuny F, et al. Cardiac imaging in infectious endocarditis. Eur Heart J, 2014, 35(10): 624–632.

[4] Erbel R, Rohmann S, Drexler M, et al. Improved diagnostic value of echocardiography in patients with infective endocarditis by transoesophageal approach. A prospective study. Eur Heart J, 1988, 9(1): 43–53.

[5] Bai AD, Steinberg M, Showler A, et al. Diagnostic accuracy of transthoracic echocardiography for infective endocarditis findings using transesophageal echocardiography as the reference standard: a meta-analysis. J Am Soc Echocardiogr, 2017, 30(7): 639–646.e8.

[6] Habib G, Badano L, Tribouilloy C, et al. Recommendations for the practice of echocardiography in infective endocarditis. Eur J Echocardiogr, 2010, 11(2): 202–219.

[7] Murphy DJ, Din M, Hage FG, et al. Guidelines in review: comparison of ESC and AHA guidance for the diagnosis and management of infective endocarditis in adults. J Nucl Cardiol, 2019, 26(1): 303–308.

[8] Salaun E, Habib G. Beyond standard echocardiography in infective endocarditis: computed

tomography, 3-dimensional imaging, and multi-imaging. Circ Cardiovasc Imag, 2018, 11(3): e007626.
[9] Entrikin DW, Gupta P, Kon ND, et al. Imaging of infective endocarditis with cardiac CT angiography. J Cardiovasc Comput Tomogr, 2012, 6(6): 399–405.
[10] Saremi F, Sanchez-Quintana D, Mori S, et al. Fibrous skeleton of the heart: anatomic overview and evaluation of pathologic conditions with CT and MR imaging. Radiographics, 2017, 37(5): 1330–1351.
[11] Feuchtner GM, Stolzmann P, Dichtl W, et al. Multislice computed tomography in infective endocarditis: comparison with transesophageal echocardiography and intraoperative findings. J Am Coll Cardiol, 2009, 53(5): 436–444.
[12] Gahide G, Bommart S, Demaria R, et al. Preoperative evaluation in aortic endocarditis: findings on cardiac CT. AJR Am J Roentgenol, 2010, 194(3): 574–578.
[13] Hryniewiecki T, Zatorska K, Abramczuk E, et al. The usefulness of cardiac CT in the diagnosis of perivalvular complications in patients with infective endocarditis. Eur Radiol, 2019, 29(8): 4368–4376.
[14] Fagman E, Perrotta S, Bech-Hanssen O, et al. ECG-gated computed tomography: a new role for patients with suspected aortic prosthetic valve endocarditis. Eur Radiol, 2012, 22(11): 2407–2414.
[15] Habets J, Tanis W, van Herwerden LA, et al. Cardiac computed tomography angiography results in diagnostic and therapeutic change in prosthetic heart valve endocarditis. Int J Cardiovasc Imag, 2014, 30(2): 377–387.
[16] Fagman E, Flinck A, Snygg-Martin U, et al. Surgical decision-making in aortic prosthetic valve endocarditis: the influence of electrocardiogram-gated computed tomography. Eur J Cardio Thorac Surg, 2016, 50(6): 1165–1171.
[17] Kim IC, Chang S, Hong GR, et al. Comparison of cardiac computed tomography with transesophageal echocardiography for identifying vegetation and intracardiac complications in patients with infective endocarditis in the era of 3-dimensional images. Circ Cardiovasc Imag, 2018, 11(3): e006986.
[18] Koo HJ, Yang DH, Kang JW, et al. Demonstration of infective endocarditis by cardiac CT and transoesophageal echocardiography: comparison with intra-operative findings. Eur Heart J Cardiovasc Imag, 2018, 19(2): 199–207.
[19] Koneru S, Huang SS, Oldan J, et al. Role of preoperative cardiac CT in the evaluation of infective endocarditis: comparison with transesophageal echocardiography and surgical findings. Cardiovasc Diagn Ther, 2018, 8(4): 439–449.
[20] Ouchi K, Sakuma T, Ojiri H. Cardiac computed tomography as a viable alternative to echocardiography to detect vegetations and perivalvular complications in patients with infective endocarditis. Jpn J Radiol, 2018, 36(7): 421–428.
[21] Sims JR, Anavekar NS, Chandrasekaran K, et al. Utility of cardiac computed tomography scanning in the diagnosis and pre-operative evaluation of patients with infective endocarditis. Int J Cardiovasc Imag, 2018, 34(7): 1155–1163.
[22] Chaosuwannakit N, Makarawate P. Value of cardiac computed tomography angiography in pre-operative assessment of infective endocarditis. J Cardiothorac Surg, 2019, 14(1): 56.
[23] Moss AJ, Dweck MR, Dreisbach JG, et al. Complementary role of cardiac CT in the assessment of aortic valve replacement dysfunction. Open Heart, 2016, 3(2): e000494.
[24] Lentini S, Monaco F, Tancredi F, et al. Aortic valve infective endocarditis: could multi-detector CT scan be proposed for routine screening of concomitant coronary artery disease before surgery? Ann Thorac Surg, 2009, 87(5): 1585–1587.
[25] Kim RJ, Weinsaft JW, Callister TQ, et al. Evaluation of prosthetic valve endocarditis by 64-row multidetector computed tomography. Int J Cardiol, 2007, 120(2): e27–e29.
[26] Hekimian G, Kim M, Passefort S, et al. Preoperative use and safety of coronary angiography for acute aortic valve infective endocarditis. Heart, 2010, 96(9): 696–700.
[27] Christiaens L, Mergy J, Franco S, et al. Aortic valvular endocarditis with mobile vegetations and intracoronary embolism: demonstration by cardiac multislice computed tomography. Eur Heart J,

2008, 29(15): 1888.

[28] Budde RP, Kluin J, Symersky P, et al. Visualization by 256-slice computed tomography of mycotic aortic root aneurysms in infective endocarditis. J Heart Valve Dis, 2010, 19(5): 623–625.

[29] Passen E, Feng Z. Cardiopulmonary manifestations of isolated pulmonary valve infective endocarditis demonstrated with cardiac CT. J Cardiovasc Comput Tomogr, 2015, 9(5): 399–405.

[30] Wilson TN, Tew K, Taranath A. Multiple mycotic aneurysms of the pulmonary arteries resolving with conservative management: multislice CT examination findings. J Thorac Imag, 2008, 23(3): 197–201.

[31] Tsai IC, Lin YK, Chang Y, et al. Correctness of multi-detector-row computed tomography for diagnosing mechanical prosthetic heart valve disorders using operative findings as a gold standard. Eur Radiol, 2009, 19(4): 857–867.

[32] Juneau D, Golfam M, Hazra S, et al. Molecular Imaging for the diagnosis of infective endocarditis: a systematic literature review and meta-analysis. Int J Cardiol, 2018, 253: 183–188.

[33] Kokalova A, Dell'aquila AM, Avramovic N, et al. Supporting imaging modalities for improving diagnosis of prosthesis endocarditis: preliminary results of a single-center experience with ^{18}F-FDG-PET/CT. Minerva Med, 2017, 108(4): 299–304.

[34] Chen W, Sajadi MM, Dilsizian V. Merits of FDG PET/CT and functional molecular imaging over anatomic imaging with echocardiography and CT angiography for the diagnosis of cardiac device infections. JACC Cardiovasc Imag, 2018, 11(11): 1679–1691.

[35] Erba PA, Lancellotti P, Vilacosta I, et al. Recommendations on nuclear and multimodality imaging in IE and CIED infections. Eur J Nucl Med Mol Imag, 2018, 45(10): 1795–1815.

[36] Tanis W, Scholtens A, Habets J, et al. CT angiography and (1)(8)F-FDG-PET fusion imaging for prosthetic heart valve endocarditis. JACC Cardiovasc Imag, 2013, 6(9): 1008–1013.

[37] Asmar A, Ozcan C, Diederichsen AC, et al. Clinical impact of ^{18}F-FDG-PET/CT in the extra cardiac work-up of patients with infective endocarditis. Eur Heart J Cardiovasc Imag, 2014, 15(9): 1013–1019.

[38] Bonfiglioli R, Nanni C, Morigi JJ, et al. ^{18}F-FDG PET/CT diagnosis of unexpected extracardiac septic embolisms in patients with suspected cardiac endocarditis. Eur J Nucl Med Mol Imag, 2013, 40(8): 1190–1196.

[39] Hohmann C, Michels G, Schmidt M, et al. Diagnostic challenges in infective endocarditis: is PET/CT the solution? Infection, 2019, 47(4): 579–587.

[40] Chen W, Kim J, Molchanova-Cook OP, et al. The potential of FDG PET/CT for early diagnosis of cardiac device and prosthetic valve infection before morphologic damages ensue. Curr Cardiol Rep, 2014, 16(3): 459.

[41] Kestler M, Munoz P, Rodriguez-Creixems M, et al. Role of ^{18}F-FDG PET in patients with infectious endocarditis. J Nucl Med, 2014, 55(7): 1093–1098.

[42] Brix G, Lechel U, Glatting G, et al. Radiation exposure of patients undergoing whole-body dual-modality ^{18}F-FDG PET/CT examinations. J Nucl Med, 2005, 46(4): 608–613.

[43] Signore A, Jamar F, Israel O, et al. Clinical indications, image acquisition and data interpretation for white blood cells and anti-granulocyte monoclonal antibody scintigraphy: an EANM procedural guideline. Eur J Nucl Med Mol Imag, 2018, 45(10): 1816–1831.

[44] Erba PA, Sollini M, Conti U, et al. Radiolabeled WBC scintigraphy in the diagnostic workup of patients with suspected device-related infections. JACC Cardiovasc Imag, 2013, 6(10): 1075–1086.

[45] Holcman K, Szot W, Rubis P, et al. ^{99}mTc-HMPAO-labeled leukocyte SPECT/CT and transthoracic echocardiography diagnostic value in infective endocarditis. Int J Cardiovasc Imag, 2019, 35(4): 749–758.

[46] Erba PA, Conti U, Lazzeri E, et al. Added value of ^{99}mTc-HMPAO-labeled leukocyte SPECT/CT in the characterization and management of patients with infectious endocarditis. J Nucl Med, 2012, 53(8): 1235–1243.

[47] Holcman K, Malecka B, Rubis P, et al. The role of ^{99}mTc-HMPAO-labelled white blood cell

scintigraphy in the diagnosis of cardiac device-related infective endocarditis. Eur Heart J Cardiovasc Imag, 2020, 21(9): 1022–1030. https://doi.org/10.1093/ehjci/jez257. PMID: 31605137.

[48] Malecka BA, Zabek A, Debski M, et al. The usefulness of SPECT-CT with radioisotope-labeled leukocytes in diagnosing lead-dependent infective endocarditis. Adv Clin Exp Med, 2019, 28(1): 113–119.

[49] Osborne MT, Hulten EA, Murthy VL, et al. Patient preparation for cardiac fluorine-18 fluorodeoxyglucose positron emission tomography imaging of inflammation. J Nucl Cardiol, 2017, 24(1): 86–99.

[50] Scholtens AM, Verberne HJ, Budde RP, et al. Additional heparin preadministration improves cardiac glucose metabolism suppression over low-carbohydrate diet alone in ^{18}F-FDG PET imaging. J Nucl Med, 2016, 57(4): 568–573.

[51] Granados U, Fuster D, Pericas JM, et al. Diagnostic accuracy of ^{18}F-FDG PET/CT in infective endocarditis and implantable cardiac electronic device infection: a cross-sectional study. J Nucl Med, 2016, 57(11): 1726–1732.

[52] Keyes Jr JW. SUV: standard uptake or silly useless value? J Nucl Med, 1995, 36(10): 1836–1839.

[53] Scholtens AM, Swart LE, Kolste HJT, et al. Standardized uptake values in FDG PET/CT for prosthetic heart valve endocarditis: a call for standardization. J Nucl Cardiol, 2018, 25(6): 2084–2091.

[54] Jimenez-Ballve A, Perez-Castejon MJ, Delgado-Bolton RC, et al. Assessment of the diagnostic accuracy of ^{18}F-FDG PET/CT in prosthetic infective endocarditis and cardiac implantable electronic device infection: comparison of different interpretation criteria. Eur J Nucl Med Mol Imag, 2016, 43(13): 2401–2412.

[55] Scholtens AM, Swart LE, Verberne HJ, et al. Confounders in FDG-PET/CT imaging of suspected prosthetic valve endocarditis. JACC Cardiovasc Imag, 2016, 9(12): 1462–1465.

[56] Mathieu C, Mikail N, Benali K, et al. Characterization of ^{18}F-fluorodeoxyglucose uptake pattern in noninfected prosthetic heart valves. Circ Cardiovasc Imag, 2017, 10(3): e005585.

[57] Roque A, Pizzi MN, Fernandez-Hidalgo N, et al. Morpho-metabolic post-surgical patterns of non-infected prosthetic heart valves by ^{18}F-FDG PET/CTA: "normality" is a possible diagnosis. Eur Heart J Cardiovasc Imag, 2020, 21(1): 24–33. https://doi.org/10.1093/ehjci/jez222. PMID: 31539031.

[58] Scholtens AM, Swart LE, Verberne HJ, et al. Dual-time-point FDG PET/CT imaging in prosthetic heart valve endocarditis. J Nucl Cardiol, 2018, 25(6): 1960–1967.

[59] Pizzi MN, Roque A, Cuellar-Calabria H, et al. ^{18}F-FDG-PET/CTA of prosthetic cardiac valves and valve-tube grafts: infective versus inflammatory patterns. JACC Cardiovasc Imag, 2016, 9(10): 1224–1227.

[60] Swart LE, Gomes A, Scholtens AM, et al. Improving the diagnostic performance of ^{18}F-fluorodeoxyglucose positron-emission tomography/computed tomography in prosthetic heart valve endocarditis. Circulation, 2018, 138(14): 1412–1427.

[61] Pijl JP, Glaudemans A, Slart R, et al. FDG-PET/CT for detecting an infection focus in patients with bloodstream infection: factors affecting diagnostic yield. Clin Nucl Med, 2019, 44(2): 99–106.

[62] Kagna O, Kurash M, Ghanem-Zoubi N, t al. Does antibiotic treatment affect the diagnostic accuracy of ^{18}F-FDG PET/CT studies in patients with suspected infectious processes? J Nucl Med, 2017, 58(11): 1827–1830.

[63] Calais J, Touati A, Grall N, et al. Diagnostic impact of ^{18}F-fluorodeoxyglucose positron emission tomography/computed tomography and white blood cell SPECT/computed tomography in patients with suspected cardiac implantable electronic device chronic infection. Circ Cardiovasc Imag, 2019, 12(7): e007188.

[64] Rouzet F, Chequer R, Benali K, et al. Respective performance of ^{18}F-FDG PET and radiolabeled leukocyte scintigraphy for the diagnosis of prosthetic valve endocarditis. J Nucl Med, 2014, 55(12): 1980–1985.

[65] Habib G, Erba PA, Iung B, et al. Clinical presentation, aetiology and outcome of infective

endocarditis. Results of the ESC-EORP EURO-ENDO (European infective endocarditis) registry: a prospective cohort study. Eur Heart J, 2019, 40(39): 3222–3232.

[66] Salomaki SP, Saraste A, Kemppainen J, et al. ^{18}F-FDG positron emission tomography/computed tomography in infective endocarditis. J Nucl Cardiol, 2017, 24(1): 195–206.

[67] Kouijzer IJE, Berrevoets MAH, Aarntzen E, et al. ^{18}F-fluorodeoxyglucose positron-emission tomography combined with computed tomography as a diagnostic tool in native valve endocarditis. Nucl Med Commun, 2018, 39(8): 747–752.

[68] de Camargo RA, Bitencourt MS, Meneghetti JC, et al. The role of ^{18}F-FDG-PET/CT in the Diagnosis of left-sided Endocarditis: native vs. prosthetic valves endocarditis. Clin Infect Dis, 2020, 70(4): 583–594. https://doi.org/10.1093/cid/ciz267. PMID: 30949690.

[69] Abou Jokh Casas E, Pubul Nunez V, Pombo Pasin MDC, et al. Advantages and limitations of 18-fluoro-2-deoxy-d-glucose positron emission tomography/computed tomography in the diagnosis of infective endocarditis. Rev Port Cardiol, 2019, 38(8): 573–580.

[70] Gomes A, Glaudemans A, Touw DJ, et al. Diagnostic value of imaging in infective endocarditis: a systematic review. Lancet Infect Dis, 2017, 17(1): e1–e14.

[71] Saby L, Laas O, Habib G, et al. Positron emission tomography/computed tomography for diagnosis of prosthetic valve endocarditis: increased valvular ^{18}F-fluorodeoxyglucose uptake as a novel major criterion. J Am Coll Cardiol, 2013, 61(23): 2374–2382.

[72] Bensimhon L, Lavergne T, Hugonnet F, et al. Whole body ^{18}F-fluorodeoxyglucose positron emission tomography imaging for the diagnosis of pacemaker or implantable cardioverter defibrillator infection: a preliminary prospective study. Clin Microbiol Infect, 2011, 17(6): 836–844.

[73] Athan E, Chu VH, Tattevin P, et al. Clinical characteristics and outcome of infective endocarditis involving implantable cardiac devices. JAMA, 2012, 307(16): 1727–1735.

[74] Mahmood M, Kendi AT, Farid S, et al. Role of ^{18}F-FDG PET/CT in the diagnosis of cardiovascular implantable electronic device infections: a meta-analysis. J Nucl Cardiol, 2019, 26(3): 958–970.

[75] Diemberger I, Bonfiglioli R, Martignani C, et al. Contribution of PET imaging to mortality risk stratification in candidates to lead extraction for pacemaker or defibrillator infection: a prospective single center study. Eur J Nucl Med Mol Imag, 2019, 46(1): 194–205.

[76] Cautela J, Alessandrini S, Cammilleri S, et al. Diagnostic yield of FDG positron emission tomography/computed tomography in patients with CEID infection: a pilot study. Europace, 2013, 15(2): 252–257.

[77] Leccisotti L, Perna F, Lago M, et al. Cardiovascular implantable electronic device infection: delayed vs standard FDG PET-CT imaging. J Nucl Cardiol, 2014, 21(3): 622–632.

[78] Memmott MJ, James J, Armstrong IS, et al. The performance of quantitation methods in the evaluation of cardiac implantable electronic device (CIED) infection: a technical review. J Nucl Cardiol, 2016, 23(6): 1457–1466.

[79] Scholtens AM, Verberne HJ. Attenuation correction and metal artifact reduction in FDG PET/CT for prosthetic heart valve and cardiac implantable device endocarditis. J Nucl Cardiol, 2018, 25(6): 2172–2173.

[80] Sarrazin JF, Philippon F, Tessier M, et al. Usefulness of fluorine-18 positron emission tomography/computed tomography for identification of cardiovascular implantable electronic device infections. J Am Coll Cardiol, 2012, 59(18): 1616–1625.

[81] Amraoui S, Tlili G, Sohal M, et al. Contribution of PET imaging to the diagnosis of septic embolism in patients with pacing lead endocarditis. JACC Cardiovasc Imag, 2016, 9(3): 283–290.

[82] Garcia-Arribas D, Vilacosta I, Ortega Candil A, et al. Usefulness of positron emission tomography/computed tomography in patients with valve-tube graft infection. Heart, 2018, 104(17): 1447–1454.

[83] Guenther SP, Cyran CC, Rominger A, Set al. The relevance of ^{18}F-fluorodeoxyglucose positron emission tomography/computed tomography imaging in diagnosing prosthetic graft infections post cardiac and proximal thoracic aortic surgery. Interact Cardiovasc Thorac Surg, 2015, 21(4): 450–458.

[84] Meyer Z, Fischer M, Koerfer J, et al. The role of FDG-PET-CT in pediatric cardiac patients and

patients with congenital heart defects. Int J Cardiol, 2016, 220: 656–660.
[85] Pizzi MN, Dos-Subira L, Roque A, et al. ^{18}F-FDG-PET/CT angiography in the diagnosis of infective endocarditis and cardiac device infection in adult patients with congenital heart disease and prosthetic material. Int J Cardiol, 2017, 248: 396–402.
[86] Akin S, Muslem R, Constantinescu AA, et al. ^{18}F-FDG PET/CT in the diagnosis and management of continuous flow left ventricular assist device infections: a case series and review of the literature. ASAIO J, 2018, 64(2): e11–e19.
[87] Bernhardt AM, Pamirsad MA, Brand C, et al. The value of fluorine-18 deoxyglucose positron emission tomography scans in patients with ventricular assist device specific infections dagger. Eur J Cardio Thorac Surg, 2017, 51(6): 1072–1077.
[88] Dell'Aquila AM, Avramovic N, Mastrobuoni S, et al. Fluorine-18 fluorodeoxyglucose positron emission tomography/computed tomography for improving diagnosis of infection in patients on CF-LVAD: longing for more 'insights'. Eur Heart J Cardiovasc Imag, 2018, 19(5): 532–543.
[89] Kim J, Feller ED, Chen W, et al. FDG PET/CT for early detection and localization of left ventricular assist device infection: impact on patient management and outcome. JACC Cardiovasc Imag, 2019, 12(4): 722–729.
[90] de Vaugelade C, Mesguich C, Nubret K, et al. Infections in patients using ventricular-assist devices: comparison of the diagnostic performance of ^{18}F-FDG PET/CT scan and leukocyte-labeled scintigraphy. J Nucl Cardiol, 2019, 26(1): 42–55.
[91] Saghir S, Ivey TD, Kereiakes DJ, et al. Anterior mitral valve leaflet aneurysm due to infective endocarditis detected by cardiac magnetic resonance imaging. Rev Cardiovasc Med, 2006, 7(3): 157–159.
[92] Vilacosta I, Gomez J. Complementary role of MRI in infectious endocarditis. Echocardiography, 1995, 12(6): 673–676.
[93] Dursun M, Yilmaz S, Yilmaz E, et al. The utility of cardiac MRI in diagnosis of infective endocarditis: preliminary results. Diagn Interv Radiol, 2015, 21(1): 28–33.
[94] Stork A, Franzen O, Ruschewski H, et al. Assessment of functional anatomy of the mitral valve in patients with mitral regurgitation with cine magnetic resonance imaging: comparison with transesophageal echocardiography and surgical results. Eur Radiol, 2007, 17(12): 3189–3198.
[95] Motwani M, Kidambi A, Herzog BA, et al. MR imaging of cardiac tumors and masses: a review of methods and clinical applications. Radiology, 2013, 268(1): 26–43.
[96] Sievers B, Brandts B, Franken U, et al. Cardiovascular magnetic resonance imaging demonstrates mitral valve endocarditis. Am J Med, 2003, 115(8): 681–682.
[97] Skoldborg V, Madsen PL, Dalsgaard M, et al. Quantification of mitral valve regurgitation by 2D and 3D echocardiography compared with cardiac magnetic resonance a systematic review and meta-analysis. Int J Cardiovasc Imag, 2020, 36(2): 279–289. https://doi.org/10.1007/s10554-019-01713-7. Epub 2019 Oct 29. PMID: 31664679.
[98] Zatorska K, Michalowska I, Duchnowski P, et al. The usefulness of magnetic resonance imaging in the diagnosis of infectious endocarditis. J Heart Valve Dis, 2015, 24(6): 767–775.
[99] Thadani SR, Dyverfeldt P, Gin A, et al. Comprehensive evaluation of culture-negative endocarditis with use of cardiac and 4-dimensional-flow magnetic resonance imaging. Tex Heart Inst J, 2014, 41(3): 351–352.
[100] Dursun M, Yilmaz S, Ali Sayin O, et al. A rare cause of delayed contrast enhancement on cardiac magnetic resonance imaging: infective endocarditis. J Comput Assist Tomogr, 2005, 29(5): 709–711.
[101] Royston AP, Gosling OE. Patient with native valve infective endocarditis and concomitant bacterial myopericarditis. BMJ Case Rep, 2018, 2018.
[102] Elagha A, Mohsen A. Cardiac MRI clinches diagnosis of Libman-Sacks endocarditis. Lancet, 2019, 393(10182): e39.
[103] Gouya H, Cabanes L, Mouthon L, et al. Severe mitral stenosis as the first manifestation of systemic lupus erythematosus in a 20-year-old woman: the value of magnetic resonance imaging

in the diagnosis of Libman-Sacks endocarditis. Int J Cardiovasc Imag, 2014, 30(5): 959–960.

[104] Schneider C, Bahlmann E, Antz M, et al. Images in cardiovascular medicine. Unusual manifestation of Libman-Sacks endocarditis in systemic lupus erythematosus. Circulation, 2003, 107(22): e202–e204.

[105] Hess A, Klein I, Iung B, et al. Brain MRI findings in neurologically asymptomatic patients with infective endocarditis. Am J Neuroradiol, 2013, 34(8): 1579–1584.

[106] Iung B, Klein I, Mourvillier B, et al. Respective effects of early cerebral and abdominal magnetic resonance imaging on clinical decisions in infective endocarditis. Eur Heart J Cardiovasc Imag, 2012, 13(8): 703–710.

[107] Jiad E, Gill SK, Krutikov M, et al. When the heart rules the head: ischaemic stroke and intracerebral haemorrhage complicating infective endocarditis. Practical Neurol, 2017, 17(1): 28–34.

[108] Garcia-Cabrera E, Fernandez-Hidalgo N, Almirante B, et al. Neurological complications of infective endocarditis: risk factors, outcome, and impact of cardiac surgery: a multicenter observational study. Circulation, 2013, 127(23): 2272–2284.

[109] Tam DY, Yanagawa B, Verma S, et al. Early vs late surgery for patients with endocarditis and neurological injury: a systematic review and meta-analysis. Can J Cardiol, 2018, 34(9): 1185–1199.

[110] Duval X, Iung B, Klein I, et al. Effect of early cerebral magnetic resonance imaging on clinical decisions in infective endocarditis: a prospective study. Ann Intern Med, 2010, 152(8): 497–504. w175.

[111] Goulenok T, Klein I, Mazighi M, et al. Infective endocarditis with symptomatic cerebral complications: contribution of cerebral magnetic resonance imaging. Cerebrovasc Dis, 2013, 35(4): 327–336.

[112] Cho SM, Marquardt RJ, Rice CJ, et al. Cerebral microbleeds predict infectious intracranial aneurysm in infective endocarditis. Eur J Neurol, 2018, 25(7): 970–975.

[113] Cho SM, Rice C, Marquardt RJ, et al. Magnetic resonance imaging susceptibility-weighted imaging lesion and contrast enhancement may represent infectious intracranial aneurysm in infective endocarditis. Cerebrovasc Dis, 2017, 44(3-4): 210–216.

[114] Sotero FD, Rosario M, Fonseca AC, et al. Neurological complications of infective endocarditis. Curr Neurol Neurosci Rep, 2019, 19(5): 23.

[115] Morelli S, Carmenini E, Caporossi AP, et al. Spondylodiscitis and infective endocarditis: case studies and review of the literature. Spine, 2001, 26(5): 499–500.

第6章

感染性心内膜炎的预防

Cansin Tulunay Kaya, Cetin Erol

Ankara University School of Medicine, Cardiology Department, Samanpazari, Ankara, Turkey

感染性心内膜炎（IE）是一种罕见但后果严重的疾病，左侧心内膜炎的院内死亡率约为20%。尽管在诊治措施上已取得长足进步，但5年死亡率仍高达40%[1]。该病的高并发症发生率和死亡率以及治疗上的困难要求我们必须制定有效的预防措施以进一步降低其发生率。但遗憾的是，由于IE发病率本身较低，因此很难获得高质量的前瞻性随机研究数据来衡量预防措施的有效性。

60多年前，美国心脏协会（AHA）最先推荐对牙科手术预防性使用抗生素[2]。在这之后的50年里，这一预防措施有所扩大，对存在各种潜在心脏问题的患者，在经历不同侵入性手术时，均会使用抗生素进行预防。1977年AHA指南对患者及手术类型进行了分层，分为高风险组和低风险组[3]；1997年，指南又将风险分型细化为高风险组、中风险组和低风险组。1997年的AHA指南建议：中、高风险组患者接受包括牙科手术在内的各种手术时需要预防性使用抗生素[4]。然而，这些推荐是基于动物实验或菌血症被认为是心内膜炎替代标志的研究。在接下来的几年里，多项研究表明，日常口腔卫生活动如刷牙、使用牙线、甚至咀嚼等行为均可出现反复的菌血症[5-7]，尤其在那些口腔卫生不良的人群中，刷牙引起菌血症的微生物与IE致病菌一致[6]。这会导致一种概念，即：在口腔卫生不良的患者中，日常口腔卫生操作存在的风险可能比零星的侵入性牙科手术风险更高。针对IE，由于缺乏关于预防性使用抗生素的有效性及抗生素潜在风险的可靠数据，为此，各主要学会在2000年中期对指南做了调整。然而，全球范围内，关于哪些患者及哪些操作需要预防性使用抗生素并未达成完全一致。欧洲心脏病学会（ESC）[8]和AHA[9]指南推荐预防性使用抗生素仅限于风险最高的患者，但英国国家健康与临床优化中心（NICE）的指南则建议完全限制预防性使用抗生素[10]。随着这一原则在英国的落实，时间趋势分析表明，在英国，预防IE的处方药量减少了，但IE病例却出现了增加[11]。对此，2016年，NICE修订了之前的推荐，针对牙科手术，将原来"不推荐预防性使用抗生素"改为"不常规推荐预防性使用抗生素"，这为医务工作者对他们认为高风险的病例开具预防性抗生素提供了一定的可操作空间[12]。另一方面，日本循环学会（JCS）指南仍建议对高风险和中风险患者进行抗生素预防[13]。

与此同时，IE 的流行病学也在发生变化。IE 更多见于与医疗操作相关的老年人群和静脉吸毒者，伴之出现了常见致病微生物的变化，由链球菌转变为葡萄球菌[14-15]。

易感心血管风险因素

高风险患者的定义是可能因 IE 导致不良结果的患者，而不是指一生中具有更高的罹患心内膜炎风险的患者。

指南中划定的高风险个体如下[8-9,16]：

·既往有 IE 病史的患者；

·人工瓣膜置换术后[包括经导管植入的瓣膜，如经导管主动脉瓣置换（TAVR）]患者，以及使用人工瓣环或人工腱索的瓣膜成形术后患者；

·发绀型先天性心脏病患者；

·先天性心脏病使用人工材料经外科手术或经导管修复术后的前 6 个月（如果术后有残余分流或瓣膜反流，则风险长期存在）。

AHA 还建议对出现心脏瓣膜反流的心脏移植患者预防性使用抗生素，但因缺乏强有力的证据，ESC 并未推荐。表 6.1 总结了易于诱发 IE 的中、高风险因素。近期的流行病学数据显示：既往 IE 史、人工瓣膜置换或修复史、先天性心脏病姑息性心内分流或导管分流史，以及发绀型先天性心脏病患者有更高的概率在 5 年内发生心内膜炎或死于心内膜炎。数据还显示：有某些中等风险疾病的患者，例如风湿性瓣膜病，发生 IE 的可能性高于发绀型心脏病，但因 IE 发生死亡的风险则低于发绀型心脏病。先天性瓣膜畸形发生 IE 或死于心内膜炎的风险与上述几种高风险类型相当。此外，对先天性心脏病使用人工材料修复的病例，目前将该类病例术后早期 6 个月列为高风险，但其发生 IE 或死亡的风险低于那些目前被认为是中风险的所有情况。而有心脏植入式电子设备（CIED）的患者虽未进行风险分层，但发生心内膜炎的风险比普通人群高出了 10 倍[17]。

表 6.1 能诱发感染性心内膜炎（IE）的高风险和中风险情况[4,8–9,13,16]

高风险
·人工心脏瓣膜置换术后（生物瓣或机械瓣）或使用人工材料进行瓣膜修复后
·未根治的发绀型先天性心脏病，包括姑息性心内分流或导管分流
·既往 IE 病史
·心内分流矫治术后的前 6 个月，如果仍有残余分流则为终生高风险
·心脏移植术后瓣膜病[a]

中风险
·风湿性瓣膜病
·任何其他形式的自体瓣膜疾病（包括二叶主动脉瓣、二尖瓣脱垂和主动脉瓣狭窄钙化）
·未能矫治的先天性心脏瓣膜异常
·肥厚型梗阻性心肌病

[a]AHA 指南分类，非 ESC 指南分类

容易导致心内膜炎的非心脏因素包括高龄、免疫力下降、血液透析、血管内留置装置、恶性肿瘤、糖尿病、慢性肝病、牙病和静脉吸毒[18]。

侵入性手术的相关风险

侵入性牙科手术

牙菌斑是细菌生物膜，可导致龋齿和软组织感染。存在于生物膜中可导致龋齿的微生物大多是草绿色链球菌（变形链球菌和血链球菌），它们可经侵入性牙科操作时的出血和牙龈黏膜破坏进入血流，引起短暂的菌血症，成为引起心内膜炎的风险因素。关于近期侵入性牙科手术与心内膜炎发生的相关性，IE病例对照或病例交叉研究得出的结果并不一致[19-23]。关于预防性使用抗生素的效果也存在类似争议[20,24]。侵入性牙科操作带来的心内膜炎发生风险似乎很低，但一旦发生，后果则非常严重。大多数指南仍保持一种谨慎的态度，继续推荐高风险患者在接受某些侵入性牙科操作时预防性使用抗生素。

对于涉及以下情况的侵入性牙科操作，建议使用抗生素进行预防：高风险人群进行牙龈组织或根尖周操作，或存在黏膜穿孔的操作[8-9]。澳大利亚指南列出了一份可能导致菌血症高发生率的牙科操作清单，要求如下操作要预防性使用抗生素[25]：

- 拔牙；
- 牙周手术、龈下刮治及根面平整术；
- 脱位牙再植；
- 其他牙科手术，例如种植体植入或根尖切除术。

对于可能引起菌血症中等程度发生率的手术，如果手术需要进行多次才能完成、手术时间长或伴有牙周病时，则需要抗生素预防。

对于菌血症可能性较低的操作，不建议使用抗生素预防，例如：

- 口腔检查；
- 局部麻醉注射；
- 牙科X线检查；
- 浅表龋齿的修复性治疗；
- 正畸矫治器的放置和调整；
- 乳牙脱落；
- 嘴唇或口腔创伤后。

人体艺术

在身体上穿孔和文身在年轻人中非常流行，这一趋势直接导致人体艺术相关IE病例的增加。舌头、耳垂和肚脐是与IE相关的常见穿孔部位，而舌头和鼻腔穿孔被证明可导致没有先天性心脏病基础的年轻人发生心内膜炎[26]。文身的风险似乎低于在身体上穿孔。2015 年的 ESC 指南建议高风险人群不要进行文身和身体穿孔[8]，相关人群及人体艺术工作从业人员应被告知 IE 的风险，如果相关人员决意行穿孔和（或）文身，应在严格无菌的条件下进行操作，但对耳朵和身体穿孔或文身不建议使用抗生素预防。

非牙科、非心脏侵入类操作

资料显示，1/4～1/3 的 IE 患者有近期就医史。与社区获得性心内膜炎相比，医源性 IE 患者群年龄较大，葡萄球菌和肠球菌感染率更高[15,27]。血管操作、外周或中心静脉置管是菌血症的主要来源，进而导致医源性 IE[28]。新近的病例交叉研究显示，一些住院和门诊侵入性操作与心内膜炎风险增加有关，包括骨髓穿刺、输血、血液透析、膀胱镜检查、支气管镜检查、胃肠内镜手术、动脉穿刺、治疗性耳鼻喉科手术、泌尿生殖系统手术、皮肤手术和伤口处理。大多数内镜检查都会增加心内膜炎的风险，无论是否进行活检。假设预防性治疗百分之百有效的话，治疗 476 例仅能预防 1 例心内膜炎，在一些更高风险的操作中，这种预防效果可能更差[29]。

ESC 和 2014 年 AHA/ACC 心脏瓣膜病重点更新诊疗指南[16]建议：在呼吸道、胃肠道、泌尿生殖系统、皮肤或肌肉骨骼手术中不常规预防性使用抗生素，除非在感染或细菌定植部位进行手术，这类手术包括局部脓肿的切开或引流，或须经感染的皮肤部位进行手术。如果病原体已知，则应进行针对性治疗。如果病原体未知，则根据感染部位常见的病原体进行经验性治疗。AHA 和 JCS 指南认为，对接受扁桃体切除术或腺样体切除术的高危患者进行抗生素预防是合理的。

心血管侵入性手术

医学的进步带来了人工心脏瓣膜和心内装置植入数量的显著增加。与之相伴，经导管瓣膜介入治疗 [如 TAVR 或经导管二尖瓣钳夹术（MitraClip）] 相关的 IE 病例也有增加[30-31]。虽因相关手术感染或死于 IE 的病例不多，但因 CIED 导致的感染发病和死亡却显著增加[17]。

早期人工瓣膜心内膜炎主要是由于围手术期人工瓣膜污染造成。中心静脉或外周静脉置管以及胸骨切口深部感染均可导致心内膜炎，金黄色葡萄球菌、表皮葡萄球菌、肠球菌、革兰氏阴性菌和真菌是术后早期人工瓣膜 IE 的主要致病菌。最近有报道，体外膜肺氧合（ECMO）管路中的加热 - 冷却装置的水箱可能在制造过程中受到污染，导致嵌合分枝杆菌感染暴发[32-33]，从加热 - 冷却装置中排出的生物气溶胶可能是潜在的感染源[34]。这一感染已导致一系列疾病，包括从手术部位感染到肺部感染，或播散性肉芽肿性疾病和人工瓣膜 IE。通过定期采样仔细检查自来水和手术室设备可能有助于预防其他一些来源的污染。

TAVR 也存在导致 IE 的风险，最常见的致病菌包括表皮葡萄球菌、金黄色葡萄球菌和肠球菌[30,35-37]。虽然外科手术置换主动脉瓣（SAVR）术后的肠球菌 IE 较葡萄球菌 IE 相对罕见，但 TAVR 术后两者的发病率相同。这一差异可能与其腹股沟操作部位的定植菌不同有关，还有一个可能是 TAVR 一般在导管室进行，那里的无菌程度低于手术室。其他一些与该手术相关的感染风险因素包括：术后瓣周漏的湍流可能成为诱发感染的原发病灶，手术操作对自体瓣叶的损伤，以及术中起搏器的使用[38]。

虽然未对 CIED 患者进行心内膜炎的风险分层，但其实际风险是普通病例的 10 倍[17]。CIED 感染是一类系列性的感染，包括从局部的囊袋感染到影响全身的 IE。CIED 感染可发生在没有其他心脏异常的患者中，病原来自植入过程中的皮肤细菌接种，或远处感染的继发播种。大多数感染与早期细菌定植和生物膜形成有关。预防围手术期的细菌定植能够预防大多数 CIED 感染。CIED 心内膜炎可累及电极导线和（或）三尖瓣，凝固酶阴性葡萄球菌和金黄色葡萄球菌是最常见的病原体[39]。与手术相关的 CIED 感染风险因素包括未做抗生素预防、手术时间过长、血肿形成、需重新调整设备以及与植入电子设备的特征相关（如双腔系统和使用腹部囊袋）[40]。

新近的欧洲心律协会（EHRA）国际共识制定了关于如何预防、诊断和治疗 CIED 感染的方案[41]。英国也就心内装置感染的诊断、预防和治疗制定了指南[42]，建议采取相关围手术期干预措施以避免 CIED 感染（表 6.2）。

在植入人工瓣膜或其他血管内及心内装置前至少 2 周，应消除牙源性脓毒症的感染源。

25%~30% 的人群是金黄色葡萄球菌的鼻腔带菌者[43-44]。对择期心脏手术或 CIED 植入病例，建议术前筛查鼻腔金黄色葡萄球菌的带菌状况，并使用莫匹罗星软膏涂抹和用氯己定肥皂清洗鼻腔以处理金黄色葡萄球菌携带者，从而防止手术部位的葡萄球菌感染以及可能由此导致的心内膜炎[45]。

表 6.2 预防心脏植入式电子设备（CIED）感染的措施

- 对有感染迹象的患者延迟手术
- 如果可能，避免使用中心静脉置管或临时起搏器
- 在完全无菌的环境中进行手术，手术室每小时换气 15 次，最好是 25 次，遵守无菌原则，限制手术室内的人数
- 由经验丰富的医生操作或监督手术
- 避免桥接抗凝，中断抗血小板药使用，以防止血肿形成
- 手术前鼻拭子筛查葡萄球菌和去定植处理
- 使用电动推剪（而非剃须刀）去除毛发
- 使用酒精氯己定（氯己定最低浓度为 2%）制剂进行皮肤准备（无法耐受者，使用酒精聚维酮碘）
- 给予预防性抗生素
- 使用抗菌封套（用于高危病例）
- 适当的伤口护理

IE 的预防措施

非药物措施

非药物手段仍然是预防 IE 最关键的干预措施。指南强调了良好的口腔和皮肤卫生习惯对预防 IE 的重要性。应教育患者保持良好的卫生习惯，根据其风险程度，推荐每年进行 1~2 次常规口腔科检查。然而，欧洲心脏调查研究的数据显示：IE 预防的教育水平仍然很低，只有一半有自体瓣膜疾病的患者接受过相关教育，只有 1/3 的人参加了常规口腔保健护理[46]。

其他非药物措施包括适当消毒伤口、积极处理特应性皮炎、减少静脉导管的使用，以及静脉导管穿刺及任何有创操作过程的无菌性防护。建议治疗皮肤和尿道的慢性细菌定植。反对患者自行使用抗生素治疗，并应告知他们：如果发热数天无缓解，应咨询心脏内科专家。

抗生素预防

·对抗生素预防的担忧

抗生素预防心内膜炎的效果一直备受争议。由于该病发病率低，因此开展以发生 IE 为研究终点的、高质量的关于预防性使用抗生素的随机试验难以实施。目前的数据多来自心内膜炎的动物实验，而临床试验是以术后菌血症作为心内膜炎的替代标志，通过病例对照及时间趋势分析试验病例在指南实施前后的变化。结果显示：预防性使用抗生素可有效减少手术相关菌血症，但术后菌血症的减少是否能够真正代表 IE 的减少目前尚不确定[47]。指南限制预防性抗生素使用后的时间趋势研究也出现了不同结果：在法国，指南变化后口腔链球菌心内膜炎病例无增加[48]；而在美国、德国、英国和加拿大，心内膜炎病例有所增加[11,49-51]。

广泛地预防性使用抗生素，除了不确定疗效之外，还存在诸多备受关注的问题，如潜在的过敏反应、抗生素耐药性以及高昂的医疗成本。英国就 2004—2014 年间使用 3g 阿莫西林出现的非致命性反应进行了报道，通常，每百万张处方中有 22.62 例非致命性反应。而每百万张 600 mg 克林霉素处方中会发生 13 例致命性反应和 149 例非致命性反应，主要是艰难梭菌的二重感染[52]。另外，预防性使用抗生素带来的是费用负担，牙科术前对存在潜在危险的患者使用抗生素导致每年相关费用高达 1.45 亿美元[53]。再者，针对 IE 预防性使用抗生素可能带来的耐药性问题尚不确定。已知口腔微生物具有很高的抗生素耐药率：在牙齿感染的人群中，45% 的变异链球菌具有耐药性，其中，对克林霉素的耐药性比对阿莫西林 - 克拉维酸的耐药性更显著[54]；而存在于生物膜中的微生物的耐药性更强[55]。在所有抗生素处方中，10% 用于治疗口腔感染。这种高耐药率的出现可能是由于反复使用抗生素造成的，而非单次大剂量的预防性使用。而口腔菌群的高耐药率可能会影响未来预防性抗生素的选择。

预防性使用抗生素的方案

• 侵入性牙科手术

预防性使用抗生素对草绿色链球菌有效。术前 30~60 min 单次口服 2 g 阿莫西林可作为预防 IE 的首选[8-9]，阿莫西林已被证明可有效减少牙科手术相关菌血症[56]。它是一种中等广谱的 β-内酰胺类抗生素，对链球菌和肠球菌有杀菌作用，因其口服生物利用度较氨苄西林高而使用更广，口服给药 1~2 h 达到峰值浓度。儿童剂量为 50 mg/kg，最大剂量为 2 g。如果不能口服，可选择肠外用药，给予 2 g 阿莫西林或氨苄西林。

口服头孢氨苄或等效第一代或第二代头孢菌素，或选择肠外注射头孢唑林或头孢曲松，则作为二线用药。

对青霉素过敏的患者，可于术前 30~60 min 给予克林霉素 600 mg。目前尚不清楚草绿色链球菌耐药率增加是否会影响未来抗生素的选择，但口腔微生物对克林霉素的耐药较为显著，在为青霉素过敏患者开具克林霉素时应考虑这一点。目前，ESC 指南推荐克林霉素作为青霉素过敏患者的唯一替代药物。而 AHA 指南还推荐了大环内酯类抗生素——阿奇霉素 500 mg 或克拉霉素 500 mg（儿童 15 mg/kg）——作为青霉素过敏的另一选择。

为确保抗生素从手术开始就具有抗菌活性，应在术前 30~60 min 使用；如果这一时间段未曾给药，则可以手术开始后的 2 h 内给药。如果手术要分次进行，则应在每次治疗时重复给药，但应尽可能减少手术的次数。

对于已经服用抗生素的患者，术前预防性用药应选择不同类别的抗生素，或手术推迟 10 d 以上，以待正常口腔菌群的恢复[9,57]。

• CIED 的植入

葡萄球菌是 CIED 心内膜炎最常见的致病菌，因此，CIED 植入前应针对性地选择预防葡萄球菌感染的药物。对甲氧西林敏感的菌株，头孢唑林已被证明可以显著减少 CIED 感染[58]，植入前给予单剂头孢唑林即可达到预防目的。但甲氧西林耐药葡萄球菌在院内感染中很常见，且不同医院的耐药率不同。当预期为甲氧西林耐药葡萄球菌感染，或青霉素过敏时，可选择万古霉素 1~1.5 g（15 mg/kg）缓慢输注[41]。英国抗微生物化疗协会指南则推荐首选替考拉宁，联合或不联合庆大霉素[42]，替考拉宁可在术前 60 min 内给予一剂 800 mg。

对于高风险 CIED 植入病例，使用米诺环素和利福平抗菌封套可降低 CIED 感染的发生率[59]。最近的指南也推荐针对接受囊袋或电极导线重置、脉冲发生器更换、系统升级或首次植入心脏再同步除颤器（CRT-D）的高危患者使用这一治疗方案[41]。不建议无益的局部使用抗生素或杀菌剂。

• TAVR

大多数接受 TAVR 的患者均服用第一代或第二代头孢菌素用于预防。头孢菌素类药物可有效预防甲氧西林敏感葡萄球菌感染。然而，瑞士 TAVR 登记处的数据和最近的系统性回顾研究表明，肠球菌正在成为 TAVR 之后早期引起 IE 的最常见微生物[37,60]。因此，预防性使用的抗生素应覆盖肠球菌和葡萄球菌。肠球菌对头孢菌素具有固有的耐药性，抗菌药敏试验显示预防性用药对 47.9% 的 TAVR 后心内膜炎病例无效，主要原因是肠球菌感染率高[60]。但肠球菌对氨苄西林耐药并不严重，临床可考虑使用阿莫西林 – 克拉维酸、氨苄西林 – 舒巴坦预防。而对青霉素过敏者，则可考虑万古霉素，这些药物在预防肠球菌方面，效果优于头孢菌素。

表 6.3 总结了针对特定情况推荐的抗生素预防方案[61]。

表 6.3　不同手术中感染性心内膜炎（IE）的抗生素预防方案[a]

	常见病原菌	药物选择	成人剂量	青霉素过敏时药物选择	成人剂量
手　术					
牙科	·草绿色链球菌	·阿莫西林 ·阿莫西林/氨苄西林 二线用药： ·头孢氨苄 ·头孢唑林/头孢曲松	2 g, po 2 g, im/iv 2 g, po 1 g, im/iv	克林霉素	600 mg
CIED 植入	·甲氧西林敏感葡萄球菌 ·甲氧西林耐药葡萄球菌	·头孢唑林 ·万古霉素[b]	1~2 g, iv 1~1.5 g	万古霉素[b]	1~1.5 g
在感染/细菌定植组织的操作					
呼吸系统	·葡萄球菌	·头孢唑林	1~2 g, iv	克林霉素 万古霉素[b]	600 mg 1~1.5 g
泌尿生殖系统/胃肠道	·肠球菌	·阿莫西林/氨苄西林	2 g, im/iv	万古霉素[b]	1~1.5 g
皮肤	·葡萄球菌 ·β – 溶血性链球菌 ·甲氧西林耐药葡萄球菌	·阿莫西林 ·头孢氨苄 头孢唑林/头孢曲松 ·万古霉素[b]	2 g, im/iv/po 2 g, po 1 g, im/iv 1~1.5 g	克林霉素 万古霉素[b]	600 mg 1~1.5 g

[a] 经许可，改编自参考文献 [61]。[b] 万古霉素应以 1 g/h 剂量缓慢输注，手术前 60～90 min 开始给药。CIED：心脏植入式电子设备；po：口服；im：肌内注射；iv：静脉注射

参考文献

[1] Bannay A, Hoen B, AEPEI Study Group, et al. The impact of valve surgery on short- and long-term mortality in left-sided infective endocarditis: do differences in methodological approaches explain previous conflicting results? Eur Heart J, 2011, 32(16): 2003–2015. https://www.ncbi.nlm.nih.gov/pubmed/19208650.

[2] Jones TD, Baumgartner L, Bellows MT, et al. Prevention of rheumatic fever and bacterial endocarditis through control of streptococcal infections. Pediatrics, 1955, 15(5): 642–626. https://www.ncbi.nlm.nih.gov/pubmed/14370902.

[3] Kaplan EL, Anthony BF, Committee on Rheumatic Fever and Bacterial Endocarditis, et al. Prevention of bacterial endocarditis. Circulation, 1977, 56(1): 139A–143A. https://www.ncbi.nlm.nih.gov/pubmed/324659.

[4] Dajani AS, Taubert KA, Wilson W, et al. Prevention of bacterial endocarditis: recommendations by the American Heart Association. Clin Infect Dis, 1997, 25(6): 1448–1458. https://www.ncbi.nlm.nih.gov/pubmed/9431393.

[5] Lockhart PB, Brennan MT, Sasser HC, et al. Bacteremia associated with toothbrushing and dental extraction. Circulation, 2008, 117(24): 3118–3125. https://www.ncbi.nlm.nih.gov/pubmed/18541739.

[6] Lockhart PB, Brennan MT, Thornhill M, et al. Poor oral hygiene as a risk factor for infective endocarditis-related bacteremia. J Am Dent Assoc, 2009, 140(10): 1238–1244. https://www.ncbi.nlm.nih.gov/pubmed/19797553.

[7] Mougeot FK, Saunders SE, Brennan MT, et al. Associations between bacteremia from oral sources and distant-site infections: tooth brushing versus single tooth extraction. Oral Surg Oral Med Oral Pathol Oral Radiol, 2015, 119(4): 430–435. https://www.ncbi.nlm.nih.gov/pubmed/25758845.

[8] Habib G, Lancellotti P, ESC Scientific Document Group, et al. 2015 ESC guidelines for the management of infective endocarditis: The Task Force for the Management of Infective Endocarditis of the European Society of Cardiology (ESC). Endorsed by: European Association for Cardio-Thoracic Surgery (EACTS), the European Association of Nuclear Medicine (EANM). Eur Heart J, 2015, 36(44): 3075–3128. https://www.ncbi.nlm.nih.gov/pubmed/26320109.

[9] Wilson W, Taubert KA, American Heart Association, et al. Prevention of infective endocarditis: guidelines from the American Heart Association: a guideline from the American Heart Association Rheumatic Fever, Endocarditis and Kawasaki Disease Committee, Council on Cardiovascular Disease in the Young, and the Council on Clinical Cardiology, Council on Cardiovascular Surgery and Anesthesia, and the Quality of Care and Outcomes Research Interdisciplinary Working Group. J Am Dent Assoc, 2008, 139(Suppl.l): 3S–24S. https://www.ncbi.nlm.nih.gov/pubmed/18167394.

[10] Prophylaxis against infective endocarditis: antimicrobial prophylaxis against infective endocarditis in adults and children undergoing interventional procedures. London: National Institute for Health and Clinical Excellence: Guidance, 2008.

[11] Dayer MJ, Jones S, Prendergast B, et al. Incidence of infective endocarditis in England, 2000-13: a secular trend, interrupted time-series analysis. Lancet, 2015, 385(9974): 1219–1228. https://www.ncbi.nlm.nih.gov/pubmed/25467569.

[12] Prophylaxis against infective endocarditis: antimicrobial prophylaxis against infective endocarditis in adults and children undergoing interventional procedures. London: National Institute for Health and Care Excellence: Clinical Guidelines, 2016.

[13] Nakatani S, Ohara T, Japanese Circulation Society Joint Working Group, et al. JCS 2017 guideline on prevention and treatment of infective endocarditis. Circ J, 2019, 83(8): 1767–1809. https://www.ncbi.nlm.nih.gov/pubmed/31281136.

[14] Olmos C, Vilacosta I, Fernandez-Perez C, et al. The evolving nature of infective endocarditis in Spain: a population-based study (2003 to 2014). J Am Coll Cardiol, 2017, 70(22): 2795–2804. https://www.ncbi.nlm.nih.gov/pubmed/29191329.

[15] Sy RW, Kritharides L. Health care exposure and age in infective endocarditis: results of a contemporary

[16] Nishimura RA, Otto CM, Bonow RO, et al. AHA/ACC focused update of the 2014 AHA/ACC guideline for the management of patients with valvular heart disease: a report of the American college of Cardiology/American Heart Association Task Force on clinical practice guidelines. Circulation, 2017, 135(25): e1159–e1195. https://www.ncbi.nlm.nih.gov/pubmed/28298458.
[17] Thornhill MH, Jones S, Prendergast B, et al. Quantifying infective endocarditis risk in patients with predisposing cardiac conditions. Eur Heart J, 2018, 39(7): 586–595. https://www.ncbi.nlm.nih.gov/pubmed/29161405.
[18] Chambers HF, Bayer AS. Native-valve infective endocarditis. N Engl J Med, 2020, 383(6): 567–576. https://www.ncbi.nlm.nih.gov/pubmed/32757525.
[19] Duval X, Millot S, EI-dents Association pour l'Etude, et la Prévention de l'Endocardite Infectieuse (AEPEI) Study Group, et al. Oral streptococcal endocarditis, oral hygiene habits, and recent dental procedures: a case-control study. Clin Infect Dis, 2017, 64(12): 1678–1685. https://www.ncbi.nlm.nih.gov/pubmed/28369398.
[20] Strom BL, Abrutyn E, Berlin JA, et al. Dental and cardiac risk factors for infective endocarditis. A population-based, case-control study. Ann Intern Med, 1998, 129(10): 761–769. https://www.ncbi.nlm.nih.gov/pubmed/9841581.
[21] Nakatani S, Mitsutake K, Committee on Guideline for Prevention and Management of Infective Endocarditis, et al, Current characteristics of infective endocarditis in Japan: an analysis of 848 cases in 2000 and 2001. Circ J, 2003, 67(11): 901–905. https://www.ncbi.nlm.nih.gov/pubmed/14578594.
[22] Chen TT, Yeh YC, Chien KL, et al. Risk of infective endocarditis after invasive dental treatments: case-only study. Circulation, 2018, 138(4): 356–363. https://www.ncbi.nlm.nih.gov/pubmed/29674326.
[23] Tubiana S, Blotiere PO, Hoen B, et al. Dental procedures, antibiotic prophylaxis, and endocarditis among people with prosthetic heart valves: nationwide population based cohort and a case crossover study. BMJ, 2017, 358: j3776. https://www.ncbi.nlm.nih.gov/pubmed/28882817.
[24] Imperiale TF, Horwitz RI. Does prophylaxis prevent postdental infective endocarditis? A controlled evaluation of protective efficacy. Am J Med, 1990, 88(2): 131–136. https://www.ncbi.nlm.nih.gov/pubmed/2301438.
[25] Infective Endocarditis Prophylaxis Expert Group TGL. Prevention of endocarditis. 2008. Melbourne.
[26] Armstrong ML, DeBoer S, Cetta F. Infective endocarditis after body art: a review of the literature and concerns. J Adolesc Health, 2008, 43(3): 217–225. https://www.ncbi.nlm.nih.gov/pubmed/18710675.
[27] Fernandez-Hidalgo N, Almirante B, Tornos P, et al. Contemporary epidemiology and prognosis of health care-associated infective endocarditis. Clin Infect Dis, 2008, 47(10): 1287–1297. https://www.ncbi.nlm.nih.gov/pubmed/18834314.
[28] Lomas JM, Martinez-Marcos FJ, Grupo Andaluz para el Estudio de las Infecciones Cardiovasculares at the Sociedad Andaluza de Enfermedades I, et al. Healthcare-associated infective endocarditis: an undesirable effect of healthcare universalization. Clin Microbiol Infect, 2010, 16(11): 1683–1690. https://www.ncbi.nlm.nih.gov/pubmed/19732086.
[29] Janszky I, Gemes K, Ahnve S, et al. Invasive procedures associated with the development of infective endocarditis. J Am Coll Cardiol, 2018, 71(24): 2744–2752. https://www.ncbi.nlm.nih.gov/pubmed/29903348.
[30] Gallouche M, Barone-Rochette G, Pavese P, et al. Incidence and prevention of infective endocarditis and bacteraemia after transcatheter aortic valve implantation in a French university hospital: a retrospective study. J Hosp Infect, 2018, 99(1): 94–97. https://www.ncbi.nlm.nih.gov/pubmed/29191610.
[31] Hermanns H, Wiegerinck EMA, Lagrand WK, et al. Two cases of endocarditis after MitraClip

[32] Achermann Y, Rossle M, Hoffmann M, et al. Prosthetic valve endocarditis and bloodstream infection due to Mycobacterium chimaera. J Clin Microbiol, 2013, 51(6): 1769–1773. https://www.ncbi.nlm.nih.gov/pubmed/23536407.

[33] van Ingen J, Kohl TA, Kranzer K, et al. Global outbreak of severe Mycobacterium chimaera disease after cardiac surgery: a molecular epidemiological study. Lancet Infect Dis, 2017, 17(10): 1033–1041. https://www.ncbi.nlm.nih.gov/pubmed/28711585.

[34] Gotting T, Klassen S, Jonas D, et al. Heater-cooler units: contamination of crucial devices in cardiothoracic surgery. J Hosp Infect, 2016, 93(3): 223–228. https://www.ncbi.nlm.nih.gov/pubmed/27101883.

[35] Rodriguez-Vidigal FF, Nogales-Asensio JM, Calvo-Cano A, et al. Infective endocarditis after transcatheter aortic valve implantation: contributions of a single-centre experience on incidence and associated factors. Enferm Infecc Microbiol Clín, 2019, 37(7): 428–434. https://www.ncbi.nlm.nih.gov/pubmed/30389267.

[36] Amat-Santos IJ, Messika-Zeitoun D, Eltchaninoff H, et al. Infective endocarditis after transcatheter aortic valve implantation: results from a large multicenter registry. Circulation, 2015, 131(18): 1566–1574. https://www.ncbi.nlm.nih.gov/pubmed/25753535.

[37] Khan A, Aslam A, Satti KN, et al. Infective endocarditis post-transcatheter aortic valve implantation (TAVI), microbiological profile and clinical outcomes: a systematic review. PloS One, 2020, 15(1): e0225077. https://www.ncbi.nlm.nih.gov/pubmed/31951610.

[38] Alexis SL, Malik AH, George I, et al. Infective endocarditis after surgical and transcatheter aortic valve replacement: a state of the art review. J Am Heart Assoc, 2020, 9(16): e017347. https://www.ncbi.nlm.nih.gov/pubmed/32772772.

[39] Hussein AA, Baghdy Y, Wazni OM, et al. Microbiology of cardiac implantable electronic device infections. JACC Clin Electrophysiol, 2016, 2(4): 498–505. https://www.ncbi.nlm.nih.gov/pubmed/29759872.

[40] Polyzos KA, Konstantelias AA, Falagas ME. Risk factors for cardiac implantable electronic device infection: a systematic review and meta-analysis. Europace, 2015, 17(5): 767–777. https://www.ncbi.nlm.nih.gov/pubmed/25926473.

[41] Blomstrom-Lundqvist C, Traykov V, Erba PA, et al. European Heart Rhythm Association (EHRA) international consensus document on how to prevent, diagnose, and treat cardiac implantable electronic device infections-endorsed by the Heart Rhythm Society (HRS), the Asia Pacific Heart Rhythm Society (APHRS), the Latin American Heart Rhythm Society (LAHRS), International Society for Cardiovascular Infectious Diseases (ISCVID), and the European Society of Clinical Microbiology and Infectious Diseases (ESCMID) in collaboration with the European Association for Cardio-Thoracic Surgery (EACTS). Eur Heart J, 2020, 41(21): 2012–2032. https://www.ncbi.nlm.nih.gov/pubmed/32101604.

[42] Sandoe JA, Barlow G, British Society for Antimicrobial Chemotherapy, et al. Guidelines for the diagnosis, prevention and management of implantable cardiac electronic device infection. Report of a joint Working Party project on behalf of the British Society for Antimicrobial Chemotherapy (BSAC, host organization), British Heart Rhythm Society (BHRS), British Cardiovascular Society (BCS), British Heart Valve Society (BHVS) and British Society for Echocardiography (BSE). J Antimicrob Chemother, 2015, 70(2): 325–359. https://www.ncbi.nlm.nih.gov/pubmed/25355810.

[43] Wertheim HF, Melles DC, Vos MC, et al. The role of nasal carriage in Staphylococcus aureus infections. Lancet Infect Dis, 2005, 5(12): 751–762. https://www.ncbi.nlm.nih.gov/pubmed/16310147.

[44] Wertheim HF, Vos MC, Ott A, et al. Risk and outcome of nosocomial Staphylococcus aureus bacteraemia in nasal carriers versus non-carriers. Lancet, 2004, 364(9435): 703–705. https://www.ncbi.nlm.nih.gov/pubmed/15325835.

[45] Bode LG, Kluytmans JA, Wertheim HF, et al. Preventing surgical-site infections in nasal carriers

of Staphylococcus aureus. N Engl J Med, 2010, 362(1): 9–17. https://www.ncbi.nlm.nih.gov/pubmed/20054045.

[46] Tornos P, Iung B, Permanyer-Miralda G, et al. Infective endocarditis in Europe: lessons from the Euro heart survey. Heart, 2005, 91(5): 571–575. https://www.ncbi.nlm.nih.gov/pubmed/15831635.

[47] Cahill TJ, Harrison JL, Jewell P, et al. Antibiotic prophylaxis for infective endocarditis: a systematic review and meta-analysis. Heart, 2017, 103(12): 937–944. https://www.ncbi.nlm.nih.gov/pubmed/28213367.

[48] Duval X, Delahaye F, AEPEI Study Group, et al. Temporal trends in infective endocarditis in the context of prophylaxis guideline modifications: three successive population-based surveys. J Am Coll Cardiol, 2012, 59(22): 1968–1976. https://www.ncbi.nlm.nih.gov/pubmed/22624837.

[49] Pant S, Patel NJ, Deshmukh A, et al. Trends in infective endocarditis incidence, microbiology, and valve replacement in the United States from 2000 to 2011. J Am Coll Cardiol, 2015, 65(19): 2070–2076. https://www.ncbi.nlm.nih.gov/pubmed/25975469.

[50] Keller K, von Bardeleben RS, Ostad MA, et al. Temporal trends in the prevalence of infective endocarditis in Germany between 2005 and 2014. Am J Cardiol, 2017, 119(2): 317–322. https://www.ncbi.nlm.nih.gov/pubmed/27816113.

[51] Garg P, Ko DT, Bray Jenkyn KM, et al. Infective endocarditis hospitalizations and antibiotic prophylaxis rates before and after the 2007 American Heart Association guideline revision. Circulation, 2019, 140(3): 170–180. https://www.ncbi.nlm.nih.gov/pubmed/31023074.

[52] Thornhill MH, Dayer MJ, Prendergast B, et al. Incidence and nature of adverse reactions to antibiotics used as endocarditis prophylaxis. J Antimicrob Chemother, 2015, 70(8): 2382–2388. https://www.ncbi.nlm.nih.gov/pubmed/25925595.

[53] Lockhart PB, Blizzard J, Maslow AL, et al. Drug cost implications for antibiotic prophylaxis for dental procedures. Oral Surg Oral Med Oral Pathol Oral Radiol, 2013, 115(3): 345–353. https://www.ncbi.nlm.nih.gov/pubmed/23265984.

[54] Loyola-Rodriguez JP, Ponce-Diaz ME, Loyola-Leyva A, et al. Determination and identification of antibiotic-resistant oral streptococci isolated from active dental infections in adults. Acta Odontol Scand, 2018, 76(4): 229–235. https://www.ncbi.nlm.nih.gov/pubmed/29160117.

[55] Mah TF. Biofilm-specific antibiotic resistance. Future Microbiol, 2012, 7(9): 1061–1072. https://www.ncbi.nlm.nih.gov/pubmed/22953707.

[56] Diz Dios P, Tomas Carmona I, Limeres Posse J, et al. Comparative efficacies of amoxicillin, clindamycin, and moxifloxacin in prevention of bacteremia following dental extractions. Antimicrob Agents Chemother, 2006, 50(9): 2996–3002. https://www.ncbi.nlm.nih.gov/pubmed/16940094.

[57] Pippi R. Antibiotic prophylaxis for infective endocarditis: some rarely addressed issues. Br Dent J, 2017, 222(8): 583–587. https://www.ncbi.nlm.nih.gov/pubmed/28428592.

[58] de Oliveira JC, Martinelli M, Nishioka SA, et al. Efficacy of antibiotic prophylaxis before the implantation of pacemakers and cardioverter-defibrillators: results of a large, prospective, randomized, double-blinded, placebo-controlled trial. Circ Arrhythm Electrophysiol, 2009, 2(1): 29–34. https://www.ncbi.nlm.nih.gov/pubmed/19808441.

[59] Tarakji KG, Mittal S, WRAP-IT Investigators, et al. Antibacterial envelope to prevent cardiac implantable device infection. N Engl J Med, 2019, 380(20): 1895–1905. https://www.ncbi.nlm.nih.gov/pubmed/30883056.

[60] Stortecky S, Heg D, Tueller D, et al. Infective endocarditis after transcatheter aortic valve replacement. J Am Coll Cardiol, 2020, 75(24): 3020–3030. https://www.ncbi.nlm.nih.gov/pubmed/32553254.

[61] Kaya CT, Erol C. How to achieve infective endocarditis prophylaxis. E-J Cardiol Pract, 2018, 16(33).

第7章
感染性心内膜炎的抗菌治疗

Abby L. Chiappelli[1], *Tamara L. Trienski*[2], *Jessica Snawerdt*[3], *Lauren B. McKibben*[1], *Ryan M. Rivosecchi*[1], *Edward T. Horn*[4]

[1]University of Pittsburgh Medical Center, Pittsburgh, PA, United States; [2]Allegheny General Hospital, Pittsburgh, PA, United States; [3]AdventHealth Celebration, Kissimmee, FL, United States; [4]University of Pittsburgh School of Pharmacy, Pittsburgh, PA, United States

引 言

感染性心内膜炎（IE）发病率持续增加，2018年，美国估计每10万人中有15例IE。革兰氏阳性球菌是最常见的致病菌，包括链球菌、葡萄球菌、肠球菌等。继发于心脏植入式电子设备（CIED）、静脉吸毒（IVDU）和医源性IE的病例数量不断增加，其中金黄色葡萄球菌最常见，约占"高收入国家"所有病例的40%[1-2]。鉴于IE的高并发症发生率和死亡率，为此，快速诊断和及时的药物治疗对于避免死亡、栓塞、脓肿、心力衰竭和感染转移等相关并发症至关重要[2]。

治疗原则

对于临床高度怀疑IE的病例，在抽血培养后，应尽早启动经验性抗菌治疗，即便血培养采集延迟也不应延误抗菌治疗。此外，抗菌治疗还可早于超声心动图检查，而不影响检查结果。治疗的主要目的是消除感染，包括对赘生物进行杀菌[2-3]。

IE的最佳抗菌药物选择和临床应用较为复杂，充满挑战。在进行经验性用药时，需要综合考虑药物在感染部位的渗透性、强效的杀菌能力、对药物的耐受性及不良反应等[4]。常用的抗生素（如β-内酰胺类和糖肽类）可能会因很多IE病例的高细菌负荷量而功效降低。表7.1回顾了用于治疗IE的常见抗菌药物的作用机制。"接种量效应"（inoculum effect）描述了这种高细菌负荷量与抗生素疗效的量效关系。此外，据报道，病原菌代谢活性降低会增加灭菌难度，因此，治疗时间需要延长数周甚至数月，才能确保感染的根除[2,11]。

药代动力学和药效学

了解抗生素的药代动力学和药效学特征对于确定适当的治疗方案是必要的。

药代动力学是指机体对药物的作用,包括吸收、分布、代谢和排泄的特性。药效学描述了药物在其作用部位对机体的作用,主要指药理或毒理作用。

根据药效学原理,抗菌药物可分为两类:时间依赖性和浓度依赖性(表7.2)。时间依赖性杀菌要求必须在至少40%~50%的给药间隔时间里抗生素浓度高于最低抑菌浓度(MIC),以有效消灭病原菌。浓度依赖性杀菌需要血清和感染部位达到最大峰值浓度才能有效杀死微生物[12]。

杀菌与抑菌

抗生素可分为杀菌剂和抑菌剂两大类(表7.3)。虽然杀菌剂的杀灭作用和抑菌剂的抑制作用从字面定义上似乎很清晰,但在理解这些药物治疗IE的特性时,还需要注意两者之间存在的细微差别。MIC是指在培养24 h时可抑制已知微生物生长的最低药物浓度。

这取决于培养条件,如培养基、温度和二氧化碳浓度。最低杀菌浓度(MBC)指可以使微生物生长减少至原来的1/1000的药物浓度。抑菌定义为MBC与MIC之比>4,杀菌定义为这一比率≤4。但如果一个抗生素可以使微生物生长减少至原来的1/1000,而在浓度<4倍MIC时无法达到这一效果,则该抗生素被定义为

表7.1 用于治疗感染性心内膜炎(IE)的抗生素的作用机制

药物类别	作用机制
β-内酰胺类	抑制细胞壁形成[5]
糖肽类	抑制细胞壁形成[6]
氨基糖苷类	抑制蛋白质合成[7]
环脂肽类	抑制蛋白质、DNA和RNA合成[8]
氟喹诺酮类	抑制DNA合成[9]
恶唑烷酮类	抑制蛋白质合成[10]

表7.2 时间依赖性与浓度依赖性杀菌抗生素

时间依赖性杀菌	浓度依赖性杀菌
碳青霉烯类	氨基糖苷类
头孢菌素	达托霉素
克林霉素	氟喹诺酮类
多西环素	脂糖肽类
利奈唑胺	甲硝唑
大环内酯类	
单环β-内酰胺类	
青霉素类	
替加环素	
万古霉素	

表 7.3　杀菌抗生素与抑菌抗生素

杀菌剂	抑菌剂
氨基糖苷类	克林霉素
碳青霉烯类	利奈唑胺 [a]
头孢菌素类	大环内酯类
达托霉素	磺胺类
氟喹诺酮类	四环素类
脂糖肽类	甲氧苄啶
甲硝唑	
青霉素	
利福平	
万古霉素	

[a] 根据生物体的不同，利奈唑胺兼具抑菌和杀菌特性

抑菌[13-14]。抑菌和杀菌的定义基于体外测定，而不是依据某些具体的临床原则。实验室对杀菌的定义为用药 24 h 时对微生物生长的抑制 > 99.9%，一些抑菌抗生素虽然对抑制细菌生长非常有效（90%～99%），但并不满足这一定义[13-15]。还有一些抗生素可以同时具有抑菌和杀菌两种特性（例如，利奈唑胺对葡萄球菌和肠球菌具有抑菌作用，但对链球菌具有杀菌作用）[15]。对于接种量较大的感染，如 IE，杀菌剂的杀菌作用可能受到抑制，而更符合抑菌的效果。

长期以来，人们一直认为杀菌性抗生素具有更高的功效。一项系统性文献综述回顾了自 1985 年以来的 56 项随机对照试验（RCT），它们使用头对头设计比较抑菌药物与杀菌药物对侵袭性细菌感染的疗效[13]。49 项试验（87.5%）发现抑菌和杀菌药物的功效没有显著差异；6 项试验（10.7%）发现抑菌剂利奈唑胺比杀菌剂头孢菌素或万古霉素效果更好。但以上研究存在一个缺憾，即所有 56 项试验均未对 IE 进行评估，因此很难将上述试验的结论推衍到 IE 患者群体并得出类似结论。

接种量效应

所谓接种量效应，就是当感染部位微生物密度增加时，某些抗菌药物的疗效因此而出现的降低。报道显示，许多抗菌药物都会出现这种现象，但报道最多的是 β - 内酰胺类[16]。MIC 的获得来自细菌药敏试验，而试验检测使用的是标准接种物（每毫升含 10^5 菌落形成单位），这可能远远低于感染部位的实际微生物密度（可高达每克组织 $10^8 \sim 10^{10}$ 菌落形成单位）[15]。微生物的高密度意味着有部分微生物可能处于静止生长期，而这会降低针对青霉素结合蛋白（PBP）的 β - 内酰胺的有效性。值得注意的是，金黄色葡萄球菌具有较高接种量，可达每克组织 $10^8 \sim 10^{11}$ 菌落形成单位[17]。

抗生素的分类

β-内酰胺类

β-内酰胺类药物由青霉素类、头孢菌素类和碳青霉烯类组成，具有抗多种革兰氏阳性和革兰氏阴性病原体的作用，可用于治疗链球菌、葡萄球菌和肠球菌等引起的感染。药剂包括水溶性青霉素 G、氨苄西林、苯唑西林、萘夫西林、头孢唑林和头孢曲松，以及联合 β-内酰胺酶抑制剂的复合制剂（例如氨苄西林-舒巴坦），这些药物常被用于 IE 的治疗[2]。其作用机制是 β-内酰胺可抑制 PBP，进而抑制肽聚糖的合成，影响细胞壁的形成[5,18]。目前已报道了多种对 β-内酰胺耐药的机制，包括 PBP 的改变导致 β-内酰胺与 PBP 结合减少或无法结合、细胞外膜的渗透性降低或完全不可渗透、主动外排泵（译者注：微生物以向胞外转运的方式产生对一种或多种药物抗性的系统）的作用和 β-内酰胺酶的产生[18-19]。因此一旦鉴定出病原体，即应尽快获取其药敏结果，以确保选择恰当的治疗方案。

β-内酰胺类药物一般都是时间依赖性的，因此需要延长输注时间，某些情况下，甚至需要连续输注以优化治疗[20]。常见不良反应包括：过敏反应，轻者表现为轻微不适，重者可能危及生命；神经毒性，表现为癫痫发作，常见于使用大剂量头孢吡肟或亚胺培南-西司他丁时；胃肠道不适，多见于阿莫西林和氨苄西林；急性间质性肾炎，最常见于萘夫西林；艰难梭菌感染风险增加[21-22]。

糖肽类

糖肽类药物包括万古霉素、奥利万星、特拉万星和达巴万星[23]。该类药物的作用机制主要是通过干扰后期肽聚糖的合成来抑制细菌细胞壁的形成[24]。其中万古霉素常作为治疗耐甲氧西林金黄色葡萄球菌（MRSA）感染的一线药物，用于治疗革兰氏阳性病原体感染，如葡萄球菌、链球菌和肠球菌。然而，目前已出现耐药现象，其中几种耐药机制已得到阐明，包括耐万古霉素金黄色葡萄球菌和耐万古霉素肠球菌（VRE）的耐药机制。VRE 的出现主要是由 *vanA* 基因介导，该基因通过改变肽聚糖的合成而影响万古霉素的作用，这一基因还可以通过质粒从肠球菌转移给葡萄球菌，从而导致耐万古霉素葡萄球菌的产生[24-25]。

肾毒性和耳毒性是万古霉素的不良反应。虽然尚未确定耳毒性是否为剂量依赖性不良反应，但肾毒性多为大剂量所致[26]；因此，出于安全性和有效性双重考虑，应监测万古霉素血清水平。24 h 内血药浓度的时间曲线下面积与最低抑菌浓度的比值（AUC/MIC）可作为药效最准确的评价参数，但一直未找到简单有效的测量方法。为此，当前 IE 指南推荐血清谷浓度为 10~15 μg/mL[2]；有些医疗机构基于谷浓度达到 400 mg/（L·h）（AUC/MIC）才能获得最佳疗效的考量，将谷浓度目标值定于 15~20 μg/mL[27]。最近，由于相关软件的开发，计算 AUC 变得切实可行。另外，AUC 可通过测定 2 份血清样本获得：一份取自输注万古霉素后至少

1 h，另一份为下次给药前的谷浓度。据此，目前指南针对严重 MRSA 感染（包括 IE）的治疗监测，推荐基于 AUC 的测定，目标值为 400～600 mg/（L·h）[28-29]。

达巴万星和奥利万星是两种新型长效脂糖肽类药物，具有对抗革兰氏阳性病原体的作用[30]。可每周或每 2 周给药一次，因此，这些药物为传统抗菌治疗提供了一种具有吸引力的替代方案，但目前指南未予推荐。

一项回顾性研究评估了达巴万星对革兰氏阳性菌 IE 的疗效，共 27 例患者被纳入分析：自体瓣膜 IE 16 例，人工瓣膜 IE 6 例，心脏植入装置相关心内膜炎 5 例。达巴万星治疗方案包括：1000 mg 负荷剂量，随后每周 500 mg；或 1500 mg 负荷剂量，随后每 2 周 1000 mg。大多数患者（88.9%）在使用达巴万星之前接受过其他抗生素治疗，无论是作为初始用药还是序贯治疗，本组病例中 25 例患者（92.6%）从微生物学和临床评估方面均效果良好[31]。

另一项回顾性研究评估了达巴万星作为革兰氏阳性菌 IE 和（或）血流感染（BSI）病例巩固性治疗的临床疗效。研究纳入了 83 名患者，59% 为 BSI，49% 为 IE（44% 为人工瓣膜 IE，32.4% 为自体瓣膜 IE，23.5% 为起搏器电极导线感染）；使用了多种剂量方案，从 500～1500 mg 不等。IE 患者经 12 个月治疗后临床有效率达 96.7%[32]。奥利万星因其更广泛的体外活性，故在治疗 VRE 感染方面可能比达巴万星更好，但迄今为止临床数据仅限于个案报道[33-34]。

虽然目前的文献显示出良好的效果，但仍需前瞻性研究以确定长效脂糖肽制剂治疗革兰氏阳性菌 IE 的有效性和安全性。

MRSA 的其他治疗方案

达托霉素是一种环脂肽类药物。其杀菌作用机制尚不完全清楚，已知该药可抑制蛋白质、DNA 和 RNA 的合成。抗菌谱覆盖金黄色葡萄球菌（包括 MRSA）、各种链球菌和肠球菌（包括 VRE），可作为多重耐药革兰氏阳性病原体感染的替代药物[8]。不良反应是可导致血清肌酸激酶升高和肌炎[35]。因此，在治疗期间应监测血清肌酸激酶基线值，并定期复查。

利奈唑胺是恶唑烷酮类的第一个药物，其作用机制是通过与 30S 和 50S 核糖体亚基的 rRNA 结合而抑制蛋白质合成，常用于治疗多重耐药革兰氏阳性菌感染，如 MRSA 和 VRE，但对其他葡萄球菌和链球菌同样有效[36]。不良反应包括周围神经病变、贫血和血小板减少、血清乳酸升高和低血糖。此外，因利奈唑胺可抑制单胺氧化酶，在与其他 5-羟色胺类制剂联用时可导致 5-羟色胺综合征[10]；因此在利奈唑胺治疗期间，应密切观察上述不良反应的体征和症状。

辅助性抗菌治疗

·氨基糖苷类

氨基糖苷类药物中最常用的是庆大霉素，还有妥布霉素、阿米卡星和链霉素。

其抗菌机制是通过细菌细胞摄取氨基糖苷并与30S核糖体亚基的16S rRNA结合而干扰蛋白质合成[7]。因其对许多革兰氏阳性（包括葡萄球菌和肠球菌）和革兰氏阴性（包括肠杆菌）病原体以及多重耐药菌均具有活性，故临床应用较广。

氨基糖苷类的杀菌作用为浓度依赖性，用药方案有两种：常规给药或延长间隔给药[37]。常规给药是将每天的药量分2~3次给予，针对革兰氏阳性菌IE联合用药时，多采用这一方案。对于肾功能正常的患者（肌酐清除率＞60 mL/min），庆大霉素的常规剂量为24 h总量3 mg/kg，分2~3次等剂量给药。针对革兰氏阴性菌IE且肌酐清除率＞30 mL/min的患者，多采用延长间隔给药方案。根据计算的肌酐清除率，庆大霉素和妥布霉素每24~48 h用量为5 mg/kg或7 mg/kg。为治疗的安全性和有效性考虑，两种方案治疗期间均需进行药物监测[38]。

在针对革兰氏阳性菌感染联合用药的常规给药时，氨基糖苷类应在静脉给药后30 min达到血清峰浓度，目标值为3~5 mg/L；而在下次给药前30 min达到谷浓度，目标值为＜1 mg/L。即便有时谷浓度降至很低或无法测出，氨基糖苷类仍具有抑制靶病原体生长的作用，这一现象称为抗生素后效应[39]。初始药物浓度一般在稳定状态下检测（通常为在第1剂或第2剂之后），之后每2周复测一次，以指导进一步的剂量调整，并在出现新稳态后追加检测。在肾功能和容量状态出现变化时，应及时检测血清药物浓度。延长给药间隔的药物监测策略包括随机测量血清药物浓度水平和使用列线图（例如Hartford列线图）[38,40]。除检测血清药物浓度外，还必须监测肾损害和耳毒性，这两者均为剂量依赖性的[37]。

· 氟喹诺酮类

氟喹诺酮类包括环丙沙星、左氧氟沙星和莫西沙星等几种药物，作用机制是通过与DNA旋转酶相互作用抑制DNA复制和转录，从而抑制拓扑异构酶Ⅱ；此外，还可抑制拓扑异构酶Ⅳ，导致细胞凋亡。由于该类抗生素中不同药物的抗菌谱不同，因此它们对革兰氏阳性和革兰氏阴性病原体的抗菌活性也存在差异[41]。

药物不良反应包括精神障碍，如定向和记忆障碍，以及低血糖、周围神经病变、主动脉破裂和撕裂、肌腱炎和肌腱断裂等。因此，对于有肌腱炎或肌腱断裂病史的患者应避免使用。另外，该药可导致重症肌无力患者症状加重[42]。

· 利福平

利福平是一种RNA聚合酶抑制剂，被推荐作为治疗由葡萄球菌引起的人工瓣膜IE的辅助药物[2,43]。这是基于利福平的杀菌机制——可杀灭葡萄球菌引起的外源性材料的感染，而在与细胞壁抑制剂联合使用时，还可产生协同作用，提高杀菌效率[44]。不良反应包括厌食等胃肠道副作用、肝毒性、骨髓抑制和流感样症状。利福平是一种细胞色素P450诱导剂，对药物代谢有较大影响，可导致多种药物之间的相互作用。在使用利福平之前，应仔细了解患者的既往用药史。由于对耐药性的担心，利福平应该在血培养明确有效后才能使用[45]。治疗IE抗菌药物的常见剂量、监测参数和临床要点见表7.4。

表 7.4 治疗感染性心内膜炎（IE）的常用抗生素[2]

抗生素	剂量（基于正常肾功能）	监测参数	临床要点
β-内酰胺类			
·水溶性青霉素 G	$(12\sim30)\times10^6$ U/24 h，静脉持续输注（首选）或每 4 h 一次	过敏反应、肾功能	剂量取决于敏感性
·氨苄西林	2 g，静脉注射，每 4 h 一次	过敏反应、肾功能、胃肠道不适	
·萘夫西林	12 g/24 h，静脉持续输注（首选）或每 4 h 一次分次给药	过敏反应、肾功能	肾功能减退时无须调整剂量，尽管可能发生急性间质性肾炎
·苯唑西林	12 g/24 h，静脉持续输注（首选）或每 4 h 一次分次给药	过敏反应	肾功能减退时无须调整剂量
·头孢唑林	2 g，静脉注射，每 8 h 一次	过敏反应	头孢唑林与其他青霉素没有共同的侧链结构，因此可考虑用于青霉素非严重过敏时（即非过敏性休克型反应）
·头孢噻肟	2 g，静脉注射，每 4~6 h 一次	过敏反应	
·头孢曲松	2 g，静脉注射，每 24 h 一次 双 β-内酰胺类联用时：2 g，静脉注射，每 12 h 一次	过敏反应	肾功能减退时无须调整剂量
氨基糖苷类			
·阿米卡星	革兰氏阴性菌：15 mg/kg，静脉注射，每 24 h 一次	肾毒性、耳毒性 ·革兰氏阳性菌协同用药：庆大霉素目标峰浓度为 3~5 μg/mL，目标谷浓度为 <1 μg/mL；链霉素目标峰浓度为 20~35 μg/mL，目标谷浓度 <10 μg/mL ·革兰氏阴性菌感染的延长间隔给药：庆大霉素、妥布霉素和阿米卡星（每个列线图的目标随机水平）[40,46]	
·庆大霉素	·革兰氏阳性菌协同用药：24 h 剂量为 3 mg/kg，静脉或肌内注射，分 2~3 次等量给药 ·草绿色链球菌或解没食子酸链球菌：3 mg/kg，静脉或肌内注射，每 24 h 一次 ·革兰氏阴性菌：5 mg/kg 或 7 mg/kg 静脉注射，每 24 h 一次		
·链霉素	革兰氏阳性菌协同用药：24 h 剂量为 15 mg/kg（理想体重），静脉或肌内注射，分 2 次等剂量		
·妥布霉素	革兰氏阴性菌：5 mg/kg 或 7 mg/kg，静脉注射，每 24 h 一次		

表 7.4（续）

抗生素	剂量（基于正常肾功能）	监测参数	临床要点
糖肽类			
·万古霉素	15~20 mg/kg，静脉注射，每 8~24 h 一次	肾毒性、耳毒性；目标谷浓度为 15~20 μg/mL，目标 AUC 为 400~600 mg/（L·h）	应在达到稳定状态后、下次用药前 30 min 获得谷浓度值
环脂肽类			
·达托霉素	葡萄球菌：>8 mg/kg，静脉注射，每 24 h 一次 肠球菌：10~12 mg/kg，静脉注射，每 24 h 一次	基线和每周的磷酸肌酸激酶（CPK）、肌肉分解/无力、肾功能	以下情况需停用达托霉素：CPK>1000 U/L（有症状）或>2000 U/L（无症状）[47]
氟喹诺酮类			
·环丙沙星	400 mg 静脉注射或 500 mg 口服，每 12 h 一次	精神状态、血糖水平、肌腱炎或肌腱断裂、肾功能、QTc 间期	避免在有肌腱炎或肌腱断裂病史的患者中使用 可能导致 QTc 间期延长，使用时建议密切监测
·左氧氟沙星	750 mg，静脉注射，每 24 h 一次		
·莫西沙星	400 mg，静脉注射，每 24 h 一次		
恶唑烷酮类			
·利奈唑胺	600 mg 静脉注射或口服，每 12 h 一次	5-羟色胺综合征、血小板减少、周围神经病变	由于会增加 5-羟色胺综合征的风险，因此不能同时使用 1 种以上的 5-羟色胺制剂
其他			
·利福平	900 mg/24 h，静脉注射或口服，分 3 次用药	胃肠道不适、骨髓抑制、肝毒性、流感样症状	利福平与许多药物之间存在相互作用，在开始治疗前，需要对患者的药物清单进行仔细评估 需要就利福平导致体液（包括眼泪和尿液）变色（红色）提供咨询

经验性用药

一旦临床怀疑 IE，就应立即开始抗生素经验性治疗。应使用广谱抗生素以覆盖所有可疑病原体，直到鉴定出病原体和得到药敏结果；此时，原治疗方案可降阶为针对性较强的窄谱抗生素。经验性治疗方案常常包括可覆盖革兰氏阳性球菌（包括 MRSA），以及革兰氏阴性杆菌（如铜绿假单胞菌）的药物。在选择适当的治疗方案时应考虑 IE 的风险因素，因此，不存在"标准的经验性治疗方案"，而是应针对每名患者制定个体化的经验性治疗方案。各种风险因素相关的病原体和相应的经验性治疗方案见表 7.5。

表 7.5　感染性心内膜炎（IE）的风险因素相关病原体和经验性抗菌方案

风险因素	相关病原体	经验性抗菌治疗方案
・静脉吸毒	金黄色葡萄球菌、凝固酶阴性葡萄球菌、β-溶血性链球菌、真菌、需氧革兰氏阴性杆菌	万古霉素 + 头孢吡肟 / 哌拉西林 - 他唑巴坦 ± 抗真菌药
・心血管内装置	金黄色葡萄球菌、凝固酶阴性葡萄球菌、真菌、需氧革兰氏阴性杆菌、棒状杆菌	万古霉素 + 头孢吡肟 / 哌拉西林 - 他唑巴坦 ± 抗真菌药
・泌尿生殖系统疾病、感染及相关操作，包括怀孕、分娩、流产	肠球菌、B 族链球菌、单核细胞增多性李斯特菌、需氧革兰氏阴性杆菌、淋球菌	哌拉西林 - 他唑巴坦 ± 万古霉素
・慢性皮肤病	金黄色葡萄球菌、β-溶血性链球菌	万古霉素 + 头孢曲松
・口腔卫生不佳、牙科操作	草绿色链球菌、营养变异链球菌、缺陷乏氧菌、颗粒链球菌、孪生球菌、HACEK	头孢吡肟 / 哌拉西林 - 他唑巴坦 ± 万古霉素
・酒精中毒、肝硬化	巴尔通体、气单胞菌、李斯特菌、肺炎链球菌、β-溶血性链球菌	头孢吡肟 / 哌拉西林 - 他唑巴坦 ± 万古霉素
・烧伤	金黄色葡萄球菌、需氧革兰氏阴性杆菌、真菌	万古霉素 ± 头孢吡肟 / 哌拉西林 - 他唑巴坦 ± 抗真菌药
・糖尿病	金黄色葡萄球菌、肺炎链球菌、β-溶血性链球菌	万古霉素 + 头孢曲松
・人工瓣膜	・植入 <1 年：凝固酶阴性葡萄球菌、金黄色葡萄球菌、需氧革兰氏阴性杆菌、真菌、棒状杆菌、军团菌 ・植入 >1 年：凝固酶阴性葡萄球菌、金黄色葡萄球菌、草绿色链球菌、肠球菌、真菌、棒状杆菌	・植入 <1 年：万古霉素 + 哌拉西林 - 他唑巴坦 + 环丙沙星 / 左氧氟沙星[48] ・植入 >1 年：万古霉素 + 哌拉西林 - 他唑巴坦 ± 抗真菌药
・接触狗、猫	巴尔通体、巴斯德菌、二氧化碳嗜纤维菌	哌拉西林 - 他唑巴坦 + 庆大霉素[49-52]
・接触受污染的牛奶、受感染的农场动物	布鲁氏菌、贝纳柯克斯体、丹毒丝菌	多西环素 + 左氧氟沙星[53-55]

表 7.5（续）

风险因素	相关病原体	经验性抗菌治疗方案
·无家可归、体虱	巴尔通体	哌拉西林 – 他唑巴坦 + 庆大霉素 [49-50]
·艾滋病	沙门氏菌、肺炎链球菌、金黄色葡萄球菌	万古霉素 + 哌拉西林 – 他唑巴坦
·肺炎、脑膜炎	肺炎链球菌	万古霉素 + 头孢曲松
·实体器官移植史	金黄色葡萄球菌、烟曲霉、肠球菌、念珠菌	万古霉素 + 哌拉西林 – 他唑巴坦 ± 抗真菌药
·胃肠道病变	解没食子酸链球菌、肠球菌、败毒梭菌	哌拉西林 – 他唑巴坦 + 万古霉素

HACEK：嗜血杆菌属、凝聚杆菌属、心杆菌属、侵蚀艾肯菌属、金氏杆菌属。改编自：L.M. Baddour, et al., Infective endocarditis in adults: diagnosis, antimicrobial therapy, and management of complications: a scientific statement for healthcare professionals from the American Heart Association. Circulation, 2015, 132(15): 1435–1486.

靶向治疗 [2]

确定感染病原体后，为减少不必要的治疗用药所带来的药物不良反应和耐药风险，必须缩小抗菌范围，针对病原菌进行靶向治疗。治疗持续时间取决于病原体、瓣膜类型和所选择的药物。表 7.6 描述了基于病原菌和瓣膜类型所制定的靶向治疗方案。

对于无法耐受 β – 内酰胺类药物的患者（例如过敏反应、无法耐受的副作用），万古霉素可作为替代治疗 [2]。但对于甲氧西林敏感金黄色葡萄球菌（MSSA）IE，应尽量不要使用万古霉素，因为万古霉素治疗 MSSA IE 效果较差 [56]。青霉素过敏虽然很常见，但并不妨碍其他 β – 内酰胺类抗生素的使用，如头孢菌素，因为青霉素和头孢菌素之间的交叉反应很少见 [57]。如果必须使用 β – 内酰胺类药物，可先行抗生素脱敏，如果这一方案不可行，再考虑使用万古霉素。另外，达托霉素也是一种替代选择，且疗效不比标准治疗方案差 [58-59]。

IE 的少见病因

革兰氏阴性菌 IE

HACEK（嗜血杆菌属、凝聚杆菌属、心杆菌属、侵蚀艾肯菌属和金氏杆菌属）是一大类对培养条件较为挑剔的革兰氏阴性杆菌，在常规血琼脂培养基中生长缓慢，是血培养阴性 IE 的常见病因。这类病原体通常对氨苄西林耐药，除非药敏试验证实其敏感，故青霉素和氨苄西林不宜用于治疗由 HACEK 引起的 IE。可使用头孢曲松或其他第三代和第四代头孢菌素以及氟喹诺酮类药物，HACEK 对这些药

表 7.6 感染性心内膜炎（IE）靶向治疗方案和治疗持续时间 [2]

病原体	瓣膜类型	治疗方案	持续时间
·草绿色链球菌	自体瓣膜	·青霉素 MIC≤0.12 μg/mL：水溶性青霉素 G[a] 或头孢曲松，在无肾功能不全的情况下考虑加用庆大霉素[b] ·青霉素 0.12 μg/mL＜MIC≤0.5 μg/mL：水溶性青霉素 G[a] 或头孢曲松 + 庆大霉素 ·青霉素 MIC＞0.5 μg/mL：青霉素 G[a] 或头孢曲松 + 庆大霉素	4 周 + 选择性 2 周庆大霉素
	人工瓣膜	·青霉素 MIC≤0.12 μg/mL：水溶性青霉素 G[a] 或头孢曲松，考虑加用庆大霉素[b] ·青霉素 MIC＞0.12 μg/mL 但＜0.5 μg/mL：水溶性青霉素 G[a] 或头孢曲松 + 庆大霉素 ·青霉素 MIC＞0.5 μg/mL：青霉素 G[a] 或头孢曲松 + 庆大霉素	· MIC ≤ 0.12 μg/mL：6 周 + 选择性 2 周庆大霉素 · MIC＞0.12 μg/mL：6 周 +6 周庆大霉素
·解没食子酸链球菌	自体瓣膜	·青霉素 MIC≤0.12 μg/mL：水溶性青霉素 G[a] 或头孢曲松，考虑加用庆大霉素 ·青霉素 MIC＞0.12 μg/mL 但＜0.5 μg/mL：水溶性青霉素 G[a] 或头孢曲松 + 庆大霉素 ·青霉素 MIC＞0.5 μg/mL：青霉素 G[a] + 庆大霉素	4 周 + 选择性 2 周庆大霉素
	人工瓣膜	·青霉素 MIC≤0.12 μg/mL：水溶性青霉素 G[a] 或头孢曲松，考虑加用庆大霉素[b] ·青霉素 MIC＞0.12 μg/mL 但＜0.5 μg/mL：水溶性青霉素 G[a] 或头孢曲松 + 庆大霉素 ·青霉素 MIC＞0.5 μg/mL：青霉素 G[a] + 庆大霉素	· MIC ≤ 0.12 μg/mL：6 周 + 选择性 2 周庆大霉素 · MIC＞0.12 μg/mL：6 周 +6 周庆大霉素
·缺陷乏养菌	自体瓣膜	水溶性青霉素 G[a]+ 庆大霉素	4 周 + 选择性 2 周庆大霉素
	人工瓣膜	水溶性青霉素 G[a]+ 庆大霉素	6 周 +6 周庆大霉素
·颗粒链球菌[c]	自体瓣膜	水溶性青霉素 G[a]+ 庆大霉素	4 周 + 选择性 2 周庆大霉素
	人工瓣膜	水溶性青霉素 G[a]+ 庆大霉素	6 周 +6 周庆大霉素
·肺炎链球菌	自体瓣膜	·无脑膜炎：水溶性青霉素 G、头孢唑林或头孢曲松 ·脑膜炎：头孢噻肟或头孢曲松 ·脑膜炎，且头孢噻肟 MIC＞2 μg/mL：头孢噻肟或头孢曲松 + 万古霉素 + 利福平	4 周

113

表 7.6（续）

病原体	瓣膜类型	治疗方案	持续时间
	人工瓣膜	· 无脑膜炎：水溶性青霉素 G、头孢唑林或头孢曲松 · 脑膜炎：头孢噻肟或头孢曲松 · 脑膜炎，且头孢噻肟 MIC>2 μg/mL：头孢噻肟或头孢曲松 + 万古霉素 + 利福平	6 周
· 化脓性链球菌	自体瓣膜或人工瓣膜	水溶性青霉素 G 或头孢曲松	4～6 周
· B、C、F 和 G 族 β-溶血性链球菌	自体瓣膜或人工瓣膜	水溶性青霉素 G 或头孢曲松，考虑加用庆大霉素	4～6 周 + 选择性>2 周庆大霉素
· 甲氧西林敏感金黄色葡萄球菌	自体瓣膜	萘夫西林或苯唑西林，如果对青霉素有非严重过敏反应，可用头孢唑林	· 无并发症的右侧 IE：2 周 · 无并发症左侧 IE 和存在共病的 IE：6 周
	人工瓣膜	萘夫西林或苯唑西林 + 利福平 + 庆大霉素	>6 周 +2 周庆大霉素
· 耐甲氧西林金黄色葡萄球菌	自体瓣膜	万古霉素或达托霉素	6 周
	人工瓣膜	万古霉素 + 利福平 + 庆大霉素	>6 周 +2 周庆大霉素
· 凝固酶阴性葡萄球菌	人工瓣膜	· 万古霉素 + 利福平 + 庆大霉素（或敏感的氨基糖苷类药物） · 考虑氟喹诺酮类药物（如果没有氨基糖苷类敏感药物）	>6 周 +2 周氨基糖苷类/氟喹诺酮类药物
· 肠球菌	自体瓣膜或人工瓣膜	· 青霉素和庆大霉素敏感：1) 水溶性青霉素 G 或氨苄西林 + 庆大霉素，或 2) 氨苄西林 + 头孢曲松 · 青霉素敏感但庆大霉素耐药：1) 氨苄西林 + 头孢曲松，或 2) 水溶性青霉素 G 或氨苄西林 + 链霉素[d]（如果敏感） · 青霉素耐药但万古霉素和庆大霉素敏感：万古霉素 + 庆大霉素 · 青霉素、氨基糖苷类和万古霉素耐药：利奈唑胺或达托霉素	· β-内酰胺类 + 氨基糖苷类：4～6 周 · β-内酰胺类 + 氨基糖苷类用于人工瓣膜：6 周 · 双 β-内酰胺类：6 周 · 万古霉素 + 庆大霉素：6 周 · 利奈唑胺或达托霉素：>6 周

[a] 在青霉素短缺的情况下，氨苄西林是合适的替代品。[b] 在金黄色葡萄球菌人工瓣膜 IE 中可加用利福平。[c] 如分离出缺陷乏养菌或颗粒链球菌，由于这类病原体根除难度较大，强烈建议请感染科会诊，以优化治疗方案及疗程。[d] 肌酐清除率<50 mL/min 的患者应避免使用链霉素。如果肠球菌菌株对庆大霉素和链霉素均敏感，则应使用庆大霉素而不是链霉素。当庆大霉素治疗不可行时，可采用双 β-内酰胺类方案（见后文）

物通常敏感。一般而言，自体瓣膜 IE 治疗时间为 4 周，人工瓣膜 IE 为 6 周。

其他革兰氏阴性杆菌（如肠杆菌和假单胞菌）同样是 IE 的罕见致病菌，通常与医疗暴露、人工瓣膜和其他血管内植入装置有关，治疗包括心脏手术和长时间抗生素治疗。美国心脏协会（AHA）指南推荐使用一种 β - 内酰胺类联合一种氨基糖苷类或氟喹诺酮类治疗 6 周。但由于存在各种耐药机制，这些病原体常可以隐蔽生存，因此应请感染科专家会诊，协助制定最佳抗生素治疗方案[2,60]。

血培养阴性 IE

血培养阳性是 IE 的主要诊断标准。然而，血培养阴性 IE 占到了所有病例的 5%~10%。血培养阴性有多种原因，包括血培养之前使用抗菌药物、病原体的培养条件苛刻和（或）微生物学检测技术不足等。血培养阴性 IE 的治疗具有挑战性，因为某些药物治疗时间延长可能具有潜在毒性。这类病例的内科治疗应视患者具体情况而定，包括既往心血管感染史、抗菌药物既往使用情况、临床病程、感染的严重程度和心外感染的部位。某些常规血培养条件下不能生长的病原体，可能需要特定的诊断技术，包括巴尔通体、贝纳柯克斯体和布鲁氏菌[2]。表 7.7 描述了血培养阴性 IE 的一些重要临床特征，以用于指导抗菌治疗。

真菌性 IE

真菌性 IE 发生率不高，但死亡率较高。其感染的风险因素包括静脉吸毒、免疫功能低下、植入有心血管装置和人工瓣膜。多种真菌可引起 IE，念珠菌和曲霉菌是最常见的病原体。真菌在常规血琼脂培养平板上生长不良，因此血培养阴性较为常见，尤其是曲霉菌。真菌性 IE 的主要治疗手段是手术修复受感染的瓣膜以及抗真菌药物治疗，通常使用两性霉素 B[2]。念珠菌 IE 推荐的初始治疗方案是脂质体两性霉素 B 3~5 mg/（kg·d），加或不加氟胞嘧啶 25 mg/kg，每天 4 次，或高剂量棘白素（卡泊芬净 150 mg/d，米卡芬净 150 mg/d，或阿尼芬净 200 mg/d）[61]。术后初始以此方案治疗至少 6 周，然后使用病原体敏感的口服唑类药物终生治疗，以抑制真菌[2,61]。

表 7.7 血培养阴性心内膜炎的临床方案

发病	瓣膜类型	相关病原体	治疗方案
急性（d）	自体瓣膜	金黄色葡萄球菌、β-溶血性链球菌和需氧革兰氏阴性杆菌	万古霉素+头孢吡肟
亚急性（周）	自体瓣膜	金黄色葡萄球菌、草绿色链球菌、HACEK 和肠球菌	万古霉素+氨苄西林-舒巴坦
瓣膜置换术后<1年	人工瓣膜	葡萄球菌、肠球菌、需氧革兰氏阴性杆菌	万古霉素+利福平+庆大霉素+头孢吡肟
瓣膜置换术后>1年	人工瓣膜	葡萄球菌、草绿色链球菌、肠球菌	万古霉素+头孢曲松

临床处理要点

头孢唑林与抗葡萄球菌青霉素对比

抗葡萄球菌青霉素（例如萘夫西林或苯唑西林）目前作为一线药物，推荐用于治疗 MSSA 菌血症和 IE。对于头孢唑林，AHA 指南推荐其仅用于青霉素非严重过敏（非过敏性休克型反应）时的替代，因为与萘夫西林或苯唑西林相比，头孢唑林可能更容易受到 A 型 blaZ 基因 β-内酰胺酶介导的水解的影响，同时还有接种量效应，可导致临床治疗失败[1,2,62]。

所有 β-内酰胺类药物均存在临床不良反应，包括过敏反应、神经系统副作用、骨髓抑制、间质性肾炎和肝毒性。与头孢唑林相比，抗葡萄球菌青霉素的不良反应（例如间质性肾炎、肝毒性、中性粒细胞减少）的发生率更高；而头孢唑林除上述不良反应较少外，还有其他一些优点，包括含钠量较低、可透析后给药和费用较低等[62]。一项回顾性队列研究对比了头孢唑林与萘夫西林治疗 MSSA 血流感染的情况，结果显示：萘夫西林组和头孢唑林组的急性肾损伤发生率分别为 26/81（32%）和 9/68（13%）（P=0.007）[63]。

一篇综述对 7 项回顾性研究（关于头孢唑林与抗葡萄球菌青霉素治疗 MSSA 菌血症的临床疗效）进行了总结，发现各研究尽管在设计上存在较大差异，但头孢唑林的疗效与抗葡萄球菌青霉素无差异。当然，这些研究也存在局限性，包括样本量小、心内膜炎病例少，5 项研究存在明显潜在的选择性偏倚，且没有研究头孢唑林的接种量效应或产生的 β-内酰胺酶类型[62]。

尽管这些研究存在局限性，但头孢唑林仍以其广谱的作用成为抗葡萄球菌青霉素之外、治疗 MSSA IE 的合理替代选择[62]。一项针对感染科临床医生的调查显示，89% 的受访者愿意使用头孢唑林作为单一药物治疗 MSSA 自体瓣膜 IE[64]。

抗菌协同作用

将具有不同作用机制的抗菌药物联合使用可以产生单一药物所不具备的杀菌效果，这种作用被称为协同作用。在 IE 常见病原体中，目前仅阐明了对肠球菌的杀菌协同作用机制。目前，AHA 心内膜炎指南推荐对青霉素和氨基糖苷类敏感的肠球菌分离株进行联合治疗，可采用双 β-内酰胺类（氨苄西林+头孢曲松）或 β-内酰胺类加氨基糖苷类方案[2]。

β-内酰胺类和氨基糖苷类药物之间的体外协同杀菌作用已被证明可将 IE 治愈率提高到 75%[65]。在没有细胞壁活性药物协同的情况下，氨基糖苷类药物进入革兰氏阳性病原体细胞受到限制。β-内酰胺可抑制细胞壁形成，协助氨基糖苷类进入细胞并抑制细菌蛋白质合成。而氨基糖苷类高耐药性的肠球菌（HLRAG）不易受到这种协同作用的影响，结果可能是对 IE 的联合用药抗感染效果下降[66]。

由于肠球菌的固有特征和不断增加的耐药性，治疗肠球菌 IE 等深部感染成为临床工作中的一大挑战。由于 β-内酰胺类药物缺乏对肠球菌的杀菌活性，需要多种药物联合才能发挥协同作用。目前 AHA 心内膜炎指南推荐针对青霉素和氨基糖苷类敏感菌株采用联合用药，可以是双 β-内酰胺类（氨苄西林+头孢曲松）或 β-内酰胺类加氨基糖苷类[2]。

由于粪肠球菌分离株中 HLRAG 越来越常见，双 β-内酰胺类方案应运而生。该组合通过氨苄西林使 PBP4 和 PBP5 部分饱和，头孢曲松使非必需的 PBP2 和 PBP3 完全饱和，从而发挥协同作用，以强化对病原体细胞壁合成的深度破坏[65]。氨苄西林和头孢曲松的组合是具有吸引力的替代治疗方案，它避免了传统方案中长期使用氨基糖苷类带来的潜在不良作用（例如肾毒性和耳毒性）。

在一项针对美国和加拿大医生的调查中，83% 的受访者倾向于首选双 β-内酰胺类方案[64]，这可能与目前肠球菌分离株中 HLRAG 的增加以及氨基糖苷类的相关毒性有关[66]。虽然从肾毒性的角度来看，氨苄西林加头孢曲松比氨基糖苷类更安全，但头孢曲松同样存在药物安全性问题，例如头孢曲松已被证明是艰难梭菌和 VRE 感染发生的独立风险因素[67-68]。

其他头孢菌素类药物，如头孢吡肟和头孢洛林，与氨苄西林联用，和单独使用氨苄西林相比，药效学研究显示出更强的抗菌活性[69]。目前尚无证据表明头孢吡肟和头孢洛林会增加 VRE 定植的风险，因此这可能是比指南推荐的治疗方案更安全的替代方案[70-71]。指南推荐的两种联合用药方案其依据均存在局限性，因此双重联合用药的必要性被提上议事日程，如果需要，最佳方案应该是怎样的？另外，针对肠球菌 IE 最安全、最有效的方案还需要进一步的研究予以证实。

口服抗生素的作用

长期以来，长时间静脉注射抗生素是 IE 的主要治疗方法。但这一方法存在诸多潜在风险，包括导管相关的血流感染、导管堵塞和血栓形成；此外，还有治疗成本高、患者安置及转运不便、给药通路的维护等不利因素[72]。为此，2015 年的 AHA 和欧洲心脏病学会（ESC）心内膜炎指南在推荐静脉注射抗生素作为整个疗程（例如 2~6 周）的一线治疗的同时，也建议针对无并发症的右侧自体瓣膜 MSSA IE、耐药肠球菌自体瓣膜或人工瓣膜 IE 以及 HACEK 引起的自体瓣膜或人工瓣膜 IE，可使用口服治疗作为替代[2,73]。

部分口服与静脉注射抗生素治疗心内膜炎试验（POET）是一项前瞻性、随机、非劣效性、多中心研究，受试者为 400 名病情稳定的患有链球菌、粪肠球菌、金黄色葡萄球菌或凝固酶阴性葡萄球菌引起的左侧 IE 成年患者。值得注意的是，该试验中没有 MRSA 患者。所有患者均接受静脉注射抗生素治疗至少 10 d，然后随机分为继续静脉注射治疗或在剩余疗程中改为口服治疗两组[74]。口服方案一般选用具有中高生物利用度的抗生素，联合使用两种具有不同作用机制的药物（表 7.8）[74-75]。需要提到的是，美国无口服夫西地酸。

主要结局是从随机分组开始到抗生素治疗完成后 6 个月期间的全因死亡率、

表 7.8　POET 试验采用的联合口服方案 [71]

- 阿莫西林 1 g（每天 4 次）+ 夫西地酸 750 mg（每天 2 次）
- 阿莫西林 1 g（每天 4 次）+ 利福平 600 mg（每天 2 次）
- 双氯西林 1 g（每天 4 次）+ 夫西地酸 750 mg（每天 2 次）
- 双氯西林 1 g（每天 4 次）+ 利福平 600 mg（每天 2 次）
- 利奈唑胺 600 mg（每天 2 次）+ 莫西沙星 400 mg（每天 1 次）
- 利奈唑胺 600 mg（每天 2 次）+ 夫西地酸 750 mg（每天 2 次）
- 利奈唑胺 600 mg（每天 2 次）+ 利福平 600 mg（每天 2 次）
- 莫西沙星 400 mg（每天 1 次）+ 克林霉素 600 mg（每天 3 次）

非计划心脏手术、栓塞事件或原发病原体菌血症复发等综合指标。共 42 名患者（10.5%）发生复合终点事件：静脉治疗组 24 例（12.1%），口服治疗组 18 例（9.0%）（OR=0.72，95%CI=0.37 ~ 1.36）。研究表明，在病情稳定的左侧 IE 患者中，改用口服抗生素并不劣于静脉注射抗生素 [74]。

一篇系统性综述研究了口服降阶方案治疗 IE 的效果。24 项研究（21 项观察性或准试验性研究和 3 项随机对照试验）纳入该研究范围，它们均将口服抗生素作为治疗方案的一部分。结果显示，没有一项研究表明静脉注射治疗比口服降阶治疗更有效。然而，确定适合采用口服降阶治疗的病例至关重要，患者应满足以下标准 [76]：①临床病情稳定；②菌血症得到清除；③口服吸收可靠；④缺乏选择静脉治疗的社会心理原因；⑤已有文献证实口服治疗方案对致病微生物敏感。

值得注意的是，大多数已发表的研究都采用联合口服治疗方案。关于口服降阶治疗方案的推荐见表 7.9 [76]。

目前已有大量关于通过口服降阶疗法而不是长期静脉注射治疗 IE 的成功报道，而正确的患者选择至关重要，这包括所选病例临床稳定和菌血症已得到清除 [76-77]。

表 7.9　口服降阶抗生素推荐 [76]

抗生素	病原菌	临床评价
阿莫西林（1 g，每天 4 次）	对青霉素高度敏感链球菌（MIC ≤ 0.12 μg/mL）	
左氧氟沙星（750 mg，每天 1 次）或莫西沙星（400 mg，每天 1 次）	敏感的革兰氏阳性菌	需要与第 2 种抗生素联合使用
利奈唑胺（600 mg，每天 2 次）	敏感的革兰氏阳性菌	单独使用或与第 2 种抗生素联合使用
复方磺胺甲恶唑（TMP-SMX）（每天 960 ~ 4800 mg，分 2 ~ 3 次服用）	金黄色葡萄球菌	仅在初始其他静脉注射药物后使用，如可能，静脉注射 TMP-SMX 联合静脉注射克林霉素

门诊肠外抗菌治疗计划

使用长疗程肠外抗菌药物是目前治疗血管内感染的标准方法。这一方案要求患者能从住院治疗过渡到门诊肠外抗菌治疗（OPAT）计划，在家或社区完成治疗。在此期间，由感染科相关医务人员、药剂师、护士和协调员组成的跨专业团队负责进行监测。OPAT 计划的目标是通过提供针对静脉抗生素用药患者的不同专业护理需求来减少住院时间、降低再入院率[78]。

决定转至门诊治疗取决于几个关键因素，包括近期静脉吸毒史、患者的自我管理能力、身边有无照护者、社会因素和保险问题等，这些都是出院前必须考虑的因素。选择居家治疗要求家庭保健护士可登门为患者注射抗菌药物，而经验丰富的护理机构或门诊输液中心更适合活动能力受限的患者。由于心内膜炎与静脉吸毒的关联性越来越强，因此对自行静脉注射抗生素的担忧包括依从性、输注管道的操作、社会心理问题和失访[78-79]。潜在的解决方案包括缩短静脉注射时间、使用口服抗生素替代，或是长效抗生素的使用，这样患者仅需每周前往输液中心就诊。这些患者常常一出院即转往成熟的护理机构。尽管没有证据表明院外操作失误的风险有所降低[78]，但起码一些社会问题可以得到解决，且临床随访得以增加。

药剂师管理的 OPAT 计划允许药剂师根据与感染科医生的合作实践协议（CPA）进行工作，以改善患者的治疗结局并减少不良反应的发生[80]。OPAT 药剂师通过评估每周实验室检查结果，并与患者或家庭保健护士沟通以评估不良反应，定期参与药物监测。根据 CPA 中对肾功能和血浆浓度的概述进行剂量调整。门诊环境为心内膜炎患者提供了独特的治疗机会，当然 OPAT 失败的潜在风险也很高，这也说明越来越需要更强有力的研究以找到更为可靠的替代方案。

对未来的思考和总结

总之，IE 的治疗应从经验性的广谱抗生素治疗开始，当明确病原体及其药敏结果后，可逐步降级至最窄谱的药物。IE 的治疗选择为深入研究抗菌药物的重要药理学特性（例如相关药物的药效学）提供了机会。抗菌治疗的持续时间可以是长期的，这主要取决于病原体和心脏瓣膜类型。最近的研究评估了多种治疗模式，包括部分口服抗菌药物治疗，以进一步改善患者的治疗体验和结局。鉴于 IE 的复杂性和较长的随访时间，强烈建议 IE 患者咨询感染科专家，尤其是多药耐药病原体引起 IE 的患者以及对多种药物过敏的患者。

参考文献

[1] Wang A, Gaca JG, Chu VH. Management considerations in infective endocarditis: a review. J Am Med Assoc, 2018, 320(1): 72–83.

[2] Baddour LM, et al. Infective endocarditis in adults: diagnosis, antimicrobial therapy, and management of complications: a scientific statement for healthcare professionals from the American heart association. Circulation, 2015, 132(15): 1435–1486.

[3] Chopra T, Kaatz GW. Treatment strategies for infective endocarditis. Expet Opin Pharmacother, 2010, 11(3): 345–360.
[4] Cahill TJ, et al. Challenges in infective endocarditis. J Am Coll Cardiol, 2017, 69(3): 325–344.
[5] Bush K, Bradford PA. beta-Lactams and beta-Lactamase Inhibitors: an Overview. Cold Spring Harb Perspect Med, 2016, 6(8).
[6] Allen NE, Nicas TI. Mechanism of action of oritavancin and related glycopeptide antibiotics. FEMS Microbiol Rev, 2003, 26(5): 511–532.
[7] Krause KM, et al. Aminoglycosides: an overview. Cold Spring Harb Perspect Med, 2016, 6(6).
[8] Heidary M, et al. Daptomycin. J Antimicrob Chemother, 2018, 73(1): 1–11.
[9] Sanders CC. Ciprofloxacin: in vitro activity, mechanism of action, and resistance. Rev Infect Dis, 1988, 10(3): 516–527.
[10] Hashemian SMR, Farhadi T, Ganjparvar M. Linezolid: a review of its properties, function, and use in critical care. Drug Des Dev Ther, 2018, 12: 1759–1767.
[11] Durack DT, Beeson PB. Experimental bacterial endocarditis. II. Survival of a bacteria in endocardial vegetations. Br J Exp Pathol, 1972, 53(1): 50–53.
[12] Levison ME, Levison JH. Pharmacokinetics and pharmacodynamics of antibacterial agents. Infect Dis Clin, 2009, 23(4): 791–815 [vii].
[13] Wald-Dickler N, Holtom P, Spellberg B. Busting the myth of "static vs cidal": a systemic literature review. Clin Infect Dis, 2018, 66(9): 1470–1474.
[14] Spellberg B. Principles of antiinfective therapy//Mandell GL, Bennett JE, Dolin R. Mandell, Douglas, and Bennett's principles and practices of infectious diseases. Philadelphia, PA: Churchill Livingstone/Elsevier, 2020: 211–221.
[15] Pankey GA, Sabath LD. Clinical relevance of bacteriostatic versus bactericidal mechanisms of action in the treatment of Gram-positive bacterial infections. Clin Infect Dis, 2004, 38(6): 864–870.
[16] Tan C, et al. The inoculum effect and band-pass bacterial response to periodic antibiotic treatment. Mol Syst Biol, 2012, 8: 617.
[17] Lenhard JR, Bulman ZP. Inoculum effect of beta-lactam antibiotics. J Antimicrob Chemother, 2019, 74(10): 2825–2843.
[18] Shahid M, et al. Beta-lactams and beta-lactamase-inhibitors in current- or potential-clinical practice: a comprehensive update. Crit Rev Microbiol, 2009, 35(2): 81–108.
[19] Pitout JD, Sanders CC, Sanders Jr WE. Antimicrobial resistance with focus on beta-lactam resistance in gram-negative bacilli. Am J Med, 1997, 103(1): 51–59.
[20] Grupper M, Kuti JL, Nicolau DP. Continuous and prolonged intravenous beta-lactam dosing: implications for the clinical laboratory. Clin Microbiol Rev, 2016, 29(4): 759–772.
[21] Gallagher JC, MacDougall C. Antibiotics simplified. 4th ed. Burlington, MA: Jones&Bartlett Learning, 2017.
[22] Burrelli CC, et al. Does the beta-lactam matter? Nafcillin versus cefazolin for methicillin-susceptible Staphylococcus aureus bloodstream infections. Chemotherapy, 2018, 63(6): 345–351.
[23] Pace JL, Yang G. Glycopeptides: update on an old successful antibiotic class. Biochem Pharmacol, 2006, 71(7): 968–980.
[24] McGuinness WA, Malachowa N, DeLeo FR. Vancomycin resistance in Staphylococcus aureus. Yale J Biol Med, 2017, 90(2): 269–281.
[25] Ahmed MO, Baptiste KE. Vancomycin-resistant enterococci: a review of antimicrobial resistance mechanisms and perspectives of human and animal health. Microb Drug Resist, 2018, 24(5): 590–606.
[26] Alvarez R, et al. Optimizing the clinical use of vancomycin. Antimicrob Agents Chemother, 2016, 60(5): 2601–2609.
[27] Rybak MJ, et al. Therapeutic monitoring of vancomycin in adults summary of consensus recommendations from the American society of health-system pharmacists, the infectious diseases society of America, and the society of infectious diseases pharmacists. Pharmacotherapy, 2009, 29(11): 1275–1279.

[28] Rybak MJ, et al. Therapeutic monitoring of vancomycin for serious methicillin-resistant Staphylococcus aureus infections: a revised consensus guideline and review by the American Society of Health-System Pharmacists, the Infectious Diseases Society of America, the Pediatric Infectious Diseases Society, and the Society of Infectious Diseases Pharmacists. Clin Infect Dis, 2020, 71(6): 1361–1364.

[29] Brown J, Brown K, Forrest A. Vancomycin AUC24/MIC ratio in patients with complicated bacteremia and infective endocarditis due to methicillin-resistant Staphylococcus aureus and its association with attributable mortality during hospitalization. Antimicrob Agents Chemother, 2012, 56(2): 634–638.

[30] Saravolatz LD, Stein GE. Oritavancin: a long-half-life lipoglycopeptide. Clin Infect Dis, 2015, 61(4): 627–632.

[31] Tobudic S, et al. Dalbavancin as primary and sequential treatment for gram-positive infective endocarditis: 2-year experience at the general hospital of vienna. Clin Infect Dis, 2018, 67(5): 795–798.

[32] Hidalgo-Tenorio C, et al. DALBACEN cohort: dalbavancin as consolidation therapy in patients with endocarditis and/or bloodstream infection produced by gram-positive cocci. Ann Clin Microbiol Antimicrob, 2019, 18(1): 30.

[33] Stein GE, et al. A pharmacokinetic/pharmacodynamic analysis of ceftaroline prophylaxis in patients with external ventricular drains. Surg Infect, 2015, 16(2): 169–173.

[34] Johnson JA, et al. Prolonged use of oritavancin for vancomycin-resistant Enterococcus faecium prosthetic valve endocarditis. Open Forum Infect Dis, 2015, 2(4): ofv156.

[35] Bliziotis IA, et al. Daptomycin versus other antimicrobial agents for the treatment of skin and soft tissue infections: a meta-analysis. Ann Pharmacother, 2010, 44(1): 97-106.

[36] Batts DH. Linezolid—a new option for treating gram-positive infections. Oncology, 2000, 14(8 Suppl. 6): 23–29.

[37] Serio AW, et al. Aminoglycoside revival: review of a historically important class of antimicrobials undergoing rejuvenation. EcoSal Plus, 2018, 8(1).

[38] Banerjee S, Narayanan M, Gould K. Monitoring aminoglycoside level. BMJ, 2012, 345: e6354.

[39] Zhanel GG, Hoban DJ, Harding GK. The postantibiotic effect: a review of in vitro and in vivo data. DICP, 1991, 25(2): 153–163.

[40] Nicolau DP, et al. Implementation of a once-daily aminoglycoside program in a large community-teaching hospital. Hosp Pharm, 1995, 30(8). pp. 674–676, 679–680.

[41] Ezelarab HAA, et al. Recent updates of fluoroquinolones as antibacterial agents. Arch Pharm, 2018, 351(9): e1800141.

[42] Administration, F.a.D. FDA updates warnings for fluoroquinolone antibiotics on risks of mental health and low blood sugar adverse reactions, 2018.

[43] Lee CY, et al. Role of rifampin for the treatment of bacterial infections other than mycobacteriosis. J Infect, 2017, 75(5): 395–408.

[44] Shrestha NK, et al. Rifampin for surgically treated staphylococcal infective endocarditis: a propensity score-adjusted cohort study. Ann Thorac Surg, 2016, 101(6): 2243–2250.

[45] Zimmerli W, Sendi P. Role of rifampin against staphylococcal biofilm infections in vitro, in animal models, and in orthopedic-device-related infections. Antimicrob Agents Chemother, 2019, 63(2).

[46] Bailey TC, et al. A meta-analysis of extended-interval dosing versus multiple daily dosing of aminoglycosides. Clin Infect Dis, 1997, 24(5): 786–795.

[47] Cubicin (Daptomycin) [package insert]. Whitehouse Station, NJ: Merck Sharp&Dohme Corporation, 2016.

[48] Brouqui P, Raoult D. Endocarditis due to rare and fastidious bacteria. Clin Microbiol Rev, 2001, 14(1): 177–207.

[49] Gould FK, et al. Guidelines for the diagnosis and antibiotic treatment of endocarditis in adults: a report of the Working Party of the British Society for Antimicrobial Chemotherapy. J Antimicrob Chemother, 2012, 67(2): 269–289.

[50] Raoult D, et al. Outcome and treatment of Bartonella endocarditis. Arch Intern Med, 2003, 163(2): 226–230.

[51] Porter RS, Hay CM. Pasteurella endocarditis: a case report and statistical analysis of the literature. Case Rep Infect Dis, 2020, 2020: 8890211.

[52] Zajkowska J, et al. Capnocytophaga canimorsus- an underestimated danger after dog or cat bite - review of literature. Przegl Epidemiol, 2016, 70(2): 289–295.

[53] Jia B, et al. Brucella endocarditis: clinical features and treatment outcomes of 10 cases from Xinjiang, China. J Infect, 2017, 74(5): 512–514.

[54] Eldin C, et al. From Q fever to Coxiella burnetii infection: a paradigm change. Clin Microbiol Rev, 2017, 30(1): 115–190.

[55] Jean S, Lainhart W, Yarbrough ML. The brief case: erysipelothrix bacteremia and endocarditis in a 59-year-old immunocompromised male on chronic high-dose steroids. J Clin Microbiol, 2019, 57(6).

[56] Cervera C, et al. Effect of vancomycin minimal inhibitory concentration on the outcome of methicillin-susceptible Staphylococcus aureus endocarditis. Clin Infect Dis, 2014, 58(12): 1668–1675.

[57] Yuson CL, Katelaris CH, Smith WB. 'Cephalosporin allergy' label is misleading. Aust Prescr, 2018, 41(2): 37–41.

[58] Carugati M, et al. High-dose daptomycin therapy for left-sided infective endocarditis: a prospective study from the international collaboration on endocarditis. Antimicrob Agents Chemother, 2013, 57(12): 6213–6222.

[59] Fowler Jr VG, et al. Daptomycin versus standard therapy for bacteremia and endocarditis caused by Staphylococcus aureus. N Engl J Med, 2006, 355(7): 653–665.

[60] Holland DJ, et al. Infective endocarditis: a contemporary study of microbiology, echocardiography and associated clinical outcomes at a major tertiary referral centre. Heart Lung Circ, 2020, 29(6): 840–850.

[61] Pappas PG, et al. Clinical practice guideline for the management of candidiasis: 2016 update by the infectious diseases society of America. Clin Infect Dis, 2016, 62(4): e1–e50.

[62] Li J, Echevarria KL, Traugott KA. Beta-lactam therapy for methicillin-susceptible Staphylococcus aureus bacteremia: a comparative review of cefazolin versus antistaphylococcal penicillins. Pharmacotherapy, 2017, 37(3): 346–360.

[63] Flynt LK, et al. The safety and economic impact of cefazolin versus nafcillin for the treatment of methicillin-susceptible Staphylococcus aureus bloodstream infections. Infect Dis Ther, 2017, 6(2): 225–231.

[64] Huang G, et al. Infective endocarditis guidelines: the challenges of adherence-a survey of infectious diseases clinicians. Open Forum Infect Dis, 2020, 7(9): ofaa342.

[65] Beganovic M, et al. A review of combination antimicrobial therapy for Enterococcus faecalis bloodstream infections and infective endocarditis. Clin Infect Dis, 2018, 67(2): 303–309.

[66] Nigo M, et al. What's new in the treatment of enterococcal endocarditis? Curr Infect Dis Rep, 2014, 16(10): 431.

[67] Owens Jr RC, et al. Antimicrobial-associated risk factors for Clostridium difficile infection. Clin Infect Dis, 2008, 46(Suppl. 1): S19–S31.

[68] Amberpet R, et al. Screening for intestinal colonization with vancomycin resistant enterococci and associated risk factors among patients admitted to an adult intensive care unit of a large teaching hospital. J Clin Diagn Res, 2016, 10(9): DC06–DC09.

[69] Luther MK, Rice LB, LaPlante KL. Ampicillin in combination with ceftaroline, cefepime, or ceftriaxone demonstrates equivalent activities in a high-inoculum Enterococcus faecalis infection model. Antimicrob Agents Chemother, 2016, 60(5): 3178–3182.

[70] Lakticova V, et al. Antibiotic-induced enterococcal expansion in the mouse intestine occurs throughout the small bowel and correlates poorly with suppression of competing flora. Antimicrob Agents Chemother, 2006, 50(9): 3117–3123.

[71] Panagiotidis G, et al. Effect of ceftaroline on normal human intestinal microflora. Antimicrob Agents Chemother, 2010, 54(5): 1811–1814.

[72] Kobayashi T, et al. Current evidence on oral antibiotics for infective endocarditis: a narrative review. Cardiol Ther, 2019, 8(2): 167–177.

[73] Habib G, et al. ESC guidelines for the management of infective endocarditis: the task force for the management of infective endocarditis of the European society of Cardiology (ESC). Endorsed by: European association for cardio-thoracic surgery (EACTS), the European association of nuclear medicine (EANM). Eur Heart J, 2015, 36(44): 3075–3128.

[74] Iversen K, et al. Partial oral versus intravenous antibiotic treatment of endocarditis. N Engl J Med, 2019, 380(5): 415–424.

[75] Boucher HW. Partial oral therapy for osteomyelitis and endocarditis—is it time? N Engl J Med, 2019, 380(5): 487–489.

[76] Spellberg B, et al. Evaluation of a paradigm shift from intravenous antibiotics to oral step-down therapy for the treatment of infective endocarditis: a narrative review. JAMA Intern Med, 2020, 180(5): 769–777.

[77] Brown E, Gould FK. Oral antibiotics for infective endocarditis: a clinical review. J Antimicrob Chemother, 2020, 75(8): 2021–2027.

[78] Norris AH, et al. 2018 infectious diseases society of America clinical practice guideline for the management of outpatient parenteral antimicrobial therapy. Clin Infect Dis, 2019, 68(1): e1–e35.

[79] Sanaiha Y, Lyons R, Benharash P. Infective endocarditis in intravenous drug users. Trends Cardiovasc Med, 2020, 30(8): 491–7.https://doi.org/10.1016/j.tcm.2019.11.007. PMID: 31870712.

[80] Chung EK, et al. Development and implementation of a pharmacist-managed outpatient parenteral antimicrobial therapy program. Am J Health Syst Pharm, 2016, 73(1): e24–e33.

第 8 章
危重感染性心内膜炎患者的术前准备

Katherine A. Giuliano, Eric W. Etchill, Glenn J.R. Whitman
Division of Cardiac Surgery, Department of Surgery, Johns Hopkins Hospital, Baltimore, MD, United States

引 言

无论是采用内科还是外科治疗，感染性心内膜炎（IE）的院内死亡率依然高达 10%~20%[1-6]，发病 6 个月时这一数值接近 30%，而 7 年左右时死亡率将超过 50%[3,7]。多种因素可导致死亡率的增加，包括高龄，以及入院时就已出现的神经或肺部并发症、栓塞事件和肾损伤[1-3,7-8]。Hasbun 等设计了一个 4 级评分系统，用于预测左侧自体瓣膜 IE 患者 6 个月内的死亡率，评分指标包括患者的精神状态、Charlson 共病评分量表、充血性心力衰竭程度、病原微生物学和治疗情况（药物治疗或手术治疗）[9]。

关于在内科或外科治愈前需要入住重症监护病房（ICU）患者的比例尚无专门研究，但在出现终末器官损伤或心力衰竭时，重症监护通常是必要的[10]。据估计，60% 的心内膜炎患者至少会发生一次严重并发症，其中 50% 需要手术干预[6,11]。毋庸置疑，需要 ICU 监护治疗的病例也就意味着高风险，住院死亡率可达 50%[12-13]。并发症通常是由感染对心脏的直接损伤、赘生物栓塞或因脓毒症或心源性休克导致的全身低灌注引起，其中，约 30% 的病例可合并全身性栓塞[14-15]。当然，抗菌治疗是重中之重，第 7 章已对此进行介绍。

本章将重点阐述危重心内膜炎病例的术前管理。首先讨论心脏相关并发症的治疗，包括瓣膜功能障碍和传导异常；随后讨论神经、肾脏、呼吸和内脏并发症的治疗（表 8.1）。下一章将讨论此类危重人群的术后管理和并发症治疗。

心脏并发症的术前处理

有超过一半的 IE 病例可出现心脏并发症，最常见的是瓣膜关闭不全及其导致的心力衰竭，以及传导异常和急性冠脉综合征（ACS）。

瓣膜关闭不全

40% 的 IE 患者可并发瓣周脓肿，进而导致急性瓣膜关闭不全。瓣周脓肿常见

表 8.1　感染性心内膜炎（IE）术前并发症总结

器官	并发症	发生率	诊断	治疗
心脏	瓣膜关闭不全	40%	超声心动图	手术
	传导异常	25%	心电图、超声心动图	手术
	急性冠脉综合征	罕见	CT、冠状动脉造影	手术
脑	栓塞性卒中	20%~40%	脑部 CT、MRI	考虑抗凝治疗
	脑出血	20%~40%	脑部 CT、MRI	支持性治疗，确保没有需要干预的真菌性动脉瘤
	真菌性动脉瘤	少见	磁共振血管造影（MRA）	神经外科手术、神经介入夹闭或弹簧圈栓塞
	脑膜炎	1%~5%	腰椎穿刺	静脉抗生素治疗
	脑脓肿	1%~5%	MRA	穿刺吸引、置管引流
	脑病	25%	临床诊断、MRI	支持性治疗、纠正营养或代谢缺陷（维生素 B_{12}、叶酸、硫胺素）
肾	急性肾损伤	30%~35%	尿液分析、尿电解质、生化检测	静脉抗生素、维持肾灌注、液体管理
	脓毒性栓塞	可达 30%	尿液分析、腹部/盆腔 CT	静脉抗生素、维持肾灌注、液体管理
	肾小球肾炎	25%	尿液分析（红细胞管型）、生化检查	静脉抗生素、维持肾灌注、液体管理
	急性间质性肾炎	10%	尿液分析（白细胞管型）、生化检测	静脉抗生素、维持肾灌注、液体管理
肺	脓毒性栓塞	5%~10%	胸部 X 线片、CT	静脉抗生素，内科治疗失败时手术切除病灶
脾	脓毒性栓塞	30%~35%	腹部 CT、实验室检查	脾切除术
骨	骨髓炎	5%	X 线检查、CT、MRI、核素骨扫描	延长静脉抗生素治疗时间

于人工瓣膜心内膜炎，其次是自体主动脉瓣心内膜炎，二尖瓣心内膜炎则相对较少。当瓣周脓肿破坏舒张期瓣膜的正常对合，或者当炎症导致自身瓣叶穿孔或撕裂等结构性破坏时，就会发生瓣膜关闭不全。约 15% 的心内膜炎病例可出现多瓣膜受累，推测可能是由于感染直接蔓延或带病原菌的瓣膜反流束引起邻近瓣膜的卫星感染病灶所致。但无论何种机制，急性瓣膜关闭不全都是一种临床急症，如果不立即处理，可能会导致急性心力衰竭、呼吸循环崩溃，甚至死亡。

左侧心脏瓣膜急性关闭不全通常表现为突发的呼吸短促和疲劳。体检常可发现明显的心动过速，伴有舒张期减弱的或全舒张期高强度杂音；有劳力性呼吸困难和双肺啰音等肺充血的证据；以及心输出量减少的表现，如低血压、四肢发凉和皮肤苍白。紧急检查应包括心肌酶和超声心动图。超声具有诊断价值，可显示瓣膜关闭不全及受累瓣膜的连枷样运动或钙化。对于并发急性肺水肿的急性主动脉瓣关闭不全，应急诊手术，内科治疗对这类肺水肿效果有限。而对于没有出现急性肺水肿或危及生命状况的病例，可先行内科保守治疗，使用广谱抗生素、优化手术条件。治疗重点是利尿、扩血管降低心脏后负荷，以纠正心力衰竭。不过这类病例最终还是需要手术治疗，这将在后续章节中讨论。

传导异常

约25%的心内膜炎病例可并发传导障碍，这是死亡率增加和预后较差的独立预测因子[16-17]。通常，房室传导阻滞或束支传导阻滞是瓣周脓肿累及传导系统的结果[16]，最常见于主动脉根部受累，原因在于解剖上主动脉瓣邻近室间隔和希氏束，结果可表现为不同程度的束支阻滞，如Ⅰ度、Ⅱ度或完全性房室传导阻滞。

传导异常通常使用心电图检查即可诊断，如果怀疑传导系统异常系心内膜炎所致，则应进行超声心动图追踪检查[17]。对于新发房室传导阻滞，如果超声心动图发现瓣环或瓣膜异常，并侵犯瓣周，应立即进行手术。多半需要进行瓣膜置换，有时还需要修复受累的瓣环或心内间隔[16]。

急性冠脉综合征

急性冠脉综合征是IE的一种罕见并发症，多发生在原有冠状动脉疾病的情况下[18]。而原有正常冠状动脉在IE病变中受累则多源于以下几种情况：可因主动脉根部脓肿引起根部形态改变以致冠脉开口直接受机械挤压变形，也可因感染蔓延至冠脉开口直接侵害而致；另一种可能是脓毒性栓塞或真菌性动脉瘤血栓形成导致的心肌梗死[19-20]；还有一种少见的原因，即可能是继发于环周或根部周围感染对冠状动脉的外压[21-22]。对这些病例的处理均需外科手术，针对感染的瓣膜或组织进行彻底清创，存在心肌缺血或冠脉开口受累的则行冠状动脉血运重建。

其他心脏并发症

其他可能出现的极具破坏性的IE心脏并发症多由瓣周脓肿向周围蔓延扩大引起，如纤维蛋白性心包炎（更常见）和化脓性心包炎、主动脉根部和心肌脓肿、心包积血、心脏压塞、主动脉瘤、夹层和邻近心腔的心内瘘[5,23]。心内瘘在人工瓣膜IE中较为常见，这与人工瓣膜的缝合环对邻近心肌组织的侵蚀作用有关[13]。心内膜炎引起的上述结构性破坏是手术的绝对指征。

非心脏并发症的术前处理

神经系统并发症

神经系统并发症是心内膜炎最常见的心外并发症，发生率为20%~40%[9,10,24-26]。最常见的神经系统并发症是短暂性脑缺血或赘生物（通常是左心）脱落栓塞引起的脑卒中,多发生于病程早期[8,15]。其他神经系统并发症包括脑出血、真菌性动脉瘤、脑膜炎、脑脓肿和脑病。任何一种神经系统并发症都会导致死亡风险的增加[1,13,24]，就如 Mourvillier 等的发现，出现神经系统并发症的 ICU 心内膜炎患者的死亡风险是普通病例的 3 倍[13]。但无论是神经系统的还是其他系统的任何 IE 并发症，早期抗感染对感染源的控制至关重要。另外，一旦启动恰当的抗感染治疗，心内膜炎相关神经系统并发症就会大幅减少[15,27]。

如果 IE 患者出现精神状态改变等神经系统缺陷，应进行脑部影像学检查。检查方式中，CT 检查更快、更普及，但 MRI 对于病变的灵敏度更高[10]，MRI 常可发现一些没有临床症状的神经系统病理改变。例如，在法国的一项研究中，所有疑似或确诊的心内膜炎病例，不论有无神经系统症状，均接受脑部 MRI 及血管造影，结果显示：82% 的病例存在脑部病变，28% 的病例因检查结果从疑似 IE 升级为确诊 IE 或改变治疗计划[28]。

虽然对于确诊为心内膜炎之前就需要抗凝的病例应延续抗凝治疗，但没有证据支持预防性抗凝可以防止 IE 病例栓塞的发生。更进一步，在面临一个缺血性卒中病例时，在考虑是否抗凝的问题上，还必须慎重权衡抗凝的获益与缺血转化为出血的风险[29]。这方面数据有限，主要文献来自人工瓣膜心内膜炎。相关证据显示，在接受抗凝治疗后，估计缺血性卒中转化为出血性卒中的比例为 10%～14%[30-31]。为预测这一风险，人们创建了一些评分系统以协助抗凝决策。虽然这些系统并非为心内膜炎特设，但根据临床参数可估测出血转化的风险程度，以指导有抗凝适应证的病例（例如静脉血栓栓塞或心房颤动）是否接受抗凝治疗。例如，出血风险分层评分（HeRS）预测，随年龄增大、梗死面积加大和肾小球滤过率降低，出血风险会增加[32]。HeRS 的附加评分系统还利用入院前的血糖、白细胞计数和华法林的使用来预测出血的风险[33]。

一项随机试验显示使用全量阿司匹林并无获益，表明抗血小板药物在预防卒中和栓塞并发症方面无效[34]。相反，该研究显示接受阿司匹林的治疗组病例有出血风险加大的趋势，其中大出血（定义为颅内出血，出血导致血红蛋白下降 ≥ 20 g/L 或需要输血，或出血进入限制性空间，如心包）或小出血（其他所有导致血红蛋白下降 < 20 g/L 的显性出血）的发生率在阿司匹林组接近 30%，而对照组的发生率只有试验组的一半[34]。

对于发生卒中同时又具备手术指征的患者，手术干预的时机至关重要，因为术中或术后早期梗死转化为出血将是灾难性的。不幸的是，这一问题尚未得到解决，仍处于争论中。通常，对这类手术的决策是个体化的，术者对手术方案的选择常缺乏完全的信心。有关手术时机和适应证的更多信息参阅第 14 章[35]。手术的决策常需权衡清除感染瓣膜（栓塞的潜在来源）带来的益处与手术可能造成进一步脑损伤的风险。目前，大多数人主张在缺血性栓塞梗死后手术应延期至少 2 周[36-37]。在这些情况下，HeRS 评分可能有助于决定手术时机，但这尚未有明确的研究结果。

真菌性动脉瘤是由脓毒性栓塞引起的异常动脉扩张，栓子导致动脉壁继发感染、破坏变薄和随后的瘤样扩张。真菌性动脉瘤是少见的神经系统并发症，通常无神经系统症候，只有当瘤体扩大引起占位效应或出现破裂时，才有临床表现。因此，对于这类无症状患者有必要利用高灵敏度的 MRI 或磁共振血管造影（MRA）进行排查[29]。鉴于该类病例较少，因此尚无标准化的治疗模式，文献报道的方案也是个体化和多样性的[38-40]。总体而言，治疗方法包括神经外科手术和介入神经放射，具体采用哪种方法取决于动脉瘤的位置和相关医疗机构已有的处理能力。通常，存在明显血肿并有占位效应的，首选手术夹闭；而对于手术操作难以暴露的真菌性动脉瘤、多发性动脉瘤或手术风险较高的病例则选用血管内弹簧圈栓塞[38]。血管腔内介入治疗的特殊优势在于能够在神经介入治疗后立即进行全身抗凝，而开颅手术需要等待更长的时间才能抗凝。一言以蔽之，与开颅患者相比，接受介入治疗的患者可以更快地接受心脏手术。

心内膜炎并发蛛网膜下腔出血时应进行真菌性动脉瘤影像排查，因为约 1.5% 的该类出血与真菌性动脉瘤有关。一旦动脉瘤诊断成立将改变治疗方案，如上所述，需要进行动脉瘤显微手术夹闭或血管内介入栓塞[41-42]。

脑膜炎和脑脓肿也较少见，在 IE 中的发病率分别为 6% 和 1% 左右[43]。与所有脑并发症一样，主要发生于左侧瓣膜病变。总体而言，心内膜炎是脑膜炎发病的一个罕见病因。荷兰的一项全国性调查发现，在 6 年的时间里，只在 2% 的社区获得性细菌性脑膜炎患者中发现了心内膜炎[44]。这一研究发现，在心内膜炎相关脑膜炎的病例中，约 60% 患者的脑脊液（CSF）检查结果预示有细菌性脑膜炎，而在其他原因引起的脑膜炎病例中这一比例为 90%[44]。尽管如此，如果出现发热、颈项强直、精神状态改变、头痛和（或）恶心等症状，应怀疑脑膜炎。需立即行腰椎穿刺检查相关指标，如脑脊液葡萄糖水平是否 <34 mg/dL（1.88 mmol/L）、脑脊液葡萄糖与血糖之比是否 <0.23、蛋白质水平是否 >220 mg/dL，或白细胞计数是否 >2000/μL[3,45]。静脉应用抗生素是主要治疗手段，治疗以脑脊液培养药敏结果为指导，在抗生素治疗的同时应静脉注射糖皮质激素，通常是地塞米松。感染病协会给出的上述建议来自几项重要的临床试验，其结果表明，地塞米松可降低细菌性脑膜炎（不特定于心内膜炎并发的脑膜炎）患者的死亡率和神经系统后遗症（如听力丧失）发生率，尤其是对于肺炎链球菌性脑膜炎[46-48]。

脑脓肿的诊断一旦成立，应尽快进行影像学检查以评估真菌性动脉瘤（如上所述），因为两者经常共存。脑脓肿的处理以引流为主，通常首选穿刺引流。与开颅手术相比，穿刺的神经系统后遗症风险较低。引流的液体应送培养以指导抗菌治疗[49]。

所有神经系统并发症都可以表现为癫痫发作，治疗方法与其他危重癫痫发作相同，静脉注射抗癫痫药物（如左乙拉西坦）。如果心内膜炎并发脑病，治疗则应侧重于支持治疗以纠正营养或代谢缺陷，如补充维生素 B_{12}、叶酸和硫胺素。通常，这类危重患者的脑病病因是多因素的，常见的有脓毒症、多器官功能障碍和谵妄；但也可由一些可调节的因素引起，如电解质异常、营养缺陷和行为问题。应针对相关因素进行治疗，尽量减少谵妄发生，以改善脑病。

肾脏并发症

肾功能障碍和急性肾损伤（AKI）可由肾局部或全肾梗死 [由脓毒性栓塞或感染性和（或）心源性休克低灌注引起]、肾小球肾炎和抗生素引起的急性间质性肾炎所致[50]。近 1/3 的心内膜炎病例可并发急性肾损伤[51]。Majumdar 等对 62 例心内膜炎患者（活检或尸检）的肾脏进行了组织学分析，发现肾局部梗死的发生率为 31%（超过一半由脓毒性栓塞引起），急性肾小球肾炎的发生率为 26%，急性间质性肾炎的发生率为 10%，脓毒性栓塞还可引起肾脓肿，所有这些肾脏并发症都会增加死亡率[1,12]。

腰痛病史可提示栓塞性肾缺血，尿液分析有助于区分出心内膜炎并发急性肾损伤的病因。无论是肉眼血尿还是镜下血尿，都提示有肾缺血，同时约 12% 的肾梗死患者还会出现蛋白尿[52]。尿沉渣中的白细胞管型提示有急性间质性肾炎，红细胞管型提示有肾小球肾炎。使用抗生素对于控制感染源至关重要，但应注意抗生素剂量以防止肾毒性，尤其是在已有肾功能障碍或急性肾损伤的情况下。维持良好的心输出量和血压可保护肾脏免于缺血性损伤和急性肾小管坏死的危害。谨慎的出入量管理同样起着重要作用，与其他出现肾损伤的疾病一样，当存在血液透析指征——最常见的有液体超负荷、电解质异常或症状性尿毒症——应立即开始透析治疗。

肺部并发症

肺栓塞并发症比脑或肾脏并发症少见，原因是它们通常只发生在右侧 IE，而右侧 IE 仅占心内膜炎的 5%～10%[53]。脓毒性栓塞通常导致细菌性肺炎或肺脓肿，通过胸部 X 线检查或灵敏度更高的胸部 CT 进行评估。胸部 CT 的特征性发现包括胸膜下外周结节和楔形外周病变[54]。如前所述，无论是出于预防还是治疗目的，立即予以抗菌治疗都至关重要。胸腔积液可能需要通过胸腔穿刺或置管进行引流，但包裹性积液则可能需要外科手术引流，就像肺脓肿可能需要外科手术引流或切除一样[55]。由于心内膜炎发生肺栓塞较为罕见，因此相关死亡率的直接数据很少。据报道，所有脓毒性肺栓塞的死亡率为 12%～30%，这包括由心内膜炎、Lemierre 综合征、感染性外周深静脉血栓等引起的肺栓塞[55-57]。

根据欧洲心脏病学会（ESC）和美国心脏协会 / 美国心脏病学会（AHA/ACC）指南[53,58]，在适当的抗生素治疗下，复发性脓毒性肺栓塞是心内膜炎手术干预的指征，详见第 14 章。

脾脏并发症

脾栓塞可引起脾梗死，进而导致脾脓肿，脓肿的形成源于感染的栓子或梗死组织继发感染。一项对 68 例心内膜炎患者的尸检报告显示，约 1/3 的患者存在脾梗死[59]。腹部 CT 是最佳诊断方法。脾梗死不需要特殊治疗，但如果患者需要全身抗凝以进行体外循环，则有出血或破裂的风险。一旦发生出血和破裂，则需进行脾切除手术[60-61]。

脾脓肿通常可引起发热、白细胞增多和左上腹痛等典型症状[62]。抗生素不能有效穿透脾脓肿，IE 并发脾脓肿内科治疗的死亡率高达 80%[61,63-65]，因此，脾切除手术是必要的治疗手段。虽然报道显示脾脓肿脾切除相关死亡率为 6%~14%，但这一发生率是否符合 IE 须脾切除这种情况还不清楚[65-66]。Robinson 等人报道了在他们 564 例心内膜炎患者中 27 例（5%）并发脾脓肿患者的预后，死亡率约 50%（13 例），其中内科治疗死亡率为 100%，而外科脾切除术后存活率超过 80%（14/17）[61]。此外还有证据表明，如果可能，应在瓣膜置换术之前进行脾切除，以避免脾内感染病灶对新植入的心内假体的污染[67-69]。也有报道使用介入引导进行经皮穿刺抽吸和（或）置管引流的方法[62]。

骨髓炎

6% 的 IE 病例可并发骨髓炎[70]。因此，针对持续的肌肉骨骼不适（例如背痛、骨痛、僵硬、关节痛）应进行相应检查。首先行 X 线平片检查，尽管 50% 的早期骨髓炎病例 X 线检查结果正常[70]，但约 2 周后，骨骼的 X 线异常表现会变得明显。为了提高检查的灵敏度，可选择 CT、MRI 或核素骨扫描。MRI 通常是首选，核素骨扫描用于对 CT 或 MRI 有禁忌的患者。抗生素治疗强调长疗程——需至少 6 周的静脉抗生素和至少 3 个月的口服治疗。如果血培养病原体阳性，则不一定需要骨活检；但在诊断不确定的情况下，可经皮或开放进行骨活检，为诊断及指导抗菌治疗提供依据[71]。

总　结

IE 的并发症和后遗症很常见，致残率和死亡率很高。心脏或心外受累多表现为瓣膜破坏或栓塞现象，病变可累及几乎全身任何一个器官系统。充分了解各种并发症和受累的器官的变化可以为拟定检查计划、做出适当诊断、给予恰当治疗提供一个总体方案。检查、治疗的结果进而可为手术必要性和时机提供判断依据。综上所述，所有针对 IE 并发症的术前恰当的处理，其目标均旨在改善这一危重人群的整体医疗质量。

参考文献

[1] Smith JM, So RR, Engel AM. Clinical predictors of mortality from infective endocarditis. Int J Surg, 2007, 5(1): 31–34.

[2] Chu VH, Cabell CH, Benjamin DK, et al. Early predictors of in-hospital death in infective endocarditis. Circulation, 2004, 109(14): 1745–1749.

[3] Wallace SM, Walton BI, Kharbanda RK, et al. Mortality from infective endocarditis: clinical predictors of outcome. Heart, 2002, 88(1): 53–60.

[4] Olaison L, Pettersson G. Current best practices and guidelines indications for surgical intervention

in infective endocarditis. Infect Dis Clin, 2002, 16(2): 453–475 [xi].

[5] Mylonakis E, Calderwood SB. Infective endocarditis in adults. N Engl J Med, 2001, 345(18): 1318–1330.

[6] Murdoch DR, Corey GR, Hoen B, et al. Clinical presentation, etiology, and outcome of infective endocarditis in the 21st century: the International Collaboration on Endocarditis-Prospective Cohort Study. Arch Intern Med, 2009, 169(5): 463–473.

[7] Netzer ROM, Altwegg SC, Zollinger E, et al. Infective endocarditis: determinants of long term outcome. Heart, 2002, 88(1): 61–66.

[8] Cabell CH, Pond KK, Peterson GE, et al. The risk of stroke and death in patients with aortic and mitral valve endocarditis. Am Heart J, 2001, 142(1): 75–80.

[9] Hasbun R, Vikram HR, Barakat LA, et al. Complicated left-sided native valve endocarditis in adults: risk classification for mortality. J Am Med Assoc, 2003, 289(15): 1933–1940.

[10] Sonneville R, Mourvillier B, Bouadma L, et al. Management of neurological complications of infective endocarditis in ICU patients. Ann Intens Care, 2011, 1(1): 10.

[11] Parsek MR, Singh PK. Bacterial biofilms: an emerging link to disease pathogenesis. Annu Rev Microbiol, 2003, 57: 677–701.

[12] Karth G, Koreny M, Binder T, et al. Complicated infective endocarditis necessitating ICU admission: clinical course and prognosis. Crit Care, 2002, 6(2): 149–154.

[13] Mourvillier B, Trouillet J-L, Timsit J-F, et al. Infective endocarditis in the intensive care unit: clinical spectrum and prognostic factors in 228 consecutive patients. Intens Care Med, 2004, 30(11): 2046–2052.

[14] Klein M, Wang A. Infective endocarditis. J Intens Care Med, 2016, 31(3): 151–163.

[15] Vilacosta I, Graupner C, San Román JA, et al. Risk of embolization after institution of antibiotic therapy for infective endocarditis. J Am Coll Cardiol, 2002, 39(9): 1489–1495.

[16] Pierre Charbel Atallah. Significance of first-degree atrioventricular block in acute endocarditis-diagnosis. JAMA Intern Med, 2013, 173(9). 726–726.

[17] Meine TJ, Nettles RE, Anderson DJ, et al. Cardiac conduction abnormalities in endocarditis defined by the Duke criteria. Am Heart J, 2001, 142(2): 280–285.

[18] Kandoussi TE, Malki HE, Masmoudi AE, et al. Infective endocarditis presenting as acute coronary syndrome. Pan Afr Med J, 2016, 23. https://doi.org/10.11604/pamj. 2016.23.230.7429.

[19] Okai I, Inoue K, Yamaguchi N, et al. Infective endocarditis associated with acute myocardial infarction caused by septic emboli. J Cardiol Cases, 2010, 1(1): e28–e32.

[20] Khiatah B, Jazayeri S, Wilde J, et al. ST-segment elevation myocardial infarction from septic emboli secondary to infective endocarditis by abiotrophia defectiva. Case Rep Cardiol, 2020, 2020. https://doi.org/10.1155/2020/8811034.

[21] Manzano MC, Vilacosta I, Román JAS, et al. Acute coronary syndrome in infective endocarditis. Rev Española Cardiol, 2007, 60(1): 24–31.

[22] Attias D, Messika-Zeitoun D, Wolf M, et al. Acute coronary syndrome in aortic infective endocarditis. Eur J Echocardiogr, 2008, 9(6): 727–728.

[23] Khalid N, Shlofmitz E, Ahmad SA. Aortic valve endocarditis. In: StatPearls. StatPearls Publishing, 2020.

[24] Pang PYK, Sin YK, Lim CH, et al. Surgical management of infective endocarditis: an analysis of early and late outcomes. Eur J Cardio Thorac Surg, 2015, 47(5): 826–832.

[25] Heiro M, Nikoskelainen J, Engblom E, et al. Neurologic manifestations of infective endocarditis: a 17-year experience in a teaching hospital in Finland. Arch Intern Med, 2000, 160(18): 2781–2787.

[26] Hoen B, Alla F, Selton-Suty C, et al. Changing profile of infective endocarditis: results of a 1-year survey in France. J Am Med Assoc, 2002, 288(1): 75–81.

[27] Dickerman SA, Abrutyn E, Barsic B, et al. The relationship between the initiation of antimicrobial therapy and the incidence of stroke in infective endocarditis: an analysis from the ICE Prospective Cohort Study (ICE-PCS). Am Heart J, 2007, 154(6): 1086–1094.

[28] Duval X, Iung B, Klein I, et al. Effect of early cerebral magnetic resonance imaging on clinical decisions in infective endocarditis: a prospective study. Ann Intern Med, 2010, 152(8): 497–504. W175.
[29] Skinner CR. Neurological complications of endocarditis: pathophysiologic mechanisms and management issues//Kwan-Leung Chan, John M Embil. Endocarditis: diagnosis and management. Switerland: Springer Cham, 2016: 375–395.
[30] Kim J-S, Yang W-I, Shim CY. Hemorrhagic transformation of ischemic stroke: severe complications of prosthetic valve endocarditis. Korean Circ J, 2011, 41(8): 490–493.
[31] Cho I-J, Kim J-S, Chang H-J, et al. Prediction of hemorrhagic transformation following embolic stroke in patients with prosthetic valve endocarditis. J Cardiovasc Ultrasound, 2013, 21(3): 123–129.
[32] Marsh EB, Llinas RH, Hillis AE, et al. Hemorrhagic transformation in patients with acute ischaemic stroke and an indication for anticoagulation. Eur J Neurol, 2013, 20(6): 962–967.
[33] Marsh EB, Llinas RH, Schneider ALC, et al. Predicting hemorrhagic transformation of acute ischemic stroke: prospective validation of the HeRS score. Medicine, 2016, 95(2): e2430.
[34] Chan K-L, Dumesnil JG, Cujec B, et al. A randomized trial of aspirin on the risk of embolic events in patients with infective endocarditis. J Am Coll Cardiol, 2003, 42(5): 775–780.
[35] AATS Surgical Treatment of Infective Endocarditis Consensus Guidelines Writing Committee Chairs, Pettersson GB, Coselli JS, et al. 2016 the American Association for Thoracic Surgery (AATS) consensus guidelines: surgical treatment of infective endocarditis: executive summary. J Thorac Cardiovasc Surg, 2017, 153(6): 1241–1258. e29.
[36] Gillinov AM, Shah RV, Curtis WE, et al. Valve replacement in patients with endocarditis and acute neurologic deficit. Ann Thorac Surg, 1996, 61(4): 1125–1129. discussion 1130.
[37] Yeates A, Mundy J, Griffin R, et al. Early and mid-term outcomes following surgical management of infective endocarditis with associated cerebral complications: a single centre experience. Heart Lung Circ, 2010, 19(9): 523–527.
[38] Ducruet AF, Hickman ZL, Zacharia BE, et al. Intracranial infectious aneurysms: a comprehensive review. Neurosurg Rev, 2010, 33(1): 37–46.
[39] Asai T, Usui A, Miyachi S, et al. Endovascular treatment for intracranial mycotic aneurysms prior to cardiac surgery. Eur J Cardio Thorac Surg, 2002, 21(5): 948–950.
[40] Peters PJ, Harrison T, Lennox JL. A dangerous dilemma: management of infectious intracranial aneurysms complicating endocarditis. Lancet Infect Dis, 2006, 6(11): 742–748.
[41] Chukwudelunzu FE, Brown RD, Wijdicks EFM, et al. Subarachnoid haemorrhage associated with infectious endocarditis: case report and literature review. Eur J Neurol, 2002, 9(4): 423–427.
[42] Hui FK, Bain M, Obuchowski NA, et al. Mycotic aneurysm detection rates with cerebral angiography in patients with infective endocarditis. J Neurointerv Surg, 2015, 7(6): 449–452.
[43] García-Cabrera E, Fernández-Hidalgo N, Almirante B, et al. Neurological complications of infective endocarditis: risk factors, outcome, and impact of cardiac surgery: a multicenter observational study. Circulation, 2013, 127(23): 2272–2284.
[44] Lucas MJ, Brouwer MC, van der Ende A, et al. Endocarditis in adults with bacterial meningitis. Circulation, 2013, 127(20): 2056–2062.
[45] Spanos A, Harrell Jr FE, Durack DT. Differential diagnosis of acute meningitis. An analysis of the predictive value of initial observations. J Am Med Assoc, 1989, 262(19): 2700–2707.
[46] Brouwer MC, McIntyre P, Prasad K, et al. Corticosteroids for acute bacterial meningitis. Cochrane Database Syst Rev, 2015, 9: CD004405.
[47] de Gans J, van de Beek D. European dexamethasone in adulthood bacterial meningitis study investigators. Dexamethasone in adults with bacterial meningitis. N Engl J Med, 2002, 347(20): 1549–1556.
[48] Tunkel AR, Hartman BJ, Kaplan SL, et al. Practice guidelines for the management of bacterial meningitis. Clin Infect Dis, 2004, 39(9): 1267–1264.
[49] Ratnaike TE, Das S, Gregson BA, et al. A review of brain abscess surgical treatment–78 years: aspiration versus excision. World Neurosurg, 2011, 76(5): 431–436.

[50] Majumdar A, Chowdhary S, Ferreira MA, et al. Renal pathological findings in infective endocarditis. Nephrol Dial Transpl, 2000, 15(11): 1782–1787.
[51] Conlon PJ, Jefferies F, Krigman HR, et al. Predictors of prognosis and risk of acute renal failure in bacterial endocarditis. Clin Nephrol, 1998, 49(2): 96–101.
[52] Oh YK, Yang CW, Kim Y-L, et al. Clinical characteristics and outcomes of renal infarction. Am J Kidney Dis, 2016, 67(2): 243–250.
[53] Habib G, Lancellotti P, Antunes MJ, et al. 2015 ESC guidelines for the management of infective endocarditis: the task force for the management of infective endocarditis of the European society of Cardiology (ESC). Endorsed by: European association for cardio-thoracic surgery (EACTS), the European association of nuclear medicine (EANM). Eur Heart J, 2015, 36(44): 3075–3128.
[54] Iwasaki Y, Nagata K, Nakanishi M, et al. Spiral CT findings in septic pulmonary emboli. Eur J Radiol, 2001, 37(3): 190–194.
[55] Goswami U, Brenes JA, Punjabi GV, et al. Associations and outcomes of septic pulmonary embolism. Open Respir Med J, 2014, 8: 28–33.
[56] Chou D-W, Wu S-L, Chung K-M, et al. Septic pulmonary embolism requiring critical care: clinicoradiological spectrum, causative pathogens and outcomes. Clinics, 2016, 71(10): 562–569.
[57] Oh HG, Cha S-I, Shin K-M, et al. Risk factors for mortality in patients with septic pulmonary embolism. J Infect Chemother, 2016, 22(8): 553–558.
[58] Nishimura RA, Otto CM, Bonow RO, et al. 2014 AHA/ACC guideline for the management of patients with valvular heart disease: executive summary: a report of the American College of Cardiology/American heart association task force on practice guidelines. Circulation, 2014, 129(23): 2440–2492.
[59] Fernández Guerrero ML, Álvarez B, Manzarbeitia F, et al. Infective endocarditis at autopsy: a review of pathologic manifestations and clinical correlates. Medicine, 2012, 91(3): 152–164.
[60] Ting W, Silverman NA, Arzouman DA, et al. Splenic septic emboli in endocarditis. Circulation, 1990, 82(5 Suppl. l): IV105–IV109.
[61] Robinson SL, Saxe JM, Lucas CE, et al. Splenic abscess associated with endocarditis. Surgery, 1992, 112(4): 781–786. discussion 786–787.
[62] Green BT. Splenic abscess: report of six cases and review of the literature. Am Surg, 2001, 67(1): 80–85.
[63] Johnson JD, Raff MJ, Barnwell PA, et al. Splenic abscess complicating infectious endocarditis. Arch Intern Med, 1983, 143(5): 906–912.
[64] Farres H, Felsher J, Banbury M, et al. Management of splenic abscess in a critically ill patient. Surg Laparosc Endosc Percutan Tech, 2004, 14(2): 49–52.
[65] Ng K-K, Lee T-Y, Wan Y-L, et al. Splenic abscess: diagnosis and management. Hepato-Gastroenterology, 2002, 49(44): 567–571.
[66] Nelken N, Ignatius J, Skinner M, et al. Changing clinical spectrum of splenic abscess. A multicenter study and review of the literature. Am J Surg, 1987, 154(1): 27–34.
[67] Baddour LM, Wilson WR, Bayer AS, et al. Infective endocarditis: diagnosis, antimicrobial therapy, and management of complications: a statement for healthcare professionals from the committee on rheumatic fever, endocarditis, and Kawasaki disease, council on cardiovascular disease in the young, and the councils on clinical Cardiology, stroke, and cardiovascular surgery and anesthesia, American Heart Association: endorsed by the Infectious Diseases Society of America. Circulation, 2005, 111(23): e394–e434.
[68] Simsir SA, Cheeseman SH, Lancey RA, et al. Staged laparoscopic splenectomy and valve replacement in splenic abscess and infective endocarditis. Ann Thorac Surg, 2003, 75(5): 1635–1637.
[69] Yoshikai M, Kamachi M, Kobayashi K, et al. Splenic abscess associated with active infective endocarditis. Jpn J Thorac Cardiovasc Surg, 2002, 50(11): 478–480.
[70] Speechly-Dick ME, Swanton RH. Osteomyelitis and infective endocarditis. Postgrad Med J, 1994, 70(830): 885–890.
[71] Schmitt SK. Osteomyelitis. Infect Dis Clin, 2017, 31(2): 325–338.

第9章

危重感染性心内膜炎患者的术后处理

Eric W. Etchill, Katherine A. Giuliano, Glenn J.R. Whitman

Division of Cardiac Surgery, Department of Surgery, Johns Hopkins Hospital,
Baltimore, MD, United States

引 言

虽然感染性心内膜炎（IE）手术死亡率高，并发症严重，入住重症监护病房（ICU）的时间和总体住院时间长；但手术患者生存率仍可达到90%以上，其中，人工瓣膜IE的手术死亡率高于自体瓣膜IE（13% vs.5.6%）[1]。对于瓣膜置换患者，无论使用哪种瓣膜，1年存活率均可达到80%[1]。IE患者术后平均住院时长为（18±2）d[2]，术后结果与术前存在的风险因素密切相关，如年龄、持续性菌血症、栓塞性卒中、充血性心力衰竭、肝硬化、肾功能不全，以及其他一些严重共病[3-4]。

除上述的术前因素外，一些IE特有的或是与IE手术修复显著相关的围手术期因素都会增加并发症的发生风险和严重程度，如长时间体外循环、脓毒症、感染组织彻底清创、大范围的瓣膜和组织重建。这些因素有可能导致严重的术后血管麻痹和低血压、混合性休克、凝血功能障碍、术后出血过多等，需要再次开胸探查止血，以解除心脏压塞[3-5]。

其他严重可致残甚至致死的并发症包括心律失常、脑血管意外、急性肾衰竭和肺炎[5]。最后，医务人员应将静脉吸毒（IVDU）者作为特殊患者群体处理，尤其是在疼痛管理和预防复发方面，以改善这一脆弱群体的治疗结局，减少复发。

术后血管麻痹

心脏手术术后易发生严重血管麻痹，发生率为5%~25%[6-7]。术后血管麻痹综合征发生于外周血管阻力明显降低时，常伴有容量反应缺乏和心脏需求增加以维持氧输送[6]。接受心脏手术治疗的IE患者发生血管麻痹综合征的风险较高[6]，这可能是多因素造成的，包括长时间体外循环、术前使用血管扩张剂、血管内皮功能失调、术前心功能不全，以及IE特有的严重炎症反应[6]。血管麻痹的初始治疗主要包括使用大剂量的α肾上腺素能药物，如肾上腺素、去甲肾上腺素、去氧肾上腺素和血管升压素。当这些一线药物无效，发生难治性血管麻痹时，可考虑使用亚甲蓝[8]。

液体管理

除因严重炎症状态和脓毒症导致的血管麻痹（以分布性休克为特征）外，IE 术后因为其他一些原因（包括心肌恢复过程中的心输出量降低）还存在低血压风险。此外，接受手术的 IE 患者容易出现肺水肿，尤其是在三尖瓣心内膜炎术后。因此，需要在术后早期密切观察患者的液体和血流动力学状态，术中经食管超声心动图（TEE）检查以及术后频繁的床旁超声评估血容量状态有助于指导复苏[9]。

尽管放置肺动脉导管（PAC）与右侧心内膜炎有关，但当心内膜炎出现混合心源性、分布性和血管麻痹性休克状态时，临床通常还是需要 PAC 用于检测[10-11]。

心律失常管理

由于 IE 术后出现心脏传导阻滞的风险较大[12-14]，因此有必要术中放置心房和心室心外膜起搏电极导线。当心动过缓需要起搏治疗时，依据房室间隔时间长短（可能会有显著延长），决定采用心房起搏还是房室顺序起搏，以维持适当的房室传导间隔时间。但对于Ⅲ度房室传导阻滞合并左心室功能不全，房室顺序起搏显然优于心室起搏[15-16]。

抗凝管理

IE 术后是否抗凝需个体化管理，应根据患者术前的抗凝要求、植入的瓣膜类型以及患者出血和血栓风险大小等因素来决定。中枢神经系统出血是人工瓣膜心内膜炎抗凝治疗病例死亡的主要原因[17]。抗凝治疗不仅不能有效预防脓毒性栓塞，相反可成为显著增加缺血性卒中出血转化或加重颅内出血的风险因素；因此对于 IE 术后患者，必须在有强烈的抗凝指征情况下，如植入机械瓣膜、深静脉血栓或肺栓塞，才开始或恢复抗凝[3]。即使如此，在启动抗凝前，还须再次权衡预防血栓或栓塞的获益和抗凝所带来的颅内出血风险，尤其是对于那些术前诊断为缺血性卒中的病例。

抗生素管理

所有患者术后均应接受抗生素治疗。以感染源得到控制为起点计算，抗生素治疗的标准疗程一般为 6 周，但疗程长短在一定程度上取决于临床整体情况、感染的侵袭性、病原体类型和是否存在植入物等[3]。一般而言，在血培养最初呈阳性的情况下，6 周疗程应从血培养呈阴性的第一天或手术当天开始计算（以日期较后者为准）（Ⅱa 类，证据级别 C 级）[18]。手术时应进行组织培养，根据培养结果选择敏感抗生素，调整用药和疗程。如果术中组织培养呈阳性，则以手术日为起始时间继续抗感染，完成整个疗程[美国心脏协会（AHA）Ⅱa类，证据级别B级][18]。如果术中组织培养为阴性，根据临床整体情况，可以将手术前抗感染治疗的天数计入总疗程中，或缩短治疗时间（如果血培养也为阴性）（Ⅱb类推荐，证据级别C级）[18-19]。手术前后还应清查菌血症的其他来源及卫星病灶，如牙齿/口腔、慢性皮肤病变或骨感染、结肠（针对解没食子酸链球菌病例）和植入式医疗装置。对于真菌性心内膜炎，由于其易复发，建议终生口服抗真菌药物以抑制感染复发。另外，开始抗生素治疗时，建议请感染科会诊，以协助确定抗生素使用类型和治疗持续时间（Ⅰ类推荐，证据级别B级）[18]。

术后镇痛

就像对其他所有心脏手术患者一样，术后疼痛管理对于心内膜炎患者至关重要。而在这当中，一个需要考虑的特殊人群就是阿片类IVDU患者，据估计，约90%的单纯右侧心内膜炎和20%的左侧心内膜炎发生在这一人群[20]。与未使用过阿片类药物的人群相比，阿片药物的滥用会产生对该类药物的耐受，这部分患者术后需要更大剂量的阿片类药物才能起到镇痛效果。此外，持续的阿片类药物使用还可导致痛觉过敏，疼痛阈值和耐受性降低，导致该人群的术后镇痛极具挑战性[21]。因此，如有可能，可邀请疼痛科会诊治疗，协助制定最佳镇痛方案。

一般而言，术后镇痛应采用多种模式用药，可使用非麻醉剂辅助，以减少麻醉剂的用量，从而最大限度地减少相关的副作用。可推荐的多模式药物包括对乙酰氨基酚、加巴喷丁、氯胺酮和右美托咪定。非甾体抗炎药（NSAID）通常禁用于心脏外科术后镇痛，这与它们潜在的肾毒性和血小板抑制作用有关[22-23]，NSAID的潜在肾毒性在心内膜炎人群中尤应重视，因为该人群近1/3的病例存在急性肾损伤（AKI）[24]。

在没有肝功能障碍的情况下，应使用对乙酰氨基酚。一项随机临床试验发现：在心脏术后的第一个24 h内静脉注射对乙酰氨基酚6次，每次1000 mg，可减少阿片类药物的用量，并提高患者对整体疼痛体验的满意度[25]。另一项研究比较了胸骨切开术后24 h使用静脉注射对乙酰氨基酚与安慰剂的效果，结果显示：对乙酰氨基酚可使疼痛强度评分显著降低，但阿片类药物的用量没有明显减少[26]。还有一些证据支持使用加巴喷丁或普瑞巴林来治疗神经性疼痛。一项针对随机对照试验的meta分析发现：4项加巴喷丁研究中的3项和4项普瑞巴林研究中的2项均显示阿片类药物用量的减少，各有3项加巴喷丁和普瑞巴林随机对照试验显示患者疼痛评分降低[27]。

氯胺酮是一种N-甲基-D-天冬氨酸（NMDA）拮抗剂，也被证明可减少心脏手术后阿片类药物的用量[28]。一项随机对照试验表明：与安慰剂盐水相比，在接受一剂氯胺酮推注再加上后续持续输注48 h的冠状动脉旁路移植术（CABG）

患者中，术后 48 h 内羟考酮的用量明显减少，患者满意度更高[29]。如果需要镇静，与丙泊酚相比，右美托咪定可降低老年患者心脏手术后谵妄的发生率，延迟谵妄发作，并缩短谵妄持续时间[30]。一项美国和加拿大的多中心研究比较了 CABG 术后在 ICU 基于右美托咪定的镇静方案和基于丙泊酚的方案，发现在接受右美托咪定的患者中，8 h 后仍在使用呼吸机者更少，吗啡的使用量也显著减少[31]。

硬膜外镇痛在心脏外科的应用也有相应评估，但这一方法禁用于持续性菌血症患者[32]。已有报道行单次注射双侧胸前神经阻滞麻醉，结果显示能显著降低疼痛评分[33]。多模式、非麻醉剂镇痛方案的有效性推动了专门针对心脏外科手术的加速康复外科（ERAS）方案的出现。该方案整合了对乙酰氨基酚、加巴喷丁、氯胺酮、右美托咪定和区域神经阻滞的应用[34]。虽然这些方案更多是针对心脏外科择期手术患者进行设计和测试，而非危重心内膜炎患者，但其中许多概念（多模式治疗、使用非麻醉辅助药物、使用非麻醉镇静剂）可推广至术后心内膜炎的管理。

术后非心脏并发症

如第 8 章所述，心内膜炎并发症通常是由感染对心脏直接侵害、赘生物栓塞、感染性或心源性休克导致的全身低灌注引起的。在心内膜炎手术时，赘生物被清除，感染组织被清创处理，相关栓塞风险随之消除。虽然栓塞风险降低了，但大型心脏手术和体外循环引起的相关血流动力学变化意味着全身低灌注并发症的风险仍然存在。

研究表明，脑血管意外是 IE 术后最常见、最致命的并发症之一[2]。术后卒中常见于主动脉瓣和（或）二尖瓣上有大的赘生物，以及术前发生过栓塞性卒中的患者。

手术虽然存在风险，但与内科治疗相比，可有效改善患者生存率，降低并发症发生率，显著降低栓塞发生率，尤其对于赘生物较大的患者。一项随机研究表明：在术前无卒中的患者中，早期手术（随机分组后 48 h 内手术）可降低死亡率和栓塞发生率（随机分组后 6 周内住院死亡和栓塞事件的复合结局指标：早期手术组为 3%，常规治疗组为 28%；P=0.02）[35]。

手术虽然具有诸多益处，但术后卒中风险仍然很高。在一项小型医疗机构的研究中，16% 的患者术后出现了脑血管意外事件，其中一例因脑水肿而需要开颅手术[2]。此外，在一项包含 1345 例左侧心内膜炎病例的多中心研究中，25% 的患者术后出现了神经系统并发症[36]：14%（188 例）为缺血性事件，6%（86 例）为脑病或脑膜炎，4%（60 例）为脑出血，1%（2 例）为脑脓肿。缺血性卒中或颅内出血导致死亡率从 24% 增加到 45%（P=0.01）。关于围手术期处理，早期抗菌治疗可显著降低神经系统并发症的发生率，但抗凝治疗作为一个不确定因素，可增加脑出血风险[37]。此外，对于颅内出血患者，如果手术需要在出血发生后 4 周内进行，死亡率会升高[37]。

虽然一些研究表明，对于并发缺血性卒中的 IE 患者，延迟手术与早期手术相比，并没有生存获益；但目前的美国胸外科医师协会（STS）指南建议，对于发生严重缺血性卒中及所有颅内出血患者，瓣膜置换术至少延迟 4 周[38-39]。推荐是基于体外循环抗凝有可能导致自发性出血风险增加，另外，心脏手术期间低血压可能加重甚至导致缺血范围扩大，而这类问题在脑血管意外发生后的最初几天到几周内最为突出[39]。对于先前发生过卒中并已接受 IE 手术修复的患者，如果随后出现神经系统状态改变，应及时排除出血性转化或脑缺血和（或）水肿恶化的可能性，并予紧急处理。

约 7% 的 IE 患者术后会出现肾衰竭，人工瓣膜的发生率显著高于自体瓣膜（11% vs. 4.4%，P=0.008）[1]。IE 术后的肾脏面临着特殊的风险，急性肾损伤和肾衰竭的潜在病因依然存在，包括术前已存在的肾小球肾炎、低灌注引起的肾梗死以及抗生素引起的急性间质性肾炎[40]。抗生素在心内膜炎治疗中至关重要，但可能存在肾毒性，因此必须用量适当，特别是在肾损伤肾小球滤过率急剧下降的情况下。与术前准备一样，维持心输出量和足够的血压可保护肾脏免于缺血性损伤和急性肾小管坏死。液体出入量管理同样重要，只要有指征，血液透析应尽早实施。

无论是人工瓣膜 IE 还是自体瓣膜 IE，术后早期其他非心脏并发症的发生率都很高，包括呼吸衰竭（17%）、脓毒症（13%）和因出血再手术（6%～9%）[1]。毋庸置疑，这一群体极易发生并发症，其原因多种多样，并发症发生率和死亡率都很高，因此，及时识别和积极治疗至关重要，这样才能改善预后，使手术治疗的总体获益最大化。

特殊人群

IVDU 是心内膜炎（尤其是右侧心内膜炎）的已知风险因素。如上所述，估计 90% 的单纯右侧心内膜炎和 20% 的左侧心内膜炎发生在 IVDU 患者中[20]。IVDU 心内膜炎的发病率估计为（1.5～3.3）/1000（人·年）[41-42]。Kaiser 等回顾性比较了因心内膜炎而需要进行瓣膜置换术的 IVDU 患者和非 IVDU 患者的术后结局[43]：手术死亡率无显著差异，IVDU 患者为 11%，非 IVDU 患者为 12%；两组的围手术期并发症发生率和年龄调整后的长期生存率也相似，但 IVDU 患者再手术发生率高（17% vs. 5%）。同样，在一项自体瓣膜心内膜炎瓣膜置换术后心内膜炎复发风险因素的研究中，Fedoruk 等发现 IVDU/ 人类免疫缺陷病毒（HIV）感染与复发需要再次手术的风险比（HR）为 12.8[44]。

一项来自美国住院患者样本的数据显示，在 2000—2010 年的研究期间，接受心内膜炎手术的 HIV 阳性患者比例从 32% 降到了 8%[45]。重要的是，在对 HIV 阳性患者的心内膜炎进行手术治疗决策时，同一项研究发现 HIV 阳性并不是手术死亡率的独立预测因素。

治疗 IVDU 心内膜炎的一个具体问题是阿片类药物的依赖性和耐受性，这可能使术后疼痛管理成为一项特殊的挑战。如前文所述，必须认识到这类患者对阿片类药物的需求量更高和痛觉过敏的可能性，应采用多模式镇痛方案，必要时可紧急请疼痛科会诊指导。

IVDU 心内膜炎的另一个问题就是需要长时间门诊静脉使用抗生素。其中一种解决方案是缩短住院抗生素疗程。IVDU 者最常发生右侧心内膜炎，最常见的病原体是金黄色葡萄球菌[46]。对于无并发症的右侧金黄色葡萄球菌心内膜炎，住院接受 2 周的 β-内酰胺类药物（联合或不联合氨基糖苷类）治疗已证明疗效良好[47-49]。然而，IVDU 患者经常发生不常见病原体的感染，例如革兰氏阴性杆菌和多种病原体混合感染[50]。在这种情况下（或在出现并发症的情况下），需要更长时间的肠外抗菌治疗，而门诊治疗极具挑战性。因为这一人群通常依从性差，且静脉输液管可能被用于 IVDU。AHA 关于 IE 的科学声明（由美国感染病学会认可）建议，IVDU 心内膜炎门诊肠外抗生素治疗时应遵循以下标准：可靠的家庭支持、方便的医院就诊、家庭输液护士的定期访视以及经验丰富的医生的定期访视[50]。

最后，对 IVDU 患者的治疗还应咨询成瘾医学专家，为其戒毒提供资源及制定治疗计划。

总　结

IE 的术后管理应包括瓣膜手术后的常规术后处理以及针对 IE 的特殊治疗，包括严重血管麻痹、感染和栓塞后遗症、急性脑损伤以及对阿片类药物耐受患者的复杂疼痛的管理。鉴于此类患者通常病情严重，并发症发生率和死亡率高，且并发症多种多样，需要经验丰富的多学科团队在重症监护条件下积极处理。即使患者进入普通病房，该团队仍须继续参与术后管理。

参考文献

[1] Manne MB, Shrestha NK, Lytle BW, et al. Outcomes after surgical treatment of native and prosthetic valve infective endocarditis. Ann Thorac Surg, 2012, 93: 489–493.

[2] Volk L, Verghis N, Chiricolo A, et al. Early and intermediate outcomes for surgical management of infective endocarditis. J Cardiothorac Surg, 2019, 14: 211.

[3] AATS Surgical Treatment of Infective Endocarditis Consensus Guidelines Writing Committee Chairs, Pettersson GB, Coselli JS, et al. 2016 the American Association for Thoracic Surgery (AATS) consensus guidelines: surgical treatment of infective endocarditis: executive summary. J Thorac Cardiovasc Surg, 2017, 153: 1241–1258. e29.

[4] Farag M, Borst T, Sabashnikov A, et al. Surgery for infective endocarditis: outcomes and predictors of mortality in 360 consecutive patients. Med Sci Mon Int Med J Exp Clin Res, 2017, 23: 3617–3626.

[5] Habib G, Lancellotti P, Antunes MJ, et al. 2015 ESC guidelines for the management of infective endocarditis: the task force for the management of infective endocarditis of the European Society of Cardiology (ESC). Endorsed by: European Association for Cardio-Thoracic Surgery (EACTS), the European Association of Nuclear Medicine (EANM). Eur Heart J, 2015, 36: 3075–3128.

[6] Mirhosseini SM, Sanjari Moghaddam A, Tahmaseb Pour P, et al. Refractory vasoplegic syndrome in an adult patient with infective endocarditis: a case report and literature review. J Tehran Heart Cent, 2017, 12: 27–31.

[7] Wittwer ED, Lynch JJ, Oliver Jr WC, et al. The incidence of vasoplegia in adult patients with right-sided

[8] Lavigne D. Vasopressin and methylene blue: alternate therapies in vasodilatory shock. Semin CardioThorac Vasc Anesth, 2010, 14: 186–189.

[9] Pourmand A, Pyle M, Yamane D, et al. The utility of point-of-care ultrasound in the assessment of volume status in acute and critically ill patients. World J Emerg Med, 2019, 10: 232–238.

[10] Rowley KM, Clubb KS, Smith GJ, et al. Right-sided infective endocarditis as a consequence of flow-directed pulmonary-artery catheterization. A clinicopathological study of 55 autopsied patients. N Engl J Med, 1984, 311: 1152–1156.

[11] van Diepen S, Katz JN, Albert NM, et al. Contemporary management of cardiogenic shock: a scientific statement from the American Heart Association. Circulation, 2017, 136: e232–e268.

[12] Brown RE, Chiaco JMC, Dillon JL. Infective endocarditis presenting as Complete heart block with an unexpected finding of a cardiac abscess and purulent pericarditis. J Clin Med Res, 2015, 7: 890–895.

[13] Brancheau D, Degheim G, Machado C. Timing for pacing after acquired conduction disease in the setting of endocarditis. Case Rep Cardiol, 2015, 2015: 471046.

[14] Jeffrey Tabas, Paul D Varosy, Gregory M Marcus, et al. Significance of first-degree atrioventricular block in acute endocarditis-diagnosis. JAMA Intern Med, 2013, 173.726–726.

[15] Samet P, Castillo C, Bernstein WH. Hemodynamic sequelae of atrial, ventricular, and sequential atrioventricular pacing in cardiac patients. Am Heart J, 1966, 72: 725–729.

[16] Durbin CG, Kopel RF. Optimal atrioventricular (AV) pacing interval during temporary AV sequential pacing after cardiac surgery. J Cardiothorac Vasc Anesth, 1993, 7: 316–320. https://doi.org/10.1016/1053-0770(93)90012-a.

[17] Carpenter JL, McAllister CK. Anticoagulation in prosthetic valve endocarditis. South Med J, 1983, 76: 1372–1375.

[18] Baddour Larry M, Wilson Walter R, Bayer Arnold S, et al. Infective endocarditis in adults: diagnosis, antimicrobial therapy, and management of complications. Circulation, 2015, 132: 1435–1486.

[19] Morris AJ, Drinkovic D, Pottumarthy S. Bacteriological outcome after valve surgery for active infective endocarditis: implications for duration of treatment after surgery. Clin Infect Dis, 2005, 41: 187–194.

[20] Moreillon P, Que Y-A. Infective endocarditis. Lancet, 2004, 363: 139–149.

[21] Chu LF, Clark DJ, Angst MS. Opioid tolerance and hyperalgesia in chronic pain patients after one month of oral morphine therapy: a preliminary prospective study. J Pain, 2006, 7: 43–48.

[22] Schafer AI. Effects of nonsteroidal antiinflammatory drugs on platelet function and systemic hemostasis. J Clin Pharmacol, 1995, 35: 209–219.

[23] Whelton A. Nephrotoxicity of nonsteroidal anti-inflammatory drugs: physiologic foundations and clinical implications. Am J Med, 1999, 106: 13S–24S.

[24] Conlon PJ, Jefferies F, Krigman HR, et al. Predictors of prognosis and risk of acute renal failure in bacterial endocarditis. Clin Nephrol, 1998, 49: 96–101.

[25] Jelacic S, Bollag L, Bowdle A, et al. Intravenous acetaminophen as an adjunct analgesic in cardiac surgery reduces opioid consumption but not opioid-related adverse effects: a randomized controlled trial. J Cardiothorac Vasc Anesth, 2016, 30: 997–1004.

[26] Mamoun NF, Lin P, Zimmerman NM, et al. Intravenous acetaminophen analgesia after cardiac surgery: a randomized, blinded, controlled superiority trial. J Thorac Cardiovasc Surg, 2016, 152: 881–889. e1.

[27] Maitra S, Baidya DK, Bhattacharjee S, et al. Perioperative gabapentin and pregabalin in cardiac surgery: a systematic review and meta-analysis. Rev Bras Anestesiol, 2017, 67: 294–304.

[28] MazzeffiM, Johnson K, Paciullo C. Ketamine in adult cardiac surgery and the cardiac surgery Intensive Care Unit: an evidence-based clinical review. Ann Card Anaesth, 2015, 18: 202–209.

[29] Lahtinen P, Kokki H, Hakala T, et al. S(+)-ketamine as an analgesic adjunct reduces opioid consumption after cardiac surgery. Anesth Analg, 2004, 99: 1295–1301 [Table of contents].

[30] Djaiani G, Silverton N, Fedorko L, et al. Dexmedetomidine versus propofol sedation reduces delirium after cardiac surgery: a randomized controlled trial. Anesthesiology, 2016, 124: 362–368.

[31] Herr DL, Sum-Ping STJ, England M. ICU sedation after coronary artery bypass graft surgery: dexmedetomidine-based versus propofol-based sedation regimens. J Cardiothorac Vasc Anesth, 2003, 17: 576–584.

[32] Guay J, Kopp S. Epidural analgesia for adults undergoing cardiac surgery with or without cardiopulmonary bypass. Cochrane Database Syst Rev, 2019, 3: CD006715.

[33] Kumar KN, Kalyane RN, Singh NG, et al. Efficacy of bilateral pectoralis nerve block for ultrafast tracking and postoperative pain management in cardiac surgery. Ann Card Anaesth, 2018, 21: 333–338.

[34] Grant MC, Isada T, Ruzankin P, et al. Results from an enhanced recovery program for cardiac surgery. J Thorac Cardiovasc Surg, 2020, 159: 1393–1402.e7.

[35] Kang D-H, Kim Y-J, Kim S-H, et al. Early surgery versus conventional treatment for infective endocarditis. N Engl J Med, 2012, 366: 2466–2473.

[36] Garcia-Cabrera E, et al. Neurological complications of infective endocardit. Anticoagulant therapy should be considered Circulation, 2013, 127: 2272–2284. https://doi.org/10.1161/CIRCULATIONAHA.112.000813/-/DC1.

[37] García-Cabrera E, Fernández-Hidalgo N, Almirante B, et al. Neurological complications of infective endocarditis: risk factors, outcome, and impact of cardiac surgery: a multicenter observational study. Circulation, 2013, 127: 2272–2284.

[38] Barsic B, Dickerman S, Krajinovic V, et al. Influence of the timing of cardiac surgery on the outcome of patients with infective endocarditis and stroke. Clin Infect Dis, 2013, 56: 209–217.

[39] Byrne JG, Rezai K, Sanchez JA, et al. Surgical management of endocarditis: the society of thoracic surgeons clinical practice guideline. Ann Thorac Surg, 2011, 91: 2012–2019.

[40] Majumdar A, Chowdhary S, Ferreira MA, et al. Renal pathological findings in infective endocarditis. Nephrol Dial Transplant, 2000, 15: 1782–1787.

[41] Reisberg BE. Infective endocarditis in the narcotic addict. Prog Cardiovasc Dis, 1979, 22: 193–204.

[42] Wilson LE, Thomas DL, Astemborski J, et al. Prospective study of infective endocarditis among injection drug users. J Infect Dis, 2002, 185: 1761–1766.

[43] Kaiser SP, Melby SJ, Zierer A, et al. Long-term outcomes in valve replacement surgery for infective endocarditis. Ann Thorac Surg, 2007, 83: 30–35.

[44] Fedoruk LM, Jamieson WRE, Ling H, et al. Predictors of recurrence and reoperation for prosthetic valve endocarditis after valve replacement surgery for native valve endocarditis. J Thorac Cardiovasc Surg, 2009, 137: 326–333.

[45] Polanco A, Itagaki S, Chiang Y, et al. Changing prevalence, profile, and outcomes of patients with HIV undergoing cardiac surgery in the United States. Am Heart J, 2014, 167: 363–368.

[46] Miró JM, del Río A, Mestres CA. Infective endocarditis and cardiac surgery in intravenous drug abusers and HIV-1 infected patients. Cardiol Clin, 2003, 21: 167–184 [v-vi].

[47] Chambers HF, Miller RT, Newman MD. Right-sided Staphylococcus aureus endocarditis in intravenous drug abusers: two-week combination therapy. Ann Intern Med, 1988, 109: 619–624.

[48] DiNubile MJ. Short-course antibiotic therapy for right-sided endocarditis caused by Staphylococcus aureus in injection drug users. Ann Intern Med, 1994, 121: 873–876.

[49] Fortún J, Navas E, Martínez-Beltrán J, et al. Short-course therapy for right-side endocarditis due to Staphylococcus aureus in drug abusers: cloxacillin versus glycopeptides in combination with gentamicin. Clin Infect Dis, 2001, 33: 120–125.

[50] Baddour LM, Wilson WR, Bayer AS, et al. Infective endocarditis: diagnosis, antimicrobial therapy, and management of complications: a statement for healthcare professionals from the Committee on Rheumatic Fever, Endocarditis, and Kawasaki Disease, Council on Cardiovascular Disease in the Young, and the Councils on Clinical Cardiology, Stroke, and Cardiovascular Surgery and Anesthesia, American Heart Association: Endorsed by the Infectious Diseases Society of America. Circulation, 2005, 111: e394–e434.

第10章
感染性心内膜炎的神经系统并发症

Lucy Q. Zhang[1], *Ken Uchino*[2], *Chun Woo Choi*[3], *Sung-Min Cho*[1,4]

[1]Division of Neurocritical Care, Departments of Neurology, Neurosurgery, Anesthesiology and Critical Care Medicine, Johns Hopkins University School of Medicine, Baltimore, MD, United States; [2]Cerebrovascular Center, Neurological Institute, Cleveland Clinic, Cleveland, OH, United States; [3]Division of Cardiac Surgery, Cardiovascular Surgical Intensive Care, Department of Surgery, Heart and Vascular Institute, Johns Hopkins University School of Medicine, Baltimore, MD, United States; [4]Neuroscience Critical Care Division, Departments of Anesthesiology and Critical Care Medicine, Neurology, and Neurosurgery, Johns Hopkins School of Medicine Baltimore, MD, United States

引 言

尽管现代医学在感染性心内膜炎（IE）的诊疗方面取得了进展，但 IE 患者的住院死亡率仍高达 15%~20%[1-3]。据报道，在出现神经系统并发症的患者中，死亡率可达 45%[4-6]。文献显示，左侧 IE 神经系统并发症的发生率为 20%~80%，这一数据因不同研究对"神经系统并发症"的定义不同而不同[7-10]。然而无论数据差异如何，神经系统并发症一旦发生，将对 IE 的治疗产生重大影响。

脑栓塞/缺血性卒中

栓塞性脑梗死是迄今为止左侧 IE 最常见的神经系统并发症，目前可预测这一并发症的因素包括赘生物位于二尖瓣前叶、长度＞10mm 及活动度很大[11-20]。金黄色葡萄球菌不仅是自体瓣膜 IE 的最常见病原体，也是 IE 相关脑梗死的最常见病原体[5,21-22]。而真菌和 β-溶血性链球菌虽是少见的 IE 病原体，但它们可以导致巨大赘生物形成，因而脑栓塞风险较大[19,23-24]。

大型队列研究发现，IE 卒中风险早在确诊之前的 40 天就已升高[5,25-26]。数据显示，29%~47% 的 IE 病例最初的表现即为卒中症状[6,27-28]。推测卒中的发生与感染引起的全身炎症有关，全身炎症促进局部炎症环境形成，加速了动脉粥样硬化和血栓栓塞的发生[29-30]。目前，抗菌治疗是减少感染性栓塞发生的最有效方法[5,21]。在一项前瞻性队列研究中，抗菌治疗将栓塞性卒中的发病率从治疗第 1 周的 4.82/1000（患者·天）降低到第 2 周的 1.71/1000（患者·天）[26]。抗血小板药物作为抗生素的辅助疗法以降低栓塞的风险。动物实验结果显示,阿司匹林可能有助于消除瓣膜赘生物[31-32]。但一项对 115 名 IE 病例的随机双盲对照研究显示:确诊 IE 后服用 325mg 阿司匹林 4 周和服用安慰剂相比,栓塞性脑梗死发生率相似,两组间颅内出血(ICH)发生率也没有差异;但与安慰剂组相比,阿司匹林组的出血并发症总体更多[33]。随后的一项回顾性研究评估了长期抗血小板治疗对栓塞的影响,发现在 IE 诊断前持续进行抗血小板治疗至少 6 个月的 IE 患者的栓塞发生率较低[34]。虽然这一研究表明长期抗血小板治疗可降低栓塞发生率,但没有提供关于抗血小板治疗与 ICH 风险的任何数据,因此,是否继续抗血小板治疗须根据患者临床病情,权衡利弊后使用。

影像表现方面,IE 引起的缺血性梗死与其他心源性梗死基本相似,大多数病例无临床症状,表现为扩散局限的单个点状病变或散布在脑实质中的多个微小病灶(图 10.1)[5,25,35]。有症状的栓塞性卒中(包括暂时性的神经功能缺损)与无症状之间存在临床差别。20%~40% 的 IE 可出现栓塞性卒中[6,36-37],其中 48%~82% 在磁共振成像(MRI)上仅为无症状梗死[8-9,22,35-36]。虽然无症状梗死定义上是临床无症状,但对瓣膜手术的紧迫性、安全性以及长期神经系统预后均有影响。另外,脓毒性栓塞可阻塞较大的颅内血管,不仅可引起病情恶化,还会导致手术计划延迟。在一项针对急性 IE 患者的最大规模脑部 MRI 研究中,25% 的患者(33/130)因大血管堵塞(LVO)而出现大的梗死病灶[9]。

再灌注治疗

美国神经疾病和卒中研究所进行的一项静脉组织纤溶酶原激活剂(IV tPA)静脉溶栓(IVT)临床试验中,早期设计并未排除心内膜炎患者入组,但登记中对 IE 引起的急性缺血性卒中的纳入并不常见[38-39]。尽管存在 IE 溶栓成功的个案报道,但相关的回顾性研究和系统性综述表明 IE 病例接受 IVT 后的疗效并非尽如人意[40-45]。使用国家住院病例样本数据库的数据,Asaithambi 等发表了迄今为止

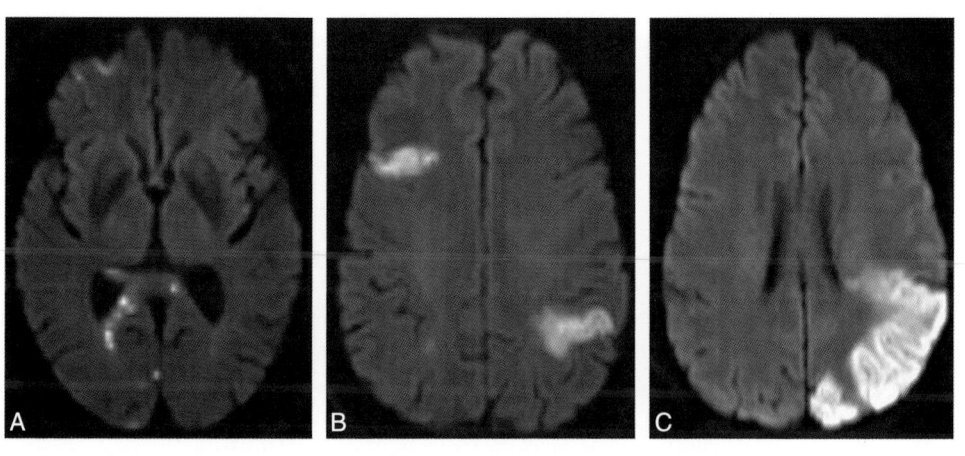

图 10.1 感染性心内膜炎(IE)并发急性缺血性梗死的扩散加权成像。A. 多点状病变。B. 多区域皮质梗死。C. 累及单血管供应区的大面积梗死

最大规模的相关研究，比较了 IE 和非 IE 溶栓后的出血发生率，警告：不要使用 IVT 治疗 IE 病例的急性缺血性卒中。他们的研究显示：接受 IVT 的 IE 急性缺血性脑梗死患者中有 20%（44/222）出现溶栓后出血，而没有 IE 者这一比例为 6.5%（8730/134 048）。系统性综述也得出与此一致的结论[44-45]，在最近的一篇综述中，Bettencourt 和 Ferro 的结论是：接受 IVT 的 IE 病例，溶栓后出血的风险是非 IE 接受 IVT 病例的 4 倍[45]。据此，美国心脏协会/美国卒中协会（AHA/ASA）不推荐静脉注射阿替普酶用于 IE 急性缺血性卒中的治疗[46]。

机械取栓（MT）对 IE 引起的近端 LVO 的疗效尚不确定。2015 年发布的 5 项 MT 随机对照试验中的 2 项，以及具有里程碑意义的晚窗口期 MT、DEFUSE 3 和 DAWN 试验，都将细菌性 IE 和可能的脓毒性栓塞明确排除在外[47-50]。但系列病例报道和系统性综述认为：MT 是 IE 相关近端 LVO 的可靠治疗手段。在评估再灌注等级和成功再通率的 2 个系列病例报道中，再通成功率按脑梗死溶栓（TICI）定义为 2B 级或以上，分别为 66% 和 83%[51-52]。已发表的系列病例和个案报道的汇总数据也表明 MT 有望成为解决 IE 相关 LVO 的一种方法。此外，就术后 ICH 而言，MT 似乎在该人群的应用也相当安全[53-56]。Marquardt 等的系统综述显示，IE 相关 LVO 在 MT 术后 ICH 的发生率明显低于 IVT[44]。虽然缺乏随机对照试验作为基础，但以上研究依然提示 MT 可能是脓毒性栓塞 LVO 有价值的解决方案。

颅内出血

IE 并发 ICH 将导致院内死亡风险显著增加[5,57]。ICH 涵盖了不同病因和不同严重程度的各种出血性脑并发症，不是单纯的一个病症，因此对其处理须非常细致。目前对 IE 引起 ICH 机制的阐明是基于对死后大脑的组织病理学分析得出的。可能机制包括：①缺血性梗死的出血性转化，而与感染并存的凝血疾病（获得性或其他原因导致）可能是诱因；②脓毒性栓子引起感染性动脉炎所致；③细菌侵入动脉壁，导致感染性颅内动脉瘤（IIA）[58-60]。这些机制中的一种或多种共同作用可能是 IE 患者脑实质出血、蛛网膜下腔出血和脑微出血的发生基础。

脑实质出血（IPH）

IE 出现 IPH 可能是梗死病灶或病灶内血凝块的出血转化[61]，也可能是原发于脑实质的血肿。本节重点讨论后者。文献报道 IE 原发性 IPH 的发生率一般在 3%~9%[5,25,57,62-63]，当然，也有发生率更高的报道，尤其是在以影像证据为基础的危重病例研究中[64-67]。实际上，IE 相关的原发性 IPH 就是脑内血管破裂及随后血肿形成导致的[38]，其发生过程与普通人群中 IPH 的形成没有什么不同[68]。差异在于引起血管破裂的机制不同：虽然 IIA 是致命 IPH 常见的病因，但它并不是 IE 人群 IPH 的主要原因；而感染性动脉炎是 IE 原发性 IPH 的常见原因[57-59]。其病理生理学已在两项研究中得以阐明：主要是动脉管腔内的脓毒性微栓子引起化脓性炎症细胞侵入动脉壁[58-59]，受累动脉被侵蚀、破裂而出血，渗出的血液引发炎症级联反应，导致周围血管进一步破裂[68]。通过这一机制，金黄色葡萄球菌 IE 可在其病程早期引发 IPH[14,58-59,70]。此外，抗血栓药物和凝血功能障碍也会促进 IE 相关 IPH 的发生[5,57-58,71]。

脑栓塞不仅是感染性动脉炎的必要基础，也是 IE 相关 IIA 的前提条件。脓毒性栓子的碎片将细菌带入脑血管或其滋养血管，由此细菌入侵动脉壁，破坏动脉壁的完整性。在动物模型中，来自滋养血管的细菌可突破外膜，也可通过内膜扩散到中间弹性层[60]，从而产生局灶性动脉瘤样扩张。IIA 是一种假性动脉瘤，可导致 IPH 和蛛网膜下腔出血，其诊断和治疗将在"感染性颅内动脉瘤"一节中单独讨论。

蛛网膜下腔出血（SAH）

据报道，IE 合并 SAH 的发病率在 1%~3%[65,70,72]，而且多出现在瓣膜感染的早期。一项研究显示：8 名患者中 6 名在急性 IE 诊断之前或同时诊断出 SAH，其余 2 名在 IE 诊断后 3~7d 确诊发生 SAH[72]。但目前尚不清楚何种程度的 IIA 破裂会引起 SAH，临床可出现小的隐匿性 IIA 破裂但找不到任何动脉瘤证据的情况，也可因未破裂的 IIA 发生血液渗漏引起 SAH[73]。同样，感染性动脉炎也可导致局灶性出血进入蛛网膜下腔[58]。精神错乱和局灶性神经功能缺损伴弥漫性头痛，是 IE 合并 SAH 的常见表现[72,74]。极少数情况下，继发于 IIA 破裂的严重 SAH，可导致癫痫发作及病情迅速恶化[75]。

脑微出血（CMB）

在活动性 IE 病例中，CMB 是 MRI 上最常见的异常发现，发生率为 50%[8,9,76]。在 T2* 加权序列上，如梯度回波和磁敏感加权成像（SWI），表现为圆形、低信号病灶[77-78]，直径通常 ≤5mm，多见于大脑皮质。CMB 可见于除 IE 以外的多种病因，且病理生理也不尽相同[79-80]，但这些不同的机制最终有一个共同的结局：血液从受损血管中渗出，随之出现的含铁血黄素被巨噬细胞吞噬[77,81]。在 IE 人群，CMB 被看作感染性微血管炎[82]，类似感染性动脉炎的病理改变，区别是其累及部位在毛细血管和微动脉。

CMB 对 IE 的意义主要在于评估出现 ICH 的临床风险。Okazaki 发现存在 ≥2 处的 CMB 病灶是 3 个月内出现症状性 ICH 的独立风险因素[67]，发生 ICH 的 IE 病例的 CMB 灶中位数为 11 个 [四分位间距（IQR）= 5~13]，而未发生 ICH 的 CMB 灶中位数为 0 个（IQR = 0~1）。值得注意的是，在本研究中，ICH 和非 ICH 两组在年龄、高血压或抗血栓治疗方面没有差异，而两组从瓣膜手术到 ICH 发生的时间间隔是否存在差异尚不清楚。在一项更大规模的研究中，Murai 认为 CMB 与瓣膜手术后症状性出血的风险增加无关[83]。Hess 等也发现他们队列中的 CMB 与 IPH 之间没有相关性[8]。尽管如此，对于具有多个 CMB 灶和神经系统缺损的 IE 病例，在决定抗凝和手术时机时仍需谨慎。

感染性颅内动脉瘤（IIA）

IIA，俗称真菌性动脉瘤，是一种可怕的 IE 并发症，可导致灾难性的 ICH。一般认为 IE 临床 IIA 的发生率为 2%～10%[84-86]，但由于脑血管造影不作为常规检查项目（因有侵入性），加之 IIA 经抗生素治疗可消退甚至治愈[86-91]，因此，IIA 的真实患病率尚不清楚。目前 IIA 的诊断主要涉及何时、何种方式才能最佳地评估 IIA，治疗方面则需要结合动脉瘤的形态、位置和临床病情进行综合处理。

如前所述，IIA 被认为是由细菌侵袭和局部炎症导致的动脉壁破裂[60]。通常体积较小（<5 mm），壁薄而脆，呈纺锤形或囊状（图 10.2）[92]，好发于大脑动脉远端，最常见于大脑中动脉的分支处[91-93]。15%～30% 的 IIA 患者在就诊时存在局灶性神经功能障碍[92-93]，还可表现为精神状态改变或癫痫发作，这些表现都预示着 IIA 有活动性血液渗漏或濒临破裂[69]。然而，IIA 通常没有临床症状，而一旦破裂则是致命的神经损伤[69,91]。

IIA 的评估从头颅 CT 平扫开始，如果显示有颅内出血，则需要进一步的血管成像检查[94]。同理，具有某些脑部 MRI 异常表现的病例也应接受 IIA 的排查。正如 Cho 等的描述，CMB 病变的强化和较大脑沟回的 SWI 病变（无论有无造影增强显影）都提示 IIA 的存在[95-96]。相反，根据 Monteleone 的研究，如果 MRI 未发现出血，则强烈提示不存在 IIA，在这种情况下，血管成像就非必需[97]。数字减影血管造影（DSA）仍然是检测 IIA 的金标准，但它通常仅用于 IE 并发 ICH 或高度

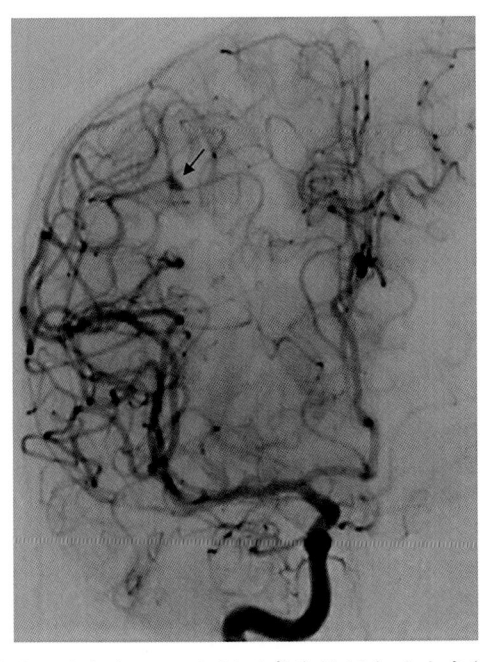

图 10.2　右侧大脑中动脉远端分支 2mm 纺锤形感染性颅内动脉瘤（IIA）（黑色箭头所示），IIA 多发于血管分叉处，但多位于分叉点近心端位置

怀疑 IIA 的病例。CT 血管造影（CTA）是一种非侵入性成像方式，具有方便易行的优点。大型单层 CTA 研究的 meta 分析显示，其灵敏度至少为 90%，特异性为 77%~86%[98-99]。而多层 CTA 则进一步提高了灵敏度和特异性，Wintermark 等的研究显示，对于 3~4mm 的 IIA，其灵敏度达到 94%，总体特异性为 95%[100]。作为 CTA 的替代方案，磁共振血管造影（MRA）的优点是可免受辐射和无须使用碘造影剂，且对颅内动脉瘤的诊断灵敏度已提升到了可与 CTA 相媲美的程度[101-102]。即便如此，没有哪种方法是绝对可靠的，诊断的准确性受动脉瘤的大小、位置、环境，使用的重建算法，以及实施和解读影像结果的医疗机构经验等多因素影响[103]。美国及欧洲心脏学会指南均推荐，当非侵入性影像结果为"阴性"，但仍然高度怀疑 IIA 时，应进行 DSA 检查[104-105]。

· IIA 的治疗注意事项

目前，IIA 尚无治疗指南，但治疗目标很明确：缩小动脉瘤、防止动脉瘤破裂。对此，不同地区和机构的做法各不相同，但普遍共识是：无论是进行血管内介入还是开放手术处理瘤体，抗生素治疗都不可缺少，使用 4~6 周的病原体特异性抗生素治疗是主要手段[69,92-93]。对大量未破裂 IIA 病例的系列研究发现，即便 IIA 体积可因治疗减小或完全消退，但 IIA 对抗生素的总体反应还是存在明显差异[86,88,106]。例如，Corr 的研究显示：他们的队列中有 1/3 完全消退，另外 1/3 的瘤体大小没有变化；此外，在影像随访中，17% 的患者在抗生素治疗期间反而出现瘤体增大的现象[88]；有些病例甚至在接受抗生素治疗期间发生动脉瘤破裂。以上这些说明单纯抗生素治疗的效果难以预测。因此，在过去 10 年，已越来越少将抗生素保守治疗作为单一治疗策略[93]，而抗生素与血管内介入或神经外科相结合的治疗已成为当今主流方案[107-108]。尽管某些情况下抗生素治疗仍是唯一的治疗选择，例如出现临床状况不稳定、严重共病以及 IIA 靠近皮质功能区等情况。对于这些患者，建议每 7~14 d 检查一次，对 IIA 进行连续动态影像学检测[88-90]。

血管内治疗的进步改变了现代 IIA 的治疗。近年来，大量的临床个案系列研究已将血管内治疗置于该领域最前沿。使用弹簧圈直接栓塞或支架分流处理 IIA 也成为当前治疗的既定策略，主要用于近端 IIA。使用正丁基氰基丙烯酸酯或乙烯-乙烯醇共聚物（Onyx®）的液体栓塞是一种新的替代方法，其安全性和有效性已得到充分证明[108-111]，可能是未来解决多发性 IIA 的一种很有前途的治疗方案，这类病例在一些大型病例系列中占比达 25%~30%[112-114]。对于位于远端或形态复杂的 IIA，可使用液体栓塞或弹簧圈来堵闭载瘤动脉，这种方法为间接方法。血管内治疗 IIA 尽管存在术中动脉瘤破裂的风险，但其创伤小于开放性神经外科手术，因此在过去 5 年，临床治疗已转向微创的血管内治疗方案（包括处理破裂的 IIA）[93]。治疗手段的改进带来了临床疗效的提升，数十年前该类疾病死亡率接近 80%，但过去几年的数据表明 IIA 破裂后的生存率显著提高，死亡率在 12%~30%[107]。

尽管如此，对于部分患者来说，开放性神经外科手术仍是一种有价值的治疗方案。这部分患者包括：病变位置易于显露的低手术风险年轻患者，已进行了充分的抗生素治疗和血管内干预、IIA 仍继续生长增大的患者；此外，接受开颅减压术清除血肿的患者，应考虑同期夹闭或切除 IIA。然而，IIA 的神经外科治疗在技术上具有挑战性：首先，涉及前循环远端分支的 IIA 在开放性手术中可能难以识别和（或）暴露[69]；其次，脆弱的壁和边界不清的动脉瘤瘤颈可能导致无法进行手术夹闭。由于缺乏随机对照试验作为依据，治疗策略将主要由专家意见和各医疗机构的实践经验决定。拥有多学科专家、大手术量样本积累的经验丰富的中心比较适宜开展 IE 并发 IIA 的治疗。

卒中对手术时机的影响

美国心脏协会和美国心脏病学会（AHA/ACA）以及美国胸外科协会（AATS）指南对于活动度较大的赘生物（直径 ≥ 10 mm）、瓣周脓肿、持续性脓毒症或反复系统性栓塞推荐手术治疗。另外，IE 继发的心力衰竭和严重瓣膜功能障碍，以及人工瓣膜 IE 也都需要手术干预[105,115-116]。然而，瓣膜手术的紧迫性和最佳手术时机尚存在诸多不确定性，其中急性缺血性或出血性卒中后瓣膜手术的时机就是一个持续存在争议的问题——需要权衡紧急或早期手术的益处与术后神经功能恶化（继发于梗死组织的出血转化）或 ICH 加重（继发于术中肝素化）的风险。

现有文献对手术时机的看法不一：从初次神经系统事件发生后 72 h 即实施手术到延迟 2~4 周不等[117-123]。在一项系统性综述中，Angstwurm 等统计了与手术时机相关的神经功能恶化风险[117]。结果发现：对于缺血性梗死，梗死后 3 d 内接受手术的神经功能恶化风险为 15%~35%，在第 4~14 天进行手术的神经功能恶化风险为 20%~50%，2 周后该风险降至 10% 以下，1 个月后降至 0.4%。Eishi 等在一项回顾性多中心研究中也发现了类似的趋势[121]：在初次缺血性卒中后第 1 周内接受手术的患者中，死亡率和神经功能恶化率分别为 31% 和 44%，而在 2 周后接受瓣膜手术的患者中该风险为 10%。Gillinov 等在 1996 年的一系列著名回顾性研究中强调了将手术推迟至少 2 周的做法，他们建议将栓塞性卒中患者的瓣膜手术推迟 2~3 周[94]；但他们的研究仅基于 34 名患者，其中近一半是静脉吸毒者。随后，García-Cabrera 等认为，这些早期研究对缺血性卒中的神经损害严重程度界定不甚明确。在他们的多中心研究中，卒中严重程度采用放射学参数进行确定[5]，中重度缺血性病变被定义为"多发性脑栓塞或单次栓塞累及 ≥ 30% 脑组织"，有 28%（15/54）的该类病例接受了瓣膜手术，其中 2 周内接受手术的病例，术后死亡率为 40%（2/5），而延迟 2 周手术的术后死亡率为 20%（2/10）。

2012 年，Kang 等人开展的具有里程碑意义的随机对照试验表明，早期手术（随机分组后 48 h 内）可降低 IE 并发缺血性卒中患者因栓塞事件或其他原因导致的死亡[124]，并对急性缺血性卒中后推迟瓣膜手术的方案提出了质疑，这与一些反对延迟瓣膜手术的相关研究意见一致。首先，Thuny 等的研究数据表明：卒中后较早接受瓣膜手术（中位时间为9 d）患者的术后神经系统并发症发生率为6.3%（4/63），明显低于之前的报道[25]；此外，术后神经系统并发症仅限于缺血性或出血性卒中患者，而不包括短暂性脑缺血发作（TIA）或无症状梗死患者；虽然IE卒中患者的总体死亡率较高，但只有1名患者直接死于卒中。他们的研究证明：卒中并非瓣膜手术的禁忌证。这当中需要强调的是：手术不必因TIA和无症状梗死而推迟，这已成为欧洲心脏病学会指南的Ⅰ类推荐[105]。其次，Barsic等对198名以缺血性卒中为主的IE患者进行了一项极具说服力的多中心前瞻性研究，发现在有指征进行瓣膜手术时推迟手术，患者并没有生存获益[125]；在调整年龄、瓣周脓肿和心力衰竭等变量影响后，缺血性卒中后1周内进行瓣膜手术并未增加住院死亡率。再次，两项基于MRI的前瞻性研究显示：其队列中无术后神经系统并发症出现，这其中1/4病例在瓣膜手术前患有急性缺血性卒中，从卒中到手术的中位时间分别为6 d和8 d[22,27]。鉴于以上研究，AHA/ACA指南于2017年进行了更新：认为对于有手术指征的IE患者，如果其缺血性卒中没有造成"广泛的神经系统损伤（Ⅱb类）"，"可以考虑"尽早进行手术[116]。

过去5年的回顾性研究也为早期手术提供了越来越多的证据。最近的研究表明：在梗死后平均4～10 d进行瓣膜手术，发生神经系统恶化和死亡的风险较低[126-130]。对于梗死体积与手术风险的关系，我们之前的研究也显示：缺血性梗死的梗死体积与术后神经系统不良预后无相关性。研究中的梗死体积中位数为12.9 cm³（IQR = 6～17 cm³），不包含点状梗死[126]。在另一项相关研究中，Oh等根据受累血管区域进行分类，比较了急性缺血性梗死后早期（IE诊断后≤7 d）和晚期手术干预的术后出血并发症和神经系统预后[131]。其中，由小的脑动脉分支供血的区域的梗死被视为"小"梗死，由主要分支动脉供血的区域受累则定义为"中度"梗死，而累及整个血管区域供应动脉的则定义为"大"梗死。研究显示：无论梗死大小，早期手术都不会导致不良神经系统结局或死亡的增加。虽然对回顾性研究应谨慎解读，但对于有迫切手术指征的患者，早期手术干预的好处可能远远大于中小型梗死相关的术后神经系统并发症的风险。

IE伴ICH术后神经系统结局的数据目前仍然很少。Angstwurm等的研究显示，在ICH后4周接受手术的患者其神经系统恶化的发生率为15%[117]。García-Cabrera等2013年的多中心研究显示：在ICH（包括IPH、出血性转化和SAH）后4周内接受手术，死亡率为75%，但4周后手术的死亡率仍高达40%。这一结果加剧了人们对IE伴ICH患者术后不良结局的担忧[5]。近5年，许多研究重新评估了ICH后瓣膜手术的安全性。在2016年的一项多中心研究中，在ICH后中位时间21 d接受瓣膜手术的IE患者的住院死亡率为5.6%[63]。2018年的研究发现，与接受保守治疗的病例相比，瓣膜手术可降低IE伴ICH患者的总体死亡率[57]，这组病例从ICH发生到手术的中位时间为34 d。这些观察性研究都存在一个显著的局限性：数据分析未考虑出血量。在我们的回顾性研究中，未发生围手术期神经系统并发症的患者的血肿大小中位数为2.8 cm³（IQR = 1.1～8.1 cm³）。另外，所有这些研究都存在病例选择上的偏倚。即便如此，这些结果提醒我们：需要重新审视当前的治疗推荐和实践指南，对于一些有强烈瓣膜手术指征的 IE 病例，将手术推迟至少 1 个月可能并不明智，而必须考虑等待手术过程中的心血管问题，特别是持续的心脏结构破坏造成的后果，例如脓肿形成、瓣膜破坏和传导阻滞。

总　结

IE 的临床病程通常因其神经系统表现而变得复杂。IE 相关脑血管并发症的异质性和复杂性需要经验丰富的中心采用多学科团队方法处理。近 10 年的研究支持早期（14 d 内）对并发卒中的 IE 病例进行瓣膜手术，而对于大面积缺血性卒中和 ICH 患者，则应谨慎行事，并需要进一步研究以确定出现此类并发症患者的最佳手术时机。治疗决策虽然有学协会和共识的指导，但应进行个体化处理。

参考文献

[1] Cabell CH, Jollis JG, Peterson GE, et al. Changing patient characteristics and the effect on mortality in endocarditis. Arch Intern Med, 2002. https://doi.org/10.1001/archinte.162.1.90.

[2] Hoen B, Alla F, Selton-Suty C, et al. Changing profile of infective endocarditis: results of a 1-year survey in France. J Am Med Assoc, 2002. https://doi.org/10.1001/jama.288.1.75.

[3] Mullany CJ, Chua YL, Schaff HV, et al. Early and late survival after surgical treatment of culture-positive active endocarditis. Mayo Clin Proc, 1995. https://doi.org/10.4065/70.6.517.

[4] Mourvillier B, Trouillet JL, Timsit JF, et al. Infective endocarditis in the intensive care unit: clinical spectrum and prognostic factors in 228 consecutive patients. Intensive Care Med, 2004. https://doi.org/10.1007/s00134-004-2436-9.

[5] García-Cabrera E, Fernández-Hidalgo N, Almirante B, et al. Neurological complications of infective endocarditis. Circulation, 2013, 127(23): 2272–2284. https://doi.org/10.1161/CIRCULATIONAHA.112.000813.

[6] Heiro M, Nikoskelainen J, Engblom E, et al. Neurologic manifestations of infective endocarditis: a 17-year experience in a teaching hospital in Finland. Arch Intern Med, 2000. https://doi.org/10.1001/archinte.160.18.2781.

[7] Hoen B, Duval X. Infective endocarditis. N Engl J Med, 2013. https://doi.org/10.1056/NEJMcp1206782.

[8] Hess A, Klein I, Iung B, et al. Brain MRI findings in neurologically asymptomatic patients with infective endocarditis. Am J Neuroradiol, 2013. https://doi.org/10.3174/ajnr.A3582.

[9] Duval X, Iung B, Klein I, et al. Effect of early cerebral magnetic resonance imaging on clinical decisions in infective endocarditis: a prospective study. Ann Intern Med, 2010. https://doi.org/10.7326/0003-4819-152-8-201004200-00006.

[10] Sonneville R, Mourvillier B, Bouadma L, et al. Management of neurological complications of infective endocarditis in ICU patients. Ann Intens Care, 2011. https://doi.org/10.1186/2110-5820-1-10.

[11] Mohananey D, Mohadjer A, Pettersson G, et al. Association of vegetation size with embolic risk in patients with infective endocarditis. JAMA Intern Med, 2018. https://doi.org/10.1001/jamainternmed.2017.8653.

[12] Tischler MD, Vaitkus PT. The ability of vegetation size on echocardiography to predict clinical complications: a meta-analysis. J Am Soc Echocardiogr, 1997. https://doi.org/10.1016/S0894-7317(97)70011-7.

[13] Martín-Dávila P, Navas E, Fortún J, et al. Analysis of mortality and risk factors associated with

native valve endocarditis in drug users: the importance of vegetation size. Am Heart J, 2005. https://doi.org/10.1016/j.ahj.2005.02.009.

[14] Weinstein L. Life-threatening complications of infective endocarditis and their management. Arch Intern Med, 1986. https://doi.org/10.1001/archinte.146.5.953.

[15] Stafford WJ, Petch J, Radford DJ. Vegetations in infective endocarditis. Clinical relevance and diagnosis by cross sectional echocardiography. Br Heart J, 1985. https://doi.org/10.1136/hrt.53.3.310.

[16] Steckelberg JM, Murphy JG, Ballard D, et al. Emboli in infective endocarditis: the prognostic value of echocardiography. Ann Intern Med, 1991. https://doi.org/10.7326/0003-4819-114-8-635.

[17] Anderson DJ, Goldstein LB, Wilkinson WE, et al. Stroke location, characterization, severity, and outcome in mitral vs aortic valve endocarditis. Neurology, 2003. https://doi.org/10.1212/01.WNL.0000094359.47929.E4.

[18] Buda AJ, Zotz RJ, LeMire MS, et al. Prognostic significance of vegetations detected by two-dimensional echocardiography in infective endocarditis. Am Heart J, 1986. https://doi.org/10.1016/0002-8703(86)90362-5.

[19] Di Salvo G, Habib G, Pergola V. Echocardiography predicts embolic events in infective endocarditis. ACC CurrJ Rev, 2001. https://doi.org/10.1016/s1062-1458(01)00382-8.

[20] Thuny F, Disalvo G, Belliard O, et al. Risk of embolism and death in infective endocarditis: prognostic value of echocardiography—a prospective multicenter study. Circulation, 2005. https://doi.org/10.1161/CIRCULATIONAHA.104.493155.

[21] Vilacosta I, Graupner C, SanRomán J, et al. Risk of embolization after institution of antibiotic therapy for infective endocarditis. J Am Coll Cardiol, 2002. https://doi.org/10.1016/S0735-1097(02)01790-4.

[22] Cooper HA, Thompson EC, Laureno R, et al. Subclinical brain embolization in left-sided infective endocarditis: results from the evaluation by MRI of the brains of patients with left-sided intracardiac solid masses (EMBOLISM) pilot study. Circulation, 2009. https://doi.org/10.1161/CIRCULATIONAHA.108.834432.

[23] Pierrotti LC, Baddour LM. Fungal endocarditis, 1995—2000. Chest, 2002. https://doi.org/10.1378/chest.122.1.302.

[24] Lefort A, Lortholary O, Casassus P, et al. Comparison between adult endocarditis due to β-hemolytic streptococci (serogroups A, B, C, and G) and Streptococcus milleri: a multicenter study in France. Arch Intern Med, 2002. https://doi.org/10.1001/archinte. 162.21.2450.

[25] Thuny F, Avierinos J-F, Tribouilloy C, et al. Impact of cerebrovascular complications on mortality and neurologic outcome during infective endocarditis: a prospective multicentre study. Eur Heart J, 2007, 28(9): 1155–1161. https://doi.org/10.1093/eurheartj/ehm005.

[26] Dickerman SA, Abrutyn E, Barsic B, et al. The relationship between the initiation of antimicrobial therapy andthe incidence of stroke in infective endocarditis: an analysis from the ICE Prospective Cohort Study (ICE-PCS). Am Heart J, 2007. https://doi.org/10.1016/j.ahj.2007.07.023.

[27] Snygg-Martin U, Gustafsson L, Rosengren L, et al. Cerebrovascular complications in patients with left-sided infective endocarditis are common: a prospective study using magnetic resonance imaging and neurochemicalbrain damage markers. Clin Infect Dis, 2008, 47(1): 23–30. https://doi.org/10.1086/588663.

[28] Corral I, Martín-Dávila P, Fortún J, et al. Trends in neurological complications of endocarditis. J Neurol, 2007, 254(9): 1253–1259. https://doi.org/10.1007/s00415-006-0512-5.

[29] Merkler AE, Chu SY, Lerario MP, et al. Temporal relationship between infective endocarditis andstroke. Neurology ,2015. https://doi.org/10.1212/WNL.0000000000001835.

[30] Elkind MSV, Luna JM, Moon YP, et al. Infectious burden and carotid plaque thickness: the northern Manhattan study. Stroke, 2010. https://doi.org/10.1161/STROKEAHA.109.571299.

[31] Kupferwasser LI, Yeaman MR, Shapiro SM, et al. Acetylsalicylic acid reduces vegetation bacterial density, hematogenous bacterial dissemination, and frequency of embolic events in

experimentalStaphylococcus aureusendocarditis through antiplatelet and antibacterial effects. Circulation, 1999. https://doi.org/10.1161/01.CIR.99.21.2791.

[32] Nicolau DP, Marangos MN, Nightingale CH, et al. Influence of aspirin on development and treatmentof experimental Staphylococcus aureus endocarditis. Antimicrob Agents Chemother, 1995. https://doi.org/10.1128/AAC.39.8.1748.

[33] Chan KL, Dumesnil JG, Cujec B, et al. A randomized trial of aspirin on the risk of embolic events in patientswith infective endocarditis. J Am Coll Cardiol, 2003. https://doi.org/10.1016/S0735-1097(03)00829–5.

[34] Anavekar NS, Tleyjeh IM, Anavekar NS, et al. Impact of prior antiplatelet therapy on risk of embolism in infective endocarditis. Clin Infect Dis, 2007. https://doi.org/10.1086/513197.

[35] Cabell CH, Pond KK, Peterson GE, et al. The risk of stroke and death in patients with aortic and mitral valve endocarditis. Am Heart J, 2001, 142(1): 75–80. https://doi.org/10.1067/mhj.2 001.115790.

[36] Topcuoglu M, Kursun O, Buonanno F, et al. Ischemic and hemorrhagic strokein infective endocarditis: features, predictors and trends over three decades. Stroke, 2017, 48: A84.

[37] Novy E, Sonneville R, Mazighi M, et al. Neurological complications of infective endocarditis: new breakthroughs in diagnosis and management. Med Maladies Infect, 2013. https://doi.org/10.1016/j.medmal.2013.09.010.

[38] The National Institute of Neurological Disorders, Stroke rt-PA Stroke Study Group. Tissue plasminogen activator for acute ischemic stroke. N Engl J Med, 1995. https://doi.org/ 10.1056/NEJM199512143332401.

[39] Hacke W, Kaste M, Bluhmki E, et al. Thrombolysis with alteplase 3 to 4.5 hours after acute ischemic stroke. N Engl J Med, 2008. https://doi.org/10.1056/NEJMoa0804656.

[40] Ong E, Mechtouff L, Bernard E, et al. Thrombolysis for stroke caused by infective endocarditis: an illustrative case and review of the literature. J Neurol, 2013. https://doi.org/10.1007/s00415-012-6802-1.

[41] Junna M, Lin CCD, Espinosa RE, et al. Successful intravenous thrombolysis in ischemic stroke caused by infective endocarditis. Neurocrit Care, 2007. https://doi.org/10.1007/s12028-007-0017-9.

[42] Sontineni SP, Mooss AN, Andukuri VG, et al. Effectiveness of thrombolytic therapy in acute embolic stroke due to infective endocarditis. Stroke Res Treat, 2010. https://doi.org/10.4061/2010/841797.

[43] Asaithambi G, Adil MM, Qureshi AI. Thrombolysis for ischemic stroke associated with infective endocarditis: results from the nationwide inpatient sample. Stroke, 2013. https://doi.org/10.1161/STROKEAHA.113.001602.

[44] Marquardt RJ, Cho SM, Thatikunta P, et al. Acute ischemic stroke therapy in infective endocarditis: case series and systematic review. J Stroke Cerebrovasc Dis, 2019. https://doi.org/10.1016/j.jstrokecerebrovasdis.2019.04.039.

[45] Bettencourt S, Ferro JM. Acute ischemic stroke treatment in infective endocarditis: systematic review. J Stroke Cerebrovasc Dis, 2020. https://doi.org/10.1016/j.jstrokecerebrovasdis.2019.104598.

[46] Demaerschalk BM, Kleindorfer DO, Adeoye OM, et al. Scientific rationale for the inclusion and exclusion criteria for intravenous alteplase in acute ischemic stroke. Stroke, 2016. https://doi.org/10.1161/str.0000000000000086.

[47] Saver JL, Goyal M, Bonafe A, et al. Stent-retriever thrombectomy after intravenous t-PA vs. t-PA alone instroke. N Engl J Med, 2015. https://doi.org/10.1056/NEJMoa1415061.

[48] Campbell BCV, Mitchell PJ, Yan B, et al. A multicenter, randomized, controlled study to investigate extending the time for thrombolysis in emergency neurological deficits with intra-arterial therapy (EXTEND-IA). Int J Stroke, 2014. https://doi.org/10.1111/ijs.12206.

[49] Albers GW, Marks MP, Kemp S, et al. Thrombectomy for stroke at 6 to 16 hours with selection by perfusion imaging. N Engl J Med, 2018. https://doi.org/10.1056/NEJMoa1713973.

[50] Nogueira RG, Jadhav AP, Haussen DC, et al. Thrombectomy 6 to 24 hours after stroke with a mismatch between deficit and infarct. N Engl J Med, 2018. https://doi.org/10.1056/NEJMoa1706442.

[51] Scharf EL, Chakraborty T, Rabinstein A, et al. Endovascular management of cerebral septic embolism: three recent cases and review of the literature. J Neurointervent Surg, 2017. https://doi.org/10.1136/neurintsurg-2016-012792.

[52] Ambrosioni J, Urra X, Hernández-Meneses M, et al. Mechanical thrombectomy for acute ischemic stroke secondary to infective endocarditis. Clin Infect Dis, 2018. https://doi.org/10.1093/cid/cix1000.

[53] Sveinsson O, Herrman L, Holmin S. Intra-arterial mechanical thrombectomy: an effective treatment for ischemic stroke caused by endocarditis. Case Rep Neurol ,2016. https://doi.org/10.1159/000452213.

[54] Cuervo G, Caballero Q, Rombauts A, et al. Mechanical thrombectomy for patients with infective endocarditis and ischemic large-vessel stroke. Clin Infect Dis, 2018. https://doi.org/10.1093/cid/ciy272.

[55] Sloane KL, Raymond SB, Rabinov JD, et al. Mechanical thrombectomy in stroke from infective endocarditis: case report and review. J Stroke Cerebrovasc Dis, 2020. https://doi.org/10.1016/j.jstrokecerebrovasdis.2019.104501.

[56] Kim J-M, Jeon J-S, Kim Y-W, et al. Forced arterial suction thrombectomy of septic embolic middle cerebral artery occlusion due to infective endocarditis: an illustrative case and review of the literature. Neurointervention, 2014. https://doi.org/10.5469/neuroint.2014.9.2.101.

[57] Salaun E, Touil A, Hubert S, et al. Intracranial haemorrhage in infective endocarditis. Arch Cardiovasc Dis, 2018. https://doi.org/10.1016/j.acvd.2018.03.009.

[58] Hart RG, Kagan-Hallet K, Joerns SE. Mechanisms of intracranial hemorrhage in infective endocarditis. Stroke, 1987. https://doi.org/10.1161/01.STR.18.6.1048.

[59] Masuda J, Yutani C, Waki R, et al. Histopathological analysis of the mechanisms of intracranial hemorrhage complicating infective endocarditis. Stroke, 1992. https://doi.org/10.1161/01.STR.23.6.843.

[60] Molinari GF, Smith L, Goldstein MN, et al. Pathogenesis of cerebral mycotic aneurysms. Neurology, 1973. https://doi.org/10.1212/wnl.23.4.325.

[61] Fiorelli M, Bastianello S, von Kummer R, et al. Hemorrhagic transformation within 36 hours of a cerebral infarct. Stroke, 1999. https://doi.org/10.1161/01.str.30.11.2280.

[62] Okazaki S, Yoshioka D, Sakaguchi M, et al. Acute ischemic brain lesions in infective endocarditis: incidence, related factors, and postoperative outcome. Cerebrovasc Dis, 2013. https://doi.org/10.1159/000346101.

[63] Okita Y, Minakata K, Yasuno S, et al. Optimal timing of surgery for active infective endocarditis with cerebral complications: a Japanese multicentre study. Eur J Cardio-thoracic Surg, 2016. https://doi.org/10.1093/ejcts/ezw035.

[64] Chakraborty T, Scharf E, DeSimone D, et al. Variable significance of brain MRI findings in infective endocarditis and its effect on surgical decisions. Mayo Clin Proc, 2019. https://doi.org/10.1016/j.mayocp.2018.09.015.

[65] Yoshioka D, Toda K, Sakaguchi T, et al. Valve surgery in active endocarditis patients complicated by intracranial haemorrhage: the influence of the timing of surgery on neurological outcomes. Eur J Cardio-thoracic Surg, 2014. https://doi.org/10.1093/ejcts/ezt547.

[66] Diab M, Guenther A, Scheffel P, et al. Can radiological characteristics of preoperative cerebral lesions predict postoperative intracranial haemorrhage in endocarditis patients? Eur J Cardio-thoracic Surg. 2016. https://doi.org/10.1093/ejcts/ezw014.

[67] Okazaki S, Sakaguchi M, Hyun B, et al. Cerebral microbleeds predict impending intracranial hemorrhage in infective endocarditis. Cerebrovasc Dis 2011. https://doi.org/10.1159/000331475.

[68] Diringer MN. Intracerebral hemorrhage: pathophysiology and management. Crit Care Med 1993. https://doi.org/10.1097/00003246-199310000-00032.

[69] Peters PJ, Harrison T, Lennox JL. A dangerous dilemma: management of infectious intracranial

aneurysms complicating endocarditis. Lancet Infect Dis, 2006. https://doi.org/10.1016/S1473-3099(06)70631-4.

[70] Pruitt AA, Rubin RH, Karchmer AW, et al. Neurologic complications of bacterial endocarditis. Medicine, 1978. https://doi.org/10.1097/00005792-197807000-00004.

[71] Tornos P, Almirante B, Mirabet S, et al. Infective endocarditis due to Staphylococcus aureus: deleterious effect of anticoagulant therapy. Arch Intern Med, 1999. https://doi.org/10.1001/archinte.159.5.473.

[72] Chukwudelunzu FE, Brown RD, Wijdicks EFM, et al. Subarachnoid haemorrhage associated with infectious endocarditis: case report and literature review. Eur J Neurol, 2002. https://doi.org/10.1046/j.1468-1331.2002.00432.x.

[73] Rinkel GJE, van Gijn J, Wijdicks EFM. Subarachnoid hemorrhage without detectable aneurysm: a review of thecauses. Stroke, 1993.https://doi.org/10.1161/01.STR.24.9.1403.

[74] Salgado AV, Furlan AJ, Keys TF. Mycotic aneurysm, subarachnoid hemorrhage, and indications for cerebral angiography in infective endocarditis. Stroke, 1987. https://doi.org/10.1161/01.STR.18.6.1057.

[75] Yanagihara C, Wada Y, Nishimura Y. Infectious endocarditis associated with subarachnoid hemorrhage, subdural hematoma and multiple brain abscesses. Intern Med, 2003. https://doi.org/10.2169/internalmedicine.42.1244.

[76] Klein I, Iung B, Labreuche J, et al. Cerebral microbleeds are frequent in infective endocarditis: a case-control study. Stroke, 2009. https://doi.org/10.1161/STROKEAHA.109.562546.

[77] Haller S, Vernooij MW, Kuijer JPA, et al. Cerebral microbleeds: imaging and clinical significance. Radiology, 2018. https://doi.org/10.1148/radiol.2018170803.

[78] Viswanathan A, Chabriat H. Cerebral microhemorrhage. Stroke, 2006. https://doi.org/10.1161/01.STR.0000199847.96188.12.

[79] Van Veluw SJ, Biessels GJ, Klijn CJM, et al. Heterogeneous histopathology of cortical microbleedsin cerebral amyloid angiopathy. Neurology, 2016. https://doi.org/10.1212/WNL.0000000000002419.

[80] Shoamanesh A, Kwok CS, Benavente O. Cerebral microbleeds: histopathological correlation of neuroimaging. Cerebrovasc Dis, 2011. https://doi.org/10.1159/000331466.

[81] Fazekas F, Kleinert R, Roob G, et al. Histopathologic analysis of foci of signal loss on gradient-echo T2*-weighted MR images in patients with spontaneous intracerebral hemorrhage: evidence of microangiopathy-related microbleeds. Am J Neuroradiol, 1999, 20(4):637–642.

[82] Klein I, Iung B, Wolff M, et al. Silent T2* cerebral microbleeds: a potential new imaging clue in infective endocarditis. Neurology, 2007. https://doi.org/10.1212/01.wnl.0000266965.04112.bc.

[83] Murai R, Kaji S, Kitai T, et al. The clinical significance of cerebral microbleeds in infective endocarditis patients. Semin Thorac Cardiovasc Surg, 2019;31(1):51–58. https://doi.org/10.1053/j.semtcvs.2018.09.020.

[84] Misfeld M, Girrbach F, Etz CD, et al. Surgery for infective endocarditis complicated by cerebral embolism: a consecutive series of 375 patients. J Thorac Cardiovasc Surg, 2014. https://doi.org/10.1016/j.jtcvs.2013.10.076.

[85] Hui FK, Bain M, Obuchowski NA, et al. Mycotic aneurysm detection rates with cerebral angiography in patients with infective endocarditis. J Neurointervent Surg, 2015. https://doi.org/10.1136/neurintsurg-2014-011124.

[86] Rice CJ, Cho S-M, Marquardt RJ, et al. Clinical course of infectious intracranial aneurysm undergoing antibiotic treatment. J Neurol Sci, 2019, 403. https://doi.org/10.1016/j.jns.2019.06.004.

[87] Baddour LM, Wilson WR, Bayer AS, et al. Infective endocarditis: diagnosis, antimicrobial therapy, and management of complications a statement for healthcare professionals from the committee on rheumatic fever, endocarditis, and Kawasaki disease, council on cardiovascular disease in the young. Circulation, 2005. https://doi.org/10.1161/CIRCULATIONAHA.105.165563.

[88] Corr P, Wright M, Handler LC. Endocarditis-related cerebral aneurysms: radiologic changes with treatment. Am J Neuroradiol, 1995.

[89] Morawetz RB, Karp RB. Evolution and resolution of intracranial bacterial (mycotic) aneurysms. Neurosurgery, 1984. https://doi.org/10.1227/00006123-198407000-00009.

[90] Nakahara I, Taha MM, Higashi T, et al. Different modalities of treatment of intracranial mycotic aneurysms: report of 4 cases. Surg Neurol, 2006. https://doi.org/10.1016/j.surneu.2006.01.021.

[91] Kannoth S, Iyer R, Thomas SV, et al. Intracranial infectious aneurysm: presentation, management and outcome. J Neurol Sci, 2007. https://doi.org/10.1016/j.jns.2007.01.044.

[92] Ducruet AF, Hickman ZL, Zacharia BE, et al. Intracranial infectious aneurysms: a comprehensive review. Neurosurg Rev, 2010. https://doi.org/10.1007/s10143-009-0233-1.

[93] Alawieh A, Chaudry MI, Turner RD, et al. Infectious intracranial aneurysms: a systematic review of epidemiology, management, and outcomes. J Neurointervent Surg, 2018. https://doi.org/10.1136/neurintsurg-2017-013603.

[94] Gillinov AM, Shah RV, Curtis WE, et al. Valve replacement in patients with endocarditis and acute neurologicdeficit. Ann Thorac Surg, 1996. https://doi.org/10.1016/0003-4975(96)00014-8.

[95] Cho S-M, Marquardt RJ, Rice CJ, et al. Cerebral microbleeds predict infectious intracranial aneurysm in infective endocarditis. Eur J Neurol, 2018, 25(7). https://doi.org/10.1111/ene.13641.

[96] Cho S-M, Rice C, Marquardt RJ, et al. Magnetic resonance imaging susceptibility-weighted imaging lesion and contrast enhancement may represent infectious intracranial aneurysm in infective endocarditis. Cerebrovasc Dis, 2017, 44(3-4). https://doi.org/10.1159/000479706.

[97] Monteleone PP, Shrestha NK, Jacob J, et al. Clinical utility of cerebral angiography in the preoperative assessment of endocarditis. Vasc Med, 2014. https://doi.org/10.1177/1358863X14557152.

[98] White PM, Teasdale EM, Wardlaw JM, et al. Intracranial aneurysms: CT angiography and MR angiography for detection—prospective blinded comparison in a large patient cohort. Radiology, 2001. https://doi.org/10.1148/radiology.219.3.r01ma16739.

[99] Van Gelder JM, Hoh BL, Ogilvy CS, et al. Computed tomographic angiography for detecting cerebral aneurysms: implications of aneurysm size distribution for the sensitivity, specificity, and likelihood ratios. Neurosurgery, 2003. https://doi.org/10.1227/01.NEU.0000080060.97293.EE.

[100] Wintermark M, Uske A, Chalaron M, et al. Multislice computerized tomography angiography in the evaluation of intracranial aneurysms: a comparison with intraarterial digital subtraction angiography. J Neurosurg, 2003. https://doi.org/10.3171/jns.2003.98.4.0828.

[101] Mine B, Pezzullo M, Roque G, et al. Detection and characterization of unruptured intracranial aneurysms: comparison of 3T MRA and DSA. J Neuroradiol, 2015. https://doi.org/10.1016/j.neurad.2014.08.002.

[102] Sailer AMH, Wagemans BAJM, Nelemans PJ, et al. Diagnosing intracranial aneurysmswith MR angiography : systematic review and meta-analysis. Stroke, 2014. https://doi.org/10.1161/STROKEAHA.113.003133.

[103] Goddard AJP, Tan G, Becker J. Computed tomography angiography for the detection and characterization ofintra-cranial aneurysms: current status. Clin Radiol, 2005. https://doi.org/10.1016/j.crad.2005.06.007.

[104] Baddour LM, Wilson WR, Bayer AS, et al. Infective endocarditis in adults: diagnosis, antimicrobial therapy, and management of complications: a scientific statement for healthcare professionals from the American Heart Association. Circulation, 2015. https://doi.org/10.1161/CIR.0000000000000296.

[105] Habib G, Lancellotti P, Antunes MJ, et al. 2015 ESC Guidelines for the management of infective endocarditis. Eur Heart J, 2015, 36(44): 3075–3128. https://doi.org/10.1093/eurheartj/ehv319.

[106] Bartakke S, Kabde U, Muranjan MN, et al. Mycotic aneurysm: an uncommon cause for intra-cranial hemorrhage. Indian J Pediatr, 2002. https://doi.org/10.1007/BF02723719.

[107] Kannoth S, Thomas SV. Intracranial microbial aneurysm (infectious aneurysm): current options for diagnosis and management. Neurocritic Care, 2009. https://doi.org/10.1007/s12028-009-9208-x.

[108] Zanaty M, Chalouhi N, Starke RM, et al. Endovascular treatment of cerebral mycotic aneurysm: a review of theliterature and single center experience. BioMed Res Int, 2013. https://doi.org/10.1155/2013/151643.

[109] Ando K, Hasegawa H, Kikuchi B, et al. Treatment strategies for infectious intracranial aneurysms: report of three cases and review of the literature. Neurol Med -Chir, 2019. https://doi.org/10.2176/nmc.oa.2019-0051.

[110] Grandhi R, Zwagerman NT, Linares G, et al. Onyx embolization of infectious intracranial aneurysms. J Neurointervent Surg, 2014. https://doi.org/10.1136/neurintsurg-2013-010755.

[111] Chalouhi N, Tjoumakaris S, Gonzalez LF, et al. Endovascular treatment of distal intracranial aneurysms with Onyx 18/34. Clin Neurol Neurosurg, 2013. https://doi.org/10.1016/j.clineuro.2013.10.018.

[112] Chapot R, Houdart E, Saint-Maurice JP, et al. Endovascular treatment of cerebral mycotic aneurysms. Radiology, 2002. https://doi.org/10.1148/radiol.2222010432.

[113] Cheng-Ching E, John S, Bain M, et al. Endovascular embolization of intracranial infectious aneurysms in patients undergoing open heart surgery using n-butyl cyanoacrylate. Interv Neurol, 2017. https://doi.org/10.1159/000455806.

[114] Phuong LK, Link M, Wijdicks E, et al. Management of intracranial infectious aneurysms: a series of 16 cases. Neurosurgery, 2002. https://doi.org/10.1097/00006123-200211000-00008.

[115] Pettersson GB, Hussain ST. Current AATS guidelines on surgical treatment of infective endocarditis. Ann Cardiothorac Surg, 2019. https://doi.org/10.21037/acs.2019.10.05.

[116] Nishimura RA, Otto CM, Bonow RO, et al. 2017 AHA/ACC focused update of the 2014 AHA/ACC guideline for the management of patients with valvular heart disease: a report of the American College of Cardiology/American heart association task force on clinical practice guidelines. Circulation, 2017. https://doi.org/10.1161/CIR.0000000000000503.

[117] Angstwurm K, Borges AC, Halle E, et al. Timing the valve replacement in infective endocarditis involving the brain. J Neurol, 2004, 251(10): 1220–1226. https://doi.org/10.1007/s00415-004-0517-x.

[118] Hosono M, Sasaki Y, Hirai H, et al. Considerations in timing of surgical intervention for infective endocarditis with cerebrovascular complications. J Heart Valve Dis, 2010.

[119] Ruttmann E, Willeit J, Ulmer H, et al. Neurological outcome of septic cardioembolic stroke after infective endocarditis. Stroke, 2006. https://doi.org/10.1161/01.STR.0000229894.28591.3f.

[120] Piper C, Wiemer M, Schulte HD, et al. Stroke is not a contraindication for urgent valve replacement in acute infective endocarditis. J Heart Valve Dis, 2001, 10(6): 703–711.

[121] Eishi K, Kawazoe K, Kuriyama Y, et al. Surgical management of infective endocarditis associated with cerebral complications. Multi-center retrospective study in Japan. J Thorac Cardiovasc Surg, 1995. https://doi.org/10.1016/S0022-5223(95)70038-2.

[122] Fukuda W, Daitoku K, Minakawa M, et al. Management of infective endocarditis with cerebral complications. Ann Thorac Cardiovasc Surg, 2014. https://doi.org/10.5761/atcs.oa.13.02265.

[123] Shang E, Forrest GN, Chizmar T, et al. Mitral valve infective endocarditis: benefit of early operation and aggressive use of repair. Ann Thorac Surg, 2009. https://doi.org/10.1016/j.athoracsur.2009.02.098.

[124] Kang D-H, Kim Y-J, Kim S-H, et al. Early surgery versus conventional treatment for infective endocarditis. N Engl J Med, 2012, 366(26): 2466–2473. https://doi.org/10.1056/NEJMoa1112843.

[125] Barsic B, Dickerman S, Krajinovic V, et al. Influence of the timing of cardiac surgery on the outcome of patients with infective endocarditis and stroke. Clin Infect Dis, 2013. https://doi.org/10.1093/cid/cis878.

[126] Zhang LQ, Cho SM, Rice CJ, et al. Valve surgery for infective endocarditis complicated by stroke: surgical timing and perioperative neurological complications. Eur J Neurol, 2020. https://doi.org/10.1111/ene.14438.

[127] Raman J, Ballal A, Hota B, et al. Reconstructive valve surgery within 10 days of stroke in endocarditis. Asian Cardiovasc Thorac Ann, 2016. https://doi.org/10.1177/0218492316652746.

[128] Kim YK, Choi CG, Jung J, et al. Effect of cerebral embolus size on the timing of cardiac surgery for infective endocarditis in patients with neurological complications. Eur J Clin Microbiol Infect

Dis, 2018. https://doi.org/10.1007/s10096-017-3148-8.

[129] Ghoreishi M, Foster N, Pasrija C, et al. Early operation in patients with mitral valve infective endocarditis and acute stroke is safe. Ann Thorac Surg, 2018. https://doi.org/10.1016/j.athoracsur.2017.06.069.

[130] Murai R, Funakoshi S, Kaji S, et al. Outcomes of early surgery for infective endocarditis with moderate cerebral complications. J Thorac Cardiovasc Surg, 2017. https://doi.org/10.1016/j.jtcvs.2016.10.074.

[131] Oh THT, Wang TKM, Pemberton JA, et al. Early or late surgery for endocarditis with neurological complications. Asian Cardiovasc Thorac Ann, 2016. https://doi.org/10.1177/ 0218492316646903.

第 11 章
静脉吸毒并发感染性心内膜炎的精神问题

Neeta Shenai, Elizabeth Hovis, Alex Israel, Priya Gopalan
University of Pittsburgh Medical Center, Pittsburgh, PA, United States

引 言

　　静脉注射阿片类药物滥用（OUD）已经成为一个社会性问题。感染性心内膜炎（IE）是与之相关的主要并发症，一旦出现则死亡风险显著增加。为此而住院治疗的患者有增加的趋势，其中在年轻人、非拉美裔白人和乡村地区这一趋势更为明显[1]。一项研究显示，42% 的该类疾病住院患者没有保险或医疗补助，面临高昂的治疗费，有必要采取预防和减少相关伤害的策略，以降低可能出现的治疗费用[2]。OUD 继发性心内膜炎患者的治疗过程非常繁杂，通常存在以下特点：需长期住院、长疗程静脉抗感染治疗、需在专业机构接受急性期后的护理、再次住院率高、合并精神疾病等问题。

　　来自医务人员的成见和患者自身的病耻感可能会影响诊疗工作，进而带来不良的临床结局。一项纳入医务人员和患者的定性研究表明，病耻感会延误治疗并导致医院内护理工作的不连续性[3]。另外一项系统性综述显示，医护人员对药物/物质滥用（SUD）的患者普遍持负面态度，认为该类患者存在暴力、积极性低、难以管理等问题[4]。许多患者认为影响他们康复的社会因素是治疗上的障碍，这也凸显出需要一种以患者为中心的诊疗方法，整合各级医疗机构的资源，并加强对医务人员的培训。

　　SUD 和精神疾病通常同时存在。美国卫生部指出，37.2% 的受困于 SUD 的患者存在严重的精神疾病史[5]。鉴于 SUD 和精神疾病的高共病率，一些人认为应将"双重"诊断治疗作为一种标准。因此，所有指南都建议对 SUD 和精神疾病均进行筛查，并采取多学科方法进行个体化管理、家庭干预、教育、自助小组、药物治疗和安置。此外，还建议采用应急管理、预防复发、动机访谈和主动式社区治疗等策略[6]。即便如此，目前只有小部分患者接受了这种综合治疗[7]。

　　本章将介绍 SUD 患者中常见的精神疾病，并在相关数据支持的情况下对 OUD 的发生状况进行具体分析；同时，回顾每种疾病的筛查、检查方法和治疗策略，讨论针对这一特殊群体的临床治疗。

抑郁症

抑郁症是SUD患者最常见的精神共病[8]。研究发现，与无抑郁症状的患者相比，伴有OUD的抑郁症患者治疗完成率较低、社会心理功能较差，且复发的可能性较高[9]。抑郁症与阿片类药物之间的关系是复杂、双向和多因素的。

流行病学

在各项研究中，OUD患者的抑郁症发生率都很高。在OUD患者中，27%的求医者符合重度抑郁症（MDD）的诊断标准；如果将不完全符合MDD标准的抑郁症状也纳入考虑，这一数字将增至57%[10]。1999—2016年，因过量使用阿片类药物而致死的人数增加了30%以上[11]，涉及阿片类药物的自杀人数从1999年的640人到2014年的1825人，人数增加了2倍[12]。一项纳入OUD退伍军人的研究发现，与患有其他精神疾病的退伍军人相比，这些人的自杀率最高（每年120/10万）[13]。另一项来自疼痛诊所的军事研究发现，抑郁症和OUD会增加自杀风险，因此，应仔细筛查OUD患者当前的自杀意念、近期的自杀行为，以及既往自杀和自伤史。

诊断标准和检查

《诊断与统计手册》第5版（DSM-5）将MDD定义为2周内至少出现5种抑郁症状，包括：情绪低落；对活动的兴趣或乐趣明显减退；在不节食的情况下体重明显下降，或体重增加，或食欲减退或增加；他人可观察到的思维迟缓和身体活动减少；几乎每天都感到疲乏或无精打采；几乎每天都有无用感，或过度或不适当的内疚感；思考或集中注意力的能力减退；反复出现死亡或自杀的念头，至少情绪低落或失去乐趣[14]。DSM-5中其他抑郁障碍还包括破坏性心境失调障碍、持续性抑郁障碍（心境恶劣）、经前期烦躁障碍、药物/物质诱发的抑郁障碍、非典型抑郁障碍以及由其他疾病引起的抑郁障碍。

目前已开发出许多经过验证的筛查工具，可用于不同环境下对抑郁的筛查。患者健康问卷（PHQ）已通过验证，可用于SUD患者的抑郁筛查，特别是静脉吸毒的患者[15]。流行病学研究中心抑郁量表（CES-D）和贝克抑郁量表也可用于此类人群的筛查，不过，美国药物滥用和精神卫生服务管理局（SAMHSA）建议对于筛查阳性的患者应进一步完善临床评估[16]。

此外，应考虑引起抑郁症或表现为抑郁症的疾病，包括感染（如脊髓脓肿、肺炎）、心脏疾病（如心肌梗死）、营养不良（如维生素B_{12}缺乏）和内分泌疾病（如甲状腺功能减退）。有些医生认为急性病引起的低活动性谵妄也可能是抑郁的一种。用药过量导致的缺氧性脑损伤和长期使用药物导致的严重神经认知障碍也可能表现为情感淡漠或缺乏动力，这些症状与抑郁症相似。更多信息参见表11.1。

表 11.1 抑郁症的鉴别诊断

躯体疾病	·感染（例如：脊髓脓肿、肺炎） ·心脏疾病（例如：心肌梗死） ·营养缺乏（例如：维生素 B_{12} 缺乏） ·内分泌疾病（例如：甲状腺功能减退症） ·肿瘤疾病（例如：胰腺癌） ·风湿疾病（例如：狼疮） ·药物诱发（例如：类固醇） ·神经系统疾病（例如：多发性硬化症、额叶肿瘤或卒中、额叶癫痫发作）
低活动性谵妄	·多种病因
缺氧性脑损伤	·药物过量（例如：阿片类药物） ·药物诱发（例如：可卡因诱发的血管痉挛，吸入阿片类药物引起的进行性白质脑病）
严重神经认知障碍	·继发于长期使用药物/物质（例如：阿片类药物、酒精、吸入药剂、可卡因/甲基苯丙胺）

治 疗

美国社区行为保健委员会与 SAMHSA 共同开发的"四象限临床整合模型"建议，在精神科、初级保健和其他医疗机构中对有精神健康需求的患者进行健康管理。对于存在精神共病的患者，美国成瘾医学协会（ASAM）建议应进行全面评估以确定其稳定性，围绕自杀意念和行为进行直接问询以降低和监控患者的自杀风险，并根据需要进行药物治疗和其他社会心理干预[17]。

选择性 5- 羟色胺再摄取抑制剂（SSRI）是用于治疗不同程度抑郁患者的一线药物。5- 羟色胺去甲肾上腺素再摄取抑制剂（SNRI）和其他抗抑郁药（如安非他酮、米氮平）也是用于治疗 OUD 患者抑郁症状的一线药物。虽然有充分证据表明三环类抗抑郁药（TCA）可用于治疗抑郁症，但对于高易冲动性且存在过量用药风险的患者，应避免使用这类药物。抗抑郁药物的选择应根据患者的个体情况而定，包括药物与药物之间的相互作用、个人用药史、家族治疗史、副作用和药代动力学等因素，同时根据患者的最大药物耐受剂量进行至少 4~8 周的调试，以确定适当的用药剂量[18]。

对于轻度抑郁障碍的患者，可考虑仅采用心理疗法；对于中度至重度抑郁障碍的患者，则应考虑心理疗法与抗抑郁药物联合治疗。已有证据证明了认知行为疗法（CBT）和接纳与承诺疗法（ACT）在 SUD 患者中的有效性。动机访谈技术可以提高患者治疗的参与度，并促进其行为的改变。此外，以正念为基础的心理干预对该类患者也有不错的疗效[10]。

焦虑症

与抑郁症类似，焦虑症也与 OUD 高度共病，并干扰对阿片类药物的戒断[20]

或戒断维持,这可能使患者对阿片类药物终生成瘾[21]。焦虑症的终生患病率与早期使用海洛因有关,且焦虑症也是导致患者阿片快速成瘾的一个因素[22]。此外,正在戒断阿片类药物或接受阿片类药物脱毒的患者可能会出现明显的焦虑症状[21]。

流行病学

一篇综述研究提示,26%~35%的OUD患者终生患有焦虑症[23]。使用阿片类药物、镇静剂和安定剂的患者合并终生焦虑症的比例高达60%[不包括创伤后应激障碍(PTSD)或强迫症(OCD)患者],这高于其他药物/物质滥用的情况[24]。在一项纳入90名滥用处方类阿片药物患者的研究中,惊恐障碍是最常见的精神共病(13.9%),其次是广泛性焦虑症(10.7%)[25]。Kidorf等人对200多名静脉吸毒患者进行的研究发现,女性更有可能被诊断患有重度焦虑症[26]。

诊断标准和检查

DSM-5将焦虑症分为分离焦虑症、选择性缄默症、特定恐惧症、社交恐惧症、惊恐症、广场恐惧症、广泛性焦虑症、物质/药物引起的焦虑症以及由其他疾病引起的焦虑症。

已得到验证的焦虑症筛查工具包括广泛性焦虑症量表(GAD7)和汉密尔顿焦虑量表(HAMA)评分。对患有OUD的患者进行焦虑症检查还需排除其他疾病引起的焦虑,如感染、代谢异常、心脏疾病(如心内膜炎、心房颤动)、肺部疾病(如肺栓塞、哮喘)和内分泌疾病(如甲状腺功能减退或亢进)等。

治 疗

OUD患者焦虑症的一线治疗包括心理治疗(如CBT、正念干预)和服用抗抑郁药物(如SSRI和SNRI)。比较恰当的用药方案通常是服用4~6周最大耐受剂量的抗抑郁药物,但由于焦虑敏感的患者对相关副作用的耐受性可能较低,因此调节用药剂量过程中不能大剂量增减,必须缓慢调试。治疗中可加以辅助用药,包括丁螺环酮、羟嗪、可乐宁、普萘洛尔,以及一些不常用的抗精神病药物[27]。

虽然苯二氮䓬类药物是治疗急性焦虑症的常用处方药,但不建议将这类药物用于长期治疗,尤其是对于合并SUD的患者。一项对寻求戒毒的患者的调查显示:44%的患者在前一个月曾使用过苯二氮䓬类药物,其中有42%是为了治疗焦虑,而有27%是为了增强另一种药物带来的欣快感[28]。由于苯二氮䓬类药物极有可能被滥用,因此不主张在OUD患者中使用苯二氮䓬类药物[29]。

双相情感障碍

双相情感障碍(BD)是一种严重的精神疾病,其特征为情绪高涨和情绪低落交替出现[14]。双相情感障碍患者约占全美总人口的2.6%,是一种复杂的疾病,可带来一系列负面影响,包括生活质量低下、整体功能减退、医疗负担加重和死亡率升高[30]。

流行病学

双相情感障碍与 SUD 共病率较高。在全美酒精及相关疾病流行病学调查中,8.9%~33.4% 的酒精滥用或依赖者患有终生躁狂症,而 3.7%~13.4% 患有终生轻躁狂[31]。一项 meta 分析研究了住院和门诊寻求治疗的双相情感障碍患者 SUD 的患病率,结果发现有 42% 的患者酗酒,20% 的患者吸食大麻,17% 的患者使用其他非法药物[32]。另一份来自转诊的阿片类依赖寻求治疗患者的单中心样本数据发现,12% 的患者在过去 12 个月中符合双相情感障碍 I 型的诊断标准[26]。

诊断标准和检查

DSM-5 将双相情感障碍 I 型定义为具有躁狂发作史,虽然患者通常表现为抑郁症,但双相情感障碍 I 型诊断标准并不需要具有重度抑郁发作。躁狂症的定义是存在 1 周(或在住院或接受治疗的情况下持续任意时长)异常和持续的情绪高涨、膨胀或易怒以及精力充沛,并伴有 ≥ 3 个相关症状,如:自大、睡眠需求减少、言语急迫、思维奔逸、注意力分散、目标导向性活动增加或行为鲁莽。双相情感障碍 II 型的定义则包含有重度抑郁发作(如上文抑郁症部分所述)和轻躁狂发作的病史。轻躁狂应能被他人观察到,但其严重程度并不足以导致社交或职业能力受损。DSM-5 中的其他双相情感障碍和相关疾病包括循环性心境障碍、药物 / 物质引起的双相障碍及相关障碍、其他疾病引起的双相障碍及相关障碍、其他特定的双相障碍及相关障碍和未分类的双相障碍及相关障碍[14]。

在筛查方面,SAMHSA 建议使用复合性国际诊断交流核心版(CIDI)筛查量表对 SUD 患者进行双相情感障碍谱系的筛查。基于 CIDI 的筛查量表可识别 67%~96% 的双相情感障碍患者[33]。将心境障碍问卷作为筛查 SUD 患者是否合并双相情感障碍的一种工具进行评估后,并未发现其有效性[34-36]。

急性中毒(尤其是可卡因或苯丙胺)、酒精或苯二氮䓬类药物戒断的表现也可能被误认为是躁狂症或轻躁狂,这就构成了对 SUD 患者进行双相情感障碍共病诊断的挑战性。当患者出现明显的躁狂症或轻躁狂时,应考虑可引起躁狂或出现躁狂(或激惹)的疾病(表 11.2)。此外,类固醇等药物也可能诱发躁狂症。与 SUD 相关的现象学因素也可能会混淆临床诊断,例如睡眠和觉醒周期的紊乱、为获得药物或酒精而采取的冒险行为,以及注意力分散或与渴求相关的目标导向行为增加。

治 疗

双相情感障碍的治疗可能很复杂,需要根据患者的症状、需求、偏好和对治疗的反应进行个体化治疗。疑似双相情感障碍的患者应转诊至心理医生,因为治

表 11.2　双相情感障碍和精神病的鉴别诊断

躯体疾病	・感染（例如：脊髓脓肿、肺炎） ・心脏疾病（例如：心肌梗死） ・营养缺乏（例如：维生素 B$_{12}$ 缺乏） ・内分泌疾病（例如：皮质醇增多症、甲状腺功能亢进症） ・肿瘤疾病（例如：胰腺癌） ・风湿疾病（例如：狼疮） ・药物诱发的疾病（例如：类固醇） ・神经系统疾病（例如：多发性硬化症、癫痫发作、卒中、创伤性脑损伤） ・自身免疫性疾病（例如：系统性红斑狼疮）
躁动型谵妄	・多种病因
药物/物质滥用	・急性中毒（例如：可卡因或苯丙胺） ・戒断综合征（例如：酒精或苯二氮䓬类药物）

疗需要包括药物治疗和社会心理治疗。治疗方式可针对躁狂症、双相抑郁症或维持心境平稳状态进行选择。心境稳定剂（如锂、丙戊酸、卡马西平和拉莫三嗪）以及抗抑郁药是主要治疗药物[37]。社会心理治疗包括 CBT、以家庭为中心的治疗以及人际和社会节奏治疗（IPSRT）[33]。

SUD 患者的精神病性障碍

精神分裂症是一种慢性或复发性的精神病性障碍，以幻觉、思维和言语混乱、阴性症状和认知障碍为特征[14]。世界卫生组织将精神分裂症列为造成全球疾病负担的十大疾病之一[38]。

流行病学

据估计，美国精神分裂症患者中终生有 SUD 的占比为 47%～59%，而普通人群的患病率为 16%[39-40]。Hunt 等人在 2018 年进行的一项系统性综述和 meta 分析中估计，在诊断为精神分裂症或首发精神病患者中 OUD 的患病率为 4.8%[41]。

诊断标准和检查

DSM-5 将精神分裂症定义为在 1 个月内出现 ≥ 2 种以下症状：妄想、幻觉、言语混乱；行为严重混乱或紧张；阴性症状（情感淡漠、嗜睡或缺乏意志力或动力）。此外，必须在 6 个月内持续出现精神障碍症状，但无须满足上述标准（例如，可仅有阴性症状，或上述症状的减弱形式）。药物/物质诱发的精神病性障碍是指在中毒、戒断或接触某种物质期间或之后很快出现妄想和（或）幻觉，且这种障碍不能用其他类型的精神病性障碍更好解释。DSM-5 精神分裂症谱系和其他精神病性障碍还包括分裂情感性障碍、妄想症、短期精神病性障碍、类精神分裂症、其他疾病导致的精神病性障碍、其他特定的精神分裂症谱系和其他精神病性障碍，以及未分类的精神分裂症谱系和其他精神病性障碍[14]。

对精神病的检查，尤其是对未确诊为精神分裂症患者的检查，范围应当广泛，包括排除可引起精神病或可表现为精神病的其他疾病（表 11.2）。急性中毒（尤其是可卡因或苯丙胺类药物）、戒酒、苯二氮䓬类药物戒断时可能会被误认为或表现为精神病。此外，类固醇等药物也可能引起精神病。

治 疗

精神分裂症的治疗包括药物治疗和社会心理治疗，其中药物治疗主要依赖抗精神病类药物。然而，在精神分裂症的治疗中，除了对难治人群使用氯氮平效果明显之外，没有任何一种抗精神病药物被证明比其他药物更有效。因此，抗精神病药物的选择要以患者的耐受性、既往治疗反应、副作用、患者的共病和患者偏好作为用药参考[42]。对精神分裂症有疗效的社会心理干预包括技能培训、家庭教育干预、认知矫正和 CBT[43]。2013 年，一项 Cochrane 系统综述和 meta 分析对同时患有严重精神病和药物 / 物质滥用的患者进行了研究，结果并未提示社会心理干预具有明确的疗效，也未能推荐任何一种干预方法[44]。尽管如此，指南仍然支持在药物治疗的基础上，对同时患有精神分裂症和 SUD 的患者进行社会心理干预[43,45]。

SUD 患者合并创伤

研究发现，不良的童年经历会增加创伤对身心健康的有害影响，自此人们对有创伤史的个体给予了更多关注。有证据表明，童年时期的创伤经历会对神经生物学的发育产生负面影响，进而导致个体日后易患精神疾病，如创伤后应激障碍（PTSD）和 SUD[46]。由于 PTSD 合并 SUD 患者的健康状况和社会功能都比单独患这两种疾病的人要差[47]，因此对已确诊 SUD 的患者进行 PTSD 筛查至关重要。

流行病学

SUD 和 PTSD 共病的现象已经得到证实。据估计，在被诊断为 SUD 的患者中，PTSD 的终生患病率为 26%～52%[48]。就 OUD 而言，多项研究的数据提示了 OUD 和 PTSD 的高共病率。此外，特定人群（包括有性创伤史的妇女）非医疗使用处方药（包括阿片类药物）的比例较高[49]。与没有潜在精神疾病的退伍军人相比，有 PTSD 的退伍军人更有可能接受阿片类处方药，并表现出更高风险的阿片类药物滥用，如剂量更大、接受多种阿片类药物和（或）同时服用镇静催眠药，以及提前重新开具阿片类处方[50]。最后，虽然创伤史和 PTSD 会增加个人罹患 OUD 的风险，但静脉吸毒的个体在获取或使用非法药物的过程中往往会面临更多的创伤经历[51]。

诊断标准和检查

DSM-5 将 PTSD 定义为一种与创伤和应激源相关的障碍，常由于患者暴露于创伤事件（包括死亡或受到死亡威胁、严重伤害或性侵害）而导致[14]。暴露的形式可以是直接经历、目睹创伤事件、得知该事件发生在家人或朋友身上，也可以是反复或极端暴露于创伤事件的细节。诊断 PTSD 需要在创伤暴露后至少 1 个月内出现以下 4 组症状：重新体验、回避、负面认知和情绪以及反应过度。PTSD 的筛查工具包括：创伤后应激障碍自评量表（PCL-C 量表）、创伤后应激障碍检查简化版量表和生活事件量表（LEC 量表）。

治 疗

PTSD 合并 SUD 的治疗依赖于利用社会心理干预、循证心理疗法和药物治疗的综合方法[47-48]。以创伤为中心的疗法是治疗 PTSD 的金标准，其他可用的方法包括长期暴露疗法、认知加工疗法、眼动脱敏和再加工疗法（EMDR）以及 CBT。关于在 PTSD 合并 SUD 的患者中采用心理疗法的有效性的数据非常有限[52]。然而，《寻求安全：创伤和药物/物质滥用治疗手册》（Seeking Safety: A Treatment Manual for Trauma and Substance Use）一书提供了一种循证治疗方法，可同时治疗 PTSD 和 SUD，并已在许多情况下发现其疗效显著，可明显改善患者的整体功能[53]。

PTSD 的一线药物治疗包括 SSRI，建议试用 4~6 周。其他可替代的抗抑郁药有 SNRI 和 TCA 等，这些药物对合并 SUD 患者的疗效尚缺乏研究证据，但可考虑用于治疗 PTSD 相关症状。哌唑嗪是 α1 受体拮抗剂，已被证明可以减轻创伤后出现的噩梦[48]。然而，最近一项针对患有慢性 PTSD 退伍军人的研究并未发现哌唑嗪能改善与创伤相关的噩梦[54]。

SUD 患者的认知和能力问题

治疗剂量的阿片类药物会影响认知，并导致一系列神经心理学上的功能障碍[55]。阿片类药物对认知功能的影响主要集中在阿片受体上，这些受体可以调节注意力、记忆力和学习能力。一项系统性综述提示，阿片类药物的使用影响了延迟情景记忆、注意力、语言、口头工作记忆、认知冲动和口头表达能力[56]。此外，过量使用阿片类药物会导致缺氧性脑损伤，造成慢性认知障碍。阿片类药物的使用会使患者暴露在危险的环境中，增加创伤性脑损伤的风险，从而导致弥漫性轴索损伤、慢性注意力和记忆力缺陷、冲动和去抑制。目前，对慢性 OUD 及其对认知影响的研究仍然不足。

阿片类药物对认知的影响可能会影响患者的医疗决策能力。因此，可能需要通过正规的筛查工具对患者的认知能力进行评估，包括蒙特利尔认知评估、简易精神状态检查表或其他经过验证的认知量表，以量化受损程度。在评估医疗决策能力之前，应向患者提供相关的临床信息，以便使其所做决定是在知情的情况下做出的。评估决策能力的四要素模型包括：①表达明确的、前后一致的选择的能力；②对相关临床信息的清晰理解；③对每种治疗方案的风险和获益的评估；④理解临床病情及所做决定的后果[57]。这种评估的实施与否依医疗决策的具体风险与获益而定。

在 OUD 住院患者中，一个常见的问题是违反医嘱要求出院，SUD 患者提出这一要求的可能性要比普通患者高出 3 倍[58]。此时需根据停止住院治疗带来的具体风险和降低风险的可用策略提出相关建议。如果患者被认为缺乏决策能力，治疗重点应放在尽可能恢复其决策能力、评估其离开医院的潜在原因和动机、降低风险以及确定代理决策者。一家专门治疗药物/物质戒断的住院部数据显示，从急诊室入院、年龄较小、戒断评分较高等因素与违反医嘱出院相关[59]。在一项定性研究中，患者过早离院的主要原因是戒断治疗不足和对药物的强烈需求、镇痛不充分、认为医护人员存在成见以及医院的活动限制（如限制离开病房）[58]。了解患者要求离开医院的理由可以防止出现负面的健康结局，而进行全面评估以确定潜在原因对于防止过早出院和疗效不佳至关重要。更多信息请参阅下面的临床情景和评估示例。

临床案例：X 女士是一名 20 岁的女性，既往有 OUD 病史，因胸痛到医院就诊，被诊断为三尖瓣心内膜炎。生命体征：血压 135/90mmHg，心率 108/min，呼吸 14/min，体温 37.0℃。给予抗生素静脉注射，同时咨询心胸外科。住院第 2 天，患者违反医嘱要求出院。医疗团队指出，如果不进行治疗，患者将面临脓毒症的高风险。决策能力评估见表 11.3。

表 11.3　临床案例：违反医嘱要求出院时患者决策能力的评估

首先，确保初级医疗团队已向患者提供了必要的信息，以便做出明智的离院决定。

标　准	临床评估提问
就患者是否做出前后一致的选择进行沟通	对于医生给出的留院治疗的建议，您做出了什么决定？
了解相关信息	您的医生诊断您患有什么疾病，推荐的治疗方法是什么？ 您的医生与您讨论了哪些治疗方案？
权衡风险和获益	是什么让您违背医生的建议选择离开医院？ 这个决定有什么风险？有什么益处？ 是什么让您认为离开医院是更好的选择？
了解临床状况的严重性	如果您没有完成抗生素疗程会发生什么？ 您认为上述风险发生的可能性有多大？ 您出院后有什么计划？

如果患者有决策能力：
・解决未满足的需求（例如，疼痛、阿片类药物戒断、尼古丁戒断）可能有助于做出决策

如果患者没有决策能力：
・确定代理决策者
・尝试通过以下方式恢复决策能力：
　— 如果患者诊断为谵妄，则评估其认知能力并识别潜在的可逆性病因
・考虑咨询精神科医生和医学伦理学专家

应评估长期服用阿片类药物患者的认知能力，特别是注意力和记忆力方面的缺陷，这对于确定功能受限至关重要。虽然任何一名了解决策能力标准的医生都可以进行这种评估，但咨询精神病学和医学伦理学专家可为高风险患者提供更多指导。

特殊人群

孕 妇

围产期心内膜炎的发病率估计为 0.6/10 万，是一种罕见但可危及生命的妊娠并发症，孕产妇和胎儿死亡率估计为 10%~15%[60-61]。2000—2009 年间，美国围产期阿片类药物的使用增加了 5 倍[62]，新生儿中确诊的 OUD 比率几乎翻了两番，从每 1000 例住院病例中的 1.5 例增至 6.5 例[63]。

多种社会决定因素与围产期阿片类药物的使用有关。具体而言，年龄较大、未婚、多胎、白人和非拉美裔、未受过大学教育、失业或社会经济地位较低，以及(或)合并多种药物使用或精神疾病的妇女更有可能在怀孕期间使用阿片类药物[64-65]。怀孕对一些妇女来说是药物使用的中断期，也为停用阿片类药物提供了强大的精神动力。但产后重新使用的风险很高，这是多因素造成的[62,66]。此外，产后发生致命性和非致命性过量服药的风险也会增加。最近的文献表明，产后 7~12 个月发生过量服药的风险更高[67]。鉴于这些数据，对以上人群建议进行药物辅助治疗（MAT）和心理干预，并进行密切随访。

妊娠期使用阿片类药物会给孕产妇和胎儿带来许多不良影响，包括产前保健中断、早产、孕产妇和新生儿住院时间延长、胎儿发育不良、胎儿死亡、胎盘早剥、早产和新生儿戒断综合征（NAS）[65,68-69]。鉴于这些潜在的并发症，建议将 SUD 筛查作为产前保健的一项常规内容，最好在第一次产前检查时进行。已得到验证的筛查工具包括：4Ps、NIDA 快速筛查和 CRAFFT 筛查（译者注：来自 6 个筛查问题中的关键词——Car、Relax、Alone、Forget、Friends、Trouble），这些可用来识别 SUD 妇女[68]。

一旦确诊为 OUD，一线治疗包括结合 MAT 和心理干预。在孕妇群体中，MAT 包括美沙酮（阿片受体完全激动剂）或丁丙诺啡（阿片受体部分激动剂）。纳曲酮（Vivitrol©）最近也在妊娠期中应用，但数据尚不完备，目前不建议将其作为一线药物。

·妊娠期药代动力学变化（剂量）

妊娠会带来生理上的巨大变化，包括母体脂肪、水分和血容量的增加，血浆蛋白的减少，以及心输出量增加、肾灌注增加和血压下降，所有这些都可能导致药物的药代动力学特性发生变化[70]。就妊娠人群的 MAT 而言，这些变化具有重大影响，包括丁丙诺啡和美沙酮的剂量调整后血浆浓度降低，可能需要增加剂量和次数才能达到足够的血浆浓度[71-72]。详见表 11.4。

表 11.4 妊娠期丁丙诺啡、美沙酮和纳曲酮（Vivitrol©）的使用

	丁丙诺啡	美沙酮	纳曲酮（Vivitrol©）
作用机制	μ 阿片受体部分激动剂	μ 阿片受体完全激动剂	非选择性阿片受体拮抗剂
对胎儿的影响	・没有生理性出生异常的证据 ・与完全阿片受体激动剂相比，NAS 的严重程度较低、持续时间较短	・NAS 症状的频率、严重程度更高，持续时间更长 ・胎儿低出生体重、低身长、小头围	・如果持续使用到分娩，则没有 NAS 的风险 ・可能会在子宫内促发胎儿戒断症状
怀孕期间的剂量	增加给药频率（每天 3~4 次），以达到足够的血浆水平，最大剂量为 24 mg/d	通常需要增加剂量或分次给药以减轻戒断症状	每天口服 50 mg，即将分娩时调整；或 380 mg 肌内注射，每 4 周 1 次，即将分娩时调整
怀孕期间的特殊考量	有限的新数据表明了丁丙诺啡-纳洛酮在妊娠期的有效性和安全性，特别是在那些希望围产期逐渐减少和（或）停用阿片类药物的围产期人群中		

NAS：新生儿戒断综合征

・新生儿戒断综合征（NAS）

建议对围产期使用阿片类药物的妇女所生的婴儿进行 NAS 症状监测[68]。虽然美沙酮和丁丙诺啡都与 NAS 有关，但有证据表明，与包括美沙酮在内的阿片受体完全激动剂相比，使用丁丙诺啡时新生儿戒断症状的严重程度较轻、持续时间较短[73]。此外，支持性非药物疗法，包括母婴同室、皮肤接触、襁褓包裹、弱光、最小刺激、轻柔唤醒和母乳喂养，这些已被证明是有效的，可减少婴儿阿片类药物的用量[74]。

・药物辅助阿片类药物戒断

药物辅助阿片类药物戒断是治疗妊娠期 OUD 的另一种方法，但由于复发风险较高，因此不推荐使用。这种方法依赖于使用美沙酮或丁丙诺啡来缓解戒断症状，然后逐渐减量并停止药物治疗。虽然有病例报道提示胎儿宫内死亡、胎粪排出羊水污染和早产的风险会增加，但目前的证据尚有限，并不支持妊娠晚期之前接受阿片类药物辅助戒断的患者会有更高的胎儿伤害风险[75-76]。这些研究表明，对于有强烈停用阿片类药物愿望的孕妇群体，在得到门诊的高度支持以及她们能够了解药物辅助戒断风险的情况下，可考虑采用药物辅助进行阿片类药物戒断。

・妊娠期精神疾病

围产期 OUD 妇女合并精神疾病的比例很高。情绪障碍和焦虑症是最常见的精神疾病，估计患病率分别高达 58% 和 42%[77]。一项关于 OUD 孕妇精神共病的系统性综述显示，PTSD 也很常见，在 3%~26% 的 OUD 孕妇中被检出。目前

有关 OUD 孕妇合并精神病、双向情感障碍、强迫症和进食障碍的患病率数据较为有限。

尽管对所有孕妇进行精神疾病筛查应该是产前护理的一项常规内容，但鉴于精神疾病在 OUD 孕妇中的高患病率，以及双重诊断后带来的长期显著影响，因此，对确诊为 OUD 的孕妇进行精神疾病的评估显得尤为重要。治疗关键在于采用多学科方法，将围产期护理与药物滥用治疗和精神科护理相结合。有证据表明，当治疗团队根据患者的特点，找到这些妇女在寻求和继续治疗时所面临的显著的外在和自身的障碍，并有针对性地提供解决方案时，治疗效果是最成功的[77]。

在开始对妊娠期抑郁和焦虑进行药物治疗时，必须考虑药物对胎儿和疾病的影响，并与患者进行讨论。治疗的一般原则包括：轻度疾病可考虑非药物治疗，排除可逆病因（如甲状腺功能减退、营养不良等），以最低治疗剂量使用既往应用证实有效的药物。妊娠期精神疾病如不及时治疗，有可能导致 SUD 复发或加重、产前护理减少（包括营养状况不良）、出现自杀念头或企图自杀，并可能影响母婴关系。当然，这些风险必须与每项治疗对胎儿存在的风险进行权衡。

LGBT 人群

尽管有关特定人群的数据有限，但男女同性恋、双性恋、跨性别者和"酷儿"（queer）（LGBTQ）群体同样存在阿片类药物滥用的问题。根据 2015 年的美国药物滥用和健康调查，过去一年中，LGB（同性恋和双性恋）群体比异性恋更有可能滥用处方镇痛药（10.4% *vs.* 4.5%）和海洛因（0.9% *vs.* 0.3%）[78]。跨性别女性使用阿片类药物的比例更高：在一项对纽约大都会区 230 名年龄在 19～59 岁的跨性别女性进行的为期 3 年的前瞻性研究中，有 3.5% 的跨性别女性使用海洛因；而在旧金山湾区一个年龄在 16～24 岁的跨性别女性队列中，有 3% 的跨性别女性使用海洛因[79-80]。

与异性恋者相比，具有 LGBTQ 特征的 SUD 患者更有可能合并精神疾病，但相关数据同样非常有限。在一项针对华盛顿州 69 525 名接受政府资助的药物治疗者的回顾性研究中，女同性恋和双性恋女性合并精神健康问题的可能性是异性恋的 2 倍多。心理异常的诊断结果（而非性取向）对男性和女性在开始治疗后 1 年内能否完成治疗有负面影响[81]。

LGBTQ 群体中 SUD 和精神疾病共病发生率的增加并没有明确的原因。Meyer 等人认为，性少数群体面临的压力，包括污名化、偏见和歧视等，形成了一个充满敌意和压力的社会环境，导致出现心理健康问题[82]。此外，Hatzenbueler 提出了一个心理调解框架，该框架认为性少数群体面临的污名化带来了更大压力，而这种压力会导致广泛的情绪失调、社会及人际问题，伴随的认知过程可引发精神病理学风险[83]。

与所有 OUD 患者一样，LGBTQ 者中既有 SUD 又有精神疾病诊断的患者需要接受 MAT、心理咨询和行为健康干预等的综合治疗。美沙酮和丁丙诺啡等阿片受体激动剂可能会与跨性别者常用的激素调节药物发生相互作用，在有严密监测的情况下可以安全使用[84]。此外，鉴于存在显著的共病率，综合护理模式（包括药物使用、行为健康和初级护理）可能会带来益处，包括减少污名化和护理的不连续性。

艾滋病和丙型肝炎患者

抑郁症和其他神经精神障碍在 HIV 感染者和艾滋病（AIDS）患者中很常见[85]，但有关 HIV 感染者和 SUD 共患人群中精神疾病的患病率数据却很少。常见的精神疾病包括：原发性精神障碍、药物引起的精神障碍、与 HIV 相关的精神障碍（包括神经认知障碍）或与 HIV 治疗药物相关的精神障碍[86]。诊断并治疗合并有精神疾病的 HIV/AIDS 患者可增加他们接受高效抗逆转录病毒治疗（HAART）的可能性，从而降低死亡率[87]。HIV 阳性患者的治疗非常复杂，在针对这类药物滥用的治疗方案中应加入对患者身体和精神的健康治疗，当部分机构无法开展这类综合治疗时，应向患者介绍可获取相关治疗的渠道或资源[86]。对 HIV 感染者治疗还有一些特殊注意事项，其中包括对抗逆转录病毒药物副作用的处理，对精神疾病药物副作用的敏感把握，以及了解抗逆转录病毒药物与精神疾病药物或 MAT 之间的相互作用[86]。

先前患有精神疾病（包括情绪和精神障碍）的人群罹患慢性丙型肝炎病毒（HCV）感染的患病率是普通人群的 3~4 倍[88]。在一个多中心队列中，HCV 患者目前的抑郁症患病率为 29.7%[89]。抑郁症一直是 HCV 接受干扰素治疗的主要排除标准，而新的直接抗病毒药物（DAA）治疗彻底改变了这一状况，因为这些药物没有干扰素带来的精神疾病风险。然而，DAA 有可能与多种精神疾病药物相互作用，造成不必要的不良反应，并间接影响治疗效果[90]。如果患者肝功能受损，也可能会限制精神疾病药物的使用。在 HCV 专科门诊中加入精神卫生的协作治疗可适度改善 HCV 患者抑郁的治疗效果[91]。

总　结

SUD 和精神疾病的共病率很高，导致患者的治疗效果和社会功能较差。因此，必须对这两种疾病进行筛查，并在适当的情况下转诊至精神科进行双重诊断治疗。

参考文献

[1] Wurcel AG, Anderson JE, Chui KKH, et al. Increasing infectious endocarditis admissions among young people who inject drugs. Open Forum Infect Dis, 2016, 3(3).

[2] Fleischauer AT, Ruhl L, Rhea S, et al. Hospitalizations for endocarditis and associated health care costs among persons with diagnosed drug dependence - North Carolina, 2010—2015. Morb Mortal Wkly Rep, 2017, 66: 569-573. https://doi.org/10.15585/mmwr.mm6622a1.

[3] Bearnot B, Mitton JA, Hayden M, et al. Experiences of care among individiuals with opioid use disorder-associated endocarditis and their healthcare providers: results from a qualitative study. J

Subst Abuse Treat, 2019, 102: 16–22.
[4] Van Boekel LC, Brouwers WB, Van Weeghel J, et al. Stigma among health professionals towards patients with substance use disorders and its consequences for healthcare delivery: systematic review. Drug Alcohol Depend, 2013, 131(1): 23–35.
[5] Department Substance Abuse and Mental Health Services Administration. Key substance use and mental health indicators in the United States: results from the 2018 national survey on drug use and health (HHS publication No. PEP19-5068, NSDUH series H-54). Rockville, MD: Center for Behavioral Health Statistics and Quality, Substance Abuse and Mental Health Services Administration, 2019. https://www.samhsa.gov/data/.
[6] Treatment Improvement Protocol (TIP) Series, No. 42. Center for substance abuse treatment. Substance abuse treatment for persons with Co-occurring disorders. Rockville (MD): Substance Abuse and Mental Health Services Administration (US), 2005. https://www.ncbi.nlm.nih.gov/books/NBK64197/.
[7] Perron BE, Bunger A, Bender K, et al. Treatment guidelines for substance use disorders and serious mental illnesses: do they address Co-occurring disorders? Subst Use Misuse, 2010, 45(7-8): 1262–1278. https://doi.org/10.3109/10826080903442836.
[8] Swendsen JD, Merikangas KR. The comorbidity of depression and substance use disorders. Clin Psychol Rev, 2000, 20(2): 173–189.
[9] Brewer DD, Catalano RF, Haggerty K, et al. A meta-analysis of predictors of continued drug use during and after treatment for opiate addiction. Addiction, 1998, 93(1): 73–92.
[10] Goldner EM, Lusted A, Roerecke M, et al. Prevalence of Axis-1 psychiatric (with focus on depression and anxiety) disorder and symptomatology among non-medical prescription opioid users in substance use treatment: systematic review and meta-analyses. Addict Behav, 2014, 39(3): 520–531. https://doi.org/10.1016/j.addbeh.2013.11.022. Epub 2013 Dec 2.
[11] Hedegaard H, Bastian BA, Trinidad JP, et al. Drugs most frequently involved in drug overdose deaths: United States, 2011—2016. Natl Vital Stat Rep, 2018, 67(no 9). Hyattsville, MD: National Center for Health Statistics.
[12] Rudd RA, Aleshire N, Zibbell JE, et al. Increases in drug and opioid overdose deaths - United States,2000—2014. Morb Mortal Wkly Rep, 2016, 64(50): 1378–1382.
[13] Bohnert ASB, Walton MA, Cunningham RM, et al. Overdose and adverse drug event experiences among adult patients in the emergency department. Addict Behav, 2018, 86: 66-72. https://doi.org/10.1016/j.addbeh.2017.11.030. Epub 2017 Nov 16. PMID: 29198490; PMCID: PMC5955832.
[14] American Psychiatric Association. Diagnostic and statistical manual of mental disorders: diagnostic and statistical manual of mental disorders. 5th ed. Arlington, VA: American Psychiatric Association, 2013.
[15] Hides L, Lubman DA, Devlin H. Reliability and validity of the kessler 10 and patient health questionnaire among injecting drug users. Aust N Z J Psychiatr, 2007, 41(2): 166–168.
[16] Urban RM, Barruth B, Frey J, et al. Managing depression symptoms in substance abuse clients during early recovery. Substance abuse and mental health services administration: TIP 48;revised. 2014. https://store.samhsa.gov/system/files/sma13-4353.pdf.
[17] American Society of Addiction Medicine. The ASAM national practice guideline for the use of medications in the treatment of addiction involving opioid use. 2015. https://www.asam.org/docs/default-source/practice-support/guidelines-and-consensus-docs/asam-national-practice-guideline-supplement.pdf.
[18] American Psychiatric Association. Practice guideline for the treatment of patients with major depressive disorder. 2010. https://psychiatryonline.org/pb/assets/raw/sitewide/practice_guidelines/guidelines/mdd.pdf.
[19] Alexander K, Kronk R, Sekula K, et al. Implementation of a mindfulness intervention for women in treatment for opioid use disorder and its effects on depression symptoms. Issues Ment Health Nurs, 2019, 40(8): 690–696. https://doi.org/10.1080/01612840.2019.1585499. Epub 2019 May 17.
[20] Franken IH, Hendriks VM. Screening and diagnosis of anxiety and mood disorders in substance

[21] Substance Abuse and Mental Health Services Administration. TIP 63 part 2. Addressing opioid use disorder in general medical settings. 2018. https://store.samhsa.gov/system/files/sma18-5063pt.2.pdf.

[22] Karsinti E, Fortias M, Dupuy G, et al. Anxiety disorders are associated with early onset of heroin use and rapid transition to dependence in methadone maintained patients. Psychiatr Res, 2016, 245: 423–426. https://doi.org/10.1016/j.psychres.2016.04.064.

[23] Fatséas M, Denis C, Lavie E, et al. Relationship between anxiety disorders and opiate dependence– a systematic review of the literature: implications for diagnosis and treatment. J Subst Abuse Treat, 2010, 38(3): 220–230. https://doi.org/10.1016/j.jsat.2009.12.003. Epub 2010 Feb 8.

[24] Conway KP, Green VR, Kasza KA, et al. Co-occurrence of tobacco product use, substance use, and mental health problems among adults: findings from Wave 1 (2013—2014) of Population Assessment of Tobacco and Health (PATH) Study. Drug Alcohol Depend, 2017, 177: 104–111. https://doi.org/10.1016/j.drugalcdep.2017.03.032.

[25] Gros DG, Milanak ME, Brady KT, et al. Frequency and severity of comorbid mood and anxiety disorders in prescription opioid dependence. Am J Addict, 2013, 22(3): 261–265. https://doi.org/10.1111/j.1521-0391.2012.12008.x.

[26] Kidorf M, Solazzo S, Yan H, et al. Psychiatric and substance use comorbidity in treatment-seeking injection opioid users referred from syringe exchange. J Dual Diagn, 2018, 14(4): 193–200.

[27] Stein MD, Kanabar M, Anderson BJ, et al. Reasons for benzodiazepine use among persons seeking opioid detoxication. J Subst Abuse Treat, 2016, 68: 57–61.

[28] Kehoe WA. Generalized anxiety disorder. ACSAP 2017 book 2. Neurologic/Psychiatric Care, 2017.

[29] Dowell D, Haegerich TM, Chou R. CDC guideline for prescribing opioids for chronic pain— United States. MMWR Recomm Rep, 2016, 65(No. RR-1): 1–49. https://doi.org/10.15585/mmwr.rr6501e1.

[30] Kessler RC, Chiu WT, Demler O, et al. Prevalence, severity, and comorbidity of 12-month DSM-IV disorders in the national comorbidity survey replication. Arch Gen Psychiatr, 2005, 62: 617–627.

[31] Conway KP, Compton W, Stinson FS, et al. Lifetime comorbidity of DSM-IV mood and anxiety disorders and specific drug use disorders: results from the National Epidemiologic Survey on Alcohol and Related Conditions. J Clin Psychiatr, 2006, 67: 247–257.

[32] Hunt GE, Malhi GS, Cleary M, et al. Prevalence of comorbid bipolar and substance use disorders in clinical settings, 1990—2015: systematic review and meta-analysis. J Affect Disord, 2016, 206: 331–349.

[33] Substance Abuse and Mental Health Services Administration. An introduction to bipolar disorder and Co-occurring substance use disorders. 2016. https://store.samhsa.gov/system/files/sma16-4960.pdf.

[34] Van Zaane J, van den Berg B, Draisma S, et al. Screening for bipolar disorders in patients with alcohol or substance use disorders: performance of the mood disorder questionnaire. Drug Alcohol Depend, 2012, 124(3): 235–241.

[35] Chiasson JP, Rizkallah É, Stavro K, et al. Is the Mood Disorder Questionnaire an appropriate screening tool in detecting bipolar spectrum disorder among substance use populations? Am J Drug Alcohol Abuse, 2011, 37(2): 79–81.

[36] Villagonzalo KA, Dodd S, Ng F, et al. The utility of the Mood Disorders Questionnaire as a screening tool in a methadone maintenance treatment program. Int J Psychiatr Clin Pract, 2010, 14(2): 150–153.

[37] Yatham LN, Kennedy SH, Parikh SV, et al. Canadian network for mood and anxiety treatments (CANMAT) and international society for bipolar disorders (ISBD) 2018 guidelines for the management of patients with bipolar disorder. Bipolar Disord, 2018, 20(2): 97–170.

[38] Murray CJL, Lopez AD. The global burden of disease. Cambridge, MA: Harvard University Press, 1996.

[39] Kendler KS, Gallagher TJ, Abelson JM, et al. Lifetime prevalence, demographic risk factors, and diagnostic validity of nonaffective psychosis as assessed in a US community sample. The National

Comorbidity Survey. Arch Gen Psychiatr, 1996, 53(11): 1022–1031.

[40] Regier DA, Farmer ME, Rae DS, et al. Comorbidity of mental disorders with alcohol and other drug abuse. Results from the Epidemiologic Catchment Area (ECA) Study. J Am Med Assoc, 1990, 264(19): 2511–2518.

[41] Hunt GE, Large MM, Cleary M, et al. Prevalence of comorbid substance use in schizophrenia spectrum disorders in community and clinical settings, 1990—2017: systematic review and meta-analysis. Drug Alcohol Depend, 2018, 191: 234–258.

[42] Buchanan RW, Kreyenbuhl J, Kelly DL, et al. The 2009 schizophrenia PORT psychopharmacological treatment recommendations and summary statements. Schizophr Bull, 2010, 36(1): 71–93.

[43] Dixon LB, Dickerson F, Bellack AS, et al. The 2009 schizophrenia PORT psychosocial treatment recommendations and summary statements. Schizophr Bull, 2010, 36(1): 48–70.

[44] Hunt GE, Siegfried N, Morley K, et al. Psychosocial interventions for people with both severe mental illness and substance misuse. Cochrane Database Syst Rev, 2013, 10: CD001088.

[45] Ziedonis DM, Smelson D, Rosenthal RN, et al. Improving the care of individuals with schizophrenia and substance use disorders: consensus recommendations. J Psychiatr Pract, 2005, 11(5): 315–339.

[46] Khoury L, Tang YL, Bradley B, et al. Substance use, childhood traumatic experience, and Post-traumatic Stress Disorder in an urban civilian population. Depress Anxiety, 2010, 27(12): 1077–1086.

[47] McCauley JL, Killeen T, Gros DF, et al. Posttraumatic stress disorder and Co-occurring substance use disorders: advances in assessment and treatment. Clin Psychol, 2012, 19(3). https://doi.org/10.1111/cpsp.12006.

[48] Substance Abuse and Mental Health Services Administration. Pharmacologic guidelines for treating individuals with post-traumatic stress disorder and Co-occurring opioid use disorders. Rockville, MD: Substance Abuse and Mental Health Services Administration, 2012. HHS Publication No. SMA-12-4688.

[49] McCauley JL, Amstadter AB, Danielson CK, et al. Mental health and rape history in relation to non-medical use of prescription drugs in a national sample of women. Addict Behav, 2009, 34(8): 641–648.

[50] Seal KH, Shi Y, Cohen G, et al. Association of mental health disorders with prescription opioids and high-risk opioid use in US veterans of Iraq and Afghanistan. J Am Med Assoc, 2012, 307(9): 940–947. https://doi.org/10.1001/jama.2012.234.

[51] Johnson SD, Striley C, Cottler LB. The association of substance use disorders with trauma exposure and PTSD among African american drug users. Addict Behav, 2006, 31(11): 2063–2073.

[52] Berenz EC, Coffey SF. Treatment of co-occurring posttraumatic stress disorder and substance use disorders. Curr Psychiatr Rep, 2012, 14(5): 469–477.

[53] Najavits LM. Seeking safety: a treatment manual for PTSD and substance abuse. New York: Guilford Press, 2002.

[54] Raskind MA, Peskind ER, Chow B, et al. Trial of prazosin for post-traumatic stress disorder in military veterans. N Engl J Med, 2018, 378: 507–517.

[55] Pask S, Dell'Olio M, Murtagh FE, et al. The effects of opioids on cognition in older adults with cancer and chronic non-cancer pain: a systematic review. J Pain Symptom Manag, 2020, 59(4). 871.e1–893.e1.

[56] Baldacchino A, Balfour DJK, Passetti F, et al. Neuropsychological consequences of chronic opioid use: a quantitative review and meta-analysis. Neurosci Biobehav Rev, 2012, 36: 2056–2068. https://doi.org/10.1016/j.neubiorev.2012.06.006.

[57] Appelbaum PS. Assessment of patients' competence to consent to treatment. N Engl J Med, 2007, 357: 1834–1840. https://doi.org/10.1056/NEJMcp074045.

[58] Simon R, Snow R, Wakeman S. Understanding why patients with substance use disorders leave the hospital against medical advice: a qualitative study. Substance Abuse, 2019. https://doi.org/10.1080/08897077.2019.1671942.

[59] Pytell JD, Rastegar DA. Who leaves early? Factors associated with against medical advice discharge during alcohol withdrawal treatment. J Addiction Med, 2018, 12(6): 447–452. https://doi.org/10.1097/ADM.0000000000000430.

[60] Kebed KY, Bishu K, Al Adham RI, et al. Pregnancy and postpartum infective endocarditis: a systematic review. Mayo Clin Proc, 2014, 89(8): 1143–1152.

[61] Yuan SM. Infective endocarditis during pregnancy. J Coll Physicians Surg Pak, 2015, 25(2): 134–139.

[62] Forray A. Substance use during pregnancy. F1000Research, 2016, 5. F1000 Faculty Rev-887.

[63] Kroelinger CD, Rice ME, Cox S, et al. State strategies to address opioid use disorder among pregnant and postpartum women and infants prenatally exposed to substances, including infants with neonatal abstinence syndrome. Morb Mortal Wkly Rep, 2019, 68(36): 777–783.

[64] Azuine RE, Ji Y, Chang HY, et al. Prenatal risk factors and perinatal and postnatal outcomes associated with maternal opioid exposure in an urban, low-income, multiethnic US population. JAMA Netw Open, 2019, 2(6): e196405.

[65] Whiteman VE, Salemi JL, Mogos MF, et al. Maternal opioid drug use during pregnancy and its impact on perinatal morbidity, mortality, and the costs of medical care in the United States. J. Pregnancy, 2014, 2014: 906723.

[66] Gopman S. Prenatal and postpartum care of women with substance use disorders. Obstet Gynecol Clin N Am, 2014, 41(2): 213–228.

[67] Schiff DM, Nielsen T, Terplan M, et al. Fatal and nonfatal overdose among pregnant and postpartum women in Massachusetts. Obstet Gynecol, 2018, 132(2): 466–474.

[68] American College of Obstetricians and Gynecologists. Opioid use and opioid use disorder in pregnancy. Committee Opinion No. 711. Obstet Gynecol, 2017, 130: e81–e94.

[69] Krans EE, Cochran G, Bogen DL. Caring for opioid-dependent pregnant women: prenatal and postpartum care considerations. Clin Obstet Gynecol, 2015, 58(2): 370–379.

[70] Constantine MM. Physiologic and pharmacokinetic changes in pregnancy. Front Pharmacol, 2014, 5(65).

[71] Caritis SN, Bastian JR, Zhang H, et al. An evidence-based recommendation to increase the dosing frequency of buprenorphine during pregnancy. Am J Obstet Gynecol, 2017, 217(4): 459.e1–e6.

[72] Shiu JR, Ensom MH. Dosing and monitoring of methadone in pregnancy: literature review. Can J Hosp Pharm, 2012, 65(5): 380–386.

[73] Jones HE, Jansson LM, O'Grady KE, et al. The relationship between maternal methadone dose at delivery and neonatal outcome: methodological and design considerations. Neurotoxicol Teratol, 2013, 39: 110–115. https://doi.org/10.1016/j.ntt.2013.05.003.

[74] Ryan G, Dooley J, Finn LG, et al. Nonpharmacological management of neonatal abstinence syndrome: a review of the literature. J Matern Fetal Neonatal Med, 2018, 32(10): 1735–1740.

[75] Terplan M, Laird H, Hand D, et al. Opioid detoxification during pregnancy: a systematic review. Obstet Gynecol, 2018, 131(5): 803–814.

[76] Bell J, Towers CV, Hennessy MD, et al. Detoxification from opiate drugs during pregnancy. Am J Obstet Gynecol, 2016, 215(3). e1–e374.e6.

[77] Arnaudo CL, Andraka-Christou B, Allgood K. Psychiatric Co-morbidities in pregnant women with opioid use disorders: prevalence, impact, and implications for treatment. Current Addiction Reports, 2017, 4(1): 1–13. https://doi.org/10.1007/s40429-017-0132-4.

[78] Medley G, Lipari RN, Bose J, et al. Sexual orientation and estimates of adult substance use and mental health: results from the 2015 national survey on drug use and health. NSDUH Data Review, 2016.

[79] Nuttbrock L, Bockting W, Rosenblum A, et al. Gender abuse, depressive symptoms, and substance use among transgender women: a 3-year prospective study. Am J Publ Health, 2014, 104(11): 2199–2206.

[80] Rowe C, Santos G-M, McFarland W, et al. Prevalence and correlates of substance use among trans female youth ages 16-24 years in the San Francisco Bay Area. Drug Alcohol Depend, 2015, 147:

160–166.

[81] Lipsky S, Krupski A, Roy-Byrne P, et al. Impact of sexual orientation and co-occurring disorders on chemical dependency treatment outcomes. J Stud Alcohol Drugs, 2012, 73(3): 401–412.

[82] Meyer IH. Prejudice, social stress, and mental health in lesbian, gay, and bisexual populations: conceptual issues and research evidence. Psychol Bull, 2003, 129(5): 674.

[83] Hatzenbuehler ML. How does sexual minority stigma "get under the skin"? A psychological mediation frame-work. Psychol Bull, 2009, 135(5): 707–730.

[84] Girouard MP, Goldhammer H, Keuroghlian AS. Understanding and treating opioid use disorders in lesbian, gay, bisexual, transgender, and queer populations. Subst Abuse, 2019, 40(3): 335–339.

[85] Colibazzi T, Hsu TT, Gilmer WS. Human immunodeficiency virus and depression in primary care: a clinical review. Prim Care Companion J Clin Psychiatry, 2006, 8(4): 201–211.

[86] Substance Abuse and Mental Health Services Administration. TIP 37. Substance abuse treatment for persons with HIV/AIDS. 2019. https://store.samhsa.gov/system/files/sma12-4137.pdf.

[87] Himelhoch S, Moore RD, Treisman G, et al. Does the presence of a current psychiatric disorder in AIDS patients affect the initiation of antiretroviral treatment and duration of therapy? J Acquir Immune Defic Syndr, 2004, 37(4): 1457–1463.

[88] Yeoh SW, Holmes ACN, Saling MM, et al. Depression, fatigue and neurocognitive deficits in chronic hepatitis C. Hepatol Int, 2018, 12(4): 294–304.

[89] Boscarino JA, Lu M, Moorman AC, et al. Predictors of poor mental and physical health status among patients with chronic hepatitis C infection: the Chronic Hepatitis Cohort Study (CHeCS). Hepatology, 2015, 61(3): 802–811.

[90] Hauser P, Kern S. Psychiatric and substance use disorders co-morbidities and hepatitis C: diagnostic and treatment implications. World J Hepatol, 2015, 7(15): 1921–1935.

[91] Kanwal F, Pyne JM, Tavakoli-Tabasi S, et al. Collaborative care for depression in chronic hepatitis C clinics. Psychiatr Serv, 2016, 67(10): 1076–1082.

第12章
心脏植入式设备相关心内膜炎

Shayna McEnteggart, Abdul Rahman Akkawi, Chukudi Onyeukwu,
N. A. Mark Estes, III, Alaa Shalaby
Heart and Vascular Institute, University of Pittsburgh Medical Center, Pittsburgh, PA, United States

引 言

心脏植入式电子设备（CIED）包括永久起搏器（PPM）、植入式心脏除颤器（ICD）、心脏再同步治疗（CRT）设备，为各种具有临床指征的心脏疾病提供了挽救生命的手段。然而，这些设备短期和长期的使用也伴随众多风险，其中一个可引起严重并发症乃至死亡的就是心脏植入式电子设备相关的感染（CIED感染）。CIED感染的临床表现包括一系列自体组织和植入材料的感染，如：浅表切口感染，囊袋感染，囊袋侵蚀，伴有或不伴囊袋感染的菌血症，以及（或）单纯超声心动图提示的电极导线感染。没有明显其他来源的隐性菌血症也被认为是可能的CIED感染。

根据血培养阳性和超声发现电极导线及（或）瓣膜赘生物可以诊断CIED相关心内膜炎（CIED-RE），但当临床表现不明显时，通常需要其他的标准来辅助诊断。近期由欧洲心律协会发布、并得到其他多个学科机构认同的指南中增加了相关标准，包括：血培养阴性但对拔除的电极导线进行培养呈阳性；超声提示存在电极导线赘生物，伴有或不伴瓣膜赘生物；^{18}F-FDG PET/CT或放射标记的白细胞SPECT/CT检测到CIED脉冲发生器和（或）电极导线周围异常的代谢活动（表12.1）[1-2]。

CIED可以作为感染灶而增加被安装者发生IE的风险，另一方面，随着相关装置技术改进、功能拓展以及临床需求的增多，这些设备的使用仍持续增加。最近的一项研究发现，在所有的IE病例中，CIED-RE占比为7%[3]。这一数据凸显了循证指南在这一领域的价值，它可以将对于这一严重并发症的预防、诊断和治疗的临床实践提升到最佳状态。本章中，我们回顾了与CIED-RE相关的各种临床问题，以便读者对上述提及的CIED感染表现的连续性形成基本的认识，还将探讨相关的流行病学、诊断及微生物学，同时也分析了现今的临床证据以及最新的CIED-RE预防和治疗指南中存在的不足。为了展示CIED-RE诊治所带来的临床挑战，让我们先来看一例虽然是假设但却是现实工作中可能遇到的典型案例。

表 12.1　Diagnosis of CIED-RE*

'Definite' CIED-RE =presence of either 2 major criteria or 1 major +3 minor criteria
'Possible' CIED-RE =presence of either 1 major +1 minor criteria or 3 minor criteria
'Rejected' CIED-RE =patients who did not meet the aforementioned criteria

Major criteria:

Microbiology:

A. Blood cultures positive for typical microorganisms found in CIED infection and/or infective endocarditis（CoNS, Staphylococcus aureus）
B. Microorganisms consistent with infective endocarditis from two separate blood cultures:
  a. Viridans streptococci, Streptococcus gallolyticus（Streptococcus bovis）, HACEK group, S. aureus; or
  b. Community-acquired enterococci, in the absence of a primary focus
C. Microorganisms consistent with infective endocarditis from persistently positive blood cultures:
  a. ≥ 2 positive blood cultures of blood samples drawn >12 h apart; or
  b. All of 3 or a majority of ≥ 4 separate cultures of blood（first and last samples drawn ≥ 1 h apart）; or
  c. Single positive blood culture for Coxiella burnetii or phase I IgG antibody titer >1:800

Imaging:

D. Echocardiogram（including ICE）positive for:
  a. CIED infection:
    i. Clinical pocket/generator infection
    ii. Lead vegetation
  b. Valvular infective endocarditis
    i. Vegetations
    ii. Abscess, pseudoaneurysm, intracardiac fistula
    iii. Valvular perforation or aneurysm
    iv. New partial dehiscence of prosthetic valve
E. [18F] FDG PET/CT（caution should be taken in case of recent implants）or radiolabeled WBC SPECT/CT detection of abnormal activity at pocket/generator site, along leads or at valve site
F. Definite paravalvular leakage by cardiac CT

Minor criteria:

a. Predisposition such as predisposing heart condition（e.g., new onset tricuspid valve regurgitation）or injection drug use
b. Fever（temperature > 38℃）
c. Vascular phenomena（including those detected only by imaging）: Major arterial emboli, septic pulmonary embolisms, infectious（mycotic）aneurysm, intracranial hemorrhage, conjunctival hemorrhages, and Janeway's lesions
d. Microbiological evidence: Positive blood culture which does not meet a major criterion as noted above or serological evidence of active infection with organism consistent with infective endocarditis or pocket culture or leads culture（extracted by noninfected pocket）

CIED, cardiac implantable electronic device; CIED-RE, cardiac implantable electronic device-related endocarditis; CT, computerized tomography; E, expert opinion; ICE, intracardiac echocardiography; SPECT, single-photon emission computed tomography; WBC, white blood cell.
Modified after with permission from: Blomstrom-Lundqvist C, Traykov V, Erba PA, Burri H, Nielsen JC, Bongiorni MG, et al. European heart rhythm association (EHRA) international consensus document on how to prevent, diagnose, and treat cardiac implantable electronic device infections-endorsed by the heart rhythm society (HRS), the Asia Pacific heart rhythm society (APHRS), the Latin American heart rhythm society (LAHRS), International Society for Cardiovascular Infectious Diseases (ISCVID) and the European Society of Clinical Microbiology and Infectious Diseases (ESCMID) in collaboration with the European Association for Cardio-Thoracic Surgery (EACTS). Europace 2019; 22(4): 515-549.
★本表因涉及第三方版权，须保留原著英文

【病例学习——早期表现】

一名 73 岁的男性患者，表现为发热、寒战。既往有主动脉瓣狭窄和缺血性心肌病病史。几年前已行冠状动脉旁路移植术（CABG）和主动脉瓣生物瓣置换术，术后不久，植入 ICD 作为一级预防，其后出现高度房室传导阻滞伴心室起搏高负荷。3 个月前，患者的射血分数降为 25%，接受了装置升级以支持 CRT 功能。相关既往史包括高血压、糖尿病、痛风和慢性肾功能不全。既往用药包括利尿剂、β 受体阻滞剂、血管紧张素受体阻滞剂，以及因左肩痛风发作服用的泼尼松（剂量已递减）。滑膜液分析证实有尿酸结晶。生命体征：体温 38.4℃，心率 100/min，血压 100/70 mmHg，呼吸 20/min。白细胞计数升高伴核左移。结合上述所有表现支持脓毒症综合征的诊断。两次血培养结果均为革兰氏阳性球菌阳性。起搏器囊袋局部轻微肿胀，但无红、热、痛的表现，切口正常，无渗出或裂开。

【病例讨论】

当我们考虑如何正确处理该患者时，应关注与潜在诊断及治疗密切相关的一些重点问题。结合该患者的临床症状和血管内存在电极导线，以及已植入人工瓣膜等情况，出现菌血症，应高度怀疑 IE。此例无论是否确定 CIED 受累，患者出现的 IE 应该考虑是 CIED-RE，即使不完全符合 IE 经典的诊断标准，高度怀疑也是恰当的。这一点我们将在本章后文讨论。

流行病学

从 1950 年到 2000 年，IE 的发病率保持相对稳定，为（3.6~7）/10 万（患者·年）[3]。但近几年来的情况有所变化，研究显示，在先前未知存在心脏易感因素的人群中 IE 的发生率出现上升[3]。这可能与侵入性操作、人工瓣膜植入、CIED 的使用增多有关。这些潜在的易感因素破坏了人体的正常屏障，导致细菌可侵入循环系统[3]。

20 世纪 60 年代 CIED 进入临床——PPM 的研发和临床应用，其后逐步拓展到 ICD 和 CRT 设备[4]。2000—2012 年，丹麦起搏器和 ICD 登记处（DPIR）报道了这一时间段 PPM 和 ICD 的植入分别激增了 158% 和 535%[5]，这一趋势源于日益增多的具备治疗指征的心脏疾病和不断提高的医疗技术，使原本受多种疾病困扰的老龄人群能得到相应治疗[5]。CIED-RE 在不同研究中发病率有所不同。首次报道出现在 20 世纪 70 年代早期，患者安装 PPM 后出现感染，此后发生率不断增加。一项研究显示，CIED-RE 约占所有 IE 患者的 10%[6-7]。这一临床常见装置与感染的相关性在一项前瞻性研究中得以证实，心脏装置感染多发生于皮下发生器囊袋，其中 10%~23% 导致 CIED-RE[8]。这与一项回顾性研究所报道的 20% 的 CIED-RE 发生率结果基本一致。近几十年来 CIED-RE 一直在增加，一项长达 30 年的纵向研究发现 CIED-RE 在过去 10 年的数量明显增加，与 CIED 植入呈平行增长趋势[7]。Carrasco 等人报道 PPM 心内膜炎占总 IE 病例的 6.1%，每 1000 个起搏器植入者中有 3.6 个出现感染[7]。不幸的是，已有多位研究者发现，CIED-RE 的发生率似乎已经超过了 CIED 的植入增长率[9-11]。

CIED-RE 最常发生在植入早期。在一个全美初次植入 CIED 的队列研究中，纳入了 43 048 例患者，随访 168 343（患者·年），结果发现：综合所有类型的植入装置出现的感染，早发型（植入后 1 年内）CIED-RE 的发生率均是晚发型的 2 倍以上[5]。早发型 CIED-RE 被定义为住院期间或出院后 3 个月内发生的感染，主要归因于植入过程中的术中污染。据报道，早发型死亡率高达 24%[7]。另一项研究发现：对未移除感染设备者，死亡率为 31%~66%；在移除感染设备并予密切监护的情况下，死亡率可降至 18%[9]。作者还认为，IE 和射血分数是 CIED 感染患者住院期间死亡率的最强预测因素。值得注意的是，已有文献提出季节性菌血症。Maille 等人报道了囊袋感染（伴有或不伴心内膜炎）的季节性变化，当然这一报道并非仅限于心内膜炎[12]。最后，包括 CIED-RE 在内的 CIED 感染显著增加了医疗经济负担[4,8]。在美国，每例患者住院期间的支出预估至少为 14.6 万美元[13]。

患者因素

过去 20 年，伴随老年及疾病人群中 CIED 使用的增加，各种各样的疾病相关因素也促进了CIED-RE的发病率升高。其中与感染高风险相关的共病包括：糖尿病、肾功能不全（尤其是终末期肾病）、恶性肿瘤、充血性心力衰竭、慢性阻塞性肺疾病（COPD）、抗凝药和（或）免疫抑制剂（尤其是糖皮质激素）[5,8,14]。

最近，一项前瞻性研究发现了以下容易诱发 CIED-RE 的宿主因素：营养不良、恶性肿瘤、糖尿病、皮肤病、类固醇和（或）抗凝药的使用[8]。其他一些研究也发现糖尿病、血液透析、维生素 K 拮抗剂的使用、既往 IE 病史、CIED 感染以及瓣膜病可增加发病风险[5,15]。另外，慢性疾病有损机体的免疫应答能力，成为发生 CIED-RE 的基础[5]。而维生素 K 拮抗剂的使用增加了术后血肿的发生率，成为 IE 发生的独立风险因素[10]。

Sohail 等人的研究发现 CIED-RE 是 CIED 感染第三常见的临床形式（16%）[16]。这一研究报道了长期透析、COPD 及皮肤疾病与 ICD 感染相关，具有统计学意义，而糖尿病、心力衰竭、恶性肿瘤或免疫抑制治疗在统计学上不构成显著风险因素[16]。

最近的一项研究显示：82% 的 ICD 感染者有囊袋感染的证据，而 18% 表现为全身感染，只有 14% 表现为电极导线和（或）瓣膜赘生物[17]。将全身感染与囊袋感染两组患者进行对比发现，股静脉置管是全身感染的风险因素[17]。此外，ICD 感染者比没有 PPM 或 ICD 感染者年龄更大[17]。

虽然一些研究发现年长的男性更容易罹患 CIED-RE，但其他研究并未发现年龄方面的显著差异[6,9,17]。Ozcan 等人在一项大型国家登记研究中发现，CABG 的 IE 风险较低[5]，这一低风险可以由 CABG 手术患者的选择偏倚来解释：因为状态更差的患者较少接受手术，而接受 CABG 的患者一般情况尚可。CIED-RE 患者与非心内植入装置感染的 IE 患者相比，多为男性、年龄较大及患有糖尿病[6]。随着有严重共病患者寿命的延长，他们可能发生的 CIED 感染和 CIED-RE 成为高风险，在 CIED 植入时评估患者的共病情况显得至关重要。

皮肤病损、口腔卫生差、留置导管、肠道炎症和肿瘤均为细菌侵入提供了突破口。耐药菌或毒力极强的微生物定植于皮肤及肠道会带来发病的危险，因为皮肤微生物是最常见的致病菌[18-20]。这也反过来提醒我们不可滥用抗生素以免耐药菌的出现和细菌永久定植。对耐甲氧西林金黄色葡萄球菌（MRSA）的鼻拭子筛查并用莫匹罗星软膏治疗携带者，具有明确的积极效果，已作为成熟的外科实践[21]。

设备因素

CIED 不光滑的表面为感染性微生物提供了理想的聚居场所，在此位置，感染微生物可形成生物膜，以有效抵挡抗微生物制剂的攻击。不同病原体形成生物膜的能力有所不同，设备和电极导线的表面对它们而言"宜居"程度也有所不同。在电子显微镜下可以看到，电极导线绝缘材料表面不规则的"沟壑"为微生物提供了一个天然的栖息地，供它们繁殖和传播。连续的生物膜为微生物沿着电极导线的迁移提供支架，使得囊袋感染常常由此向血管内的电极导线延伸[22]，以致微生物不会只存在于一根电极导线上而不影响其他。从 CIED 感染中最常分离出的是革兰氏阳性菌（70%～90%）。尽管凝固酶阴性葡萄球菌（CoNS）通常是无害的皮肤正常定植菌，但一旦黏附在设备上，就会大量繁殖并造成侵袭性感染。葡萄球菌属是引起菌血症的最常见病原体，这当中，甲氧西林耐药菌株和敏感菌株几乎各占一半，但近年来出现的甲氧西林耐药株感染致病率增加的趋势令人担忧。相较于包裹发生器的金属（通常是钛）材料，包裹电极导线的绝缘材料更容易给微生物提供寄生环境[23-24]。

其他影响患者发生 CIED-RE 风险的设备因素包括设备类型、设备尺寸以及电极导线特征。公认的增加感染风险的设备因素包括 ICD 的植入而非 PPM，植入两根或更多电极导线，以及术中临时起搏器的使用[25-28]。

设备因素，例如塑料聚合物的种类、不规则表面及形状都可能影响细菌的附着[6]。塑料聚合物的疏水性随着疏水程度增加而增加细菌的黏附性。聚氯乙烯相比于聚四氟乙烯，聚乙烯相比聚氨酯，硅胶相比聚四氟乙烯，乳胶相比硅胶都更利于附着；一些金属（例如不锈钢）比其他金属（例如钛）更利于附着[6]。除了涂层之外，不规则的设备表面比光滑表面更利于微生物黏附。

手术操作因素

术者的经验也会影响 CIED-RE 的发生。这是一个显而易见的风险因素。例如，再次打开囊袋、置换或翻修（包括脉冲发生器更换、CIED升级）、手术时间延长等都会增加细菌进入囊袋的概率[25,27-29]。此外，一些术者和医院因素也与感染有关，包括未接受过电生理学培训的术者，植入手术经验较少的术者，在非教学医院开展植入，在不进行CABG手术的医院植入，以上均与高感染风险有关。另外，由完成植入手术量居于该专业人群下四分位数的医生操作的手术具有更高的感染风险[6,27]，一位术者操作相比两位术者操作具有更高的后续感染风险[27]。

目前，对可直接降低感染风险的相关数据知之甚少。一些研究[30-31]认为，新系统的植入和围手术期抗生素预防可以降低感染风险[6]。还有一些小规模研究[6,32-34]提示，胸部经静脉放置装置比经腹或开胸手术植入带来的CIED感染率明显更低。这意味着经胸入路不仅侵入性较小且感染风险更低。然而，Prutkin等人发现，不管是经静脉放置左心室电极导线于冠状窦还是经心外膜放置电极导线，感染风险无差异[28]。在最近发表的系统性综述中，多项研究表明：无论是腹部囊袋，还是放置心外膜电极导线，都会增加感染风险[35]。

总之，较长的手术时间、手术复杂、短时间内的再次手术、术者手术数量少、经验缺乏等均与高感染风险有关。这些因素也就决定了ICD和CRT设备植入比起搏器植入更容易出现感染[5]。

相反，一些简单的干预措施，诸如术前鼻拭子筛查，局部耐甲氧西林葡萄球菌治疗，术前12h的皮肤清洁以及使用碘浸渍的敷料膜等，已被证明在降低术中感染性微生物播散风险方面具有重要价值[21,36]。符合安全植入标准的前提条件包括：切皮前1h内预防性静脉使用抗生素，遵守手术室的环境标准（无菌、空气湿度和换气）[37]。精湛的外科技术可最大限度地减少组织损伤并确保准确止血，这具有重要意义，因为血肿的形成可导致术后感染风险增加数倍[38]。研究显示，临床出现明显血肿的患者，7.6%的病例在随后1年内出现装置感染[39]。血肿不仅为细菌生长提供了合适的基质，还导致囊袋张力增加，引起装置周围的组织坏死或切口缝线开裂，从而使皮肤定植菌有机会进入囊袋。这不仅影响了组织愈合，还为皮肤定植菌提供了持续进入的通道。此外，为清除血肿而进行的再次手术实际上也增加了感染的风险，临床上，早期再手术的最常见原因通常都是血肿和电极导线脱位。鉴于此类原因，围手术期抗凝决策就显得十分重要。尽管传统观念提倡术前停止抗凝药物并使用肝素桥接，但近期的研究及个案经验表明：延续使用华法林抗凝和口服直接抗凝剂可提升手术安全性[38-40]；而使用普通肝素进行桥接可能会带来抗凝的波动及相关安全问题。低分子量肝素会显著增加血肿的发生率，应避免使用。目前支持新型抗凝剂最佳管理方法的证据仍有限，需要积极深入研究。虽然许多医生目前在临床继续使用阿司匹林和（或）其他抗血小板药物，但这些药物带来的风险会因同时进行的抗凝治疗而加剧。

使用抗生素进行囊袋冲洗是标准的外科方法。在近期一项随机对照研究中，高风险患者采用可吸收抗生素释放封套后感染风险较低，不过对照组的感染率也低于预期假设（基于既往研究中的对照组数据）。该封套在第 1 周释放米诺环素和利福平，并预计在 9 周内完全吸收[41]。尽管使用封套可能是降低 CIED 感染风险的有效措施，但这一方法是不是最适当的且最具成本 – 效益的方式尚存疑问[42]。对术后全身抗生素治疗仍然存在争议，鉴于最近的随机试验结果为阴性，不应继续推行。

【病例学习——诊断】

考虑患者已明确 CIED 感染的诊断并可能存在心内膜炎，在等待培养结果之前首先静脉使用万古霉素，并邀请感染科专家会诊。为明确诊断，还进行了相关检查：胸部 X 线影像显示双侧肺充血及肺实质受累；经食管超声心动图（TEE）提示射血分数明显降低（约为 20%），右心室电极导线周围高度活动的强回声团块，以及中度三尖瓣反流，电极导线相关赘生物最大直径为 21 mm，人工主动脉瓣功能正常且未见赘生物；CT 增强扫描显示双肺野多发脓肿（图 12.1）。

诊 断

CIED-RE 的确诊需要结合临床、微生物学及超声心动图各方面的检查结果[3]。不论患者有无 CIED，临床都应对 IE 存在的可能性保持高度警觉。正如在美国和其他发达国家，许多亚急性或慢性 IE 患者并不会表现出典型症状和栓塞特征，很多时候，急性心内膜炎患者也可能只表现为非特异性症候、呼吸系统症状、肌肉骨骼征象，有时发热可能是唯一表现[3,43]。任何一个有 CIED 并伴有孤立性发热或葡萄球菌菌血症的患者都应高度怀疑 CIED-RE[3,43]。

对于疑似 IE，应以改良 Duke 标准作为临床评估的主要诊断方案[44]。改良 Duke 标准是目前诊断 IE 的共识，它将患者区分为确诊、疑似和排除心内膜炎诊断三大类。确诊 IE 定义为符合 2 个主要标准，或 1 个主要标准及 3 个次要标准，或 5 个次要标准[44]，而疑似及排除 IE 诊断的条件在本章中不再赘述。

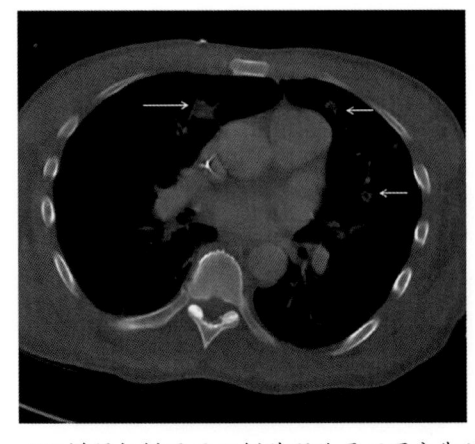

图 12.1 病例学习：CT 增强扫描显示双侧肺野处于不同分期的多发脓肿（箭头）

对于所有疑似 CIED-RE 的病例，在开始抗微生物治疗前的初次评估中，应至少抽取两组血培养[6]。另外，疑似 IE 病例的诊断还应包括一次超声心动图检查[6]。尽管改良 Duke 标准对 IE 具有灵敏度和特异性，但在 CIED-RE 中的应用尚缺乏针对性研究[45-47]。目前的临床实践及研究，对于已安装有 CIED 的病例，许多 CIED-RE 确诊的依据仍旧延续改良 Duke 标准。尽管如此，由于在这类人群中灵敏度较低，改良 Duke 标准在此应用不太适合[43]。针对这一临床困境，近期已提出了 Duke 标准的修正条款，修改了原主要标准，加入了包括电极导线赘生物的存在[2,45]、局部装置感染[45]作为主要标准，或增加了其他额外的标准（例如，在血培养阴性情况下取出的电极导线培养阳性）[2]。尽管血培养是 IE 和 CIED-RE 诊断的基石，但改良 Duke 标准尚未解决 TEE 或经胸超声心动图（TTE）是否适用于确诊 CIED-RE 的问题。

2007 年，美国心脏病学会基金会、美国心脏超声学会和其他关键的亚专业小组制定了相应标准，用于评估不同患者使用 TEE 和（或）TTE 检查的适用性水平，其中包括 IE 病例。在这一研究中，对于具有中高预测率（例如菌血症，尤其是葡萄球菌或真菌血症）的心内膜炎，以及 CIED 安装术后持续发热的病例，TEE 的使用在诊断和治疗心内膜炎中获得了适用性水平的最高评分[48]。

TEE 在诊断 CIED-RE 时的作用还得到其他研究的进一步支持，这些研究表明，在任何植入永久性心脏装置的患者中，TTE 作为唯一的影像学手段是不够的[3,49]。TEE 比 TTE 更灵敏且在检测赘生物和并发症中优于 TTE，例如脓肿形成[6,29,44,48]，在大多数情况下推荐使用，特别是当 TTE 图像质量较差或存在 CIED 时[48]。对于怀疑 CIED 感染的患者，无论血培养结果是阳性还是阴性，只要在血培养前接受过抗生素治疗，都应进行 TEE 检查以评估 CIED 感染或心脏瓣膜心内膜炎[6]。最后一点就是，只要没有明确禁忌证，所有植入了 CIED 的患者都应该考虑 TEE 检查[48]。从成本 – 效益角度来看，TEE 应作为疑似 IE 病例的首选影像学检查，尤其是有葡萄球菌菌血症时，因为这种情况下存在心内膜炎的可能性很大[3,6,29,44]。

尽管 TEE 是首选影像学检查，能提供清晰的心内结构影像，但也存在一些限制性因素：例如由于患者进食无法进行检查前的麻醉，或一些医疗机构不能开展 TEE 检查项目[50]。当临床上无法进行 TEE 或必须推迟时，应尽早行 TTE 检查[44]。虽然 TTE 不能明确排除赘生物或脓肿，但同样也能检测到许多 TEE 的发现，可用于极高危患者的鉴别诊断，使多数患者尽快得以确诊，用以指导早期治疗[44]。对于 TTE 结果阴性、TTE 图像质量极佳、无人工装置的植入且 IE 可能性较低的患者，推迟进行 TEE 并采用其他替代诊断手段是合理的。然而，除此临床情况外，由于对自体和人工瓣膜 IE 均具有非常好的诊断效果，TEE 仍是备受推崇的检查手段[48]。

TEE 虽然在诊断 CIED-RE 上优于 TTE，但也有其明显的局限性，即无法获得高清晰度的右心室图像，原因是右心室和食管内探头之间的距离较大（远场限制）[45]。这一局限性增加了部分患者确诊的难度，尤其是有 CIED 的老年患者，他们更容易发生与电极导线相关的三尖瓣心内膜炎[6,48]。虽然 TEE 对于检测赘生物和 IE 的其他心内结构比 TTE 更灵敏，尤其是在有人工瓣膜的情况下，但由于上述原因，TTE 对于右侧心内膜炎的灵敏度还是最高的[3,45]。因此，对于三尖瓣赘生物或右心室流出道的异常，TTE 相比 TEE 可获得更好的图像用于诊断，同时也表明 CIED-RE 的诊断还需要其他影像学方法予以补充佐证[3]。此外，人工瓣膜和起搏器电极导线还可导致声学伪像，限制了 TEE 对感染赘生物的检测，导致成像效果不佳[45,48]。基于上述原因，TEE 可能无法看清黏附在电极导线上的赘生物，从而不能排除可能存在的电极导线感染[6]。

最近有研究建议，使用其他影像学检查作为 TTE 和 TEE 的替代方案。心内超声心动图（ICE）是选择之一，可用于确诊瓣膜受累的 CIED-RE。它具有 TTE 所不具备的高清分辨率，同时又有 TEE 所不具备的检测右侧瓣膜的优势，操作前准备相对简单，无麻醉镇静和食管插入探头等风险[45,48]。但 ICE 的高昂费用及可能出现的假阳性妨碍了其推广使用[45,48]。

其他影像学方法，例如 ^{18}F-FDG PET/CT，已作为诊断 CIED-RE 及相关并发症的补充手段[43]。当怀疑 CIED 囊袋或电极导线感染时，^{18}F-FDG PET/CT 可以提供诊断所需的补充证据[29]。然而，虽然其对囊袋感染的灵敏度和特异性非常高（分别为 87% 和 100%），但对心内膜炎诊断的灵敏度和特异性分别只有 31% 和 62%[29]。

微生物学

随着人群风险因素的改变，IE 的相关微生物学也出现改变[3]。金黄色葡萄球菌是 IE 病例中最常见的致病微生物[3]。美国超过 7000 万次住院记录显示，与其他致病菌相比，金黄色葡萄球菌心内膜炎发病率显著上升[44]。葡萄球菌属是所有 CIED 感染中的主要病原菌，仅金黄色葡萄球菌和 CoNS 就占了所有病例的 60%~80%[10]。Aydin 等研究显示，金黄色葡萄球菌和 CoNS 分别占 CIED 感染的 41% 和 24%[9]。现已在 CIED 感染中发现了多种 CoNS[6]。此外，该研究显示，其他细菌类病原体在 CIED 感染中则相对少见，如棒状杆菌属、痤疮皮肤杆菌（之前被称为痤疮丙酸杆菌）和革兰氏阴性杆菌[6]。真菌感染导致的 CIED 感染也少有报道[9]。

CIED 感染的微生物可能有两条来源途径——通过患者皮肤来源的内源性途径，也可以是通过医疗环境和设备的接触或医院工作人员的手部来源的外源性途径[6]。感染率增加可能继发于不断增加的医疗服务（如静脉输液、手术伤口、人工假体装置和血液透析）[6]。引起 CIED-RE 的主要致病微生物包括常见的皮肤菌群，如金黄色葡萄球菌和 CoNS，尤其是表皮葡萄球菌[16,51-53]。此外，其他微生物包括革兰氏阴性杆菌、非葡萄球菌革兰氏阳性菌和布鲁氏菌也有报道[51-53]。

Sohail 等的研究显示，CIED-RE 是 ICD 感染的第二常见形式[16]。在另一篇由 Sohail 等发表的文献中，金黄色葡萄球菌、CoNS、真菌和革兰氏阴性杆菌引起的

CIED-RE 分别占 41%、41%、5% 和 5%[52]。在 Carrasco 等的研究中，葡萄球菌是主要的致病菌（占 84%），其次是肠球菌（占 12%）[7]。不同研究报道的金黄色葡萄球菌抗生素耐药性有所不同[10,51]，因此，在 CIED 感染的情况下，可以合理地假设所有表皮葡萄球菌和大多数金黄色葡萄球菌致病菌都具有耐药性，以指导经验性抗生素治疗[10,51]。

【病例学习——治疗与预后】

为从血管路径取出 CIED 相关组件，须做好前期准备工作。首先是在杂交室手术期间，确保有胸心外科手术团队保驾护航；此外，还需做好其他紧急干预的准备，例如出现心脏或大静脉撕裂的情况，需准备 2U 的交叉配型浓缩红细胞。准备好全身麻醉，并安排术中 TEE 监测。动脉穿刺持续监测动脉血压，并确保有大口径的静脉通道。手术顺利完成时，留置临时经静脉起搏器，直至菌血症得以根治，方可在远离上次放置部位重新植入新的永久性 CIED。

治 疗

2010 年美国心脏协会 / 美国心律协会（AHA/HRS）关于 CIED 感染及处理的科学声明在此后基本没有更新，主要是 2019 年欧洲心律协会（EHRA）在补充过去 10 年公布的临床数据后更新了指南，并得到了 HRS 认同。成功处理 CIED-RE 的总体方案应包括装置和电极导线的清除，以及适当抗生素覆盖治疗。

2019 年的 EHRA 指南建议清除装置的所有组件，包括装置本身以及所有正在使用的、废弃的组件和（或）心外电极导线，以确保成功治疗所有 CIED 感染。其他所有的经静脉硬件，如血管端口或永久性血液透析导管，均应清除。这一建议还适用于患有 IE 但没有明确累及 CIED 装置或硬件的患者[1]。

针对由金黄色葡萄球菌、CoNS、痤疮皮肤杆菌和念珠菌引起的隐性菌血症，即使没有电极导线和（或）瓣膜明确受累的情况，或是菌血症复发但没有明确的感染源的情况，EHRA 均推荐移除 CIED[1]。这主要是因为可能存在潜在的未检测到的装置感染；然而，这一做法仍需临床研究证实。一个需注意的例外是非假单胞菌、沙雷菌或肺炎球菌引起的菌血症，由于这些病原体感染导致 CIED 受累的可能性较低，因此不建议移除装置[1,6]。

经静脉取出电极是移除 CIED 组件的首选方法，与手术移除相比，其并发症发生率和死亡率较低[1,6,54-55]。研究发现，在入院后 3 d 内进行经静脉电极导线移除可以显著降低住院死亡率，并缩短住院时间[56]。开放手术仅用于经静脉取出失败，仍有较多残留组件的患者。一个例外情况是电极导线上存在 >20 mm 的赘生物，此时可能需要结合其他一些临床资料，用以选择适当的组件移除方法[1,29,43]。对于这类患者，使用经静脉移除电极导线的方法，可能引起巨大赘生物脱落，导致严重的肺动脉栓塞，引发血流动力学不稳定，并可能成为持续性脓毒症的根源。对此难题，只有结合进一步的临床资料才能界定其解决方式，否则，选择开放手术还是经静脉清除电极导线应个体化处理。近期引入了一种经皮抽除大的电极导线赘生物的新方法，该方法利用带内置过滤器的静脉-静脉体外回路以避免栓塞发生，但有待循证医学的证实[1,57-58]。

CIED-RE 的抗菌起始用药以经验为主，通常包括万古霉素与第三代头孢菌素或庆大霉素联合使用[1]，待血培养及药敏结果返回，则应依据检查结果针对性调整抗菌治疗方案。抗生素治疗的持续时间取决于 IE 的类型，包括是自体瓣膜感染、人工瓣膜感染还是单独的电极导线赘生物[1]。有关适当抗生素的选择和持续时间已在第 7 章详述。彻底清创设备囊袋、切除纤维包膜、移除所有不可吸收缝线材料、无菌生理盐水冲洗干净，以上措施对确保控制感染至关重要[1,6]。对于寿命有限、拒绝移除设备的患者，或因其他原因不适合手术或经皮移除 CIED 的患者，可考虑长期抗生素治疗。但在抗生素使用方式上，较为便利的口服用药对于控制 CIED 感染仍有困难[6]。

在移除设备和电极导线之前，应对临床情况进行全面评估来决定是更换还是移除 CIED。据估计，1/3～1/2 的患者在设备移除后不再需要更换[6]，出现这种需求变化的原因包括：病情逆转需继续使用原来的设备，临床病情发生变化，其他替代治疗方式的出现，首次植入设备时缺乏合适的指征等。当需要更换设备时，优先考虑将新设备放置在原位置的对侧。如果临床情况不适合放置对侧，可选择腹部皮下（经隧道植入静脉电极导线），或心外膜植入[6]。对于再次植入的最佳时间，目前尚无共识，主要根据医生的经验和患者的临床病情决定[1]。在植入新的 CIED 前，常规需反复血培养送检，保证至少连续 72 h 的结果阴性。但在瓣膜感染时，推荐 CIED 移除后至少 2 周以上再植入新的静脉电极导线[6]。尤应关注 PPM 依赖患者，他们使用临时心脏起搏器无法出院，可考虑通过主动电极导线连接外部起搏发生器或除颤器，进行临时起搏，直到可以安全植入新的 PPM。主动电极导线放置在之前去除设备的同侧，同时避免使用之前含有感染电极导线的静脉，原则上保留对侧位置以供未来新设备的植入[1,6]。

更换 CIED 之前可能的替代方式还有无电极导线起搏器和 S-ICD（全皮下植入式除颤器）。Nanostim 无电极导线心脏起搏器是一个独立的右心室起搏器，目前尚未用于临床。而 Micra 经导管起搏系统则是一个在去除 CIED 感染设备/电极导线后，可替代的安全的临床选择[1,59-60]。对于只需要除颤功能的病例，更换时植入 S-ICD 即可满足这一功能，同时还可降低新发感染的风险。即使出现感染，S-ICD 的风险也较低，通常不会引起危及生命的全身性感染。EFFORTLESS S-ICD 注册研究对 S-ICD 进行了 3 年的随访，主要评估其安全性，结果显示 2.4% 的感染需要移除设备，但无心内膜炎的报道[1,61-62]。

并发症

CIED-RE 近期和远期并发症发生率都很高，因此，制定恰当的预防和应急处理指南至关重要，以避免高并发症发生率和死亡率。最近一项前瞻性研究明确了以下相关并发症：瓣膜受累（37.2%）、心力衰竭（15.3%）和住院期间持续菌血症（15.8%）[8]。另一项研究纳入了近30年关于 CIED-RE 急性处理的病例，显示高达72%的患者出现了严重并发症。住院期间的主要并发症包括持续性脓毒症（最常见）、心脏并发症（如心力衰竭）、卒中和脓肿形成[7]。这类患者均接受抗生素治疗，如果包括已移除或未移除 CIED 的所有病例，其早期院内死亡率为24%，而取出 CIED 并接受抗生素治疗的病例死亡率为21%。感染性并发症（如脓毒症和肺炎）占这些死亡病例的一半，其余病例的死亡原因则与心血管因素相关（如心源性休克和室性心律失常）。值得注意的是，94%的 CIED 移除通过外科手术进行，这可能是导致高死亡率的原因[7]。电极导线取出相关的并发症包括脓毒性肺栓塞、持续性脓毒症、心律失常、操作引起的心血管结构穿透性损伤需急诊开胸、动静脉瘘及三尖瓣损害[1]。需提醒的一点是，12%的迟发性死亡（定义为出院3个月以后发生）与心内膜炎或心血管并发症无关。另外，那些经初始住院治疗和紧急处理存活下来的 CIED-RE 病例，无 CIED-RE 复发的报道[7]。

如上述研究所证实的，CIED-RE 患者的设备移除并非没有风险，而再次植入 CIED 也不能排除感染复发的可能。然而，再次植入之前进行适当的抗生素治疗并确认72 h内血培养阴性（瓣膜受累者除外），是降低风险的关键措施[1]。

结 果

CIED 感染的院内死亡率为5%~8%，但与 CIED-RE 相关的死亡率更高，最近一项回顾性研究显示可达29%[1,56]。而那些未能移除 CIED 并需要长期抗生素控制治疗的患者，无论是院内还是远期死亡率，都是这类患者人群中最高的[1]。

临床结果的解读要关注一点，CIED 患者具有与 CIED-RE 相似的不良心脏风险特征，可能出现两者混淆的临床结果。通常，CIED 植入者都是高龄，糖尿病等共病很常见。最近的一项前瞻性研究揭示了发生率较高的并发症，其中并发瓣膜感染尤为常见。此外，这类患者近期和远期死亡率均较高，尤其是瓣膜受累者。虽然移除 CIED 未能提高住院期间的生存率，但移除后的患者具有较高的1年生存率[8]。

关于远期结果，近来有证据表明，CIED 感染的类型是1年死亡率的强预测因素：具有血管内感染临床特征的患者，在 CIED 取出后第1年内死亡率是单纯囊袋感染者的2倍[1,63]。另一项回顾性研究表明，与囊袋感染（伴或不伴菌血症）相比，CIED-RE 的死亡风险要翻倍[1,64]。

在各类 CIED 感染中，可导致死亡率增加的因素包括全身栓塞、中重度三尖瓣反流、右心室功能异常、肾功能异常[6,65]。而电极导线是否有赘生物、赘生物大小和活动度并不是死亡的独立预测因素，由此推断，继发于电极导线赘生物的肺栓塞并不能成为解释血管内感染病例死亡率增加的原因[6,63,65]。

预　防

由于 CIED-RE 发生率的增加，相关并发症发生率和死亡率以及电极导线移除的需求也在不断增加[3,45]。CIED-RE 的预防对改善 CIED 植入患者的长期健康状况和生活质量至关重要。一些预防措施已经过验证并推荐用于预防 CIED-RE，分为 CIED 植入前、术中及植入后预防。并非所有建议都专属于预防 CIED-RE 的范畴，但它们的推广应用可起到降低 CIED 相关感染率的作用。基于 CIED 与 CIED-RE 之间的强相关性，这些建议对两者都是适用的。

CIED 植入前

在装置植入前，须确保患者没有感染。如果存在感染迹象，则应延迟植入[8,29]。排除了全身性感染后，下一步就是预防性使用抗生素，这可以显著降低装置感染的风险[29]。最常用的是第一代头孢菌素，如头孢唑林，应在术前 1h 内给药。万古霉素是可替代的选择，用于有 MRSA 暴露的患者（例如 MRSA 鼻拭子阳性）或对青霉素过敏者，应在术前 2 h 内给药[29]。对万古霉素过敏者，可选择克林霉素或利奈唑胺[27]。对于植入后的 CIED 需要进行侵入性操作，同样建议抗生素预防。术前手术部位的消毒准备应十分细致。

CIED 植入中

手术过程中，严格遵循无菌原则[27]。如果患者皮下组织薄弱和（或）营养不良，出现皮肤组织愈合不良的风险较高，则应考虑胸肌后囊袋以减少感染的发生[44]。血肿的预防重在术中，措施包括：精心烧灼出血部位，在植入电极导线时用浸有抗生素的海绵填塞囊袋，抗凝的患者局部使用凝血酶，以及（或）冲洗囊袋引流持续性出血。低分子量肝素易导致血肿形成，应避免使用。如果出现血肿，且血肿皮肤张力较高，建议清除血肿以避免皮肤菌群进入囊袋[44]。

围手术期抗生素使用和抗菌封套的新进展可进一步降低感染的发生，这些还未成为临床常规，但已展现出较好的初步结果。为确定围手术期增加抗生素用量可否有效减少 CIED 感染，有学者进行了心律失常设备感染预防试验（PADIT）。试验中，术前给予头孢唑林加万古霉素，术中杆菌肽（bacitracin）冲洗囊袋，术后口服头孢氨苄 2 d。虽然结果无统计学差异，但治疗组的感染率有所降低[66]。利用非吸收性抗菌封套包裹装置发生器的新技术已证实可显著减少 CIED 感染[25,67]，特别是 TYRX 抗菌封套用于 ICD 和 CRT 植入时，显示 CIED 感染率非常低，且无血肿发生率增高的风险[67]。Wrap-IT 试验是最近进行的一项随机对照试验，用以评估可吸收的抗生素释放封套预防 CIED 感染的安全性和有效性。结果显示：与单纯采用标准抗感染策略相比，附加使用抗菌封套可显著降低主要 CIED 感染的发生率，且未增加并发症的发生率[41]。与对照组相比，虽然治疗组的囊袋感染较少，但 IE 的发生率较高，这使得抗菌封套在预防 CIED-RE 方面的适用性受到质疑。

CIED 植入后

目前没有证据支持术后抗生素治疗，由于可能增加药物不良事件、诱发耐药菌产生、增加医疗费用，故不推荐术后使用抗生素[29]。

保持口腔卫生和抗生素预防性使用是以往实施侵入性手术时的常规做法，当然也是预防 CIED 感染和 CIED-RE 的重要措施。预防工作聚焦口腔卫生，主要原因是草绿色链球菌是口腔正常菌群，据报道由其导致的 IE 约占 IE 总病例的 20%。AHA 和其他一些主要学会的指南曾推荐，对于存在基础心脏病的患者，在进行口腔手术前预防性使用抗生素，以防止心内膜炎的发生[3]。然而，如前所述，最新证据显示，导致 CIED 感染的致病菌以葡萄球菌为主，因此在口腔操作前进行抗生素预防的价值微乎其微。在口腔病原菌引起装置感染的罕见情况中，最可能的原因是口腔卫生不佳和牙周疾病引起的菌血症，常见于刷牙、使用牙线或咀嚼食物等日常事件，与口腔操作无关[3,44]。

最近不再推荐口腔操作前预防性使用抗生素[29]。现在的建议是所有植入 CIED 的患者须保持良好的口腔卫生。法国 IE 预防指南大幅减少了预防性指征，英国国家卫生与临床优化研究所建议对所有口腔、消化道、泌尿生殖道或呼吸道操作无须进行心内膜炎预防[3]，ESC 和 AHA 的指南也提供了进一步的规范条款。2015 年 ESC 指南建议只针对 IE 最高风险人群进行口腔预防性治疗。2007 年 AHA 指南推荐口腔预防性治疗限于 4 种心脏情况：人工瓣膜置换术后或使用了瓣膜材料、既往 IE 病史、某些先天性心脏病亚型以及心脏移植术后的心脏瓣膜病[3]。

许多研究显示，以上措施实施后，IE 的发病率和（或）死亡率显著增加，但也有研究报道了心内膜炎病例的减少[3,68-72]。无论如何，过去 5 年的数据提示了病例数的回升，已恢复到了实施更新指南前的水平[73-74]，表明这些严格的条款可能需要进一步调整[3]。然而，这些相关的随访研究并未提供病原体流行病学的数据，也未做清晰分层，使得最近增加的病例是否是由于正常口腔菌群或其他病原体导致的感染成为一个未解的问题[3,75]。2015 年 AHA 指南支持在植入 CIED 后保持健康的口腔卫生，以显著降低未来发生 IE 的可能性。最终，AHA 推荐平时注意保持口腔卫生，而在口腔手术前进行心内膜炎预防[44]。

如果患者遵守以下 4 项措施，几乎可以完全预防牙齿疾病，也有助于减少菌血症的发生和随后 IE 复发的风险。这些措施包括：①保持牙齿清洁，避免牙菌斑的形成；②采取膳食措施，如减少或不摄入糖和其他精制碳水化合物；③定期与家庭牙医进行随访，密切关注口腔卫生情况，早期发现和消除口腔疾病；④每天使用高浓度氟化物牙膏[44]。

除以上措施外，预防血管内置管过程中相关菌血症也可以减少医疗相关 IE 的发生。这可以通过提升干预措施的质量来实现，例如医疗组合或建立医疗流程，其中包括严格的手部卫生、在插入中心导管时使用完全无菌化的防护措施，用氯己定（洗必泰）消毒穿刺部位，在可能的情况下避免股动脉穿刺，并清除任何不必要的导管[3]。

总　结

过去 20 年，随着 CIED 一级和二级预防适应证不断扩大，一些装置、患者及手术操作相关因素的相互作用导致了 CIED-RE 发病率的显著增加。对 CIED-RE 的早期预防、及时诊断及良好的处理，为防止这一高龄、心血管状况不佳及存在大量共病的人群出现严重并发症和死亡提供了有利条件。装置清除辅以抗生素治疗是治疗 CIED-RE 的关键。然而，随机对照试验的相关数据非常缺乏，目前各治疗指南多建立在观察性研究和专家共识之上。这一临床窘境需要更多的随机对照试验，以优化临床策略，减少 CIED-RE 发生，改善相关预后。

参考文献

[1] Blomstrom-Lundqvist C, Traykov V, Erba PA, et al. European heart rhythm association (EHRA) international consensus document on how to prevent, diagnose, and treat cardiac implant-able electronic device infections-endorsed by the heart rhythm society (HRS), the Asia Pacific heart rhythm society (APHRS), the Latin American heart rhythm society (LAHRS), International Society for Cardiovascular Infectious Diseases (ISCVID) and the European Society of Clinical Microbiology and Infectious Diseases (ESC-MID) in collaboration with the European Association for Cardio-Thoracic Surgery (EACTS). Europace, 2019, 22(4): 515–549.

[2] Bongiorni MG, Burri H, Deharo JC, et al. 2018 EHRA expert consensus statement on lead extraction: recommendations on definitions, endpoints, research trial design, and data collection requirements for clinical scientific studies and registries: endorsed by APHRS/HRS/LAHRS. Europace, 2018, 20: 1217.

[3] Holland TL, Baddour LM, Bayer AS, et al. Infective endocarditis. Nat Rev Dis Primers, 2016, 2: 16059.

[4] Polewczyk A, Janion M, Kutarski A. Cardiac device infections: definition, classification, differential diagnosis, and management. Pol Arch Med Wewn, 2016, 126: 275–283.

[5] Ozcan C, Raunso J, Lamberts M, et al. Infective endocarditis and risk of death after cardiac implantable electronic device implantation: a nationwide cohort study. Europace, 2017, 19: 1007–1014.

[6] Baddour LM, Epstein AE, Erickson CC, et al. Update on cardiovascular implantable electronic device infections and their management: a scientific statement from the American Heart Association. Circulation, 2010, 121: 458–477.

[7] Carrasco F, Anguita M, Ruiz M, et al. Clinical features and changes in epidemiology of infective endocarditis on pacemaker devices over a 27-year period (1987—2013). Europace, 2016, 18: 836–841.

[8] Athan E, Chu VH, Tattevin P, et al. Clinical characteristics and outcome of infective endocarditis involving implantable cardiac devices. Jama, 2012, 307: 1727–1735.

[9] Aydin M, Yildiz A, Kaya Z, et al. Clinical characteristics and outcome of cardiovascular implantable electronic device infections in Turkey. Clin Appl Thromb Hemost, 2016, 22: 459–464.

[10] Baddour LM, Cha YM, Wilson WR. Clinical practice. Infections of cardiovascular implantable

electronic devices. N Engl J Med, 2012, 367: 842–849.

[11] Voigt A, Shalaby A, Saba S. Rising rates of cardiac rhythm management device infections in the United States:1996 through 2003. J Am Coll Cardiol, 2006, 48: 590–591.

[12] Maille B, Koutbi L, Resseguier N, et al. Seasonal variations in cardiac implantable electronic device infections. Heart Ves, 2019, 34: 824–831.

[13] Ferguson Jr TB, Ferguson CL, Crites K, et al. The additional hospital costs generated in the management of complications of pacemaker and defibrillator implantations. J Thorac Cardiovasc Surg, 1996, 111: 742-51. discussion 751–742.

[14] Sohail MR, Uslan DZ, Khan AH, et al. Management and outcome of permanent pacemaker and implantable cardioverter-defibrillator infections. J Am Coll Cardiol, 2007, 49: 1851–1859.

[15] Lin YS, Hung SP, Chen PR, et al. Risk factors influencing complications of cardiac implantable electronic device implantation: infection, pneumo-thorax and heart perforation: a nationwide population-based cohort study. Medicine (Baltim), 2014, 93: e213.

[16] Sohail MR, Hussain S, Le KY, et al. Risk factors associated with early- versus late-onset implantable cardioverter-defibrillator infections. J Intervent Card Electrophysiol, 2011, 31: 171–183.

[17] Cengiz M, Okutucu S, Ascioglu S, et al. Permanent pacemaker and implantable cardioverter defibrillator infections: seven years of diagnostic and therapeutic experience of a single center. Clin Cardiol, 2010, 33: 406–411.

[18] Darouiche RO. Treatment of infections associated with surgical implants. N Engl J Med, 2004, 350: 1422–1429.

[19] Chamis AL, Peterson GE, Cabell CH, et al. Staphylococcus aureus bacteremia in patients with permanent pacemakers or implantable cardioverter-defibrillators. Circulation, 2001, 104: 1029–1033.

[20] Fowler Jr VG, Miro JM, Hoen B, et al. Staphylococcus aureus endocarditis: a consequence of medical progress. Jama, 2005, 293: 3012–3021.

[21] Bode LG, Kluytmans JA, Wertheim HF, et al. Preventing surgical-site infections in nasal carriers of Staphylococcus aureus. N Engl J Med, 2010, 362: 9–17.

[22] Darouiche RO. Device-associated infections: a macroproblem that starts with microadherence. Clin Infect Dis, 2001, 33: 1567–1572.

[23] Hussein AA, Baghdy Y, Wazni OM, et al. Microbiology of cardiac implantable electronic device infections. JACC Clin Electrophysiol, 2016, 2: 498–505.

[24] Sandoe JA, Barlow G, Chambers JB, et al. Guidelines for the diagnosis, prevention and management of implantable cardiac electronic device infection. Report of a joint working party project on behalf of the British society for antimicrobial chemotherapy (BSAC, host organization), British heart rhythm society (BHRS), British cardiovascular society (BCS), British heart valve society (BHVS) and British society for echocardiography (BSE). J Antimicrob Chemother, 2015, 70: 325–359.

[25] Mittal S, Shaw RE, Michel K, et al. Cardiac implantable electronic device infections: incidence, risk factors, and the effect of the AigisRx antibacterial envelope. Heart Rhythm, 2014, 11: 595–601.

[26] Chung MK, Holcomb RG, Mittal S, et al. REPLACE DARE (Death after Replacement Evaluation) score: determinants of all-cause mortality after implantable device replacement or upgrade from the REPLACE registry. Circ Arrhythm Electrophysiol, 2014, 7: 1048–1056.

[27] Gould PA, Gula LJ, Yee R, et al. Cardiovascular implantable electrophysiological device-related infections: a review. Curr Opin Cardiol, 2011, 26: 6–11.

[28] Prutkin JM, Reynolds MR, Bao H, et al. Rates of and factors associated with infection in 200 909 Medicare implantable cardioverter-defibrillator implants: results from the National Cardiovascular Data Registry. Circulation, 2014, 130: 1037–1043.

[29] Kusumoto FM, Schoenfeld MH, Wilkoff BL, et al. 2017 HRS expert consensus statement on cardiovascular implantable electronic device lead management and extraction. Heart Rhythm, 2017, 14: e503–e551.

[30] Sohail MR, Uslan DZ, Khan AH, et al. Risk factor analysis of permanent pacemaker infection.

Clin Infect Dis, 2007, 45: 166–173.
[31] Klug D, Balde M, Pavin D, et al. Risk factors related to infections of implanted pacemakers and cardioverter-defibrillators: results of a large prospective study. Circulation, 2007, 116: 1349–1355.
[32] Mela T, McGovern BA, Garan H, et al. Long-term infection rates associated with the pectoral versus abdominal approach to cardioverter- defibrillator implants. Am J Cardiol, 2001, 88: 750–753.
[33] Trappe HJ, Pfitzner P, Klein H, et al. Infections after cardioverter-defibrillator implantation: observations in 335 patients over 10 years. Br Heart J, 1995, 73: 20–24.
[34] Lai KK, Fontecchio SA. Infections associated with implantable cardioverter defibrillators placed transvenously and via thoracotomies: epidemiology, infection control, and management. Clin Infect Dis, 1998, 27: 265–269.
[35] Polyzos KA, Konstantelias AA, Falagas ME. Risk factors for cardiac implantable electronic device infection: a systematic review and meta-analysis. Europace, 2015, 17: 767–777.
[36] Webster J, Alghamdi A. Use of plastic adhesive drapes during surgery for preventing surgical site infection. Cochrane Database Syst Rev, 2015, 2015(4): Cd006353.
[37] Da Costa A, Kirkorian G, Cucherat M, et al. Antibiotic prophylaxis for permanent pacemaker implantation: a meta-analysis. Circulation, 1998, 97: 1796–1801.
[38] Essebag V, Verma A, Healey JS, et al. Clinically significant pocket hematoma increases long-term risk of device infection: BRUISE CONTROL INFECTION study. J Am Coll Cardiol, 2016, 67: 1300–1308.
[39] Birnie DH, Healey JS, Wells GA, et al. Pacemaker or defibrillator surgery without interruption of anticoagulation. N Engl J Med, 2013, 368: 2084–2093.
[40] Birnie DH, Healey JS, Wells GA, et al. Continued vs. interrupted direct oral anticoagulants at the time of device surgery, in patients with moderate to high risk of arterial thrombo-embolic events (BRUISE CONTROL-2). Eur Heart J, 2018, 39: 3973–3979.
[41] Tarakji KG, Mittal S, Kennergren C, et al. Antibacterial envelope to prevent cardiac implantable device infection. N Engl J Med, 2019, 380: 1895–1905.
[42] Shariff N, Eby E, Adelstein E, et al. Health and economic outcomes associated with use of an antimicrobial envelope as a standard of care for cardiac implantable electronic device implantation. J Cardiovasc Electrophysiol, 2015, 26: 783–789.
[43] Habib G, Lancellotti P, Antunes MJ, et al. 2015 ESC guidelines for the management of infective endocarditis: the task force for the management of infective endocarditis of the European society of Cardiology (ESC). Endorsed by: European association for cardio-thoracic surgery (EACTS), the European association of nuclear medicine(EANM). Eur Heart J, 2015, 36: 3075–3128.
[44] Baddour LM, Wilson WR, Bayer AS, et al. Infective endocarditis in adults: diagnosis, antimicrobial therapy, and management of complications: a scientific statement for healthcare professionals from the American heart association. Circulation, 2015,132: 1435–1486.
[45] Narducci ML, Pelargonio G, Russo E, et al. Usefulness of intracardiac echocardiography for the diagnosis of cardiovascular implantable electronic device-related endocarditis. J Am Coll Cardiol, 2013, 61: 1398–1405.
[46] Habib G, Hoen B, Tornos P, et al. Guidelines on the prevention, diagnosis, and treatment of infective endocarditis (new version 2009): the task force on the prevention, diagnosis, and treatment of infective endocarditis of the European society of Cardiology (ESC). Endorsed by the European society of clinical microbiology and infectious diseases (ESCMID) and the international society of chemotherapy (ISC) for infection and cancer. Eur Heart J, 2009, 30: 2369–2413.
[47] Baddour LM, Wilson WR, Bayer AS, et al. Infective endocarditis: diagnosis, antimicrobial therapy, and management of complications: a statement for healthcare professionals from the committee on rheumatic fever, endocarditis, and kawasaki disease, council on cardiovascular disease in the young, and the councils on clinical cardiology, stroke, and cardiovascular surgery and anesthesia, American heart association: Endorsed by the infectious diseases society of America. Circulation, 2005, 111: e394–e434.

[48] Sedgwick JF, Burstow DJ. Update on echocardiography in the management of infective endocarditis. Curr Infect Dis Rep, 2012, 14: 373–380.

[49] Holland TL, Arnold C, Fowler Jr VG. Clinical management of Staphylococcus aureus bacteremia: a review. Jama, 2014, 312: 1330–1341.

[50] Ali S, George LK, Das P, et al. Intracardiac echocardiography: clinical utility and application. Echocardiography, 2011, 28: 582–590.

[51] Le KY, Sohail MR, Friedman PA, et al. Impact of timing of device removal on mortality in patients with cardiovascular implantable electronic device infections. Heart Rhythm, 2011, 8: 1678–1685.

[52] Sohail MR, Uslan DZ, Khan AH, et al. Infective endocarditis complicating permanent pacemaker and implantable cardioverter-defibrillator infection. Mayo Clin Proc, 2008, 83: 46–53.

[53] Osmonov D, Ozcan KS, Erdinler I, et al. Cardiac device-related endocarditis: 31-years' experience. J Cardiol, 2013, 61: 175–180.

[54] Patel D, Khan F, Shah H, Bhattacharya S, Adelstein E, Saba S. Cardiac implantable electronic device lead extraction in patients with underlying infection using open thoracotomy or percutaneous techniques. Cardiol J, 2015, 22: 68–74.

[55] Rusanov A, Spotnitz HM. A 15-year experience with permanent pacemaker and defibrillator lead and patch extractions. Ann Thorac Surg, 2010, 89: 44–50.

[56] Viganego F, O'Donoghue S, Eldadah Z, Shah MH, Rastogi M, Mazel JA, Platia EV. Effect of early diagnosis and treatment with percutaneous lead extraction on survival in patients with cardiac device infections. Am J Cardiol, 2012, 109: 1466–1471.

[57] Schaerf RHM, Najibi S, Conrad J. Percutaneous vacuum-assisted thrombectomy device used for removal of large vegetations on infected pacemaker and defibrillator leads as an adjunct to lead extraction. J Atr Fibrillation, 2016, 9: 1455.

[58] Starck CT, Eulert-Grehn J, Kukucka M, Eggert-Doktor D, Dreizler T, Haupt B, Falk V. Managing large lead vegetations in transvenous lead extractions using a percutaneous aspiration technique. Expet Rev Med Dev, 2018, 15: 757–761.

[59] Beurskens NEG, Tjong FVY, Dasselaar KJ, Kuijt WJ, Wilde AAM, Knops RE. Leadless pacemaker implantation after explantation of infected conventional pacemaker systems: a viable solution? Heart Rhythm, 2019, 16: 66–71.

[60] El-Chami MF, Johansen JB, Zaidi A, Faerestrand S, Reynolds D, Garcia-Seara J, Mansourati J, Pasquie JL, McElderry HT, Roberts PR, Soejima K, Stromberg K, Piccini JP. Leadless pacemaker implant in patients with pre-existing infections: results from the Micra postapproval registry. J Cardiovasc Electrophysiol, 2019, 30: 569–574.

[61] Brouwer TF, Yilmaz D, Lindeboom R, Buiten MS, Olde Nordkamp LR, Schalij MJ, Wilde AA, van Erven L, Knops RE. Long-term clinical outcomes of subcutaneous versus transvenous implantable defibrillator therapy. J Am Coll Cardiol, 2016, 68: 2047–2055.

[62] Boersma L, Barr C, Knops R, Theuns D, Eckardt L, Neuzil P, Scholten M, Hood M, Kuschyk J, Jones P, Duffy E, Husby M, Stein K, Lambiase PD. Implant and midterm outcomes of the subcutaneous implantable cardioverter-defibrillator registry: the EFFORTLESS study. J Am Coll Cardiol, 2017, 70: 830–841.

[63] Tarakji KG, Wazni OM, Harb S, Hsu A, Saliba W, Wilkoff BL. Risk factors for 1-year mortality among patients with cardiac implantable electronic device infection undergoing transvenous lead extraction: the impact of the infection type and the presence of vegetation on survival. Europace, 2014, 16: 1490–1495.

[64] Lee DH, Gracely EJ, Aleem SY, Kutalek SP, Vielemeyer O. Differences of mortality rates between pocket and nonpocket cardiovascular implantable electronic device infections. Pacing Clin Electrophysiol, 2015, 38: 1456–1463.

[65] Baman TS, Gupta SK, Valle JA, Yamada E. Risk factors for mortality in patients with cardiac device-related infection. Circ Arrhythm Electrophysiol, 2009, 2: 129–134.

[66] Krahn AD, Longtin Y, Philippon F, Birnie DH, Manlucu J, Angaran P, Rinne C, Coutu B, Low

RA, Essebag V, Morillo C, Redfearn D, Toal S, Becker G, Degrace M, Thibault B, Crystal E, Tung S, LeMaitre J, Sultan O, Bennett M, Bashir J, Ayala-Paredes F, Gervais P, Rioux L, Hemels MEW, Bouwels LHR, van Vlies B, Wang J, Exner DV, Dorian P, Parkash R, Alings M, Connolly SJ. Prevention of arrhythmia device infection trial: the PADIT trial. J Am Coll Cardiol, 2018, 72: 3098–3109.

[67] Henrikson CA, Sohail MR, Acosta H, et al. Antibacterial envelope is associated with low infection rates after implantable cardioverter-defibrillator and cardiac resynchronization therapy device replacement: results of the citadel and centurion studies. JACC Clin Electrophysiol, 2017, 3: 1158–1167.

[68] Thornhill MH, Dayer MJ, Forde JM, et al. Impact of the NICE guideline recommending cessation of antibiotic prophylaxis for prevention of infective endocarditis: before and after study. Br Med J, 2011, 342: d2392.

[69] Pasquali SK, He X, Mohamad Z, et al. Trends in endocarditis hospitalizations at US children's hospitals: impact of the 2007 American heart association antibiotic prophylaxis guidelines. Am Heart J, 2012, 163: 894–899.

[70] Lockhart PB, Hanson NB, Ristic H, et al. Acceptance among and impact on dental practitioners and patients of American heart association recommendations for antibiotic prophylaxis. J Am Dent Assoc, 2013, 144: 1030–1035.

[71] Duval X, Hoen B. Prophylaxis for infective endocarditis: let's end the debate. Lancet, 2015, 385: 1164–1165.

[72] Centre for Clinical Practice at National Institute for Health and Clinical Excellence. Prophylaxis against infective endocarditis: antimicrobial prophylaxis against infective endocarditis in adults and children undergoing interventional procedures. London: National Institute for Health and Clinical Excellence (UK), 2008.

[73] Dayer MJ, Jones S, Prendergast B, et al. Incidence of infective endocarditis in England, 2000-13: a secular trend, interrupted time-series analysis. Lancet, 2015, 385: 1219–1228.

[74] Pant S, Patel NJ, Deshmukh A, et al. Trends in infective endocarditis incidence, microbiology, and valve replacement in the United States from 2000 to 2011. J Am Coll Cardiol, 2015, 65: 2070–2076.

[75] Pericas JM, Falces C, Moreno A, et al. Neglecting enterococci may lead to a misinterpretation of the consequences of last changes in endocarditis prophylaxis American Heart Association guidelines. J Am Coll Cardiol, 2015, 66: 2156.

第13章
感染性心内膜炎患者的门诊随访与处理

A. Dahl[1,2], M. Hernandez-Meneses[1], J. Ambrosioni[1], J.M. Pericàs[1], C. Falces[3], E. Quintana[3], B. Vidal[3], A. Perissinotti[4], M. Almela[5], D. Fuster[4], E. Sandoval[3], J.M. Tolosana[3], C. García de la Maria[1], D. García-Pares[1,6], A. Moreno[1], N.E. Bruun[7], J.M. Miro[1], the Hospital Clinic Endocarditis Team Investigators[8]

[1]Infectious Diseases Service, Hospital Clinic-IDIBAPS, University of Barcelona, Barcelona, Spain; [2]Department of Cardiology, Herlev Gentofte University Hospital, Herlev, Denmark; [3]Cardiovascular Institute, Hospital Clinic-IDIBAPS, University of Barcelona, Barcelona, Spain; [4]Nuclear Medicine Service, Hospital Clinic-IDIBAPS, University of Barcelona, Barcelona, Spain; [5]Microbiology Service, Hospital Clinic-IDIBAPS, University of Barcelona, Barcelona, Spain; [6]Internal Medicine Service, Clinica Sagrada Familia, Barcelona, Spain; [7]Department of Cardiology, Zealand University Hospital, Roskilde, Denmark; [8]See Appendix

引 言

感染性心内膜炎（IE）患者的治疗在过去几十年取得了长足进步。从仅能靠留院长期静脉注射抗生素进行保守治疗，转变成以心脏手术治疗为主，结合院内外使用静脉和口服抗生素进行联合治疗。

本章主要探讨心内膜炎患者出院后的治疗及随访管理。当IE患者可以出院时，相应的门诊随访计划也应得到落实。出院IE患者一般可分为3大类：①患者的感染已治愈，可在出院前停止抗生素（痊愈）；②患者在抗生素治疗完成前病情稳定，可以出院，因此抗生素疗程将继续在门诊完成（好转）；③由于年龄、共病和IE病情严重等因素，认为患者感染无法治愈，出院接受个体化治疗，可计划终生抗生素治疗，或仅实施姑息性治疗（未愈）。

本章将阐述出院后在家中完成抗生素疗程的标准，包括口服或者静脉给药。此外，还将讨论临床、微生物学和外科随访，以及这些相关领域的研究前景。

门诊抗生素治疗

院外完成抗生素治疗有几个好处。首先，患者可早些从紧张的医院环境中解脱出来，享受家中的舒适。其次，患者暴露于医院获得性感染风险的时间缩短[1]。

第三，减少住院天数，可降低相关的医疗费用，成就更好的社会效益[2]。另一方面，在抗生素疗程完成前让患者出院也可能存在一些弊端：一个缺点是在家中进行的抗生素治疗可能不像在院内那么严格按计划执行，可能导致治疗失败；另一个挑战是，与在医院相比，患者出院后的病情评估次数会减少，这可能会延误诊断，导致病情恶化[3]。当然，所有患者都能在家完成治疗将是一种理想的方式，但这并不现实。现实需回答的关键问题是"在哪些情况下，院外治疗是安全的？"。为了回答这一问题，医疗界酝酿了几种不同的标准。下文将这些标准分为静脉治疗（本章中称为"门诊肠外抗生素治疗"）和口服治疗（本章中称为"部分口服心内膜炎治疗"）进行阐述。

门诊肠外抗生素治疗（OPAT）

早在 1980 年左右，OPAT 已用于治疗病情稳定的 IE 或骨、皮肤和软组织感染[4-5]。20 世纪 90 年代，多项研究调查了链球菌 IE 的 OPAT，为简化和减少单纯链球菌 IE 的治疗提供了证据[6-8]。1997 年，Graninger 等在门诊每周使用 3 次替考拉宁治疗 10 例葡萄球菌 IE 患者，20% 的病例需再次入院治疗[9]。这些早期的研究与 OPAT 试验的临床经验相结合，促成 Andrews 和 Reyn 制定了一套全面的标准来指导 IE 患者的 OPAT[10]。由于 OPAT 治疗和早期出院可能会带来一些致命的问题，故他们制定标准时，为安全考虑，采用了相对选择性的策略（表 13.1）。Andrews 和 Reyn 认为治疗的最初 2 周最为关键，IE 并发症最多出现在这个阶段，因此首选住院治疗。在接下来的几周（第 2 ~ 4 周或第 2 ~ 6 周），他们建议 OPAT 可用于病情稳定的患者，即在转为 OPAT 时无发热、血培养结果阴性、心电图结果稳定。然而，根据他们提出的排除标准，很大一部分患者并不建议使用 OPAT。排除标准包括：主动脉瓣疾病、人工瓣膜疾病、急性 IE（发病时间 <2 周）、IE 并发症（心力衰竭、脓肿、传导异常、精神状态改变）或由金黄色葡萄球菌、肺炎链球菌、流感嗜血杆菌、脑膜炎奈瑟菌、淋病奈瑟菌、B 族链球菌、革兰氏阴性菌或真菌引起的 IE[10]。从 2001 年至今，美国和欧洲的 IE 治疗指南仍然在强调这些严格的选择标准[11-12]。然而值得注意的是，美国和欧洲的指南都建议对该标准做出修改，不再将特定的细菌病因、急性 IE、主动脉瓣或人工瓣膜疾病作为 OPAT 的排除标准[11-12]。

尽管提出了上述严格标准，但在随后的几年中，来自不同地区的病例系列还是纳入了大量人工瓣膜 IE、主动脉瓣 IE 和金黄色葡萄球菌 IE 患者接受了 OPAT，这也成为当时的一个显著特征[2,13-19]。2019 年，Pericàs 等人总结了这些发现，他们将 2001 年标准用于核实已发表的 OPAT 病例系列，发现不到一半的病例符合 2001 年标准[20]。在同一篇论文中，他们公布了一项多中心前瞻性队列研究的结果，其中包括 429 例接受 OPAT 治疗的患者，成功地将平均住院时间减少了 10 d[20]。该研究还发现，即便符合 2001 年标准，很多患者实际上还是接受了住院抗生素治疗，而非 OPAT，因此并不能以此来严格区分两组患者（接受住院抗生素治疗组

表 13.1　2001 年提出的感染性心内膜炎（IE）门诊肠外抗生素治疗（OPAT）标准

治疗阶段	指导方针
关键阶段 （0~14 d）	大多数 IE 并发症发生于这一阶段，及时诊断对于获得良好的结果非常重要 首选治疗方法：住院 2 周抗生素治疗 例外情况：满足以下 3 个条件的可在 1 周后考虑 OPAT 　1）草绿色链球菌 IE 　2）病情稳定，无发热，血培养阴性，出院时心电图稳定 　3）无 IE 并发症，不属于高危人群（见下文 a 和 b）
延续阶段 （第 2~4 周 或第 2~6 周）	大多数未出现 IE 并发症的患者在剩余的治疗期间可能会保持稳定，但肠外抗生素治疗的副作用仍可能发生 首选治疗方法：大多数病情稳定的患者都可以考虑 OPAT（见上文第 2 点） 例外情况：合并以下任何一项的患者一般不应使用 OPAT 　a）发生 IE 并发症，如充血性心力衰竭、传导异常、精神状态改变或 TEE 显示瓣周脓肿 　b）属高危亚组，如急性 IE、主动脉瓣 IE、人工瓣膜 IE 或由金黄色葡萄球菌或肺炎链球菌、流感嗜血杆菌、淋病奈瑟菌、B 族链球菌、革兰氏阴性菌和真菌等致病菌引起的 IE
OPAT 计划的 基本要素	向患者宣教 IE 的并发症，了解与医生或 IE 医护团队联系的指征和方式。患者和家属需可靠性强、依从性好，并住在医院附近。出院后的常规评估包括：OPAT 期间每 2 周一次门诊访视或由 IE 医护小组家访。对于再次发热或出现新症状的患者，IE 医护小组成员应在当天对其进行评估

改编自：M.M. Andrews, C.F. von Reyn. Patient selection criteria and management guidelines for outpatient parenteral antibiotic therapy for native valve infective endocarditis. Clin Infect Dis, 2001, 33（2）: 203–209.

有 23.3% 符合标准 vs. OPAT 组有 21.7% 符合标准，P=0.465）。根据以上分析，Pericàs 等认为，如果 IE 的病原体不是高度难治的，不存在发病后短时间难以消除的临床确诊、超声心动图发现或者术后出现的并发症，这类病例实施 OPAT 是可行的。为此，基于他们国家的指南要求[21]和他们自己的研究推荐，对 OPAT 的使用可采用相对宽松的纳入标准（表 13.2）[20]。与 2001 年的标准相比，他们的新标准做了几处修改。首先，对于大多数病情不复杂病例，最短住院时间从 14 d 缩短到 10 d 可以接受，症状的急缓（急性与慢性）不再作为决定因素。其次，2019 年的标准并没有排除导致 IE 的所有微生物，仅排除了需要静脉注射抗生素联合治疗的高度难治的微生物，这些微生物多存在多种药物耐药性，另外，潜在的抗生素毒性也需要在医院进行密切监测。再次，新标准并未排除主动脉瓣 IE 和人工瓣膜 IE，而是强调在改用 OPAT 前应进行经食管超声心动图（TEE）检查，以排除严重的主动脉瓣反流和人工瓣膜功能障碍，包括瓣周并发症[20]。

据估计，美国每年有超过 25 万人因各种感染性疾病接受 OPAT[22]。但迄今尚无 OPAT 与住院治疗 IE 比较性随机临床试验，不同的指南和标准是根据专家共识和有关 IE 并发症的观察数据制定的。虽然无法确定哪个标准最好，但临床的实际情况似乎更接近于较为宽松的 2019 年标准，而不是 2001 年标准。当然，选择

表 13.2　2019 年更新的感染性心内膜炎（IE）门诊肠外抗生素治疗（OPAT）标准

IE 类型	建　议	适应证	要　求
自体瓣膜	·快速转为 OPAT（入院/术后>10 d）	除 HDTTM[a] 外的任何病原菌引起的 IE，患者无严重临床并发症，患者接受或未接受心脏手术	72 h 内所有血培养均为阴性，无严重并发症，无抗凝问题，TEE 排除了严重的主动脉瓣反流和人工瓣膜功能障碍
	·延迟转为 OPAT（入院/术后>3 周）	患者起病时有严重并发症，患者非常虚弱，或接受心脏手术或其他治疗时存在严重共病	与上述标准相同，附加：无严重后遗症及临床并发症，无须频繁和（或）复杂的治疗
人工瓣膜	·快速转为 OPAT（入院>10 d）	由草绿色链球菌或牛链球菌或肠球菌引起的 IE，且患者未接受心脏手术	与自体瓣膜 IE 的快速转换相同
	·延迟转为 OPAT（入院/术后>3 周）	患者接受了心脏手术、非 HDTTM 感染且无严重并发症	与自体瓣膜 IE 的延迟转换相同
CIED	·快速转为 OPAT（装置取出/重新植入后>7 d）	无严重临床并发症且非 HDTTM 感染的病例，早期顺利拔除电极导线的病例（入院<1 周）	新装置在电生理团队调试下功能正常 无囊袋感染迹象，再植入后 72 h 内多次血培养阴性，TEE 正常
	·延迟转为 OPAT（装置取出/重新植入后>2 周）	伴有右侧 IE，赘生物>2 cm 的左侧 IE，有临床并发症，电极导线取出较晚，或取出过程较为复杂	与上述标准相同，附加：无严重后遗症及临床并发症，无须频繁和（或）复杂的治疗
排除 OPAT	肝硬化（Child B 或 C）、严重中枢神经系统栓塞（多发>3 处、大小>2 cm、出血性或有固定的神经功能缺损）的患者。存在未引流的巨大脾或肾脓肿、需要神经外科手术的椎体脓肿、瓣周并发症或其他严重病情需要手术治疗但存在手术禁忌证[b]。严重的术后并发症、HDTTM 感染和静脉吸毒者		

[a]HDTTM= 高度难治、需要静脉联合使用抗生素的微生物，这些联合使用的抗生素不能通过 OPAT 给药，或者由于其具有潜在毒性、安全浓度范围窄，需要严格监测血液或其他体液中的药物浓度（例如，耐甲氧西林金黄色葡萄球菌或耐万古霉素肠球菌，同时也对达托霉素和利奈唑胺等替代药物耐药；耐多种药物或广泛耐药的革兰氏阴性杆菌；高度耐青霉素的草绿色链球菌；念珠菌以外的真菌）。[b]在与患者和（或）亲属仔细讨论并达成一致意见后，可以将患者转至家中或其他门诊场所进行姑息治疗。CIED：心脏植入式电子设备；HDTTM：高度难治性微生物；TEE：经食管超声心动图。改编自：S.J.M.Perià, J.Llopis, V.González-Ramallo, et al. Outpatient parenteral antibiotic treatment for infective endocarditis: a prospective cohort study from the games cohort. Clin Infect Dis, 2019, 69 (10): 1690–1700.

OPAT 的患者会比必须在医院完成治疗的患者一般状况要好，因此，OPAT 组在观察性研究中的死亡率相对较低。但如果他们在医院内接受治疗，死亡率是否会更低，目前还无法知晓。在获得进一步的临床证据前，OPAT 成功的秘诀似乎是对国际指南（美国和欧洲）相对开放的解读，以及结合 IE 团队的丰富临床经验。

除了选择合适的患者进行 OPAT 外，执行 OPAT 所需的后勤保障也至关重要，包括患者的宣教和组织良好的多学科团队。应全面告知患者 IE 的并发症和治疗失败可能出现的症状，以及如何在事发当天联系 IE 小组及时进行评估[10]。OPAT 管理应由熟练的 IE 护士执行，检查是否出现导管感染等并发症。患者每周应至少 2 次门诊访视或接受主治医生的探访，评估病情的进展情况，并排除新发 IE 并发症的征兆[10,20]。

部分口服心内膜炎治疗（POET）

POET 的定义是在心内膜炎治疗后期改用口服抗生素治疗。原则上，口服治疗可以在医院进行，但 POET 的目标是使患者尽早出院，以获得前文 OPAT 中提到的优势。另外，与 OPAT 相比，POET 的优势在于无须医务人员协助静脉给药，减少了静脉置管的留置时间，从而可降低发生导管相关感染的风险[23]。

二十世纪八九十年代，多项研究在治疗链球菌和葡萄球菌 IE 过程中阐述了 POET 治疗的概念[6,24-29]。Parker 等治愈了 35 例由葡萄球菌引起的 IE，平均静脉给药时间 16 d，随后口服抗生素，平均用药时间 26 d，主要使用的药物是双氯西林或苯唑西林[24]。有两项规模较小的观察性研究（分别纳入了 15 名和 11 名患者）在治疗单纯左侧自体瓣膜链球菌 IE 时，分别采用了单纯口服氨苄西林 6 周和联合肌内注射链霉素 2 周的疗法，但效果仍值得商榷[25-26]。然而，直接口服治疗可能存在很大风险。Stamboulian 等人在一项链球菌 IE 随机临床试验中，比较了 15 例患者单纯接受 4 周静脉滴注头孢曲松与 15 例接受 2 周静脉滴注头孢曲松后再口服 2 周氨苄西林的疗效，所有患者均治愈[6]。Dworkin 等人通过静脉注射环丙沙星 1 周，然后口服环丙沙星 3 周，再联合口服利福平 4 周，治愈了 13 名静脉吸毒右侧自体瓣膜金黄色葡萄球菌 IE 中的 10 名[27]。1996 年，Heldman 等也做了上述类似的研究，成功完成了一项针对静脉吸毒右侧金黄色葡萄球菌 IE 的随机临床试验：对 19 名患者进行了为期 4 周的环丙沙星和利福平口服治疗，对 25 名患者进行了为期 4 周的氧氟沙星或万古霉素联合庆大霉素静脉注射治疗，两种方法的疗效相同[29]。10 余年后，Demonchy 等人将 19 名患者（12 名葡萄球菌 IE 和 7 名链球菌 IE）在静脉注射抗生素平均 18 d 后转为口服治疗，结果发现无一人死亡[30]。迄今为止最大的一项回顾性研究发表于 2016 年，共纳入 426 例 IE 患者，这些患者具有不同的细菌学特征（主要是链球菌、葡萄球菌和肠球菌）和所有类型的 IE（右侧和左侧 + 自体瓣膜和人工瓣膜 + 心脏植入式电子设备）[31]。在整个回顾性队列中，有 214 名患者在接受平均 21d 的静脉注射抗生素治疗后转为口服治疗，在多变量分析中，未发现静脉治疗转口服治疗是不良预后的独立风险因素。

2018 年，Iversen 等发表了一项期待已久的前瞻性随机多中心 POET 研究的结果。试验包括 400 例左侧 IE 病例，整个疗程接受常规静脉治疗或在疗程中转为口服治疗[32]。病原体有链球菌、肠球菌、金黄色葡萄球菌或凝固酶阴性葡萄球菌，所有患者对静脉注射抗生素治疗（至少 10 d 和心脏手术后至少 7d）反应良好，经初始治疗病情稳定（表 13.3）。该研究旨在证明 POET 在全因死亡、计划外心脏手术、出现症状的栓塞事件和菌血症复发（<6 个月）等主要复合终点中的非劣效性。据预测，10%（5%~13%）的患者会出现主要复合终点事件，效能计算以 10 个百分点的绝对风险差异（100% 的相对风险差异）作为临床相关差异的非劣效界值。静脉注射组有 12.1% 的患者出现复合终点，口服组有 9.0% 的患者出现复合终点，组间绝对差异为 3.1 个百分点（95% CI = −3.4~9.6，P=0.40），达到了非劣效性目标。因此，口服治疗的结果令人满意，且风险可控：在支持采用静脉注射的假设下，口服组出现复合终点事件的比例与静脉组差异仅为 3.4 个百分点（相对风险差异约为 30%）。在安全性方面，两组的抗生素不良反应相似（6% vs.5%）。POET 试验的一大优势在于其严格的纳入标准，因此可作为在 IE 治疗过程中患者转为口服治疗的临床指南（表 13.3）。

在确定患者符合改用口服治疗的标准后，下一步就是选择口服抗生素方案以完成治疗。根据 POET 试验的纳入标准，在改为口服抗生素治疗前，患者必须接受至少 10 d 的静脉抗生素治疗。而在选择使用哪种抗生素方案之前，还要扩大药敏试验的药物范围，以确保口服治疗的疗效。表 13.4 根据 POET 试验的实际使用

表 13.3　部分口服心内膜炎治疗（POET）的纳入标准

标　准	特别说明
由链球菌、金黄色葡萄球菌、粪肠球菌或凝固酶阴性葡萄球菌引起的成人左侧心内膜炎	≥ 18 岁
适当的初始肠外抗生素治疗	静脉抗生素治疗 ≥ 10 d（适当） 心脏瓣膜手术后静脉抗生素治疗 ≥ 7 d
对治疗反应良好	体温 <38.0℃至少 2 d C- 反应蛋白 <峰值水平的 25% 或 <20 mg/L 白细胞 <15 × 10^9/L
经胸和经食管超声心动图	在改用口服抗生素后 48 h 内进行 没有需要手术的脓肿或瓣膜异常等征象
不存在使口服治疗无效的因素	BMI<40 kg/m^2 没有引起吸收减少的腹部疾病 不存在依从性差的问题
没有其他需要静脉使用抗生素的感染	无其他需要长期静脉使用抗生素的指征
细菌药敏试验	细菌对两种不同类型的口服抗生素敏感[a]

[a] 建议的口服抗生素方案见表 13.4。BMI：体重指数。参考自：K. Iversen, N. Ihlemann, S.U. Gill, et al. Partial oral versus intravenous antibiotic treatment of endocarditis. N Engl J Med, 2019, 380 (5): 415–424.

表 13.4　POET 研究中用于部分口服心内膜炎治疗（POET）的口服抗生素组合

青霉素和甲氧西林敏感性金黄色葡萄球菌和 CoNS	甲氧西林敏感性金黄色葡萄球菌和 CoNS	耐甲氧西林 CoNS	粪肠球菌	链球菌（青霉素 MIC < 1 mg/L）	链球菌（青霉素 MIC > 1 mg/L）
阿莫西林 1g × 4[a] 利福平 600mg × 2	双氯西林 1g × 4 利福平 600mg × 2	利奈唑胺 600mg × 2 夫西地酸 750mg × 2	阿莫西林 1g × 4 莫西沙星 400mg × 1	阿莫西林 1g × 4 利福平 600mg × 2	利奈唑胺 600mg × 2 利福平 600mg × 2
阿莫西林 1g × 4 夫西地酸 750mg × 2	双氯西林 1g × 4 夫西地酸 750mg × 2	**利奈唑胺 600mg × 2 利福平 600mg × 2**	阿莫西林 1g × 4 利奈唑胺 600mg × 2	阿莫西林 1g × 4 莫西沙星 400mg × 1	莫西沙星 400mg × 1 利福平 600mg × 2
莫西沙星 400mg × 1 利福平 600mg × 2	莫西沙星 400mg × 1 利福平 600mg × 2		阿莫西林 1g × 4 利福平 600mg × 2	阿莫西林 1g × 4 利奈唑胺 600mg × 2	利奈唑胺 600mg × 2 莫西沙星 400mg × 1
利奈唑胺 600mg × 2 利福平 600mg × 2	利奈唑胺 600mg × 2 利福平 600mg × 2		利奈唑胺 600mg × 2 莫西沙星 400mg × 1	利奈唑胺 600mg × 2 利福平 600mg × 2	
利奈唑胺 600mg × 2 夫西地酸 750mg × 2	利奈唑胺 600mg × 2 夫西地酸 750mg × 2		利奈唑胺 600mg × 2 利福平 600mg × 2	利奈唑胺 600mg × 2 莫西沙星 400mg × 1	

[a] 在 POET 研究中最常用的疗法首先提及，并用粗体标出。CoNS：凝固酶阴性葡萄球菌；MIC：最小抑菌浓度。参考自：K. Iversen, N. Ihlemann, S.U. Gill, et al. Partial oral versus intravenous antibiotic treatment of endocarditis. N Engl J Med, 2019, 380 (5): 415–424.

情况列出了推荐的口服联合疗法。

在 POET 试验随机分配到口服治疗的病例中，80% 的患者在改用口服抗生素后平均 3 d（IQR=1~10 d）出院，院外完成疗程。出院前患者必须病情稳定，无心力衰竭或有临床影响的心律失常，无入院时的神经系统改变或栓塞引起的临床改变，也没有其他影响在家治疗的共病或功能障碍。此外，在改用口服治疗前，患者应进行 TEE 评估，以排除 IE 并发症。门诊患者每天测量自己的体温，若体温超过 38℃，则与科室联系。门诊患者每周 3 次到病区接受临床评估和药片清点以确保治疗依从性，并接受包括感染指标在内的血液检查。POET 研究队列的长期随访（中位数为 3.5 年）表明，改用口服方案与治疗延迟导致治疗失败无关[33]。

POET 标准作为指南在临床实施并无障碍，但对于患者的纳入标准一定程度上限制了 POET 结果的推广应用。只有最常见病因的 IE 病例才被纳入，其中，链球菌 IE 被纳入的频率是肠球菌和金黄色葡萄球菌 IE 的 2 倍[34-35]。没有纳入静脉吸毒患者，也没有纳入耐甲氧西林金黄色葡萄球菌 IE 病例。此外，196 例链球菌 IE 患者中只有 2 例（1%）感染了青霉素 MIC 值升高（>1 mg/L）的菌株。

临床随访

随着 IE 疗程的结束，患者进入治疗后阶段，这一阶段需要注意以下几点（表 13.5）。首先，指南建议这一阶段完善临床检查和经胸超声心动图（TTE）检查，以获得心功能、瓣膜形态和功能的新基线状态[11-12]。在完成疗程的第 1 年，建议对患者进行定期随访，反复进行临床检查和 TTE 检查。最新版指南没有明确规定就诊频率，但早前曾建议在完成治疗后的 1、3、6 和 12 个月后对患者进行密切随访和会诊[36-37]。然而这种大规模密集的随访是否有益尚无实据，因此新指南建议根据患者病情制定个体化的随访计划。两项新的观察性研究表明，密切随访对残留赘生物（>5 mm）或瓣膜功能不全的患者尤为重要，因为这些患者发生卒中和心力衰竭的风险会增加[38-39]。

其次，既往 IE 病史是 IE 新发的一个已知风险因素，因此对于这类病例可认为他们是 IE 风险增加人群[40]。对于这一状况，应对相关人员进行有关 IE 症状和体征的宣教，尤其应关注发热和感染出现时的一些征象[11-12]。当怀疑感染时，在

表 13.5 美国心脏协会（AHA）对感染性心内膜炎（IE）患者随访的建议

治疗及随访的阶段	建 议
治疗前或治疗结束时	·建立超声心动图新基线 ·为静脉吸毒患者提供戒毒治疗 ·对患者进行宣传教育，使其了解心内膜炎复发的征兆，以及在进行某些牙科、外科、侵入性手术时进行抗生素预防的必要性 ·如果尚未进行牙科评估和治疗，则应进行详尽的牙科评估和治疗 ·完成抗菌治疗后尽快清除静脉置管
短期随访	·出现任何发热疾病且未开始抗生素治疗前，至少从不同部位进行 3 组血液培养 ·体格检查以明确是否存在心力衰竭 ·评估当前及之前抗菌药物治疗的毒性
长期随访	·出现任何发热疾病且未开始抗生素治疗前，至少从不同部位进行 3 组血液培养 ·评估瓣膜和心室功能（超声心动图） ·注意口腔卫生，经常去牙科诊所就诊

改编自：L.M. Baddour, W.R. Wilson, A.S. Bayer, et al. Infective endocarditis in adults: diagnosis, antimicrobial therapy, and management of complications: a scientific statement for healthcare professionals from the American Heart Association. Circulation, 2015, 132(15): 1435–1486.

开始抗生素治疗之前，必须进行包括感染指标在内的血液检测和多次血液培养。尽量避免对未确定发热原因的病例进行经验性抗生素治疗，除非患者是脓毒症或其他需要立即开始抗生素治疗的情况[11]。

再次，如果患者有既往 IE 病史，同时伴有人工心脏瓣膜置换和发绀型先天性心脏病，即被认为是 IE 的高危人群。针对这一人群，在进行一些医疗操作时，应考虑使用抗生素预防治疗。如在处理牙龈或根周，或需穿破口腔黏膜的侵入性口腔科手术时，即应使用阿莫西林预防。但在非感染组织注射局部麻醉剂和简单治疗浅表龋齿时则无须预防性使用抗生素[12]。进行非牙科侵入性操作时，如呼吸道、泌尿生殖道或胃肠道，只有操作区域存在活动性感染时才建议进行预防。在这些操作中，预防性用药应涵盖进行操作的感染区域的典型细菌谱。对于中心静脉置管血液透析患者的预防，目前尚无统一意见，但这类患者属于 IE 高风险病例，需密切关注[41]。

最后，有必要找到原发感染病灶的位置，如果治疗前尚未明确，则应在治疗后继续查找。这包括对解没食子酸链球菌感染患者进行结肠镜检查，同理，粪肠球菌感染也应考虑结肠镜检查；如果是口腔链球菌感染，则应进行广泛的牙科检查，彻底清除口腔感染的活动性来源[42-43]。

微生物学随访

如上所述，IE 治疗后的关键是防止感染复发。IE 的微生物学治愈是指抗生素治疗结束后没有再次发生菌血症。随着时间推移，人们在评估 IE 复发时提出了不同的间隔时长[44]。最常用的描述是将复发定义为在上次治愈后的 6 个月内新出现的任何 IE，病原体与上次 IE 相同[12,45]。而再感染的定义是：感染了另一种病原体（在任何时间），或感染了同一种病原体但是在上次病愈 6 个月后再次发生的 IE。目前，多数 IE 病例都能通过抗生素治愈，必要时还可辅以手术治疗。复发和再感染率为 2%～6%，这取决于微生物和患者的特征[12,44,46-47]。复发的原因可能是首次发病时治疗时间不足、抗生素选择欠佳、微生物顽固难治或感染原发病灶问题未解决[12]。作为 IE 的第三大常见病因，粪肠球菌导致的复发占了很大比例，一项系统性综述也表明了这一点：粪肠球菌 IE 的平均复发率为 6%[48]。根据国际心内膜炎协作组织（ICE）的研究，Alagna 等发现，血液透析、静脉吸毒和 IE 既往史（在索引病例之前）是 IE 复发的独立风险因素[44]。Heiro 等也发现，血液透析、静脉吸毒和糖尿病与 IE 复发独立相关[49]。ESC 指南指出，人工瓣膜 IE 和 IE 瓣周受累与 IE 复发风险增加有关[12]。但目前证据并不支持这一观点——事实上，指南所参考的关于瓣周受累的研究[50]得出结论认为两者之间并无明显关联；而关于人工瓣膜的研究，也只是描述了在近一半的复发病例中发现患有人工瓣膜 IE，这些病例在平均 45 个月（$s=46$ 个月）后出现重复感染[51]。因此，在获得进一步证据之前，将 IE 复发的已知风险因素限制在 ICE 队列中发现的风险因素范围内是合理的[44]。

心脏外科随访

　　IE 的门诊管理应包括治疗后的心脏外科随访。这类患者一般包括两个不同的群体：①在 IE 病程中接受瓣膜置换手术者；② IE 经药物已治愈，但遗留瓣膜严重破坏者（通常是瓣膜关闭不全）。手术患者应根据植入的瓣膜类型（生物瓣 vs. 机械瓣）相关的常规指南进行随访。各地的指南可能有所不同。ESC 对生物瓣的建议是在术后 30 d 用超声心动图测量跨瓣压差，1 年后再测量一次，之后每年一次[52]。对于机械瓣，除非临床症状变化或出现瓣膜功能障碍相关表现，该指南并未规定其他情况下需要重复进行超声心动图检查[53]。在手术治疗患者出院前，应告知相关不良事件出现的征兆，如呼吸困难、晕厥和发热，这些不良事件可能由积液（心包积液、胸膜腔积液或因心力衰竭）、心律失常和感染引起。

　　早些时候，推迟 IE 手术并不少见，如果患者病情足够稳定，可以等待抗生素治疗结束后再手术。IE 的晚期手术率已逐渐降至 3%~8%[46-47,49]。对于有明显瓣膜反流的未手术患者，也应根据常规的瓣膜治疗临床指南进行随访[52-53]。对于无症状的重度主动脉瓣反流患者，至少每年进行一次 TTE（每 6~12 个月）；如果出现左心室功能恶化或左心室逐渐扩张的迹象，应缩短为每 3~6 个月进行一次 TTE，且患者的情况应在有心脏外科医生在内的多学科专家会议上进行讨论[52-53]。对于无症状的原发性重度二尖瓣反流且左心室功能正常的患者，建议每 6~12 个月进行一次 TTE；如果左心室开始扩张，则应增加检测频次[52-53]。对于中度主动脉瓣或二尖瓣反流患者，建议每 1~2 年进行一次 TTE 检查[52-53]。

研究前景

　　进行 POET 试验的同时[32]，在法国，还同期开展了 IE 病程最后阶段口服治疗的两项随机临床试验：RODEO1 试验研究了金黄色葡萄球菌 IE 改用左氧氟沙星和利福平口服联合疗法的情况（clinicaltrials.gov 识别码：NCT02701608），RODEO2 试验研究了药物敏感的链球菌和肠球菌 IE 改用口服阿莫西林单药疗法的情况（clinicaltrials.gov 识别码：NCT02701595）。每项研究旨在纳入 324 名患者，RODEO1 研究中的这一数字几乎是 POET 试验纳入的金黄色葡萄球菌 IE 病例数（$n=87$）的 4 倍[54]。

　　POET 试验表明，口服治疗在 IE 疗程的后半段是有效的，这自然而然产生了新的问题：这部分治疗是否可以缩短或完全省略？如果 IE 患者已经接受了 2 周的静脉抗生素治疗（术后至少 1 周），且各方面情况稳定，那么可能就不需要继续抗生素治疗。这一想法促使 POET 研究人员启动了一项名为"心内膜炎加速治疗（POET Ⅱ）"的新的随机对照试验[55]。该研究将比较标准治疗和加速治疗（即将标准治疗缩短到 2~3 周），目标是在 2019—2023 年间纳入 750 名链球菌、葡萄球菌和肠球菌 IE 病例（clinicaltrials.gov 识别码：NCT03851575）。而一项名为"革兰氏阳性球菌 IE 的短期抗生素治疗"的类似研究也相继在西班牙马德里筹划开展。

这项试验计划纳入约 300 名革兰氏阳性球菌 IE 病例，随机分组进行 2 周静脉治疗与标准的 4~6 周静脉治疗（clinicaltrials.gov 识别码：NCT04222257），以比较疗效。

对于 OPAT，尽管这一方案目前在临床应用已相当广泛，尤其是在美国，但至今仍缺乏一项随机临床试验对 OPAT 与传统住院治疗的效果进行比较。而西班牙一项名为"门诊口服抗菌药与肠外抗菌药治疗 IE 试验"的新研究旨在纳入 360 名链球菌、葡萄球菌和粪肠球菌 IE 病例，以比较在疗程最后阶段 OPAT 治疗和口服治疗的效果。患者的纳入和口服治疗方案均以 POET Ⅰ试验为基础。

未来研究的另一个有趣视角是针对革兰氏阳性菌的长效抗生素（延长半衰期）的应用。新一代脂糖肽类抗生素如达巴万星和奥利万星可以每周给药一次，使其成为门诊治疗的理想选择。到目前为止，这些药物还没有在 IE 中进行充分的检测，不能作为常规治疗使用。未来将这些抗生素用于门诊治疗的对照试验将会具有非常重要的临床意义。

至于后治疗阶段，有关 IE 出院后患者教育和康复的研究还不多。两项基于问卷调查的研究表明，在后治疗阶段，IE 患者认为自己生活得不够好，自述健康状况较差，并且经常再入院[56-57]。在这方面，我们正在等待名为"哥本哈根 IE 患者的心脏综合康复治疗"（clinicaltrials.gov 识别码：NCT01512615）的随机对照试验的结果（最后一次审查是 2021 年 3 月 1 日）。该研究于 2012—2019 年进行，共纳入 117 名 IE 患者，他们被随机分配为标准护理组或专业康复组，包括体育训练（每周 3 次，为期 12 周）和心理教育护理（为期 6 个月，共 5 次），旨在改善身体素质和心理健康。

总　结

在 IE 患者的门诊治疗中，在院外完成抗生素治疗对患者和社会而言收益都是最大的。但问题的关键在于哪些人群适合在门诊接受疗程中最后阶段的治疗。静脉和口服抗生素治疗都取得了良好的效果，尤其是具有里程碑意义的 POET 试验表明，在 IE 疗程的最后阶段，口服治疗的效果并不差。最新的 OPAT 标准相当宽松，为选择病情稳定的患者接受 OPAT 奠定了良好基础。不过，这些标准和国际指南的措辞相对宽泛，使用了"非常虚弱"和"严重并发症"等表述，因此需要一个经验丰富的 IE 团队来把控这些标准的实施。而 POET 标准则更为严格，更易于应用。POET 标准面临的挑战是，除了纳入如同随机临床试验病情相同的那类非常稳定的患者外，迄今为止还无法推广到其他患者群体。如果用于判定 IE 患者病情是否足够稳定以接受门诊治疗的标准在 OPAT 和 POET 之间是相同的，则更有意义。转为门诊治疗（无论是口服还是静脉注射）的关键点在于，应避免漏诊可能即将发生的脓肿或严重心功能不全等心内灾难性并发症。因此，本章的关键信息之一就是，在转为门诊治疗时，一定要按照 OPAT 和 POET 的建议进行 TEE 检查（图 13.1）。

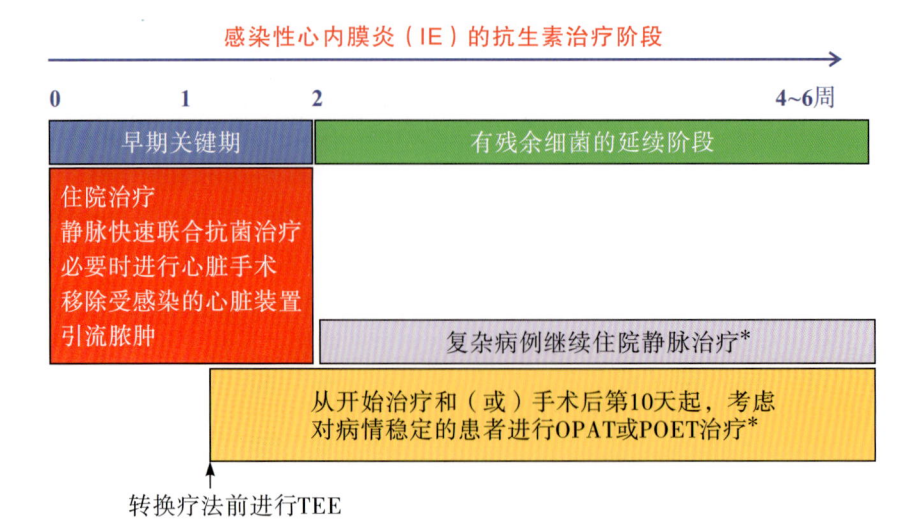

```
感染性心内膜炎（IE）的抗生素治疗阶段
                                                                →
 0        1        2                              4~6周
          早期关键期        有残余细菌的延续阶段

          住院治疗
          静脉快速联合抗菌治疗
          必要时进行心脏手术              复杂病例继续住院静脉治疗*
          移除受感染的心脏装置
          引流脓肿
                          从开始治疗和（或）手术后第10天起，考虑
                          对病情稳定的患者进行OPAT或POET治疗*
     ↑
  转换疗法前进行TEE
```

图 13.1 IE 的抗生素治疗阶段与 OPAT 和 POET 治疗的关系。OPAT：门诊肠外抗生素治疗；POET：部分口服心内膜炎治疗；TEE：经食管超声心动图。* 转用 OPAT 或 POET 治疗的标准见表 13.1 至表 13.3

在后治疗阶段，患者教育是最重要的。应让患者了解有关反复感染和心力衰竭的体征和症状，并指导预防性抗生素的应用。通过以上全面的信息教育，使患者自己成为早期识别复发和其他不良事件的最重要一环。为支持患者教育方面的工作，后治疗阶段的另一个核心是在第 1 年内通过临床检查和超声心动图进行密切随访。应特别关注 IE 复发高风险群体，如滥用药物者和血液透析患者。

对于 IE 病程中接受瓣膜置换手术的患者应在术后接受新瓣膜的首次超声心动图检查以进行评估，而后根据人工瓣膜的标准指南对患者进行随访。而 IE 病程中未接受手术、仍有严重瓣膜功能不全的心内膜炎患者，则应根据瓣膜疾病的标准指南进行随访。

如前所述，下一步是巩固门诊治疗中的积极成果，并研究在治疗效果最好、病情最稳定的患者中能否缩短治疗时间。

附 录

Members of the Hospital Clínic Endocarditis Team Investigators: Jose M. Miró, Marta Hernández-Meneses, Juan Ambrosioni, Anders Dahl, Alberto Cozar, Adrian Téllez, D. García-Parés, Juan M. Pericàs, Asuncion Moreno (Infectious Diseases Service); Cristina García de la Mària, Maria Alexandra Cañas, Javier García-González (Experimental Endocarditis Laboratory); Manel Almela, Climent Casals, Francisco-Javier Morales, Francesc Marco, Jordi Vila (Microbiology Service); Eduard Quintana, Elena Sandoval, Carlos Falces, Daniel Pereda, Manel Azqueta, Merçe Roque, Marta Sitges, Barbara Vidal, Rut Andrea, José L. Pomar, Manuel Castella, José M. Tolosana, José Ortiz (Cardiovascular Institute); Irene Rovira (Anesthesiology Department); Andrés Perissinotti, David Fuster (Nuclear Medicine Service); Jose Ramírez (Pathology Department); Mercè Brunet (Toxicology Service); Dolors Soy (Pharmacy Service); Pedro Castro (Intensive Care Unit) and Jaume Llopis (Genetics and Biostatistics Department, Faculty of Biology, University of Barcelona).

资助及致谢

JMM received a personal 80:20 research grant from Institut d'Investigacions Biomèdiques August Pi i Sunyer (IDIBAPS), Barcelona, Spain, during 2017—2019. AD received postdoctoral grants for his stay at the Hospital Clinic of Barcelona from the Lundbeck Foundation and the European Society of Cardiology.

Financial disclosures: JMM has received consulting honoraria and/or research grants from Angelini, Contrafect, Cubist, Genentech, Gilead Sciences, Jansen, Lysovant; Medtronic, MSD, Novartis, Pfizer, and ViiV Healthcare, outside the submitted work. Other authors, no conflicts.

参考文献

[1] Umscheid CA, Mitchell MD, Doshi JA, et al. Estimating the proportion of healthcare-associated infections that are reasonably preventable and the related mortality and costs. Infect Control Hosp Epidemiol, 2011, 32(2): 101-114.

[2] Lacroix A, Revest M, Patrat-Delon S, et al. Outpatient parenteral antimicrobial therapy for infective endocarditis: a cost-effective strategy. Med Maladies Infect, 2014, 44(7): 327-330.

[3] Dahl A, Hansen TF, Bruun NE. Staphylococcus aureus endocarditis with fast development of aortic root abscess despite relevant antibiotics. Heart Lung, 2013, 42(1): 72-73.

[4] Kind AC, Williams DN, Persons G, et al. Intravenous antibiotic therapy at home. Arch Intern Med, 1979, 139(4): 413-415.

[5] Rehm SJ, Weinstein AJ. Home intravenous antibiotic therapy: a team approach. Ann Intern Med, 1983, 99(3): 388-392.

[6] Stamboulian D, Bonvehi P, Arevalo C, et al. Antibiotic management of outpatients with endocarditis due to penicillin-susceptible streptococci. Rev Infect Dis, 1991, 13(Suppl. 2): S160-S163.

[7] Francioli P, Etienne J, Hoigné R, et al. Treatment of streptococcal endocarditis with a single daily dose of ceftriaxone sodium for 4 weeks. Efficacy and outpatient treatment feasibility. J Am Med Assoc, 1992, 267(2): 264-267.

[8] Sexton DJ, Tenenbaum MJ, Wilson WR, et al. Ceftriaxone once daily for four weeks compared with ceftriaxone plus gentamicin once daily for two weeks for treatment of endocarditis due to penicillin-susceptible streptococci. Endocarditis Treatment Consortium Group. Clin Infect Dis, 1998, 27(6): 1470-1474.

[9] Graninger W, Presterl E, Wenisch C, et al. Management of serious staphylococcal infections in the outpatient setting. Drugs, 1997, 54(Suppl. 6): 21-28.

[10] Andrews MM, von Reyn CF. Patient selection criteria and management guidelines for outpatient parenteral antibiotic therapy for native valve infective endocarditis. Clin Infect Dis, 2001, 33(2): 203-209.

[11] Baddour LM, Wilson WR, Bayer AS, et al. Infective endocarditis in adults: diagnosis, antimicrobial therapy, and management of complications: a scientific statement for healthcare professionals from the American heart association. Circulation, 2015, 132(15): 1435-1486.

[12] Habib G, Lancellotti P, Antunes MJ, et al. 2015 ESC guidelines for the management of infective endocarditis: the task force for the management of infective endocarditis of the European society of cardiology (ESC). Endorsed by: European association for cardio-thoracic surgery (EACTS), the European association of nuclear medicine (EANM). Eur Heart J, 2015, 36(44): 3075-3128.

[13] McMahon JH, O'keeffe JM, Victorian HITH Outcomes Study Group, et al. Is hospital-in-the-home (HITH) treatment of bacterial endocarditis safe and effective? Scand J Infect Dis, 2008, 40(1): 40-43.

[14] Larioza J, Heung L, Girard A, et al. Management of infective endocarditis in outpatients: clinical experience with outpatient parenteral antibiotic therapy. South Med J, 2009, 102(6): 575-579.

[15] Cervera C, del Río A, García L, et al. Efficacy and safety of outpatient parenteral antibiotic therapy for infective endocarditis: a ten-year prospective study. Enferm Infecc Microbiol Clín, 2011, 29(8): 587-592.

[16] Partridge DG, O'Brien E, Chapman ALN. Outpatient parenteral antibiotic therapy for infective endocarditis: a review of 4 years' experience at a UK centre. Postgrad Med, 2012, 88(1041): 377–381.

[17] Duncan CJA, Barr DA, Ho A, et al. Risk factors for failure of outpatient parenteral antibiotic therapy (OPAT) in infective endocarditis. J Antimicrob Chemother, 2013, 68(7): 1650–1654.

[18] Htin AKF, Friedman ND, Hughes A, et al. Outpatient parenteral antimicrobial therapy is safe and effective for the treatment of infective endocarditis: a retrospective cohort study. Intern Med J, 2013, 43(6): 700–705.

[19] Goenaga MA, Kortajarena X, Ibarguren O, et al. Outpatient parenteral antimicrobial therapy (OPAT) for infectious endocarditis in Spain. Int J Antimicrob Agents, 2014, 44(1): 89–90.

[20] Pericà SJM, Llopis J, González-Ramallo V, et al. Outpatient parenteral antibiotic treatment for infective endocarditis: a prospective cohort study from the games cohort. Clin Infect Dis, 2019, 69(10): 1690–1700.

[21] López Cortés LE, Mujal Martínez A, Fernández Martínez de Mandojana M, et al. Executive summary of outpatient parenteral antimicrobial therapy: guidelines of the Spanish society of clinical microbiology and infectious diseases and the Spanish domiciliary hospitalisation society. Enferm Infecc Microbiol Clín, 2019, 37(6): 405–409.

[22] Kobayashi T, Ando T, Streit J, et al. Current evidence on oral antibiotics for infective endocarditis: a narrative review. Cardiol Ther, 2019, 8(2): 167–177.

[23] Iversen K, Høst N, Bruun NE, et al. Partial oral treatment of endocarditis. Am Heart J, 2013, 165(2): 116–122.

[24] Parker RH, Fossieck BE. Intravenous followed by oral antimicrobial therapy for staphylococcal endocarditis. Ann Intern Med, 1980, 93(6): 832–834.

[25] Pinchas A, Lessing J, Siegman-Igra Y, et al. Oral treatment of bacterial endocarditis. Isr J Med Sci, 1983, 19(7): 646–648.

[26] Chetty S, Mitha AS. High-dose oral amoxycillin in the treatment of infective endocarditis. S Afr Med J, 1988, 73(12): 709–710.

[27] Dworkin RJ, Lee BL, Sande MA, et al. Treatment of right-sided Staphylococcus aureus endocarditis in intravenous drug users with ciprofloxacin and rifampicin. Lancet, 1989, 2(8671): 1071–1073.

[28] Chayakul P, Yipintsoi T. Intravenous followed by oral antimicrobial therapy for staphylococcal endocarditis. J Med Assoc Thai, 1993, 76(10): 559–563.

[29] Heldman AW, Hartert TV, Ray SC, et al. Oral antibiotic treatment of right-sided staphylococcal endocarditis in injection drug users: prospective randomized comparison with parenteral therapy. Am J Med, 1996, 101(1): 68–76.

[30] Demonchy E, Dellamonica P, Roger PM, et al. Audit of antibiotic therapy used in 66 cases of endocarditis. Med Maladies Infect, 2011, 41(11): 602–607.

[31] Mzabi A, Kernéis S, Richaud C, et al. Switch to oral antibiotics in the treatment of infective endocarditis is not associated with increased risk of mortality in non-severely ill patients. Clin Microbiol Infect, 2016, 22(7): 607–612.

[32] Iversen K, Ihlemann N, Gill SU, et al. Partial oral versus intravenous antibiotic treatment of endocarditis. N Engl J Med, 2019, 31; 380(5): 415–424.

[33] Bundgaard H, Ihlemann N, Gill SU, et al. Long-term outcomes of partial oral treatment of endocarditis. N Engl J Med, 2019, 04; 380(14): 1373–1374.

[34] Østergaard L, Bruun NE, Voldstedlund M, et al. Prevalence of infective endocarditis in patients with positive blood cultures: a Danish nationwide study. Eur Heart J, 2019; 40(39): 3237–3244.

[35] Dahl A, Iversen K, Tonder N, et al. Prevalence of infective endocarditis in Enterococcus faecalis bacteremia. J Am Coll Cardiol, 2019, 74(2): 193–201.

[36] Botelho-Nevers E, Thuny F, Casalta JP, et al. Dramatic reduction in infective endocarditis-related mortality with a management-based approach. Arch Intern Med, 2009, 169(14): 1290–1298.

[37] Habib G, Hoen B, Tornos P, et al. Guidelines on the prevention, diagnosis, and treatment of infective endocarditis (new version 2009): the task force on the prevention, diagnosis, and treatment of infective endocarditis of the European society of cardiology (ESC). Endorsed by the European society of clinical microbiology and infectious diseases (ESCMID) and the international society of chemotherapy (ISC) for infection and cancer. Eur Heart J, 2009, 30(19): 2369-2413.

[38] Østergaard L, Dahl A, Fosbøl E, et al. Residual vegetation after treatment for left-sided infective endocarditis and subsequent risk of stroke and recurrence of endocarditis. Int J Cardiol, 2019, 293: 67-72.

[39] Østergaard L, Dahl A, Bruun NE, et al. Valve regurgitation inpatients surviving endocarditis and the subsequent risk of heart failure. Heart, 2020, 106(13): 1015-1022.

[40] Østergaard L, Valeur N, Ihlemann N, et al. Incidence of infective endocarditis among patients considered at high risk. Eur Heart J, 2018, 39(7): 623-629.

[41] Chaudry MS, Carlson N, Gislason GH, et al. Risk of infective endocarditis inpatients with end stage renal disease. Clin J Am Soc Nephrol, 2017, 12(11): 1814-1822.

[42] Pericàs JM, Corredoira J, Moreno A, et al. Relationship between Enterococcus faecalis infective endocarditis and colorectal neoplasm: preliminary results from a cohort of 154 patients. Rev Esp Cardiol, 2017, 70(6): 451-458.

[43] Lockhart PB, Brennan MT, Thornhill M, et al. Poor oral hygiene as a risk factor for infective endocarditis-related bacteremia. J Am Dent Assoc, 2009, 140(10): 1238-1244.

[44] Alagna L, Park LP, Nicholson BP, et al. Repeat endocarditis: analysis of risk factors based on the international collaboration on endocarditis—prospective cohort study. Clin Microbiol Infect, 2014, 20(6): 566-575.

[45] Chu VH, Sexton DJ, Cabell CH, et al. Repeat infective endocarditis: differentiating relapse from reinfection. Clin Infect Dis, 2005, 41(3): 406-409.

[46] Martínez-Sellés M, Muñoz P, Estevez A, et al. Long-term outcome of infective endocarditis in non-intravenous drug users. Mayo Clin Proc, 2008, 83(11): 1213-1217.

[47] Fernández-Hidalgo N, Almirante B, Tornos P, et al. Immediate and long-term outcome of left-sided infective endocarditis. A 12-year prospective study from a contemporary cohort in a referral hospital. Clin Microbiol Infect, 2012, 18(12): E522-E5230.

[48] Dahl A, Bruun NE. Enterococcus faecalis infective endocarditis: focus on clinical aspects. Expert Rev Cardiovasc Ther, 2013, 11(9): 1247-1257.

[49] Heiro M, Helenius H, Hurme S, et al. Long-term outcome of infective endocarditis: a study on patients surviving over one year after the initial episode treated in a Finnish teaching hospital during 25 years. BMC Infect Dis, 2008, 8: 49.

[50] Fedoruk LM, Jamieson WRE, Ling H, et al. Predictors of recurrence and reoperation for prosthetic valve endocarditis after valve replacement surgery for native valve endocarditis. J Thorac Cardiovasc Surg, 2009, 137(2): 326-333.

[51] Heiro M, Helenius H, Mäkilä S, et al. Infective endocarditis in a Finnish teaching hospital: a study on 326 episodes treated during 1980—2004. Heart, 2006, 92(10): 1457-1462.

[52] Baumgartner H, Falk V, Bax JJ, et al. ESC/EACTS Guidelines for the management of valvular heart disease. Eur Heart J, 2017, 38(36): 2739-2791.

[53] Nishimura RA, Otto CM, Bonow RO, et al. AHA/ACC guideline for the management of patients with valvular heart disease: executive summary: a report of the American college of cardiology/American heart association task force on practice guidelines. Circulation, 2014, 129(23): 2440-2492.

[54] Lemaignen A, Bernard L, Tattevin P, et al. Oral switch versus standard intravenous antibiotic therapy in left-sided endocarditis due to susceptible staphylococci, streptococci or enterococci (RO-DEO): a protocol for two open-label randomised controlled trials. BMJ Open, 2020, 10(7): e033540.

[55] Østergaard L, Pries-Heje MM, Hasselbalch RB, et al. Accelerated treatment of endocarditis-The

POET II trial: rationale and design of a randomized controlled trial. Am Heart J, 2020, 227: 40–46.

[56] Rasmussen TB, Zwisler A-D, Moons P, et al. Insufficient living: experiences of recovery after infective endocarditis. J Cardiovasc Nurs, 2015, 30(3): E11–E19.

[57] Rasmussen TB, Zwisler A-D, Thygesen LC, et al. High readmission rates and mental distress after infective endocarditis—results from the national population-based CopenHeart IE survey. Int J Cardiol, 2017, 235: 133–140.

第 14 章

手术时机与手术指征

Makoto Mori, Andrea Amabile, Gabe Weininger, Arnar Geirsson
Division of Cardiac Surgery, Yale School of Medicine, New Haven, CT, United States

概 述

感染性心内膜炎（IE）的手术指征和时机复杂而微妙。决定一个患者是否需要及何时实施手术主要是从以下方面入手，包括：病变累及的是左心还是右心系统、病变对血流动力学的影响、栓塞并发症发生的风险，以及因控制感染源而需要进行侵入性治疗的可能性。最后一点涉及抗生素治疗的效果和感染病原体的类型，这些因素也决定了手术的指征和时机。其他需要考虑的特殊因素包括吸毒史、近期卒中史以及疾病是否需要实施高风险的重建手术（如 Commando 手术）。新技术的应用，如经皮血栓抽吸清除装置越来越多地用于右心系统赘生物的清除，虽然相关长期疗效的研究仍十分有限，也应纳入手术指征考虑范畴。其他如患者的基本临床状况、共病以及预期的近期和远期生存情况也将影响手术的决策。本章总结了各种情况下手术适应证的现有证据。

左心系统心内膜炎的手术指征和时机

总体而言，左心心内膜炎的手术适应证主要涉及 3 个方面：①解决血流动力学异常和心力衰竭；②控制感染源；③预防血栓栓塞的并发症。与右心心内膜炎相比，涉及二尖瓣或主动脉瓣的左心系统心内膜炎手术适应证更明确。鉴别右心和左心系统受累具有重要临床意义，因为两者的性质差别很大。例如，主动脉瓣和二尖瓣与左心室功能密切相关，任何一个瓣膜受损都会比右侧瓣膜病变的临床症状更明显，此外，左心心内膜炎发生全身血栓栓塞事件的风险比右侧高很多。区别自体瓣膜心内膜炎（NVE）还是人工瓣膜心内膜炎（PVE）关系到手术风险，PVE 的手术死亡风险更高[1]，而目前还没有针对 PVE 的临床指南。

目前对于最佳的手术时机并没有明确的定论，各个心脏学会的指南对"早期手术"或"急诊手术"的定义各不相同。2015 年欧洲心脏病学会（ESC）指南将择期手术定义为可在 2 周内对患者进行的手术，将限期手术定义为诊断后需在几天内进行的手术，"急诊手术"定义为需在 24 h 内进行的手术[2]。相比之下，2014 年美国心脏协会和美国心脏病学会（AHA/ACC）指南区分了心内膜炎应在一次住院期间治疗还是可在分次住院时治疗[3]。2012 年发表的一项对左心心内膜炎进行外科干预的随机对照试验中，将患者随机分组后以 48 h 作为区分早期和晚期手术的分界[4]。在这项试验中，76 名具有高栓塞风险的左心 NVE 患者被随机分配到 48 h 内或 48 h 后进行手术。6 个月后，早期手术组的死亡或栓塞综合事件发生率为 3%，晚期手术组为 28%（$P=0.02$）。因此，在手术具备可行性的条件下，早期手术可能是有益的。

血流动力学异常和心力衰竭

心内膜炎的并发症，例如严重的急性主动脉瓣或二尖瓣反流、梗阻，以及因内瘘造成分流导致的心源性休克和肺水肿是急诊手术的明确指征。这种因心脏结构性损伤而导致血流动力学障碍的严重病例，药物治疗是徒劳的，如果不接受手术治疗，预后极差。当血流动力学损害不那么严重时（即有心力衰竭症状但无休克），对该类患者可限期手术。根据 2015 年 ESC 指南[2]，以上两种情况都属于 I 类手术指征。

心力衰竭在心内膜炎中很常见，在住院病例中占比 40%~60%[5,6]。当临床出现心力衰竭症状或超声心动图发现血流动力学异常时，则表明该病例已有手术适应证[2,7]。与二尖瓣病变相比，主动脉瓣病变更常出现有症状的心力衰竭[8]。该类心力衰竭起病多为急性，与瓣叶破坏或穿孔、赘生物干扰瓣膜正常对合或腱索断裂有关。当心力衰竭需要外科干预时，感染状况（培养阴性）相对而言并不成为手术的重要依据，血流动力学损害的严重程度才是决定是否行限期或急诊手术的关键考量。需要强调的是，即使病情严重到出现心源性休克，但只要血流动力学损害与心内膜炎引起的瓣膜病变有关，即应进行手术治疗。这种严重的急性血流动力学损害是心内膜炎需要进行急诊手术的唯一指征[2]，而其他临床表现则可进行限期或择期手术。

无法控制的感染

使用抗生素后若感染仍未得到控制，为了控制感染源，手术常常是解决这一难题的手段。持续感染通常是由高耐药性和高致病性的病原微生物所致，而对持续感染的定义不尽相同，通常以抗生素治疗 7~10 d 后培养仍呈阳性为标准。心内感染源常常累及瓣周，而这往往需要手术进行清创。感染累及瓣周临床可表现为瘘管、脓肿或假性动脉瘤，这类感染的扩散可能非常迅速，对此，需要外科早期干预。由于传导系统位于该区域，而心律失常成为感染累及这一区域的常见临床表现。PVE 常累及瓣周，需要进行更复杂的心内结构重建，这也就造成了 PVE 手术相关的高死亡率和高并发症发生率[9]。

如果局部感染未得到控制，表现为脓肿、假性动脉瘤、瘘管或不断增大的赘生物，则需要紧急进行手术干预。必须注意的是，感染局部侵犯和组织破坏是一个动态过程，瘘管和根部脓肿可能会进一步造成对纤维支架和其他心内结构的严重破坏，导致灾难性的血流动力学受损[10]。因此，一旦临床出现这些表现都是紧急手术干预的指征，应在确诊后 2~3 d 进行手术。同样，耐药菌感染或单靠抗菌药物治疗难以控制的感染也是手术控制病源的指征，包括耐甲氧西林金黄色葡萄球菌（MRSA）、耐万古霉素肠球菌、革兰氏阴性菌感染，以及由葡萄球菌或非 HACEK 革兰氏阴性菌引起的 PVE[11-12]。

预防血栓栓塞并发症

血栓栓塞并发症很常见，且左心系统的血栓栓塞和右心的血栓栓塞临床注意事项也有所不同。与右心来源的脓毒性肺栓塞相比，左侧来源的全身性血栓栓塞往往带来更为严重的危害，包括卒中和终末器官梗死。需注意：相当一部分此类栓塞事件没有任何征兆，即没有临床表现，只有通过影像学检查才能发现。导致栓塞风险的因素包括：抗生素治疗开始后 2 周内、赘生物较大且活动幅度大。因此，手术指征需根据是否存在以上栓塞事件发生的风险因素而定。

赘生物大小与卒中风险之间似乎存在量效关系，通常以 > 10 mm 为界限。如果伴有瓣膜反流或狭窄，则更建议进行手术干预。在没有任何其他瓣膜异常，仅单独存在赘生物的情况下，建议将赘生物 > 15 mm 作为接受手术清创的界限（Ⅱb 类建议）。有一种算法可根据临床特征计算出栓塞事件的发生风险[13]。

右心心内膜炎的手术指征和时机

右心 IE（RSIE）占所有 IE 病例的 5%~10%，其流行病学随阿片类药物在美国的滥用而出现变化[14]。大多数情况下，RSIE 多累及三尖瓣，常见于有静脉吸毒史[15]、心内装置（如 ICD 和起搏器）[16-17]和先天性心脏病的患者。在过去 20 年中，所有这些风险因素在美国都变得越来越普遍[14-15]，尽管如此，对于 RSIE 最佳治疗时机和手术方式的研究仍然有限。

外科治疗：指征与时机

多达 1/3 的 RSIE 患者需要接受手术治疗[18-19]，手术适应证的实施原则与左心心内膜炎相同，即治疗心力衰竭、控制感染和预防血栓栓塞事件。但 RSIE 的手术干预指征"阈值"可能高于左心心内膜炎，部分原因是右心系统的疾病更容易耐受，全身性栓塞的风险明显较低[2]。而出现以下情况时，则应考虑对三尖瓣心内膜炎进行手术治疗：

1. 尽管进行了充分的抗生素治疗，但菌血症持续阳性超过 7 d，或一些难以根除的微生物血培养呈现阳性（例如真菌或多重耐药微生物）；

2. 继发于重度三尖瓣反流的右心衰竭，利尿剂治疗无效；

3. 三尖瓣赘生物 > 20 mm，赘生物导致反复肺栓塞并持续存在，无论右心室功能如何。

在 Yanagawa 等人的一项 meta 分析中，RSIE 接受手术的最常见原因是出现脓毒性肺栓塞、合并左心 IE、右心衰竭和持续菌血症[20]，常用的 3 种手术方式包括三尖瓣切除、三尖瓣修复和三尖瓣置换[21]。其他的手术技术还包括三尖瓣瓣环成形、三尖瓣二瓣化、单纯赘生物切除。

早期干预可防止栓塞事件和瓣叶的进一步破坏[22]。然而，RSIE 的最佳干预时机仍不明确。一些学者建议根据以下几点评估手术的最佳时机[23]：从病因入手（对病情较重的心内装置相关 IE 或人工三尖瓣 IE 限期手术），从致病微生物入手（对病情较重的真菌、假单胞菌属、MRSA 感染限期手术），另外，合并左心系统 IE、抗生素治疗的效果差及存在抗生素相关肝肾毒性风险、存在相关并发症（如脓肿、瘘管）也是手术的时机。还有学者建议，如果同时存在房间隔缺损、感染的导管、电极导线或人工瓣膜，应考虑限期手术[22]。

推荐左心 IE 和右心 IE 手术治疗流程图，参见图 14.1 和图 14.2。

改变指征或时机的特殊因素

影响手术指征和手术时机的其他因素包括静脉吸毒相关的感染性心内膜炎（IVDU-IE）、近期是否存在卒中史、术者是否具备大范围重建手术的丰富经验。决定是否为 IVDU-IE 患者进行手术仍是一个有争议的问题，取决于外科医生的不同理念。近期是否发生卒中是一个备受争议的话题，相关证据十分有限，且来自小型观察性研究。目前主要的担心是对于该类患者行早期手术治疗是否会增加出

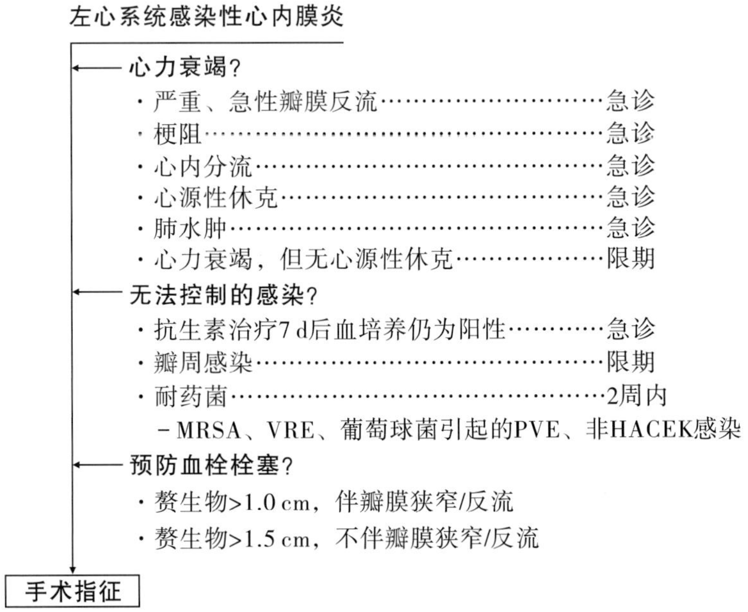

左心系统感染性心内膜炎
├── 心力衰竭？
│   · 严重、急性瓣膜反流……………………急诊
│   · 梗阻……………………………………急诊
│   · 心内分流………………………………急诊
│   · 心源性休克……………………………急诊
│   · 肺水肿…………………………………急诊
│   · 心力衰竭，但无心源性休克…………限期
├── 无法控制的感染？
│   · 抗生素治疗7 d后血培养仍为阳性………急诊
│   · 瓣周感染………………………………限期
│   · 耐药菌…………………………………2周内
│   – MRSA、VRE、葡萄球菌引起的PVE、非HACEK感染
├── 预防血栓栓塞？
│   · 赘生物>1.0 cm，伴瓣膜狭窄/反流
│   · 赘生物>1.5 cm，不伴瓣膜狭窄/反流
└── 手术指征

图 14.1　左心系统感染性心内膜炎的手术指征流程图。HACEK：副流感嗜血杆菌、嗜血杆菌、流感嗜血杆菌、凝聚杆菌、人心杆菌、侵蚀艾肯菌、金氏金氏菌和反硝化金氏金氏菌；MRSA：耐甲氧西林金黄色葡萄球菌；PVE：人工瓣膜心内膜炎；VRE：耐万古霉素肠球菌

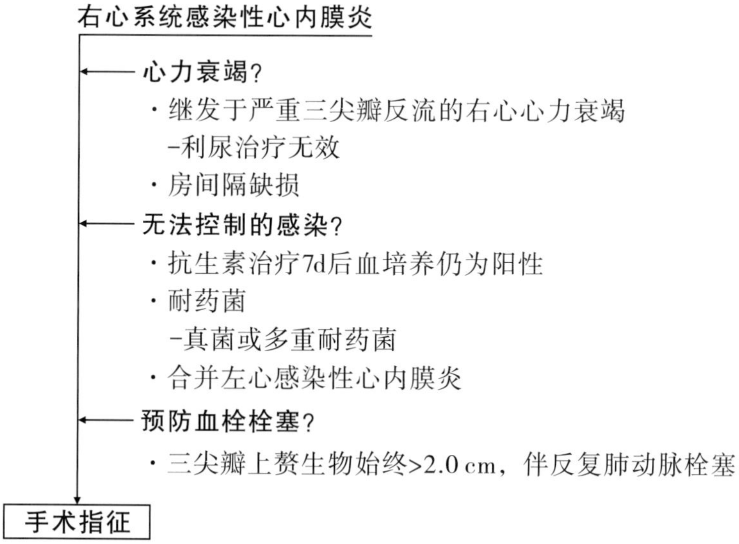

```
右心系统感染性心内膜炎
        │
        ├──── 心力衰竭?
        │       ·继发于严重三尖瓣反流的右心心力衰竭
        │         -利尿治疗无效
        │       ·房间隔缺损
        ├──── 无法控制的感染?
        │       ·抗生素治疗7d后血培养仍为阳性
        │       ·耐药菌
        │         -真菌或多重耐药菌
        │       ·合并左心感染性心内膜炎
        ├──── 预防血栓栓塞?
        │       ·三尖瓣上赘生物始终>2.0 cm,伴反复肺动脉栓塞
        ▼
   ┌─────────┐
   │ 手术指征 │
   └─────────┘
```

图 14.2 右心系统感染性心内膜炎的手术指征流程图

血转化的风险。外科医生的专业经验是一个重要的考虑因素,因为外科医生可能会认为该类患者属于禁止手术的高风险病情,尤其是当出现二尖瓣–主动脉瓣垂幕受累这样广泛性病变需要进行复杂的高风险手术(如 Commando 术)时。

静脉吸毒相关的感染性心内膜炎

欧洲指南建议,鉴于 IVDU-IE 患者的预后较差且再感染风险较高[26-27],应修改该类患者的手术适应证,因为即便集中资源进行治疗可能也是徒劳的[24-25]。与此相反,美国的指南倾向于采用外科手术治疗,同时也承认在该类患者中获得良好预后的难度[26]。

瓣膜置换术以及未来可能的再手术费用极其昂贵。美国医疗系统为该类患者再次手术的单次住院费用支付超过 5 万美元[28]。虽然 IVDU-IE 患者再次感染的风险更高,而且其接受复杂的再次手术死亡率也更高[29],但手术往往仍是控制感染源、恢复心脏功能或控制血栓栓塞并发症风险的唯一选择。对此类患者进行手术的决定是微妙的,主要取决于外科医生的理念。有些外科医生在决定是否手术时不考虑未来复发的可能性,他们认为"配给医疗"(仅给一些经过选择的患者实施手术)不是外科医生的职责,但也有一些外科医生只给那些积极配合、努力把复发风险降至最低的患者实施手术[30]。

影响 IVDU-IE 患者预后的最重要因素是他们是否会再次吸毒[31],因此最大限度地降低复吸风险对这些患者的侵入性治疗意义重大。戒毒治疗,包括丁丙诺啡、美沙酮和纳曲酮[32-33]等药物辅助治疗是非常有价值的。重要的是,完成全面的戒毒治疗和后续的护理计划是预测患者是否会再次吸毒的重要指标[34-35]。因此,我们建议,IVDU-IE 患者只要愿意接受全面的戒毒治疗,就应该与其他 IE 患者一样接受手术治疗。外科医生应发挥积极作用,强调完成戒毒的重要性。涉及心脏外科、感染科、成瘾医学和社会工作的多学科讨论是 IVDU-IE 患者所需的综合治疗策略的重要组成部分。成功的戒毒治疗应包括考虑使用丁丙诺啡或美沙酮进行药物辅助治疗，对患者进行持续监测，认识到导致复发的社会决定因素，以及社会支持、戒毒顾问的参与 [33,36-38]。

近期脑卒中和真菌性动脉瘤

IE 卒中多由赘生物脱落栓塞脑血管引起，关于卒中后心脏手术的时机尚有争议。随机对照研究对于评估这种情况下的手术时机具有安全挑战性，而从观察性研究中得出的推论也很有局限性，因为其推导出的手术时机往往源于不同患者的选择 [39-40]。判定手术时机的主要考虑因素取决于心脏手术的风险 – 获益：权衡尽早手术减少心内膜炎并发症的获益和体外循环所需的大量肝素可能会增加脑出血风险两者之间的关系 [41]。因此，指南建议：对于颅内出血的患者若病情稳定，可将手术时间推迟 1 个月 [42-43]；而对于有神经系统症状的缺血性卒中患者，则应将手术时间推迟 2 周 [2]。

如果只是影像学提示脑栓塞而无神经系统症状，则患者可以立即接受手术治疗 [44]。因此，对于无神经系统表现的患者，不需要常规进行 CT 或 MRI；但对于有卒中症状或体检结果提示为卒中的患者，则必须进行上述检查。然而，当 CT 发现蛛网膜下腔或脑实质内出血时，需要进行血管造影以排除真菌性动脉瘤。当脑卒中患者的血流动力学不稳定时需要急诊手术或限期手术，否则需要延迟手术，神经外科团队应密切参与围手术期护理。对于昏迷、有严重共病或神经功能恢复前景不佳的患者不建议手术 [2]。

由于缺乏数据，关于真菌性动脉瘤患者的手术时机仍存在争议。如果血流动力学条件允许，未破裂的真菌性动脉瘤患者应接受抗生素治疗和系列影像学检查，以监测其消退情况。如果是破裂、增大或有症状的真菌性动脉瘤，建议在心脏手术前进行神经外科开放性手术或腔内治疗 [28]。

复杂心脏损害重建手术的心脏中心经验

与心内膜炎手术复杂程度相关的手术风险范围很广，从无须修复瓣膜的赘生物简单清除到瓣膜置换，再到复杂的瓣间纤维垂幕的重建和多瓣膜置换。因此，在某些心脏中心，进行这类复杂、大范围病变的手术可能会被认为是一种禁忌，但在另一些中心，同一病例却可能得到手术治疗。Commando 手术和其他极其复杂的心内膜炎重建手术只在特定中心提供，这就要求医疗机构或相关医务人员在宣布此类复杂病理的患者不能手术之前，必须咨询相关经验丰富的中心以确保患者有机会接受手术治疗。这凸显了不同疾病状况下手术适应证的不确定性，正如 IE 的手术适应证一样，缺乏清晰的界定。然而，应该注意：即使在很优秀的心脏医疗中心，Commando 手术后的院内死亡率也高达 24%，其中 70% 以上的患者是因 PVE 而接受手术的 [22]。

可能改变手术适应证和时机的有争议性术式

三尖瓣切除术

瓣膜切除术即单纯切除感染瓣膜，不进行瓣膜置换。主要考虑是如果立即植入人工瓣膜，会显著增加 PVE 的发生风险。这只适用于右侧瓣膜，主要是三尖瓣。但在决定是否进行瓣膜切除术前，必须考虑这一术式可能导致严重的术后右心衰竭，尤其是有肺动脉高压的患者 [2]。由于这种手术很少实施，因此相关的长期随访数据很少 [45]。瓣膜切除术后，如果再感染的风险较低，可考虑更换瓣膜。这种方法可能适用于正在吸毒的患者，他们需要通过手术暂时控制感染，并在完成戒毒治疗后进行瓣膜置换。

经皮导管抽吸技术

AngioVac 导管（AngioDynamics，Latham，NY）是传统手术的介入替代方法，用于清除 RSIE 中的血管内物质。该导管由两个管道（静脉引流管和静脉回流管）组成，这两个管道连接到体外循环泵设备上，体外循环设备中有一个能过滤气泡和赘生物的过滤器。血液经吸入引流管进入体外循环，经过过滤后再回流到患者体内。小样本研究表明，这种方法在三尖瓣 IE 中具有一定的安全性和有效性 [46-50]。然而，这种方法无法直接观察和检查瓣周结构，治疗时疾病程度可能会被低估。由于不可能完全清除所有受感染的结构或材料，因此感染复发的长期风险仍然是一个严重的问题。目前还缺少相关数据证实这种方法的实用性。

参考文献

[1] Mori M, Bin Mahmood SU, Schranz AJ, et al. Risk of reoperative valve surgery for endocarditis associated with drug use. J Thorac Cardiovasc Surg, 2019. https://doi.org/10.1016/j.jtcvs.2019.06.055.

[2] Habib G, Lancellotti P, Antunes MJ, et al. 2015 ESC guidelines for the management of infective endocarditis: the Task Force for the Management of Infective Endocarditis of the European Society of Cardiology (ESC). Endorsed by: European Association for Cardio-Thoracic Surgery (EACTS), the European Association of Nuclear Medicine (EANM). Eur Heart J, 21, 2015; 36(44): 3075–3128. https://doi.org/10.1093/eurheartj/ehv319.

[3] Nishimura RA, Otto CM, Bonow RO, et al. 2014 AHA/ACC guideline for the management of patients with valvular heart disease: a report of the American College of Cardiology/American Heart Association Task Force on practice guidelines. Practice guideline review. J Thorac Cardiovasc Surg, 2014, 148(1): e1–e132. https://doi.org/10.1016/j.jtcvs.2014.05.014.

[4] Kang DH, Kim YJ, Kim SH, et al. Early surgery versus conventional treatment for infective endocarditis. N Engl J Med June, 28, 2012, 366(26): 2466–2473. https://doi.org/10.1056/NEJMoa1112843.

[5] Nadji G, Rusinaru D, Rémadi JP, et al. Heart failure in left-sided native valve infective endocarditis: characteristics, prognosis, and results of surgical treatment. Eur J Heart Fail, 2009, 11(7): 668–675.

https://doi.org/10.1093/eurjhf/hfp077.

[6] Olmos C, Vilacosta I, Fernández C, et al. Comparison of clinical features of left-sided infective endocarditis involving previously normal versus previously abnormal valves. Am J Cardiol, 2014, 114(2): 278-283. https://doi.org/10.1016/j.amjcard.2014.04.036.

[7] Habib G, Tribouilloy C, Thuny F, et al. Prosthetic valve endocarditis: who needs surgery? A multicentre study of 104 cases. Heart, 2005, 91(7): 954-959. https://doi.org/10.1136/hrt.2004.046177.

[8] Hasbun R, Vikram HR, Barakat LA, et al. Complicated left-sided native valve endocarditis in adults: risk classification for mortality. J Am Med Assoc, 2003, 289(15): 1933-1940. https://doi.org/10.1001/jama.289.15.1933.

[9] Baddour LM, Wilson WR, Bayer AS, et al. Infective endocarditis: diagnosis, antimicrobial therapy, and management of complications: a statement for healthcare professionals from the Committee on Rheumatic Fever, Endocarditis, and Kawasaki disease, Council on Cardiovascular disease in the Young, and the Councils on Clinical Cardiology, Stroke, and Cardiovascular Surgery and Anesthesia, American Heart Association: Endorsed by the Infectious Diseases Society of America. Circulation, 2005, 111(23): e394-e434. https://doi.org/10.1161/CIRCULATIONAHA.105.165564.

[10] Tingleff J, Egeblad H, Gøtzsche CO, et al. Perivalvular cavities in endocarditis: abscesses versus pseudoaneurysms? A transesophageal Doppler echocardiographic study in 118 patients with endocarditis. Am Heart J, 1995, 130(1): 93-100. https://doi.org/10.1016/0002-8703(95)90241-4.

[11] Ellis ME, Al-Abdely H, Sandridge A, et al. Fungal endocarditis: evidence in the world literature, 1965—1995. Clin Infect Dis, 2001, 32(1): 50-62. https://doi.org/10.1086/317550.

[12] Remadi JP, Habib G, Nadji G, et al. Predictors of death and impact of surgery in Staphylococcus aureus infective endocarditis. Ann Thorac Surg, 2007, 83(4): 1295-1302. https://doi.org/10.1016/j.athoracsur.2006.09.093.

[13] Hubert S, Thuny F, Resseguier N, et al. Prediction of symptomatic embolism in infective endocarditis: construction and validation of a risk calculator in a multicenter cohort. J Am Coll Cardiol, 2013, 62(15): 1384-1392. https://doi.org/10.1016/j.jacc.2013.07.029.

[14] Shmueli H, Thomas F, Flint N, et al. Right-sided infective endocarditis 2020: challenges and updates in diagnosis and treatment. J Am Heart Assoc, 2020, 9(15): e017293. https://doi.org/10.1161/JAHA.120.017293.

[15] Wurcel AG, Anderson JE, Chui KK, et al. Increasing infectious endocarditis admissions among young people who inject drugs. Open Forum Infect Dis, 2016, 3(3): ofw157. https://doi.org/10.1093/ofid/ofw157.

[16] Rennert-May E, Chew D, Lu S, et al. Epidemiology of cardiac implantable electronic device infections in the United States: a population-based cohort study. Heart Rhythm, 2020, 17(7): 1125-1131. https://doi.org/10.1016/j.hrthm.2020.02.012.

[17] Chrissoheris MP, Libertin C, Ali RG, et al. Endocarditis complicating central venous catheter bloodstream infections: a unique form of health care associated endocarditis. Clin Cardiol, 2009, 32(12): E48-E54. https://doi.org/10.1002/clc.20498.

[18] Gottardi R, Bialy J, Devyatko E, et al. Midterm follow-up of tricuspid valve reconstruction due to active infective endocarditis. Ann Thorac Surg, 2007, 84(6): 1943-1948. https://doi.org/10.1016/j.athoracsur.2007.04.116.

[19] Weber C, Gassa A, Eghbalzadeh K, et al. Characteristics and outcomes of patients with right-sided endocarditis undergoing cardiac surgery. Ann Cardiothorac Surg, 2019, 8(6): 645-653. https://doi.org/10.21037/acs.2019.08.02.

[20] Yanagawa B, Elbatarny M, Verma S, et al. Surgical management of tricuspid valve infective endocarditis: a systematic review and meta-analysis. Ann Thorac, 2018, 106(3): 708-714. https://doi.org/10.1016/j.athoracsur.2018.04.012. 09.

[21] Gaca JG, Sheng S, Daneshmand M, et al. Current outcomes for tricuspid valve infective endocarditis surgery in North America. Ann Thorac Surg, 2013, 96(4): 1374-1381. https://doi.org/10.1016/j.athoracsur. 2013.05.046.

[22] Hussain ST, Witten J, Shrestha NK, et al. Tricuspid valve endocarditis. Ann Cardiothorac Surg, 2017, 6(3): 255–261. https://doi.org/10.21037/acs.2017.03.09.

[23] Akinosoglou K, Apostolakis E, Koutsogiannis N, et al. Right-sided infective endocarditis: surgical management. Eur J Cardio Thorac Surg, 2012, 42(3): 470–479. https://doi.org/10.1093/ejcts/ezs084.

[24] Hull SC, Jadbabaie F. When is enough enough? The dilemma of valve replacement in a recidivist intravenous drug user. Ann Thorac Surg , 2014, 97(5): 1486–1487. https://doi.org/10.1016/j.athoracsur.2014.02.010.

[25] DiMaio JM, Salerno TA, Bernstein R, et al. Ethical obligation of surgeons to noncompliant patients: can a surgeon refuse to operate on an intravenous drug-abusing patient with recurrent aortic valve prosthesis infection? Ann Thorac Surg, 2009, 88(1): 1–8. https://doi.org/10.1016/j.athoracsur.2009.03.088.

[26] Wahba A, Nordhaug D. What are the long-term results of cardiac valve replacements in left sided endocarditis with a history of i.v. drug abuse? Interact Cardiovasc Thorac Surg, 2006, 5(5): 608–610. https://doi.org/10.1510/icvts.2006.135947.

[27] Østerdal OB, Salminen PR, Jordal S, et al. Cardiac surgery for infective endocarditis in patients with intravenous drug use. Interact Cardiovasc Thorac Surg, 2016, 22(5): 633–640. https://doi.org/10.1093/icvts/ivv397. 05.

[28] Fleischauer AT, Ruhl L, Rhea S, et al. Hospitalizations for endocarditis and associated health care costs among persons with diagnosed drug dependence - North Carolina, 2010—2015. MMWR Morb Mortal Wkly Rep, 2017, 66(22): 569–673. https://doi.org/10.15585/mmwr.mm6622a1.

[29] Mori M, Bin Mahmood SU, Schranz AJ, et al. Risk of reoperative valve surgery for endocarditis associated with drug use. J Thorac Cardiovasc Surg, 2020, 159(4): 1262–1268. https://doi.org/10.1016/j.jtcvs.2019.06.055. e2.

[30] Abby Goodnough. Injecting drugs can ruin a heart. How many second chances should a user get? The New York Times, 2018, 4(30).

[31] Nguemeni Tiako MJ, Mori M, Bin Mahmood SU, et al. Recidivism is the leading cause of death among intravenous drug users who underwent cardiac surgery for infective endocarditis. Semin Thorac Cardiovasc Surg, 2019, 31(1): 40–45. https://doi.org/10.1053/j.semtcvs.2018.07.016.

[32] Weinmeyer R. Needle exchange programs' status in US politics. AMA J Ethics, 2016, 18(3): 252–257. https://doi.org/10.1001/journalofethics.2016.18.3.hlaw1-1603.

[33] Suzuki J. Medication-assisted treatment for hospitalized patients with intravenous-drug-use related infective endocarditis. Am J Addict, 2016, 25(3): 191–194. https://doi.org/10.1111/ajad.12349.

[34] Miller NS, Flaherty JA. Effectiveness of coerced addiction treatment (alternative consequences): a review of the clinical research. J Subst Abuse Treat, 2000, 18(1): 9–16. https://doi.org/10.1016/s0740-5472(99)00073-2.

[35] Dugosh K, Abraham A, Seymour B, et al. A systematic review on the use of psychosocial interventions in conjunction with medications for the treatment of opioid addiction. J Addiction Med, 2016, 10(2): 93–103. https://doi.org/10.1097/ADM.0000000000000193.

[36] Gray ME, Rogawski McQuade ET, Scheld WM, et al. Rising rates of injection drug use associated infective endocarditis in Virginia with missed opportunities for addiction treatment referral: a retrospective cohort study. BMC Infect Dis, 2018, 18(1): 532. https://doi.org/10.1186/s12879-018-3408-y.

[37] Englander H, Weimer M, Solotaroff R, et al. Planning and designing the improving addiction care team (IMPACT) for hospitalized adults with substance use disorder. J Hosp Med, 2017, 12(5): 339–342. https://doi.org/10.12788/jhm.2736. 05.

[38] Priest KC, McCarty D. Role of the hospital in the 21st century opioid overdose epidemic: the addiction medicine consult service. J Addiction Med, 2019, 13(2): 104–112. https://doi.org/10.1097/ADM.0000000000000496.

[39] Anyanwu AC. The vagaries of patient selection in cardiovascular surgery. J Thorac Cardiovasc

[40] Sy RW, Bannon PG, Bayfield MS, et al. Survivor treatment selection bias and outcomes research: a case study of surgery in infective endocarditis. Circ Cardiovasc Qual Outcomes, 2009, 2(5): 469–474. https://doi.org/10.1161/CIRCOUTCOMES.109.857938.

[41] Barsic B, Dickerman S, Krajinovic V, et al. Influence of the timing of cardiac surgery on the outcome of patients with infective endocarditis and stroke. Clin Infect Dis, 2013, 56(2): 209–217. https://doi.org/10.1093/cid/cis878.

[42] Yoshioka D, Sakaguchi T, Yamauchi T, et al. Impact of early surgical treatment on postoperative neurologic outcome for active infective endocarditis complicated by cerebral infarction. Ann Thorac Surg, 2012, 94(2): 489–495. https://doi.org/10.1016/j.athoracsur.2012.04.027. Discussion 496.

[43] Eishi K, Kawazoe K, Kuriyama Y, et al. Surgical management of infective endocarditis associated with cerebral complications. Multi-center retrospective study in Japan. J Thorac Cardiovasc Surg, 1995, 110(6): 1745–1755. https://doi.org/10.1016/S0022-5223(95)70038-2.

[44] Thuny F, Beurtheret S, Mancini J, et al. The timing of surgery influences mortality and morbidity in adults with severe complicated infective endocarditis: a propensity analysis. Eur Heart J, 2011, 32(16): 2027–2033. https://doi.org/10.1093/eurheartj/ehp089.

[45] Protos AN, Trivedi JR, Whited WM, et al. Valvectomy versus replacement for the surgical treatment of tricuspid endocarditis. Ann Thorac Surg, 2018, 106(3): 664–669. https://doi.org/10.1016/j.athoracsur.2018.04.051.

[46] George B, Voelkel A, Kotter J, et al. A novel approach to percutaneous removal of large tricuspid valve vegetations using suction filtration and veno-venous bypass: a single center experience. Cathet Cardiovasc Interv, 2017, 90(6): 1009–1015. https://doi.org/10.1002/ccd.27097.

[47] Parmar YJ, Basman C, Kliger C, et al. Tricuspid valve vegetectomy using percutaneous aspiration catheter. Eur Heart J Cardiovasc Imaging, 2018, 19(6): 709. https://doi.org/10.1093/ehjci/jey017. 06.

[48] Patel N, Azemi T, Zaeem F, et al. Vacuum assisted vegetation extraction for the management of large lead vegetations. J Card Surg, 2013, 28(3): 321–324. https://doi.org/10.1111/jocs.12087.

[49] Jones BM, Wazni O, Rehm SJ, et al. Fighting fungus with a laser and a hose: management of a giant Candida albicans implantable cardioverter-defibrillator lead vegetation with simultaneous AngioVac aspiration and laser sheath lead extraction. Cathet Cardiovasc Interv, 2018, 91(2): 318–321. https://doi.org/10.1002/ccd.27153. 02.

[50] Schaerf RHM, Najibi S, Conrad J. Percutaneous vacuum-assisted thrombectomy device used for removal of large vegetations on infected pacemaker and defibrillator leads as an adjunct to lead extraction. J Atr Fibrillation, 2016, 9(3): 1455. https://doi.org/10.4022/jafib.1455.

第15章
右心感染性心内膜炎的外科治疗

Paul Brocklebank, Maxwell Kilcoyne, Arman Kilic

Division of Cardiothoracic Surgery, Medical University of South Carolina, Charleston, SC, United States

引 言

右心感染性心内膜炎（RSIE）最常发生于静脉吸毒（IVDU）者。随着阿片类药物的流行，静脉注射海洛因的人数不断增加，RSIE 手术的重要性也日益凸显[1-2]。与左心感染性心内膜炎（LSIE）相比，RSIE 的外科治疗受到的关注较少，但由于 IVDU 者较高的复吸率和心内膜炎复发率，RSIE 的外科治疗面临独特的挑战[1,3-4]。RSIE 的手术方法必须在两个矛盾的关键点中寻求平衡：①通过有效的瓣膜重建最大限度地提高疗效；②限制人工材料的植入以最大限度地降低 IE 复发的风险。本章中，我们将概述 RSIE 在流行病学、临床表现和诊断方面的特点，并确定手术干预的适应证。我们还将讨论治疗 RSIE 的主要手术技术以及术前、术中和术后的重要注意事项。

流行病学

RSIE 的发病率明显低于 LSIE，仅占 IE 病例总数的 5%~10%[1,5-6]。虽然 RSIE 可发生在右心心内膜的任何部位，但 90% 的病例发生在三尖瓣，其余 10% 发生在心脏植入电子设备（CIED）和肺动脉瓣[7]。RSIE 最常见的风险因素是 IVDU[1]。在一项研究中，34.5% 的 RSIE 患者有 IVDU 史[8]。此外，即使在 IVDU 者中，与 HIV 阴性的 IVDU 相比，HIV 阳性的 IVDU 者患 IE 的比值比（OR）为 2.31[6]。心脏起搏器、植入式心律转复除颤器（ICD）等 CIED 及中心静脉导管可作为细菌定植的原发灶，这也是导致 RSIE 的另一种机制[1]。未纠正的先天性右心畸形也会使患者易患 RSIE[9]。就致病微生物而言，金黄色葡萄球菌占 RSIE 的 60%~90%，但耐甲氧西林金黄色葡萄球菌（MRSA）、铜绿假单胞菌和多微生物混合感染 RSIE 的发病率都在上升[1,5-7]。在与人工瓣膜和 CIED 相关的 RSIE 中，凝固酶阴性葡萄球菌（CoNS）是主要的致病菌[1,7]。

与手术相关的流行病学关注点主要集中在 RSIE 手术占比的增加，以及 RSIE 和 LSIE 患者之间的人口统计学差异上。总体而言，5%~40% 的 RSIE 患者需要手术干预[7-8]。然而，在阿片类药物流行期间，IVDU（尤其是注射海洛因）的人数增加了1倍多，随着这一激增，IE的发病率也显著增加[2,10]。此外，CIED的使用也越来越常见，尤其是在老年人中，这是IE发病率增加的另一个原因[11]，这种发病率的增加自然也就意味着相关手术量的增加[2]。在短短6年内（2011—2017年），三尖瓣心内膜炎的手术占比增加了5倍[2,12]。RSIE和LSIE的人口统计学差异也反映了IVDU与RSIE的相关性。RSIE患者多为年轻男性，共病较少，这也反映了IVDU者的特征[8,13-14]。IVDU的高复吸率（27%）也导致RSIE患者心内膜炎复发的比例（12%~32%）高于LSIE患者[3,5,13-14]。最后，外科医生在评估影像学检查和进行修复、置换手术时应认识到，37.9%的RSIE患者的病情因同时合并LSIE而变得复杂[8]。

临床表现

RSIE通常会出现全身症状，主要为发热，以及因脓毒性肺栓塞导致的呼吸道症状[6,15-16]。然而，由于RSIE的心脏杂音往往不明显且无特异性，因此诊断可能会被延误，导致后期出现胸腔积液、咯血、气胸或肺梗死、肺脓肿和肺水肿等更严重的呼吸系统表现[6,14]。RSIE的心脏表现与三尖瓣受累的严重程度有关。引起严重三尖瓣反流的赘生物可导致右心房扩张，并可能促使室上性心律失常和心力衰竭[6,16]。如果存在卵圆孔未闭，则可能出现全身栓塞，并因栓塞发生部位的不同而出现不同症状，但这种情况比LSIE少得多[17-18]。

诊 断

RSIE具有独特的诊断难点，即便如此，包括RSIE在内的所有IE都可以通过病理或临床标准进行诊断[19]。长期以来，Duke标准被认为是诊断IE的金标准，其主要临床标准是：①血培养持续阳性；②超声心动图显示心内膜受累[19]。然而，Duke标准主要针对LSIE而设计，免疫学和血管征象等次要临床标准不太适用于RSIE[20]。对Duke标准提出的改良强调了经食管超声心动图（TEE）的作用，并由此提高了该标准检测RSIE的能力[21]。通常，由于经胸超声心动图（TTE）的超声探头接近右心前部结构，因而成为疑似RSIE患者的首选影像学诊断方式[22]。然而，多项研究表明，与TTE相比，TEE诊断RSIE的灵敏度与之相当或更高[23-25]。这点在CIED相关的RSIE中得到了最明确的证实，在该类患者中TTE的灵敏度特别低，尤其是对位于右心房顶部起搏器电极导线的检测[26]。现已证明，TEE可将CIED相关RSIE的检测灵敏度提高60%，因此在此类病例中必须使用TEE[22,27-28]。心内超声心动图在TTE和TEE无法得出结论的情况下非常有用，具有较高的灵敏度，但缺点是具有侵入性[29]。CT在RSIE中可用于检测脓毒性肺梗死和脓肿[1]。

内科治疗

静脉使用抗生素是治疗 RSIE 的基础[1]。一旦临床怀疑发生 IE，就应立即进行血培养，并间隔 30 min 重复采血，共进行 3 次培养[5]。对于血流动力学不稳定的疑似 RSIE 患者，应在抽血培养后立即开始经验性静脉抗生素治疗[30]。经验性抗生素的抗菌谱范围应始终包括金黄色葡萄球菌，并可根据 IVDU 使用毒品的类型及感染部位进一步指导治疗[5,7,31]。根据培养和药敏结果，应针对致病菌使用敏感的抗生素[7,30]。在三尖瓣感染性心内膜炎（TVIE）中，70%~85% 的病例可通过适当的抗生素治疗有效清除菌血症[7]。然而，还有一些卫星病灶引起的菌血症仍然需要其他干预手段解决，例如，使用胸膜剥脱术治疗胸膜脓肿或脓毒性肺栓塞引起的脓胸[32]。为此，作者主张采用逐步升级有创程度的方法来治疗 RSIE，即优先考虑使用创伤程度小的方法，在这些处理无法消除菌血症时，才考虑瓣膜手术。

手术指征

手术治疗 RSIE 的指征是药物治疗失败、未来存在发生不良事件的风险、患者病情恶化或上述因素的综合。如果在使用适当的抗生素治疗 5~7d 后出现持续发热或菌血症，则应进行手术清除赘生物[5,14,33-34]。这种情况下，手术还可破坏生物膜，使残留的病原体暴露于正在进行的抗生素治疗和免疫反应中[34]。同样，在治疗由真菌等引起的 RSIE 病例时，也可能需要进行手术，因为这些病原仅靠抗菌药物很难根除[5,7,14]。赘生物的大小和活动度也是决定手术与否的重要因素，大于 2 cm、活动度大且有相应栓塞风险的赘生物应予手术清除[5,7,14,34]。虽然文献和作者的经验表明，肺部栓塞本身不应成为手术指征[14]；但脓毒性肺栓塞是 RSIE 的不良并发症，也就是说，反复出现的脓毒性肺栓塞会导致肺血管阻力增加，降低右心泵血的能力，在三尖瓣反流容量负荷增加情况下，进一步加重反流引起的心力衰竭[34]。

重度三尖瓣反流导致的心力衰竭是手术的独立指征，尤其是在利尿剂难以缓解症状的情况下[5,7,14,33]。瓣周脓肿和破坏性穿透病变也需要手术治疗，这些病变在人工瓣膜 RSIE 中较为常见[14,33,35]。此外，如果心内膜炎或相关炎症扩散到右心的传导系统，发生心脏传导阻滞时必须进行赘生物清除以及可能的起搏器植入[33,36]。当同时存在 LSIE 时，一般 LSIE 的情况决定是否手术[34,37]。一旦确定需要手术，手术应在 48 h 内进行，因为早期手术可改善预后[34,38]。

手术技术

一旦确定手术治疗 RSIE，就必须选择合适的手术方法。主要有 3 种手术方法：瓣膜切除、瓣膜修复和瓣膜置换。由于三尖瓣是 RSIE 最常涉及的结构，本章将重点讨论 TVIE 的手术方法。

瓣膜切除

在三尖瓣切除术中，应切除三尖瓣瓣叶、腱索及所有相关赘生物[39]。瓣膜切除术可作为一种终极性治疗方法，也可作为后续瓣膜置换术的过渡手术（IVDU患者先接受戒毒治疗）[39-41]。与瓣膜修复相比，瓣膜切除的主要优点是消除了瓣膜本身作为未来心内膜炎原发灶的可能性。瓣膜切除也不会像瓣膜置换那样为再感染创造一个新的人工原发灶。鉴于IVDU的高复吸率和高心内膜炎复发率，减少心内膜表面积带来的获益在IVDU者中最为明显[39,41]。在最近的一项meta分析中，与瓣膜置换相比，瓣膜切除确实降低了复发性心内膜炎的发生率，但趋势并不显著[39]。与瓣膜修复和置换相比，瓣膜切除的另一个优点是可降低引起心脏传导阻滞的概率[42]。此外，瓣膜切除无须术后抗凝治疗，这也符合IVDU者可能依从性较差无法坚持抗凝治疗的特点[30,39]。

然而，瓣膜切除术的优点会被其并发症所抵消。可以预见，瓣膜切除术后都要经历三尖瓣反流这一病理改变[43]，然而，仅有27%的患者在术后出现心力衰竭，一些学者认为这与该群体长期存在心内膜炎相关三尖瓣反流引发的心脏代偿有关[39,41]。但对于存在肺动脉高压的患者，肺血管阻力的增加将导致严重的无法耐受的三尖瓣反流，这些患者不适合进行瓣膜切除[44-45]。瓣膜切除术的早期死亡率为12%~13%，虽然这是一种旧式、技术简单的手术方式，但与瓣膜修复和置换相比，其死亡率并没有显著增加[39,42]。

瓣膜修复

对于需要手术的TVIE患者，一般推荐瓣膜修复术[5,34,46-47]。某些情况下，可考虑单纯清除赘生物，无须对瓣膜做修复操作，以尽量减少可能引起血栓形成和（或）再感染的人工材料的植入[48]。只有在彻底清除赘生物，并需要连带清除导致严重三尖瓣反流的感染瓣膜组织时，才考虑瓣膜修复[30-49]。三尖瓣修复有3种主要方法：①补片植入；②瓣环成形；③腱索重建[30]。每种方法又包含多种术式，而切除感染灶的位置和程度决定了手术方式的选择[30]。

自体心包补片修复是处理三尖瓣单瓣叶赘生物清除后组织缺损的首选方法，特别适合环形切除赘生物后残留的较小瓣叶孔[30,50]。补片的大小应足够大，以避免直接缝在炎症受累较为脆弱的组织上[50]。出于同样的目的，清创时应尽可能多地保留健康瓣叶组织[50]。

如果三尖瓣受到赘生物更广泛的损伤时，则可能需要对瓣环进行修复。当需要近乎完全切除后瓣叶时，可行Kay二瓣化成形术（瓣环成形术），并在必要时放置补片，这是环状瓣环成形术的一种非人工材料植入替代方法[30,50-51]。在Kay二瓣化成形术中，与后叶相对应的瓣环被缝合，重塑瓣环以允许前瓣和隔瓣在收缩期对合[30,50,52-53]。如果前瓣或隔瓣被切除，则可采用De Vega瓣环成形术[30,50,53-54]。在De Vega手术中，沿三尖瓣瓣环从三尖瓣后-隔交界到前-隔交界逆时针方向做荷包缝合[30,50,53-54]。收紧荷包可缩小瓣环，使剩余的瓣叶得以对合[30,50]。最后，关于瓣环成形术，可以将人工瓣环缝合至原本的瓣环上，从而恢复瓣环的形状，并结合补片以减少反流[50]。对于植入人工瓣环可能增加感染的担忧，有研究通过与单纯瓣环缝合成形进行了比较，发现前者并未增加感染风险[55-56]。

三尖瓣修复中腱索重建有助于瓣膜更接近自体原有功能。人工腱索（又称新腱索）是仿照自身腱索的功能来修复的[57-59]。人工腱索采用膨体聚四氟乙烯制成，一端固定在右心室乳头肌上，另一端固定在三尖瓣修复补片上[50,59-60]。使用生理盐水注水试验，以模拟收缩和瓣膜关闭状态，外科医生可由此判断人工腱索的适当长度[59]。Tarola及其同事在一组12例严重TVIE患者中证实，使用补片修复和人工腱索植入可有效减少反流[59]。

瓣膜置换

IVDU者的心内膜炎复发率很高，人工瓣膜心内膜炎导致的死亡率也很高，这突显了在RSIE手术中避免使用人工瓣膜的优势[5,13-14,61]。然而，在某些病例中，心内膜炎对三尖瓣的损害可能非常严重，无法进行修复，瓣膜置换在所难免[30]，这也是修复失败的病例可以考虑的治疗方法[62]。此外，伴随三尖瓣修复难度的增加，相应需要更丰富的手术经验和专业知识，而这并非所有的医疗机构都能提供[46]。因此，尽管瓣膜置换术并非理想之选，但在TVIE的外科治疗中仍发挥着重要作用。

无论置换的是人工生物瓣膜还是机械瓣膜，三尖瓣置换术的手术技巧基本保持不变[63]。在置入人工瓣膜之前，应切除自体瓣叶（包括所有赘生物），以清除心内膜炎的原发灶并防止将来发生右心室流出道（RVOT）梗阻[53]。在切除瓣叶时，应保留隔瓣位置的缝合缘[53,63]，这一缝边可确保缝瓣线在缝合Koch三角顶点这一位置时完全缝合在瓣叶组织上，从而减少缝线引起的房室传导阻滞[63]。剩余的腱索应在靠近乳头肌附着处横断[53]。人工瓣膜大小的选择和方向的放置对于防止瓣膜损伤RVOT和（或）室间隔至关重要[53,64]。作为额外的抗感染措施，可以用抗生素溶液浸泡人工瓣膜并擦拭瓣环[64]。

TVIE是选择生物瓣还是机械瓣膜应结合患者的生理、并发症和依从性等因素。与左心相比，右心系统压力较低、血流速度较低、抗血栓前列环素水平较低[53,64-66]，这些因素共同导致了右心机械瓣膜血栓风险的增加[53,64-66]，而IVDU者对术后抗凝治疗依从性差，又是这类病例易于出现血栓的另一个关注点[30]。最近的一项meta分析证实，植入机械瓣膜的患者发生血栓事件的概率增加[67]。然而，机械瓣膜血栓形成增加的临床意义也受到质疑，因为与生物瓣膜相比，机械瓣膜血栓形成并未导致5年瓣膜故障率或再次手术率的升高，即便出现这种情况，血栓也可以通过溶栓成功治疗[67-68]。在IVDU人群心内膜炎的复发率方面，生物瓣和机械瓣没有明显差异[69]。存活率方面，最近的一项meta分析发现，生物瓣和机械瓣的近期或远期死亡率没有明显差异[67]。还有一个考虑因素是，机械瓣的设计不允许右心室起搏电极的放置，而生物瓣则更适合那些将来可能植入起搏器的患者[64]。

修复术和置换术对比

作为治疗 TVIE 的两种主要手术方法，我们需要对修复术和置换术的主要结局进行比较。在接受手术治疗的 RSIE 患者中，49%～59% 的病例接受了修复术，41%～46% 的病例接受了置换术[46,69]。修复术和置换术在围手术期死亡率（6% vs.11%）、晚期存活率或主要并发症发生率（17% vs. 25%）方面没有明显差异[46,69]。不过，接受修复术的患者术后更容易出现中重度反流[46]。与置换术相比，修复术的反流率增加，但复发性心内膜炎、再次手术、心脏传导阻滞和起搏器植入的可能性显著降低，从而抵消了反流率增加的负面影响[42,46]。

停搏手术与非停搏手术

三尖瓣修复术和置换术都需要体外循环辅助[70-73]，两种手术方式在不停搏和主动脉阻断停搏下都可以实施，即便存在卵圆孔未闭[70-74]。心脏不停搏下手术的优点是可减少心肌缺血和再灌注损伤，并可以立即发现和去除导致房室传导阻滞的缝线[70-71]。停搏下手术的优点主要是有利于瓣膜的显露，静止状态的手术视野有利于术者的操作[70]。作者基于尽量减少心肌缺血的考虑，倾向于不停搏下进行修复和置换，就结果而言，不停搏和停搏下的三尖瓣修复和置换术具有相似的手术和短期死亡率[70-73]。大多数研究发现两种方式术中的体外循环时间或手术时间总体上没有显著差异[70-73]。但停搏下心脏传导阻滞发生率略高，永久起搏器的安装也就偏多[70-73]。

CIED 相关的心内膜炎

与 CIED 相关的心内膜炎最常见于永久起搏器或植入式除颤器的感染[11]。CIED 感染指的是微生物定植局限在发生器囊袋[7,11]。CIED 感染有别于 CIED 相关性心内膜炎，但也可能发展为 CIED 相关性心内膜炎，一旦后者出现，则可在装置的电极导线和（或）三尖瓣上见到赘生物[11]。两个概念内涵的不同也带来了临床手术方法的差别，相对而言，CIED 相关性心内膜炎的手术治疗更复杂[11,75]。一般情况下，CIED 感染经皮经静脉取出电极导线即可；而 CIED 相关性心内膜炎则需要手术治疗，以便在进行三尖瓣修复的同时，降低赘生物肺栓塞的风险[11,75]。而且，CIED 相关性心内膜炎需要彻底清除植入装置的所有部件，以防止残留部分成为复发性心内膜炎的原发灶[76]。有趣的是，由于只有 1/3～1/2 的患者需要进行再手术植入新装置来替换已被取出的装置，而对 CIED 相关性心内膜炎的手术就为评估当年植入装置后心脏目前的状况，以及是否需要再次植入同一装置提供了机会[75-76]。

手术注意事项

术前注意事项

TTE 和 TEE 对于手术计划的制定至关重要。经验丰富的超声心动图医生可定位瓣膜赘生物、评估瓣膜结构受累情况、识别是否存在卵圆孔未闭，并根据瓣膜受损程度提供是否可以进行修复的初步建议[23,77]。如果超声心动图显示是轻微的 RSIE，则可考虑采用微创方法[78]。鉴于 IVDU 在 RSIE 中的普遍性，一些医疗机构的常见做法是要求进行术前咨询，患者必须签署一份协议，承诺今后不再 IVDU 并参加戒毒治疗[79]。对这种做法虽然存在争议，但强调了成瘾治疗作为药物和手术治疗的辅助手段在 RSIE 治疗中的重要性[34,80-81]。此外，还建议患者在术前接受积极的利尿治疗，以控制三尖瓣反流。手术患者必须接受抗生素治疗，理想的情况是，至少术前一周已开始使用抗生素[34,50]。针对 CIED-IE，术前还必须考虑好在取出原有装置后过渡时期的替代装置[11,76]。

术中注意事项

正中胸骨切开是心内膜炎手术的首选入路，尤其是在怀疑邻近结构受累或合并左心系统病变时。与任何瓣膜手术一样，术中 TEE 是评估修复效果和瓣周漏的必要手段[22]。此外，术中 TEE 还可发现术前未被发现的瓣膜赘生物[22]。术中需要仔细探查彻底清创，以清除感染和坏死组织，同时不损伤正常的组织或传导系统[34]。然而，由于传导系统可能受到损伤，所有患者都应植入临时起搏电极导线。如果在手术过程中出现任何心脏传导阻滞的迹象，则应在皮下隧道中植入永久性心外膜电极导线，并放置于皮下囊袋中，以便电生理学家在术后放置起搏器[34]。

在清除感染组织时，细菌毒素会释放到血液循环中，可引起血流动力学波动，对于这类情况的预测及应对显得非常重要。作者建议短时使用大剂量的血管升压药来对抗脓毒性休克。清创也可能引起肺部脓栓，使患者难以脱离体外循环。因此，作者建议右颈静脉和右股静脉备好插管位置，需要时可紧急建立体外膜肺氧合（VV-ECMO）。清创完成后和瓣膜重建前，必须进行大量冲洗、更换所有器械和手套，以确保术中无菌环境。

术后注意事项

心脏传导阻滞是 RSIE 手术的主要并发症，术后必须密切监测。手术创伤引起的炎症可导致瓣环肿胀，并可能在术后 48 h 内发展为心脏传导阻滞。这种类型的心脏传导阻滞不一定会在手术中出现，因此所有患者都必须植入临时起搏器。由于疼痛和阿片类药物耐受导致的麻醉剂疗效降低，IVDU 患者常出现术后高血压和心动过速。由于存在加重心脏传导阻滞的风险，因此不建议使用 β 受体阻滞剂来控制高血压。还应避免使用其他作用于房室结的药物，如胺碘酮。术后标准抗生素治疗持续 6 周，并应根据培养和药敏结果进行调整。对于真菌性心内膜炎的术后患者，大多数学者建议终生抗真菌治疗[34]。

总　结

与 LSIE 相比，RSIE 历来受到的关注较少，因为它在 IE 病例中所占的比例相对较小。然而，随着 IVDU 和 CIED 使用的增加，RSIE 手术治疗的重要性也随之增加。当抗生素无法消除菌血症、超声心动图显示有大的赘生物，或严重三尖瓣反流导致心力衰竭时，RSIE 的手术治疗就显得尤为重要。出于对心内膜炎复发的担忧，手术中应有意识地尽量减少假体材料的使用，为此，近 60% 的 RSIE 手术都使用瓣膜修复方式。对于严重的瓣膜破坏，瓣膜置换可能是唯一的选择，虽然心内膜炎复发的风险会增加，但置换后的存活率与修复后的存活率相当。术前进行 TEE 以指导 RSIE 手术计划的制定，使用血管升压药和机械支持控制术中预期的血流动力学波动，积极放置临时起搏装置以处理术后可能出现的心脏传导阻滞。

参考文献

[1] Shmueli H, Thomas F, Flint N, et al. Right-sided infective endocarditis 2020: challenges and updates in diagnosis and treatment. J Am Heart Assoc, 2020, 9(15): e017293. https://doi.org/10.1161/JAHA.120.017293.

[2] Wallen TJ, Szeto W, Williams M, et al. Tricuspid valve endocarditis in the era of the opioid epidemic. J Card Surg, 2018, 33(5): 260–264. https://doi.org/10.1111/jocs.13600.

[3] Rosenthal ES, Karchmer AW, Theisen-Toupal J, et al. Suboptimal addiction interventions for patients hospitalized with injection drug use-associated infective endocarditis. Am J Med, 2016, 129(5): 481–485. https://doi.org/10.1016/j.amjmed.2015.09.024.

[4] Rodger L, Shah M, Shojaei E, et al. Recurrent endocarditis in persons who inject drugs. Open Forum Infect Dis, 2019, 6(10): ofz396. https://doi.org/10.1093/ofid/ofz396.

[5] Habib G, Lancellotti P, Antunes MJ, et al. 2015 ESC guidelines for the management of infective endocarditis: the task force for the management of infective endocarditis of the European Society of Cardiology (ESC). Endorsed by: European Association for Cardio-thoracic Surgery (EACTS), the European Association of Nuclear Medicine (EANM). Eur Heart J, 2015, 36(44): 3075–3128. https://doi.org/10.1093/eurheartj/ehv319.

[6] Akinosoglou K, Apostolakis E, Marangos M, et al. Native valve right sided infective endocarditis. Eur J Intern Med, 2013, 24(6): 510–519. https://doi.org/10.1016/j.ejim.2013.01.010.

[7] Hussain ST, Witten J, Shrestha NK, et al. Tricuspid valve endocarditis. Ann Cardiothorac Surg, 2017, 6(3): 255–261. https://doi.org/10.21037/acs.2017.03.09.

[8] Weber C, Gassa A, Eghbalzadeh K, et al. Characteristics and outcomes of patients with right-sided endocarditis undergoing cardiac surgery. Ann Cardiothorac Surg, 2019, 8(6): 645–653. https://doi.org/10.21037/acs.2019.08.02.

[9] Lee MR, Chang SA, Choi SH, et al. Clinical features of right-sided infective endocarditis occurring in non-drug users. J Kor Med Sci, 2014, 29(6): 776–781. https://doi.org/10.3346/jkms.2014.29.6.776.

[10] Sanaiha Y, Lyons R, Benharash P. Infective endocarditis in intravenous drug users. Trends Cardiovasc Med, 2020, 30(8): 491–497. https://doi.org/10.1016/j.tcm.2019.11.007.

[11] Koutentakis M, Siminelakis S, Korantzopoulos P, et al. Surgical management of cardiac implantable electronic device infections. J Thorac Dis, 2014, 6(Suppl. 1): S173–S179. https://doi.org/10.3978/j.issn.2072-1439.2013.10.23.

[12] Slaughter MS, Badhwar V, Ising M, et al. Optimum surgical treatment for tricuspid valve infective endocarditis: an analysis of the Society of Thoracic Surgeons national database. J Thorac Cardiovasc Surg, 2021, 161(4). https://doi.org/10.1016/j.jtcvs.2019.10.124. 1227.e1-1235.e1.
[13] Kim JB, Ejiofor JI, Yammine M, et al. Surgical outcomes of infective endocarditis among intravenous drug users. J Thorac Cardiovasc Surg, 2016, 152(3). https://doi.org/10.1016/j.jtcvs.2016.02.072. 832.e1-841.e1.
[14] Moss R, Munt B. Injection drug use and right sided endocarditis. Heart, 2003, 89(5): 577–581. https://doi.org/10.1136/heart.89.5.577.
[15] Revilla A, López J, Villacorta E, et al. Isolated right-sided valvular endocarditis in non-intravenous drug users. Rev Española Cardiol, 2008, 61(12): 1253–1259. https://doi.org/10.1016/S1885-5857(09)60052-9.
[16] Ortiz C, López J, García H, et al. Clinical classification and prognosis of isolated right-sided infective endocarditis. Medicine (Baltim), 2014, 93(27). https://doi.org/10.1097/MD.0000000000000137. e137.
[17] Patti R, Gupta SS, Kupfer Y. Right sided infective endocarditis and systemic emboli. QJM, 2019, 112(1): 57–58. https://doi.org/10.1093/qjmed/hcy187.
[18] McCaughan J, Purvis J, Sharkey R. Embolisation of vegetation to the liver in right sided infective endocarditis. Eur J Intern Med, 2008, 20(2): e32–e33. https://doi.org/10.1016/j.ejim.2008.08.008.
[19] Durack DT, Lukes AS, Bright DK. New criteria for diagnosis of infective endocarditis: utilization of specific echocardiographic findings. Duke Endocarditis Service. Am J Med, 1994, 96(3): 200–209. https://doi.org/10.1016/0002-9343(94)90143-0.
[20] Prendergast BD. Diagnostic criteria and problems in infective endocarditis. Heart, 2004, 90(6): 611–613. https://doi.org/10.1136/hrt.2003.029850.
[21] Li JS, Sexton DJ, Mick N, et al. Proposed modifications to the Duke criteria for the diagnosis of infective endocarditis. Clin Infect Dis, 2000, 30(4): 633–638. https://doi.org/10.1086/313753.
[22] Bruun NE, Habib G, Thuny F, et al. Cardiac imaging in infectious endocarditis. Eur Heart J, 2014, 35(10): 624–632. https://doi.org/10.1093/eurheartj/eht274.
[23] Mihos CG, Nappi F. A narrative review of echocardiography in infective endocarditis of the right heart. Ann Transl Med, 2020, 8(23): 1622. https://doi.org/10.21037/atm-20-5198.
[24] Román JS, Vilacosta I, Zamorano J, et al. Transesophageal echocardiography in right-sided endocarditis. J Am Coll Cardiol, 1993, 21(5): 1226–1230. https://doi.org/10.1016/0735-1097(93)90250-5.
[25] Herrera CJ, Mehlman DJ, Hartz RS, et al. Comparison of transesophageal and transthoracic echocardiography for diagnosis of right-sided cardiac lesions. Am J Cardiol, 1992, 70(9): 964–966. https://doi.org/10.1016/0002-9149(92)90751-j.
[26] Le Dolley Y, Thuny F, Mancini J, et al. Diagnosis of cardiac device-related infective endocarditis after device removal. JACC Cardiovasc Imag, 2010, 3(7): 673–681. https://doi.org/10.1016/j.jcmg.2009.12.016.
[27] Victor F, De Place C, Camus C, et al. Pacemaker lead infection: echocardiographic features, management, and outcome. Heart, 1999, 81(1): 82–87. https://doi.org/10.1136/hrt.81.1.82.
[28] Vilacosta I, Sarria C, San Roman JA, et al. Usefulness of transesophageal echocardiography for diagnosis of infected transvenous permanent pacemakers. Circulation, 1994, 89(6): 2684–2687. https://doi.org/10.1161/01.CIR.89.6.2684.
[29] Narducci ML, Pelargonio G, Russo E, et al. Usefulness of intracardiac echocardiography for the diagnosis of cardiovascular implantable electronic device-related endocarditis. J Am Coll Cardiol, 2013, 61(13): 1398–1405. https://doi.org/10.1016/j.jacc.2012.12.041.
[30] Akinosoglou K, Apostolakis E, Koutsogiannis N, et al. Right-sided infective endocarditis: surgical management. Eur J Cardio Thorac Surg, 2012, 42(3): 470–479. https://doi.org/10.1093/ejcts/ezs084.
[31] Cherubin CE, Sapira JD. The medical complications of drug addiction and the medical assessment of the intravenous drug user: 25 years later. Ann Intern Med, 1993, 119(10): 1017–1028. https://

doi.org/10.7326/0003-4819-119-10-199311150-00009.

[32] Nalos M, Huang SJ, Ting I, et al. Diagnoses of right-sided empyema complicating tricuspid valve endocarditis during transesophageal echocardiography. J Am Soc Echocardiogr, 2004, 17(5): 464–465. https://doi.org/10.1016/j.echo.2003.12.021.

[33] Nishimura RA, Otto CM, Bonow RO, et al. 2014 AHA/ACC guideline for the management of patients with valvular heart disease: executive summary: a report of the American College of Cardiology/American Heart Association task force on practice guidelines. Circulation, 2014, 129(23): 2440–2492. https://doi.org/10.1161/CIR.0000000000000029.

[34] Pettersson GB, Hussain ST. Current AATS guidelines on surgical treatment of infective endocarditis. Ann Cardiothorac Surg, 2019, 8(6): 630–644. https://doi.org/10.21037/acs.2019.10.05.

[35] Weber C, Rahmanian PB, Nitsche M, et al. Higher incidence of perivalvular abscess determines perioperative clinical outcome in patients undergoing surgery for prosthetic valve endocarditis. BMC Cardiovasc Disord, 2020, 20(1): 47. https://doi.org/10.1186/s12872-020-01338-y.

[36] Sato M, Harada K, Watanabe T, et al. Right-sided infective endocarditis with coronary sinus vegetation causing complete atrioventricular block. Eur Heart J Cardiovasc Imag, 2020, 21(3). https://doi.org/10.1093/ehjci/jez244. 345.

[37] Witten JC, Hussain ST, Shrestha NK, et al. Surgical treatment of right-sided infective endocarditis. J Thorac Cardiovasc Surg, 2019, 157(4). https://doi.org/10.1016/j.jtcvs.2018.07.112. 1418.e14-1427. e14.

[38] Jamil M, Sultan I, Gleason TG, et al. Infective endocarditis: trends, surgical outcomes, and controversies. J Thorac Dis, 2019, 11(11): 4875–4885. https://doi.org/10.21037/jtd.2019.10.45.

[39] Luc JGY, Choi JH, Kodia K, et al. Valvectomy versus replacement for the surgical treatment of infective tricuspid valve endocarditis: a systematic review and meta-analysis. Ann Cardiothorac Surg, 2019, 8(6): 610–620. https://doi.org/10.21037/acs.2019.11.06.

[40] Arbulu A, Asfaw I. Tricuspid valvulectomy without prosthetic replacement. J Thorac Cardiovasc Surg, 1981, 82(5): 684–691. https://doi.org/10.1016/S0022-5223(19)39263-3.

[41] Protos AN, Trivedi JR, Whited WM, et al. Valvectomy versus replacement for the surgical treatment of tricuspid endocarditis. Ann Thorac Surg, 2018, 106(3): 664–669. https://doi.org/10.1016/j.athoracsur.2018.04.051.

[42] Gaca JG, Sheng S, Daneshmand M, et al. Current outcomes for tricuspid valve infective endocarditis surgery in North America. Ann Thorac Surg, 2013, 96(4): 1374–1381. https://doi.org/10.1016/j.athoracsur.2013.05.046.

[43] Robin E, Thomas NW, Arbulu A, et al. Hemodynamic consequences of total removal of the tricuspid valve without prosthetic replacement. Am J Cardiol, 1975, 35(4): 481–486. https://doi.org/10.1016/0002-9149(75)90830-9.

[44] Arbulu A, Holmes RJ, Asfaw I. Surgical treatment of intractable right-sided infective endocarditis in drug addicts: 25 years experience. J Heart Valve Dis, 1993, 2(2): 129–139.

[45] Borkhetaria N, Howsare M, Cavallazzi R. A 30-year-old woman with tricuspid valvectomy presents with shock. Chest, 2019, 155(1): e5–e7. https://doi.org/10.1016/j.chest.2018.08.1090.

[46] Yanagawa B, Elbatarny M, Verma S, et al. Surgical management of tricuspid valve infective endocarditis: a systematic review and meta-analysis. Ann Thorac Surg, 2018, 106(3): 708–714. https://doi.org/10.1016/j.athoracsur.2018.04.012.

[47] Baddour LM, Wilson WR, Bayer AS, et al. Infective endocarditis in adults: diagnosis, antimicrobial therapy, and management of complications: a scientific statement for healthcare professionals from the American Heart Association. Circulation, 2015, 132(15): 1435–1486. https://doi.org/10.1161/CIR.0000000000000296.

[48] Miró JM, Moreno A, Mestres CA. Infective endocarditis in intravenous drug abusers. Curr Infect Dis Rep, 2003, 5(4): 307–316. https://doi.org/10.1007/s11908-003-0007-9.

[49] Morokuma H, Minato N, Kamohara K, et al. Three surgical cases of isolated tricuspid valve infective endocarditis. Ann Thorac Cardiovasc Surg, 2010, 16(2): 134–138.

[50] Brescia AA, Watt TMF, Williams AM, et al. Tricuspid valve leaflet repair and augmentation for infective endocarditis. Operat Tech Thorac Cardiovasc Surg, 2019, 24(4): 206–218. https://doi.org/10.1053/j.optechstcvs.2019.09.002.

[51] Ghanta RK, Chen R, Narayanasamy N, et al. Suture bicuspidization of the tricuspid valve versus ring annuloplasty for repair of functional tricuspid regurgitation: midterm results of 237 consecutive patients. J Thorac Cardiovasc Surg, 2007, 133(1): 117–126. https://doi.org/10.1016/j.jtcvs.2006.08.068.

[52] Kay JH, Maselli-Campagna G, Tsuji KK. Surgical treatment of tricuspid insufficiency. Ann Surg, 1965, 162(1): 53–58. https://doi.org/10.1097/00000658-196507000-00009.

[53] Belluschi I, Del Forno B, Lapenna E, et al. Surgical techniques for tricuspid valve disease. Front Cardiovasc Med, 2018, 5: 118. https://doi.org/10.3389/fcvm.2018.00118.

[54] De Vega NG, De Rábago G, Castillón L, et al. A new tricuspid repair. Short-term clinical results in 23 cases. J Cardiovasc Surg, 1973: 384–386.

[55] Hata H, Fujita T, Miura S, et al. Long-term outcomes of suture vs. Ring tricuspid annuloplasty for functional tricuspid regurgitation. Circ J, 2017, 81(10): 1432–1438. https://doi.org/10.1253/circj.CJ-17-0108.

[56] Tang GHL, David TE, Singh SK, et al. Tricuspid valve repair with an annuloplasty ring results in improved long-term outcomes. Circulation, 2006, 114(1). https://doi.org/10.1161/CIRCULATIONAHA.105.001263. I577–I581.

[57] Bortolotti U, Tursi V, Fasoli G, et al. Tricuspid valve endocarditis: repair with the use of artificial chordae. J Heart Valve Dis, 1993, 2(5): 567–570.

[58] Marin D, Ramadan K, Hamilton C, et al. Tricuspid valve repair with artificial chordae in a 72-year-old woman. Thorac Cardiovasc Surg, 2011, 59(8): 495–497. https://doi.org/10.1055/s-0030-1250724.

[59] Tarola CL, Losenno KL, Chu MWA. Complex tricuspid valve repair for infective endocarditis: leaflet augmentation, chordae and annular reconstruction. Multimed Manual Cardiothorac surg, 2015; 2015. https://doi.org/10.1093/mmcts/mmv006. mmv006.

[60] Boyd JH, Edelman JJB, Scoville DH, et al. Tricuspid leaflet repair: innovative solutions. Ann Cardiothorac Surg, 2017, 6(3): 248–254. https://doi.org/10.21037/acs.2017.05.06.

[61] Manne MB, Shrestha NK, Lytle BW, et al. Outcomes after surgical treatment of native and prosthetic valve infective endocarditis. Ann Thorac Surg, 2012, 93(2): 489–493. https://doi.org/10.1016/j.athoracsur.2011.10.063.

[62] Veen KM, Etnel JRG, Takkenberg JJM. Tricuspid valve disease: surgical outcome//Soliman OI, ten Cate FJ. Practical Manual of tricuspid valve diseases. Cham: Springer International Publishing, 2018. https://doi.org/10.1007/978-3-319-58229-0.

[63] Doty JR, Doty DB. Tricuspid valve replacement. Operat Tech Thorac Cardiovasc Surg, 2003, 8(4): 193–200. https://doi.org/10.1016/S1522-2942(03)80007-7.

[64] De Bonis M, Del Forno B, Nisi T, et al. Tricuspid valve disease: surgical techniques//Soliman OI, ten Cate FJ. Practical Manual of tricuspid valve diseases. Cham: Springer International Publishing, 2018. https://doi.org/10.1007/978-3-319-58229-0.

[65] Kaplan M, Kut MS, Demirtas MM, et al. Prosthetic replacement of tricuspid valve: bioprosthetic or mechanical. Ann Thorac Surg, 2002, 73(2): 467–473. https://doi.org/10.1016/S0003-4975(01)03128-9.

[66] Hwang HY, Kim K-H, Kim K-B, et al. Propensity score matching analysis of mechanical versus bioprosthetic tricuspid valve replacements. Ann Thorac Surg, 2014, 97(4): 1294–1299. https://doi.org/10.1016/j.athoracsur.2013.12.033.

[67] Negm S, Arafat AA, Elatafy EE, et al. Mechanical versus bioprosthetic valve replacement in the tricuspid valve position: a systematic review and meta-analysis. Heart Lung Circ, 2021, 30(3): 362–371. https://doi.org/10.1016/j.hlc.2020.03.011.

[68] Shapira Y, Sagie A, Jortner R, et al. Thrombosis of bileaflet tricuspid valve prosthesis: clinical spectrum and the role of nonsurgical treatment. Am Heart J, 1999, 137(4): 721–725. https://doi.

org/10.1016/S0002-8703(99)70229-2.

[69] Di Mauro M, Foschi M, Dato GMA, et al. Surgical treatment of isolated tricuspid valve infective endocarditis: 25-year results from a multicenter registry. Int J Cardiol, 2019, 292: 62–67. https://doi.org/10.1016/j.ijcard.2019.05.020.

[70] Pfannmüller B, Davierwala P, Misfeld M, et al. Postoperative outcome of isolated tricuspid valve operation using arrested-heart or beating-heart technique. Ann Thorac Surg, 2012, 94(4): 1218–1222. https://doi.org/10.1016/j.athoracsur.2012.05.020.

[71] Baraki H, Saito S, Ahmad AA, et al. Beating heart versus arrested heart isolated tricuspid valve surgery. Int Heart J, 2015, 56(4): 400–407. https://doi.org/10.1536/ihj.14-423.

[72] Hasde Aİ, Özçınar E, Çakıcı M, et al. Comparison of aortic cross-clamping versus beating heart surgery in tricuspid valve repair. Turk Gogus Kalp Damar Cerrahisi Derg, 2018, 26(4): 519–527. https://doi.org/10.5606/tgkdc.dergisi.2018.16229.

[73] Flagiello M, Grinberg D, Connock M, et al. Beating versus arrested heart isolated tricuspid valve surgery: an 11-year experience in the current era. J Card Surg, 2021, 36(3): 1020–1027. https://doi.org/10.1111/jocs.15390.

[74] Salinas GEG, Ramchandani M. Tricuspid valve replacement on a beating heart via a right minithoracotomy. Multimed Manual Cardiothorac surg, 2013; 2013. https://doi.org/10.1093/mmcts/mmt006. mmt006-mmt006.

[75] Tarakji KG, Wilkoff BL. Cardiac implantable electronic device infections: facts, current practice, and the unanswered questions. Curr Infect Dis Rep, 2014, 16(9): 425. https://doi.org/10.1007/s11908-014-0425-x.

[76] Baddour LM, Epstein AE, Bolger AF, et al. Update on cardiovascular implantable electronic device infections and their management: a scientific statement from the American heart association. Circulation, 2010, 121(3): 458–477. https://doi.org/10.1161/CIRCULATIONAHA.109.192665.

[77] Mahmoud AN, Elgendy IY, Agarwal N, et al. Identification and quantification of patent foramen ovale-mediated shunts: echocardiography and transcranial Doppler. Interv Cardiol Clin, 2017, 6(4): 495–504. https://doi.org/10.1016/j.iccl.2017.05.002.

[78] Zhigalov K, Sá MPBO, Kadyraliev B, et al. Surgical treatment of infective endocarditis in the era of minimally invasive cardiac surgery and transcatheter approach: an editorial. J Thorac Dis, 2020, 12(3): 140–142. https://doi.org/10.21037/jtd.2020.01.59.

[79] Vlahakes GJ. "Consensus guidelines for the surgical treatment of infective endocarditis": the surgeon must lead the team. J Thorac Cardiovasc Surg, 2017, 153(6): 1259–1260. https://doi.org/10.1016/j.jtcvs.2016.10.041.

[80] Hussain ST, Gordon SM, Streem DW, et al. Contract with the patient with injection drug use and infective endocarditis: surgeons perspective. J Thorac Cardiovasc Surg, 2017, 154(6): 2002–2003. https://doi.org/10.1016/j.jtcvs.2017.08.004.

[81] Wurcel AG, Yu S, Pacheco M, Warner K. Contracts with people who inject drugs following valve surgery: unrealistic and misguided expectations. J Thorac Cardiovasc Surg, 2017, 154(6). https://doi.org/10.1016/j.jtcvs.2017.07.020. 2002.

第16章
自体二尖瓣心内膜炎的外科治疗

Cayley Bowles, William Hiesinger
Department of Cardiothoracic Surgery, Stanford University School of Medicine,
Stanford, CA, United States

流行病学

自体瓣膜感染性心内膜炎（IE）相对罕见，多项研究显示，其发病率为（2~10）/10万（人·年）[1-2]；但由于其较高的并发症发生率和死亡率，给临床带来了较高的医疗负担。IE患者的院内死亡率约为20%，可伴有卒中、栓塞和心力衰竭等多种并发症[2-4]。心内膜炎广义上通常分为自体瓣膜心内膜炎（NVE）和人工瓣膜心内膜炎（PVE）。一项纳入2781名心内膜炎患者的前瞻性队列研究发现，72%的患者为NVE，其中41%的患者为二尖瓣心内膜炎[3]。

心内膜炎的风险因素可分为心源性和非心源性。心源性风险因素包括人工瓣膜、起搏器电极导线、先天性心脏病和后天性瓣膜疾病。非心源性风险因素包括静脉吸毒和不良口腔卫生[1-2,5]。虽然静脉吸毒以前被认为仅是少数心内膜炎的病因，但由于近来阿片类药物的滥用，此病因已发生变化。多项研究表明，自2005年以来，美国和加拿大静脉吸毒和与之相关的心内膜炎病例均呈增加趋势[6-7]。

二尖瓣心内膜炎的特异性风险因素包括风湿性和退行性二尖瓣疾病。一项回顾性研究通过分析患者的超声心动图图像发现，60%的二尖瓣心内膜炎伴有二尖瓣环钙化（MAC），作者由此认为，二尖瓣钙化可能是引发感染的根源[8]。

发病机制

二尖瓣心内膜炎的起病需要：①有足够数量的细菌进入血液；②细菌在不易被宿主免疫系统发现的心脏表面定植。细菌定植和复制的机制前面章节已充分阐明。瓣膜的损伤可因先天缺陷或后天畸形导致的血液湍流、退行性二尖瓣疾病引起的慢性炎症，或静脉吸毒时反复暴露于固体颗粒而产生[2]。

当瓣膜内皮受损后，内皮下胶原蛋白会暴露出来，导致血小板和纤维蛋白附着在瓣膜表面，这一结构很容易被血液循环中的细菌黏附，进一步导致血小板和纤维蛋白的聚集，从而形成一种被称为赘生物的三维结构。由于它是多层结构，导致宿主防御系统和抗生素都较难穿透这一结构，难以攻击其中隐藏的细菌[1-2,9]。

诊 断

目前，IE 的诊断是基于本书前文所述的改良 Duke 标准。二尖瓣心内膜炎有两个重要的特殊考虑因素：首先，体格检查时，二尖瓣心内膜炎常伴有新杂音的出现，或原有杂音的加重，表现为二尖瓣反流特征性的全收缩期杂音；其次，由于二尖瓣位于左心系统，因此需要重点进行神经系统检查以评估潜在的脑部并发症。其他体格检查和实验室检查与前面讨论过的一般心内膜炎相同。

影像学

超声心动图是 IE 的主要影像学检查手段。许多患者在检查过程中都会同时接受经胸超声心动图（TTE）和经食管超声心动图（TEE）检查。一般而言，所有高度怀疑有心内膜炎的患者都应接受 TTE 检查。如果 TTE 无法确诊，而临床仍高度怀疑心内膜炎，则应接受 TEE 检查[2-3,10]。IE 超声心动图的影像学表现在不同病例间会有差异，其中 90% 可表现为赘生物，60% 为瓣膜反流，20% 可发现瓣膜脓肿[2]。早在 1986 年，有研究就报道了 TTE 和彩色多普勒对二尖瓣心内膜炎并发症如瓣叶穿孔等的诊断能力[11]。近期，Yuan 等研究显示，他们机构的 69 名 IE 患者术前 TTE 超声检查影像表现与术中大体病理所见没有差异。因此，TTE 能够有效识别赘生物的大小、数量和位置，以及瓣膜穿孔、瓣膜脱垂和腱索断裂等病变[12]。

对任何有神经症状的患者都应邀请神经科会诊，并做相应的脑部影像学检查。即使没有症状，二尖瓣心内膜炎（或其他任何左心系统感染病变）都应进行脑部影像学检查[10]。脑部并发症是心脏外科医生的一个重要考虑因素，因为相关并发症的出现会影响手术时机，这一点将在下文讨论。

内科治疗

无论手术与否，药物治疗都是有效治疗心内膜炎必不可少的环节。治疗包括长期静脉注射足量抗生素以控制感染源。治疗方案的选择通常以病原体结果为基础，与感染病小组协商后做出。但在病原菌培养和药敏结果报告之前，可根据经验使用万古霉素和头孢曲松，结果出来之后，则根据结果适当调整抗菌药物的使用。针对多数病原体的常用方案是青霉素 G 加庆大霉素，当然还有其他多种选择[1]。

外科治疗

二尖瓣心内膜炎通常需要手术治疗。公认的手术指征包括心力衰竭、无法控制的感染和全身性栓塞[1,2,5,10]。二尖瓣心内膜炎的心力衰竭多因瓣膜功能障碍或穿孔导致的严重二尖瓣反流引起；无法控制的感染通常因抗生素无法穿透脓肿或赘生物所致；而全身性栓塞则来自赘生物碎片脱落进入血流，对于左心感染病变，就可能会出现上述的脑部栓塞情况。

当然，业界对二尖瓣心内膜炎的手术时机仍有争议[1]。不过，最新的美国胸外科协会（AATS）共识指南建议，一旦确定有手术指征，应尽快手术[10]。Kang等（2012年）的一项研究将76名患者随机分为早期手术和常规治疗两组，结果发现：早期手术可降低6周时的院内死亡和栓塞风险。这些患者中60%患有二尖瓣心内膜炎，提示早期二尖瓣手术的安全性，甚至可能有益于患者的早期恢复[13]。

心脏内、外科专家一致认为，当出现神经系统并发症时，必须与神经内科共同会商决定手术时间。目前的AATS指南建议非出血性脑卒中延期1～2周行心脏手术，而出血性脑卒中则等待3～4周后手术[10]。

手术的目的是切除所有感染和坏死组织以控制感染源、修复病变组织缺损[10]。针对二尖瓣心内膜炎，外科医生面临的最常见问题是手术方式的选择——是实施二尖瓣置换还是二尖瓣修复。早在1992年，Hendren等发表了一项研究：22名患者因二尖瓣心内膜炎导致瓣膜关闭不全而成功接受了二尖瓣修复术；他们介绍了多种不同的修复技术，包括直接缝合或补片修复瓣叶穿孔、腱索缩短或转移、瓣叶切除和缝合、瓣环成形[14]。作者指出，二尖瓣修复术对年轻患者尤为有益，这一群体对抗凝治疗依从性较差。虽然这篇论文样本量较小，但为二尖瓣修复术在心内膜炎中的应用提供了理论依据。

从那时起，多项研究显示，在可能的情况下，修复术比置换术更有益处，包括提高短期和长期存活率、减少IE复发和降低并发症发生率[15-18]。鉴于有大量研究显示二尖瓣修复术的益处，AATS指南建议只要条件许可，应尽可能行二尖瓣修复术[10]。这些数据的唯一局限性是，我们不知道接受二尖瓣修复的患者是否与接受置换的患者病情相似。接受瓣膜置换的患者可能病变更广泛，因此实施修复技术上不可行。尽管如此，仍然存在一种共识，即修复术是安全的，即使要置换，也应该是尝试修复失败后进行。

在作者医院，只要有可能，我们都会进行瓣膜修复。在此，我们列举一个病例说明。患者是一个新出现全收缩期杂音的病例，经检查发现其患有二尖瓣心内膜炎。TTE显示二尖瓣严重关闭不全，前后瓣叶上均有赘生物。患者经微创右侧前胸入路进行手术，术中对二尖瓣前后瓣叶进行了广泛清创（图16.1和图16.2）。

与二尖瓣关闭不全行瓣膜修复疗效类似，现有证据表明，如果在大手术量心脏中心进行心内膜炎的二尖瓣修复，患者存活效果更好。Lee等比较了二尖瓣修复与置换治疗心内膜炎的效果，他们发现二尖瓣修复组的患者存活率更高，但如果二尖瓣修复是在手术量最低的医院进行，则不存在这种获益[16]。Toyoda等的研究也得出同样结论：由高二尖瓣手术量的外科医生进行的修复术在1年内需要再次手术的概率是低手术量外科医生的1/5[19]。该文章引发了克利夫兰诊所一个研究小组的社论，强调二尖瓣手术的总体手术量对二尖瓣内膜炎的治疗效果非常重要[20]。

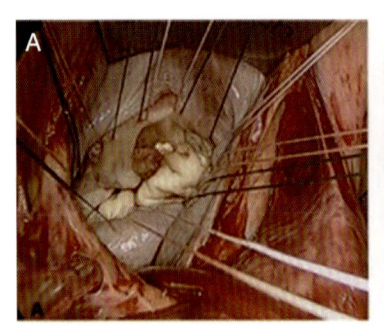

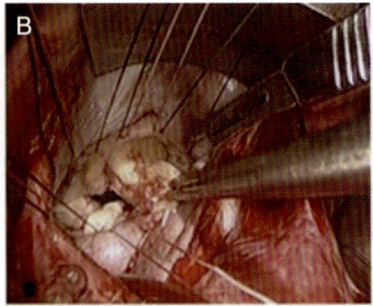

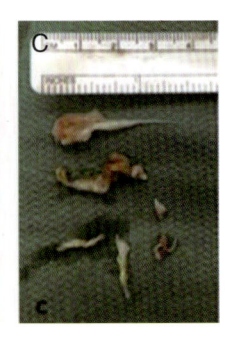

图 16.1 A. 可见二尖瓣病变，已放置瓣环缝线。B. 二尖瓣清创。C. 切除的二尖瓣感染病变组织。清创后，使用 Gore-Tex 线重建腱索、P2 切除和瓣环成形修复瓣膜

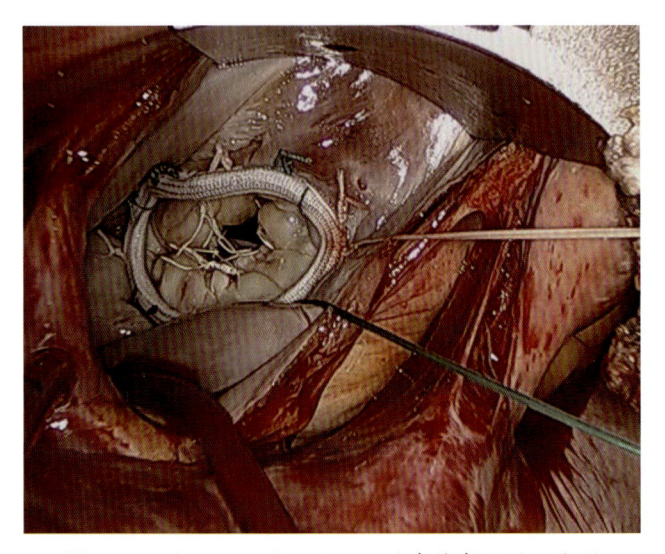

图 16.2 使用人工瓣环和人工腱索修复后的二尖瓣

如果二尖瓣病变范围过大，无法进行修复，则应进行二尖瓣置换术，其原则与退行性病变的置换相同。关于机械瓣还是生物瓣在避免心内膜炎复发中更有优势，这方面一直存在争议[21-23]。有多项重要研究显示，使用机械瓣与生物瓣在感染复发率上没有差异[24-26]。因此，IE 的瓣膜选择原则与其他类型瓣膜手术大致相同。唯一需要特别考虑的是，如果患者存在神经系统并发症，可能无法安全抗凝，这种情况则须使用生物瓣。

参考文献

[1] Chambers HF, Bayer AS. Native-valve infective endocarditis. N Engl J Med, 2020, 383(6): 567–576. https://doi.org/10.1056/NEJMcp2000400.

[2] Hoen B, Duval X. Infective endocarditis. N Engl J Med, 2013, 368(15): 1425–1433. https://doi.org/10.1056/NEJMcp1206782.

[3] Murdoch DR. Clinical presentation, etiology, and outcome of infective endocarditis in the 21st century. Arch Intern Med, 2009, 169(5): 463. https://doi.org/10.1001/archinternmed.2008.603.

[4] Mostaghim AS, Lo HYA, Khardori N. A retrospective epidemiologic study to define risk factors,

[5] Vincent LL, Otto CM. Infective endocarditis: update on epidemiology, outcomes, and management. Curr Cardiol Rep, 2018, 20(10). https://doi.org/10.1007/s11886-018-1043-2.

[6] Silverman M, Slater J, Jandoc R, et al. Hydromorphone and the risk of infective endocarditis among people who inject drugs: a population-based, retrospective cohort study. Lancet Infect Dis, 2020, 20(4): 487–497. https://doi.org/10.1016/S1473-3099(19)30705-4.

[7] Bates MC, Annie F, Jha A, et al. Increasing incidence of IV-drug use associated endocarditis in southern West Virginia and potential economic impact. Clin Cardiol, 2019, 42(4): 432–437. https://doi.org/10.1002/clc.23162.

[8] Pressman GS, et al. Mitral annular calcification as a possible nidus for endocarditis: a descriptive series with bacteriological differences noted. J Am Soc Echocardiogr, 2017, 30(6): 572–578. https://doi.org/10.1016/j.echo.2017.01.016.

[9] Pettersson GB, et al. Infective endocarditis: an atlas of disease progression for describing, staging, coding, and understanding the pathology. J Thorac Cardiovasc Surg, 2014, 147(4). https://doi.org/10.1016/j.jtcvs.2013.11.031.

[10] Pettersson GB, Hussain ST. Current AATS guidelines on surgical treatment of infective endocarditis. Ann Cardiothorac Surg, 2019, 8(6): 630–644. https://doi.org/10.21037/acs.2019.10.05.

[11] Miyatake K, et al. Diagnosis of mitral valve perforation by real-time two-dimensional Doppler flow imaging technique. J Am Coll Cardiol, 1986, 8(5): 1235–1239. https://doi.org/10.1016/S0735-1097(86)80407-7.

[12] Yuan XC, et al. Diagnosis of infective endocarditis using echocardiography. Medicine, 2019, 98: 38. https://doi.org/10.1097/MD.0000000000017141.

[13] Kang DH, et al. Early surgery versus conventional treatment for infective endocarditis. N Engl J Med, 2012, 366(26): 2466–2473. https://doi.org/10.1056/NEJMoa1112843.

[14] Hendren WG, et al. Mitral valve repair for bacterial endocarditis. J Thorac Cardiovasc Surg, 1992, 103(1): 124–129. https://doi.org/10.1016/s0022-5223(19)35074-3.

[15] Harky A, Hof A, Garner M, et al. Mitral valve repair or replacement in native valve endocarditis? Systematic review and meta-analysis. J Card Surg, 2018, 33(7): 364–371. https://doi.org/10.1111/jocs.13728.

[16] Lee HA, et al. Nationwide cohort study of mitral valve repair versus replacement for infective endocarditis. J Thorac Cardiovasc Surg, 2018, 156(4): 1473–1483.e2. https://doi.org/10.1016/j.jtcvs.2018.04.064.

[17] Tepsuwan T, et al. Comparison between mitral valve repair and replacement in active infective endocarditis. Gen Thorac Cardiovasc Surg, 2019, 67(12): 1030–1037. https://doi.org/10.1007/s11748-019-01132-4.

[18] Perrotta S, Fröjd V, Lepore V, et al. Surgical treatment for isolated mitral valve endocarditis: a 16-year single-centre experience. Eur J Cardio-thoracic Surg, 2018, 53(3): 576–581. https://doi.org/10.1093/ejcts/ezx416.

[19] Toyoda N, et al. Real-world outcomes of surgery for native mitral valve endocarditis. J Thorac Cardiovasc Surg, 2017, 154(6): 1906e9–1912e9. https://doi.org/10.1016/j.jtcvs.2017.07.077.

[20] Hussain ST, Blackstone EH, Pettersson GB. Tell it like it is: experience in mitral valve surgery does matter for improved outcomes in mitral valve infective endocarditis. J Thorac Cardiovasc Surg, 2017, 154(6): 1904e1–1905e1. https://doi.org/10.1016/j.jtcvs.2017.09.036.

[21] Reul GJ, Sweeney MS. Bioprosthetic versus mechanical valve replacement in patients with infective endocarditis. J Card Surg, 1989, 4(4): 348–351. https://doi.org/10.1111/j.1540-8191.1989.tb00302.x.

[22] Cohn LH. Valve replacement for infective endocarditis: an overview. J Card Surg, 1989, 4(4): 321–323. https://doi.org/10.1111/j.1540-8191.1989.tb00298.x.

[23] Agnihotri AK, McGiffin DC, Galbraith AJ, et al. The prevalence of infective endocarditis after

aortic valve replacement. J Thorac Cardiovasc Surg, 1995, 110(6): 1708–1724. https://doi.org/10.1016/S0022-5223(95)70035-8.

[24] Flynn CD, et al. Systematic review and meta-analysis of surgical outcomes comparing mechanical valve replacement and bioprosthetic valve replacement in infective endocarditis. Ann Cardiothorac Surg, 2019, 8(6): 587–599. https://doi.org/10.21037/acs.2019.10.03.

[25] Moon MR, et al. Treatment of endocarditis with valve replacement: the question of tissue versus mechanical prosthesis. Ann Thorac Surg, 2001: 1164–1171.

[26] Toyoda N, Itagaki S, Tannous H, et al. Bioprosthetic versus mechanical valve replacement for infective endocarditis: focus on recurrence rates. Ann Thorac Surg, 2018, 106(1): 99–106. https://doi.org/10.1016/j.athoracsur.2017.12.046.

第 17 章
自体主动脉瓣心内膜炎的外科治疗

Silvia Solari[1], *Laurent de Kerchove*[1,2]

[1]Division of Cardiothoracic and Vascular Surgery, Cliniques Universitaires Saint-Luc, Brussels, Belgium; [2]Pôle de Recherche Cardiovasculaire, Institut de Recherche Expérimentale et Clinique (IREC), Université Catholique de Louvain, Brussels, Belgium

引 言

心脏瓣膜感染是一种非常罕见的病理现象，其在正常人群的年发病率为（3~10）/10 万，死亡率为 15%~30%（根据不同的临床情况和感染病原体而有所不同）[1-2]。因此这种病症仍然是一种危及生命的疾病，同时也会导致显著的并发症发生率。

随着在感染性心内膜炎（IE）诊治方面取得的巨大进步，近几十年来 IE 的流行病学特征发生了变化，EURO-ENDO 登记处的数据也显示了这一点。EURO-ENDO 研究者 2019 年发表的论文数据显示[3]，现今 IE 更多地影响着自身有共病的老年患者（主要是 > 60 岁的男性）。人工瓣膜 IE、心内装置相关 IE、医源性感染、葡萄球菌和肠球菌性心内膜炎的发病率也越来越高。

此外，口腔链球菌性心内膜炎不常见。即便自 2009 年和 2015 年限制预防性使用抗生素的适应证实施以来，其发病率也并未增加。这些因素帮助我们勾勒出 IE 病患的总体概况。

心内膜炎团队

2015 年的指南强烈建议医院成立"心内膜炎团队"来管理这一复杂的病症[4]。该小组由心脏外科医生、心脏内科医生、麻醉医生、感染科医生、微生物学家组成，必要时，可邀请瓣膜病专家、先天性心脏病专家、电生理专家、超声心动图和其他心脏成像技术专家、神经内科医生、神经外科医生和神经介入放射科医生加入。该团队除了在院内对患者进行诊疗外，还应根据最新的指南建议组织正确的评估和随访，并参与患者教育计划。正如 Davierwala 及其同事在 2019 年发表的论文中所述，组建心内膜炎团队有助于早期诊断、实施综合治疗策略，并做出适当的决策，在降低该病的高并发症发生率和死亡率方面发挥重要作用[5]。

手术时机

据估计，约半数 IE 患者需要接受手术治疗，以防出现如心力衰竭、无法控制的感染和栓塞等严重的并发症[6]。因此，所有美国和欧洲的指南都一致认为在患者有手术指征时应尽早进行手术[4,7-8]。

早期手术指的是"在初次住院治疗期间，抗生素疗程结束之前"进行手术[7]。对于可能引起心力衰竭的瓣膜功能不全、多重耐药微生物感染（金黄色葡萄球菌、真菌或其他），以及并发脓肿、心脏传导阻滞或深层结构破坏，在适当的抗生素治疗后持续菌血症和（或）发热超过 5~7 d 的患者，均应尽早手术。早期手术的其他适应证还有赘生物 > 1 cm 和反复器官栓塞。对于赘生物较大且不稳定的个别病例，应考虑进行急诊手术（48 h 内）。如果患者出现心源性休克，也应进行急诊手术（24 h 内）[4]。

虽然对上述病例的处理所给出的建议非常直接，但还存在一些棘手的情况需要心内膜炎团队协商处理。这包括那些有症状的神经系统并发症，占所有 IE 的 15%~30%，其他无症状的并发症更常见。心内膜炎团队应该如何处理这些情况呢？关于并发卒中的最佳心脏手术时机尚未达成共识，但最近的研究大多倾向于在条件允许的情况下尽早手术。如果通过影像学检查和临床评估排除了明显的脑出血，且神经系统功能未受严重损害，则无须推迟手术。这种情况下，心血管手术相关神经系统并发症风险较低（3%~6%），术后神经系统完全康复的可能性很大[9-10]。相反，如果患者合并颅内出血且神经系统预后较差，手术最好推迟 2~4 周进行[11-12]。

手术治疗计划

术前对病变瓣膜的分析和评估是选择最佳术式的重要环节。经食管超声心动图（TEE）评估除为心内膜炎团队确定最佳的手术时机外，还能为手术方式提供相关信息，准确识别瓣膜赘生物、瓣周受累情况，揭示自体瓣膜的退行性和先天性病变[如钙化、二叶主动脉瓣（BAV）]。遗憾的是，有文献报道，术前超声心动图评估对 IE 脓肿的检出灵敏度仅为 80.5%[13]。对于外科医生来说，脓肿的存在是一个棘手但又常见的情况。事实上，在我们的经验中，在 43.9% 的自体瓣膜 IE 术中发现了脓肿，如果是人工瓣膜 IE，这一比例更是高达 65.2%[14]。

因此，我们对瓣膜解剖结构的最终评估以及恰当手术方法的选择，必须要在术中对病变瓣膜彻底探查后才能做出。

手术技术

瓣膜评估和手术清创

通常，主动脉瓣手术可通过胸骨正中切口入路，但对于感染明显局限于主动脉瓣叶的简单 IE 病例也可采用胸骨小切口入路。仔细评估主动脉瓣和病变范围至关重要。病变破坏的全部范围一般只有在仔细清创后才会显现出来。原则上，如果考虑对主动脉瓣进行修复，则在切除感染组织时就应注意保留所有健康的瓣膜和主动脉壁组织。对局限于瓣叶的感染，则重点评估瓣叶缺损的大小、受累瓣叶的数量以及残留组织的质量，穿孔部位可能非常明显，也可能会被赘生物遮挡。

单纯瓣膜受累的 IE

在过去的 30 年中，主动脉瓣修复技术已被广泛应用于临床并取得了良好的中长期疗效[15-16]。在一些心脏专科中心，这一技术已经有选择地用于主动脉瓣感染的病例[15,17-18]。这类病患多为年轻人，病变局限，为避免人工材料的植入和机械瓣或生物瓣置换的长期并发症而使用这一技术。

瓣膜修复技术使用与否取决于病变的位置和剩余瓣叶组织的质和量。在 IE 病例中，瓣叶穿孔是最常见的发现；即使没有穿孔，当完全切除赘生物后也会造成类似穿孔的瓣叶缺损。理想情况下，为了便于瓣叶修复，清创过程中应保留缺损的实性边缘，尤其是应尽可能保留瓣叶游离缘的完整性。在对缺损边缘彻底清创的同时，尽可能保留健康组织，以便缝合补片。如果缺损很小（<3~4 mm）则可直接缝合。极少数情况下，赘生物切除后瓣叶几乎完整保留，此时可能除了需要进行瓣环成形外不需要其他修复方式。当穿孔较大时，技术上添加补片是唯一可行的修复方案。正如我们团队以前所描述的[19]，使用补片技术修复瓣叶穿孔是将补片修剪成与瓣叶缺损相似的形状，并将其尺寸额外增加 2 mm 以避免补片缝合植入后出现瓣叶受牵拉收缩变形的问题。如图 17.1 所示，使用 5-0 或 6-0 Prolene 缝线连续缝合，将补片固定在瓣叶的主动脉侧。

补片的大小至关重要。事实上，过小的补片可能会牵拉瓣叶并导致继发性主动脉瓣反流，过大的补片则会在瓣膜下心室侧鼓起，增加瓣叶和缝线的应力。根据我们的经验，不同类型的心包补片（如异种心包、新鲜或戊二醛处理的自体心包）用于修复，这些补片在修复耐久性方面没有明显差异[19]。自 2015 年起，继自体心包补片之后，我们使用了脱细胞异种心包补片。与上一代异种心包补片相比，这种材料的组织重塑效果更好，钙化变性更少[20]。根据我们采用补片技术修复主动脉瓣的经验，其院内及长期生存率与接受瓣膜置换患者基本一致[17]。此外，基于修复术良好的生存率以及无再次感染，其他相关文献也主张有选择地使用修复手术[21-22]。

补片修复技术也可用于纠正瓣叶交界处的缺损或涉及瓣叶游离缘的缺损[23]。然而，补片修复技术在这些病变中的应用更为复杂。因为它们不仅需要精确地重建瓣叶游离缘，且长期稳定性也未得到充分验证。由于补片材料可能随着时间的推移发生重塑，导致新游离缘发生收缩，存在诱发主动脉瓣反流的风险。因此，一些专家建议，累及游离缘的病变应避免使用补片重建瓣叶[24]。此外，如果单个瓣叶完全损毁或两个以上的瓣叶发生穿孔，则不推荐在 IE 治疗中使用瓣膜修复手

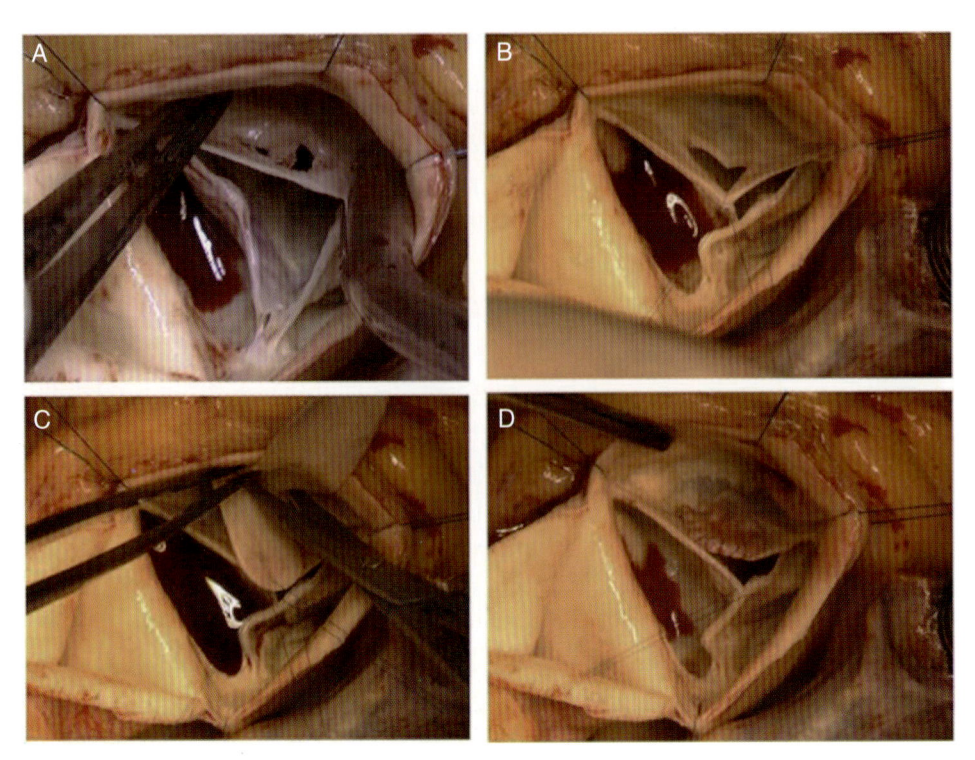

图17.1 单瓣叶受累的局限性感染性心内膜炎。A.右冠瓣受累的心内膜炎（穿孔）。B.彻底清创后对瓣膜进行评估，以选择更好的手术技术。C.修剪补片，使其形状与目前的缺损相似。D.连续缝合固定补片

术。瓣叶修补术后，为了增加瓣膜的对合面，部分病例推荐使用瓣环成形技术。对慢性主动脉瓣反流，由于瓣环扩大，建议施行瓣环成形术以提高修复的耐久性[16,25-26]。但对IE引起的急性主动脉瓣反流，主动脉瓣环大小多半正常，一般无须处理瓣环。对于活动性IE，如果瓣叶修复后瓣叶缺少或完全没有中央对合面，则应进行瓣环成形。对这些病例，可使用心包扣而不是Teflon扣进行2～3个瓣柱交界的Cabrol瓣环环缩（也称为交界下瓣环成形）[27]，以避免使用假体材料。对于需要手术治疗主动脉瓣反流的IE痊愈患者，如果瓣环扩张（>26mm），可以考虑行全瓣环成形术（即外置瓣环或保留主动脉瓣的再植术）。

对于涉及BAV的活动性IE，经验提示，瓣膜修复并非长久之计[19,21]（图17.2）。实际上，感染性病变和BAV特异性病变（融合瓣脱垂、融合嵴纤维化或钙化、瓣环扩张、升主动脉血管病变）相结合，使修复手术变得非常复杂。

此外，尽管对于IE行主动脉瓣修复的优势之一是避免使用假体材料，但事实上，大多数BAV修复术都需要植入假体材料（即人工成形环、保留瓣膜的再植术或单纯窦置换术）来稳定修复效果，有时还需要治疗主动脉病变[28]。

基于上述原因，目前瓣膜置换术是我们治疗BAV IE的唯一选择。

对于瓣叶损坏严重，或IE发生在钙化的主动脉瓣上，则必须进行机械瓣或生物瓣置换（图17.3）。现有文献显示，只要在彻底清除感染组织后进行置换，机

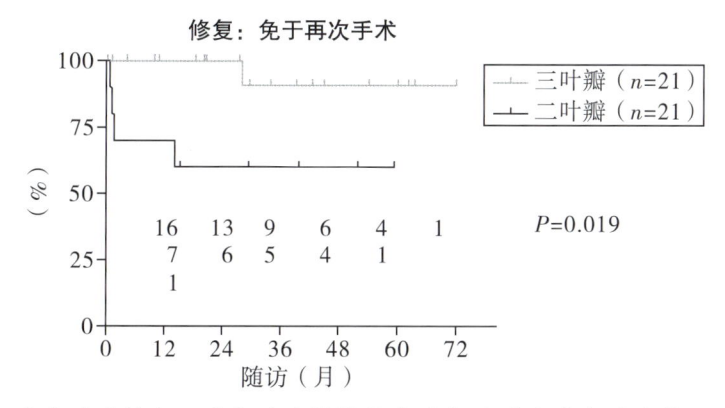

图 17.2 三叶主动脉瓣和二叶主动脉瓣修复术后免于再次手术的比较。Credits Mayer K, Aicher D, Feldner S, et al. Repair versus replacement of the aortic valve in active infective endocarditis. Eur J Cardio thoracic Surg, 2012, 42(1): 122–127. https://doi.org/10.1093/ejcts/ezr276, Figure number 5, page 125, Oxford University Press.

械瓣或生物瓣在再感染或存活率方面并没有明显差异[29-31]。

当前的临床指南并没有给出选择人工瓣膜的统一方案。在选择合适的人工瓣膜时，应权衡抗凝并发症的风险和因瓣膜结构破坏而再次手术的风险，同时考虑患者的生活方式和个人偏好，以及感染的受累范围。

瓣环受累的 IE

当感染蔓延至主动脉瓣环及其周围组织时（即瓣周脓肿或瓣环脓肿），保留原有主动脉瓣结构几乎不可能。在此情况下，一般需要主动脉瓣置换，必要时结合主动脉瓣环重建和主动脉根部置换。

对感染或坏死组织的手术清创必须彻底，可能情况下应整体清除（图17.4）。创面使用大量生理盐水冲洗干净，并在脓肿部位涂抹稀释的聚维酮碘。使用心包补片重建主动脉瓣环、二尖瓣-主动脉瓣连接处，最后重建左、右心室壁。

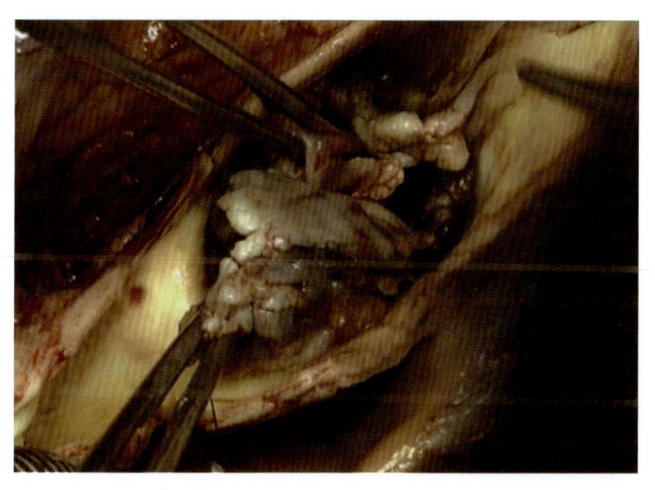

图 17.3 巨大赘生物累及所有主动脉瓣叶，但无瓣周脓肿

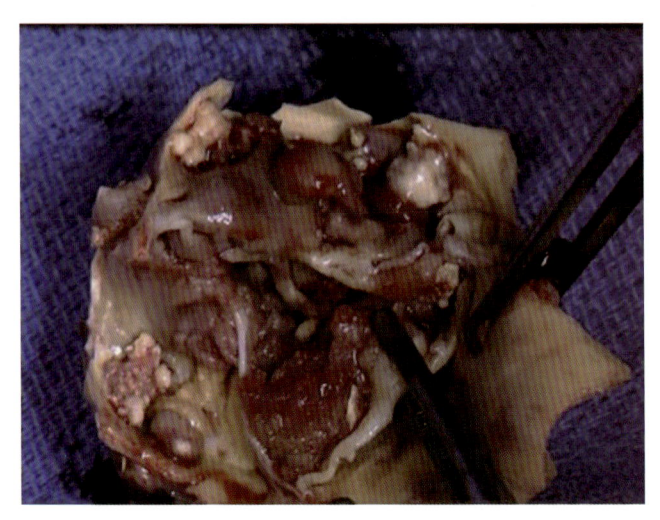

图 17.4 主动脉瓣、主动脉根部和心室 – 主动脉连接整体切除，进行瓣周脓肿清创

在极少数情况下，如果出现二尖瓣 – 主动脉瓣连接处的孤立性穿孔，可以用补片缝合，如果主动脉瓣结构是正常的，则保留主动脉瓣。如果主动脉瓣环脓肿较小并伴有瓣膜破坏或钙化，可在清创后使用心包补片修复主动脉瓣环，并在补片上安装机械瓣或生物膜。如果在清创过程中不得不切除主动脉根部血管，则必须进行根部置换手术。

对于根部病变，多个医疗中心推荐使用 Freestyle 生物瓣（Medtronic inc., Minneapolis, Mn），该瓣膜采用主动脉瓣和主动脉根部整体生物学设计，仅附带极少量的假体材料，特别适用于不同类型的主动脉根部损毁性心内膜炎病变。Heinz 等的研究[32]表明，这种无支架的生物瓣膜即使在 60 岁以下的患者中也展现出良好的耐久性[33]。

除以上使用的人工机械瓣和生物瓣以外，对于主动脉根部局部蔓延的心内膜炎，尤其是二尖瓣 – 主动脉瓣连接处受累和存在根部脓肿的病例，专家意见以及许多中心（包括我们机构）标准化的治疗策略就是使用同种异体移植物，而非其他人工瓣膜行根部置换[14,30,34]。

事实上，与有支架瓣膜相比，同种瓣更容易植入炎症严重且质地脆弱的组织中，并且同种瓣随带的二尖瓣前瓣叶可用于重建因脓肿受损的二尖瓣－主动脉瓣连接，使修复变得更为简单[35]（图 17.5）。

尽管主动脉瓣同种异体移植技术的复杂性和随着时间推移结构退化的风险限制了其应用，但根据我们的经验，在急性 IE 中使用同种主动脉瓣，感染复发的风险非常低，长期存活率也令人满意。然而，值得注意的是，接受该技术的患者 10 年后因瓣膜结构退化而需再次手术的风险显著上升，特别是对于年轻的患者。我们认为，对于这部分患者，Ross 手术是一个备选方案，因为它不仅可以提供同种瓣相同的抗感染复发能力，还具有更好的耐久性。

遗憾的是，在组织损伤和瓣环破坏严重的情况下，我们不建议采用这种手术，

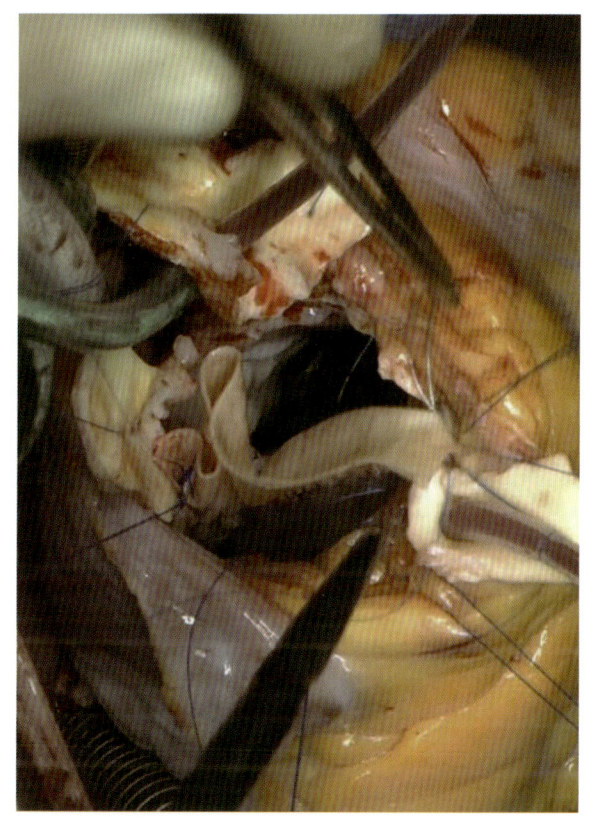

图 17.5　同种瓣植入左心室流出道

因为此类病例根部严重损毁导致局部缺乏解剖学支持，可能会导致自体肺动脉瓣因心室 - 主动脉交界处的早期扩张而出现瓣膜反流。

总　结

自体瓣膜心内膜炎的手术指征和时机是由多学科团队根据患者病情做出的个性化决策。在保留正常组织的前提下进行细致而彻底的清创是最佳手术治疗的先决条件。手术技术要根据感染病灶的范围和位置进行调整。瓣膜病变局限的年轻患者可以从瓣膜修复术中获益。

参考文献

[1] García-Cabrera E, Fernández-Hidalgo N, Almirante B, et al. Neurological complications of infective endocarditis risk factors, outcome, and impact of cardiac surgery: a multicenter observational study. Circulation, 2013, 127(23): 2272–2284. https://doi.org/10.1161/CIRCULATIONAHA.112.000813.

[2] Leone S, Ravasio V, Durante-Mangoni E, et al. Epidemiology, characteristics, and outcome of infective endocarditis in Italy: the Italian study on endocarditis. Infection, 2012, 40(5): 527–535. https://doi.org/10.1007/s15010-012-0285-y.

[3] Habib G, Erba PA, Iung B, et al. Clinical presentation, aetiology and outcome of infective endocarditis. Results of the ESC-EORP EURO-ENDO (European infective endocarditis) registry: a

prospective cohort study. Eur Heart J, 2019, 40(39): 3222–3232B. https://doi.org/10.1093/eurheartj/ehz620.

[4] Medicine N, Task A, Members F, et al. 2015 ESC guidelines for the management of infective endocarditis. Eur Heart J, 2015, 36. https://doi.org/10.1093/eurheartj/ehv319.

[5] Davierwala PM, Marin-Cuartas M, Misfeld M, et al. The value of an "endocarditis team". Ann Cardiothorac Surg, 2019, 8(6): 621–629. https://doi.org/10.3978/16659.

[6] Naber CK, Erbel R, Baddour LM, et al. New guidelines for infective endocarditis: a call for collaborative research. Int J Antimicrob Agents, 2007, 29(6): 615–616. https://doi.org/10.1016/j.ijantimicag.2007.01.016.

[7] Nishimura RA, Otto CM, Bonow RO, et al. 2014 AHA/ACC guideline for the management of patients with valvular heart disease: executive summary: a report of the American College of Cardiology/American Heart Association task force on practice guidelines. J Am Coll Cardiol, 2014, 129(23): e521–e643. https://doi.org/10.1016/j.jacc.2014.02.537.

[8] Pettersson GB, Hussain ST. Current AATS guidelines on surgical treatment of infective endocarditis. Ann Cardiothorac Surg, 2019, 8(6): 630–644. https://doi.org/10.3978/16669.

[9] Ruttmann E, Willeit J, Ulmer H, et al. Neurological outcome of septic cardioembolic stroke after infective endocarditis. Stroke, 2006, 37(8): 2094–2099. https://doi.org/10.1161/01.STR.0000229894.28591.3f.

[10] Thuny F, Avierinos J-F, Tribouilloy C, et al. Impact of cerebrovascular complications on mortality and neurologic outcome during infective endocarditis: a prospective multicentre study. Eur Heart J, 2007, 28(9): 1155–1161. https://doi.org/10.1093/eurheartj/ehm005.

[11] Yoshioka D, Sakaguchi T, Yamauchi T, et al. Impact of early surgical treatment on postoperative neurologic outcome for active infective endocarditis complicated by cerebral infarction//The Society of Thoracic Surgeons, Southern Thoracic Surgical Association. Annals of thoracic surgery. NEW YORK: Elsevier, 2012: 489–496. https://doi.org/10.1016/j.athoracsur.2012.04.027.

[12] Wilbring M, Irmscher L, Alexiou K, et al. The impact of preoperative neurological events in patients suffering from native infective valve endocarditis. Interact Cardiovasc Thorac Surg, 2014, 18(6): 740–747. https://doi.org/10.1093/icvts/ivu039.

[13] Aguado JM. Perivalvular abscesses associated with endocarditis. Clinical features and diagnostic accuracy of two-dimensional echocardiography. Chest J, 1993, 104(1): 88. https://doi.org/10.1378/chest.104.1.88.

[14] Solari S, Mastrobuoni S, De Kerchove L, et al. Over 20 years experience with aortic homograft in aortic valve replacement during acute infective endocarditis. Eur J Cardio Thorac Surg, 2016, 73: ezw175. https://doi.org/10.1093/ejcts/ezw175.

[15] Boodhwani M, de Kerchove L, Glineur D, et al. Repair-oriented classification of aortic insufficiency: impact on surgical techniques and clinical outcomes. J Thorac Cardiovasc Surg, 2009, 137(2): 286–294. https://doi.org/10.1016/j.jtcvs.2008.08.054.

[16] Lansac E, Di Centa I, Sleilaty G, et al. Long-term results of external aortic ring annuloplasty for aortic valve repair. Eur J Cardio thoracic Surg, 2016, 50(2): 350–360. https://doi.org/10.1093/ejcts/ezw070.

[17] Solari S, Tamer S, Aphram G, et al. Aortic valve repair in endocarditis: scope and results. Indian J Thorac Cardiovasc Surg, 2020, 36(1): 104–112. https://doi.org/10.1007/s12055-019-00831-0.

[18] Boodhwani M, El Khoury G. Aortic valve repair: indications and outcomes. Curr Cardiol Rep, 2014, 16(6): 490. https://doi.org/10.1007/s11886-014-0490-7.

[19] Nezhad ZM, De Kerchove L, Hechadi J, et al. Aortic valve repair with patch in non-rheumatic disease: indication, techniques and durability. Eur J Cardio thoracic Surg, 2014, 46(6): 997–1005. https://doi.org/10.1093/ejcts/ezu058.

[20] Bell D, Prabhu S, Betts K, et al. Durability of tissue-engineered bovine pericardium (CardioCel) for a minimum of 24 months when used for the repair of congenital heart defects. Interact Cardiovasc Thorac Surg, 2018: 1–7. https://doi.org/10.1093/icvts/ivy246.

[21] Mayer K, Aicher D, Feldner S, et al. Repair versus replacement of the aortic valve in active infective

endocarditis. Eur J Cardio thoracic Surg, 2012, 42(1): 122–127. https://doi.org/10.1093/ejcts/ezr276.

[22] Zhao D, Zhang B. Are valve repairs associated with better outcomes than replacements in patients with native active valve endocarditis? Interact Cardiovasc Thorac Surg, 2014, 19(6): 1036–1039. https://doi.org/10.1093/icvts/ivu296.

[23] Vohra HA, Dekerchove L, Rubay J, et al. A simple technique of commissural reconstruction in aortic valve-sparing surgery. J Thorac Cardiovasc Surg, 2013, 145(3): 882–886. https://doi.org/10.1016/j.jtcvs.2012.11.021.

[24] Schäfers HJ. The 10 commandments for aortic valve repair. Innovat Tech Tech CardioThorac Vasc Surg, 2019, 14(3): 188–198. https://doi.org/10.1177/1556984519843909.

[25] Arabkhani B, Mookhoek A, Di Centa I, et al. Reported outcome after valve-sparing aortic root replacement for aortic root aneurysm: a systematic review and meta-analysis. Ann Thorac Surg, 2015, 100(3): 1126–1131. https://doi.org/10.1016/j.athoracsur.2015.05.093.

[26] de Kerchove L, El Khoury G. Anatomy and pathophysiology of the ventriculoaortic junction: implication in aortic valve repair surgery. Ann Cardiothorac Surg, 2013, 2(1): 57–64. https://doi.org/10.3978/j.issn.2225-319X.2012.12.05.

[27] Cabrol C, Cabrol A, Guiraudon G, et al. Treatment of aortic insufficiency by means of aortic annuloplasty. Arch des Mal du coeur des Vaiss, 1966, 59(9): 1305–1312.

[28] De Kerchove L, Boodhwani M, Glineur D, et al. Valve sparing-root replacement with the reimplantation technique to increase the durability of bicuspid aortic valve repair. J Thorac Cardiovasc Surg, 2011, 142(6): 1430–1438. https://doi.org/10.1016/j.jtcvs.2011.08.021.

[29] Jassar AS, Bavaria JE, Szeto WY, et al. Graft selection for aortic root replacement in complex active endocarditis: does it matter? Ann Thorac Surg, 2012, 93(2): 480–487. https://doi.org/10.1016/j.athoracsur.2011.09.074.

[30] Klieverik LM a, Yacoub MH, Edwards S, et al. Surgical treatment of active native aortic valve endocarditis with allografts and mechanical prostheses. Ann Thorac Surg, 2009, 88(6): 1814–1821. https://doi.org/10.1016/j.athoracsur.2009.08.019.

[31] Toyoda N, Itagaki S, Tannous H, et al. Bioprosthetic versus mechanical valve replacement for infective endocarditis: focus on recurrence 326 rates. Ann Thorac Surg, 2018, 106(1): 99–106. https://doi.org/10.1016/j.athoracsur.2017.12.046.

[32] Heinz A, Dumfarth J, Ruttmann-Ulmer E, et al. Freestyle root replacement for complex destructive aortic valve endocarditis. J Thorac Cardiovasc Surg, 2014, 147(4): 1265–1270. https://doi.org/10.1016/j.jtcvs.2013.05.014.

[33] Christ T, Grubitzsch H, Claus B, et al. Stentless aortic valve replacement in the young patient: long-term results. J Cardiothorac Surg, 2013, 8(1): 1–7. https://doi.org/10.1186/1749-8090-8-68.

[34] Musci M, Weng Y, Hübler M, et al. Homograft aortic root replacement in native or prosthetic active infective endocarditis: twenty-year single-center experience. J Thorac Cardiovasc Surg, 2010, 139(3): 665–673. https://doi.org/10.1016/j.jtcvs.2009.07.026.

[35] David TE, Gavra G, Feindel CM, et al. Surgical treatment of active infective endocarditis: a continued challenge. J Thorac Cardiovasc Surg, 2007, 133(1): 144–149. https://doi.org/10.1016/j.jtcvs.2006.08.060.

第18章
主动脉根部脓肿的外科治疗

Tyler J. Wallen[1], George J. Arnaoutakis[2]

[1]Division of Thoracic and Cardiac Surgery, Geisinger Health System, Wilkes-Barre, PA, United States; [2]Division of Thoracic and Cardiovascular Surgery, University of Florida, Gainesville, FL, United States

引 言

感染性心内膜炎（IE）可引起多种临床和解剖并发症，其中包括主动脉根部脓肿。主动脉根部脓肿的定义是主动脉根部、瓣环出现感染坏死组织，乃至出现主动脉－左心室的分离。本章将讨论心内膜炎并发主动脉根部脓肿的临床表现、诊断和手术治疗。

临床表现和诊断

心内膜炎的确诊是基于临床症状、超声心动图和微生物学检查结果的综合分析。大多数临床医生在诊断心内膜炎时都采用 Durack 等人提出的改良 Duke 标准。据报道该标准诊断的灵敏度和特异性均超过 80%[1]。

主要标准包括（但不限于）血培养阳性、超声心动图发现新的心脏瓣膜赘生物或反流、心脏内活动性团块、人工瓣膜瓣周部分开裂以及脓肿。主动脉根部脓肿感染蔓延累及周围结构可导致一些症状，从而促发患者就诊。相关表现包括传导系统受累导致心律失常或心脏传导阻滞、冠状动脉受压导致急性冠脉综合征、假性动脉瘤形成导致胸痛和（或）邻近结构受压等。在极端情况下，脓肿会侵蚀邻近的心腔，形成心内瘘管。通常，如果出现血培养阳性合并上述超声心动图或影像学任何一项表现，就要考虑心脏手术的可能性。

据估计，多达 14% 的 IE 患者并发心内脓肿[2-3]。金黄色葡萄球菌是最常见的致病菌，约占 1/3，其他致病菌还包括嗜血杆菌、肠球菌、β－溶血性链球菌、拟杆菌等[4]。

经胸超声心动图（TTE）常作为疑似心内膜炎患者的首选诊断检查。然而，TTE 检出新发瓣膜赘生物的能力仅为 50%，相比之下，经食管超声心动图（TEE）对瓣膜赘生物的检出灵敏度可达 90%~100%（图 18.1）。如果将 TTE 和 TEE 结合，则可检出 90% 的心内膜炎患者的赘生物。此外，TEE 还是主动脉根部脓肿以及心

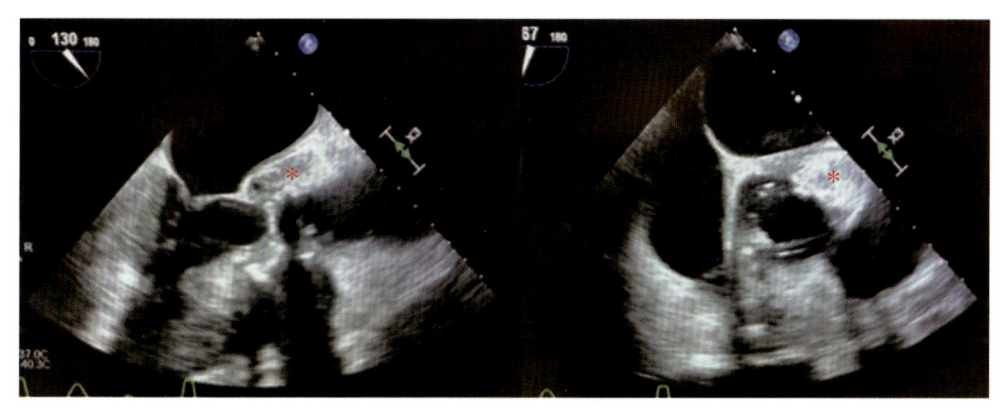

图 18.1　经胸超声心动图显示主动脉瓣心内膜炎伴主动脉根部脓肿。"*"表示脓肿区域

内瘘管和分流的首选诊断检查[5-6]。

临床上，我们建议对 IE 患者脑部、胸部、腹部和骨盆进行 CT 检查，以筛查可能存在的脑部、肺部和脾脏脓毒性栓子，并评估是否存在假性动脉瘤及其范围。通过 CT 还可详细勾勒出主动脉根部的解剖结构，为制定手术方案提供依据，例如对主动脉根部夹层假性动脉瘤的分析（图 18.2 和图 18.3）。

左心导管检查也有助于制定手术计划，如果超声心动图未发现主动脉瓣上较大的活动性赘生物，则可以安全地进行左心导管检查。

术前处理

针对心内膜炎并发主动脉根部脓肿，首先是要组建一个多学科团队，包括心脏内科、心脏外科、重症监护和感染科的临床专家，处理的核心包括根治感染（如血培养阴性）以及预防进一步的心脏损伤和全身并发症。

微生物学数据显示，约 80% 的主动脉根部脓肿的致病菌为葡萄球菌和链球菌。值得注意的是，在这些病原体中，金黄色葡萄球菌相关感染的发病率正在上升，而草绿色链球菌的发病率正在下降。在真菌性病原体中最常见的是白色念珠菌，其次是曲霉菌[4]。

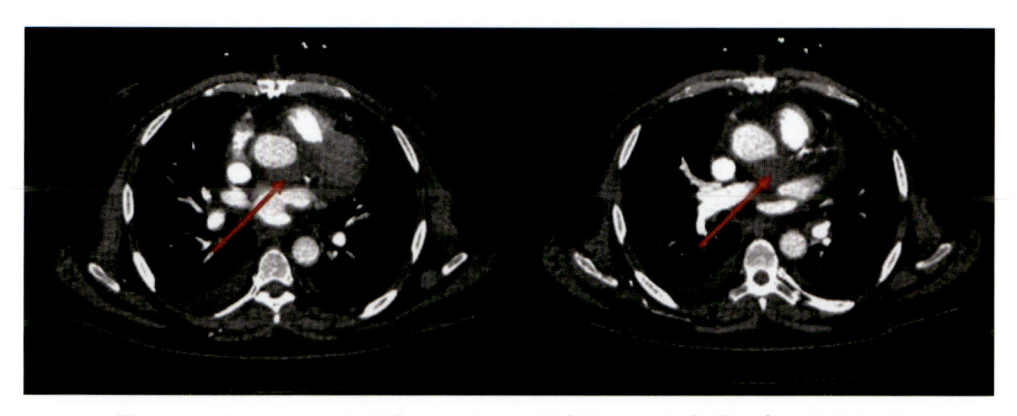

图 18.2　轴位 CT 扫描图像显示主动脉根部脓肿，红色箭头表示脓肿区域

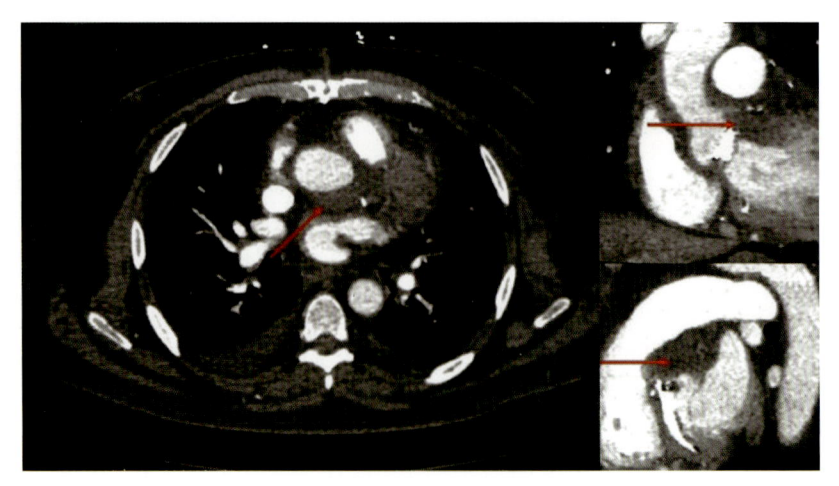

图 18.3 多平面 CT 扫描图像显示主动脉根部脓肿。红色箭头表示脓肿区域

一旦临床怀疑是 IE，就需要及时使用抗生素治疗。初始治疗应使用广谱抗生素，然后根据血培养和药敏情况进行调整。

手术指征

当感染在主动脉瓣周蔓延，表现为主动脉根部脓肿或瘘管时，即是早期手术的指征。其他指征包括充血性心力衰竭、持续性菌血症、脓毒性栓塞、心律失常等，这通常与新发的主动脉瓣和（或）二尖瓣反流或人工瓣膜瓣周裂和（或）卡瓣有关[7]。

全身性栓塞也是手术干预的一个指征，其中脑血管并发症，包括无症状的和短暂性脑缺血发作，都是栓塞表现的一部分。但如果是颅内出血，则发病 1 个月内相对禁忌手术，除非采取神经外科手术降低后续出血的风险。然而，对于病情危重的主动脉根部脓肿患者，应衡量等待手术与尽早手术的风险和获益，如果手术获益大于等待风险，则应早期手术[7-8]。

最后，持续性脓毒症，即在接受适当的抗生素治疗 5~7 d 后仍持续发热和（或）血培养阳性，是手术治疗的指征[7]。

少部分患者可以不进行手术治疗，包括脓肿<1 cm、无心脏传导阻滞、人工瓣膜瓣环无撕裂或无瓣膜关闭不全，以及那些在接受抗生素治疗期间病情没有进展的病例。如果采取非手术治疗，我们建议在发病后 2 周、4 周和 8 周复查超声心动图[9]。

外科手术原则

一旦决定手术治疗，针对主动脉根部脓肿，须遵循以下几项原则，以确保手术顺利。尽管主动脉根部脓肿没有"标准"的术式，但所有患者都应以同样的方式做好准备，包括在手术室进行详细完善的术中 TEE 检查。此外，考虑到很多患者先前接受过心脏手术，且该疾病本身进展过程中也易于形成组织粘连，因此对组织分离困难应做好充分准备。有时术中可能需要快速建立体外循环,针对这一状况,谨慎的做法是在锯开胸骨之前先期准备股动脉通路。双下肢进行消毒铺巾准备,以备需要桥血管进行冠状动脉旁路移植。

有多种安全再次开胸的技术方式。虽然外科医生可以根据各自喜好选择他们最熟悉的方式,但股动脉入路的重要性无论怎么强调都不为过。完成胸骨正中切开后,可使用主动脉插管和腔静脉二级插管建立标准体外循环,不过,对于这类复杂的根部手术,我们更倾向于使用上、下腔静脉插管。这一插管方式在右心房面严重粘连或右侧心脏存在瘘管口,需要打开右心房时尤为适用;其次,这种方式还能大大改善主动脉根部的暴露,尤其是在有广泛粘连的情况下。另外,主动脉根部脓肿往往伴有主动脉瓣关闭不全,经右上肺静脉放置左心室引流应为常规操作。

一旦体外循环开始,在心肌保护的问题上,我们倾向于先使用心脏停搏液逆行灌注,在主动脉切开后则经冠状动脉开口直接顺行灌注。鉴于这些复杂的根部或多瓣膜重建术体外循环和心肌缺血时间较长,通常全身降温至 30℃,以降低代谢,为心脏提供额外保护。

心脏停搏后,通常横断主动脉,暴露感染区域,探查受累范围。彻底探查在此非常重要,可评判根部所需重建范围。为达到良好的近远期修复效果,另一个需要坚持的原则就是彻底清除所有感染及坏死组织。清创结束后,我们常规使用浸泡过利福平的棉签擦拭主动脉瓣环和左心室,以对该区域进行消毒。

最后,在手术结束时,我们常规在纵隔感染区域放置冲洗管。术后 5~7d 使用抗生素溶液持续局部灌注冲洗,灌洗导管通常选用一根单腔 16 F 导管,去除管尖,置于纵隔内。导管由胸骨右侧第 2 或第 3 肋间隙穿过胸壁进入纵隔。虽然将利福平浸泡的棉签擦拭心脏和纵隔灌洗相结合的方式尚未被证实能改善预后,但我们发现它在实践中非常有用,尤其对革兰氏阳性菌感染。

瓣膜的选择

对于因心内膜炎并发主动脉根部脓肿而需要进行瓣膜置换和左心室流出道(LVOT)重建的患者,文献中并未明确显示哪种人工瓣膜最适合[10-11]。根据患者的年龄、共病和瓣环损毁的程度,如果能使用补片修复清创后组织缺损,同时采用机械瓣或生物瓣进行瓣膜置换,这可能是最佳选择。生物瓣或机械瓣带瓣管道、无支架异种瓣、同种主动脉瓣或自体肺动脉瓣对于部分病例也可能是合适的选择。很多研究都对这些选择的相关结果进行了阐述,并对相关结果进行了两两比较,但这些研究样本量较小,且多为单中心研究,因此,对这些数据的解读存在一定困难,解读结果也不一定准确。迄今为止,尚无令人信服的数据表明一种移植材料的选择比另一种在预防感染复发方面更有优势。Jassar 等在一项比较带瓣管道(生物瓣和机械瓣)与同种主动脉瓣的研究中指出,所选择的管道或瓣膜类型对院内或长期死亡率没有显著影响[12]。Avierinos 等在一项相似的研究中也得出了类似结论[13]。

每种人工材料都有相对的优缺点，后文将进一步讨论。

许多外科医生将保留二尖瓣前叶的同种主动脉瓣作为主动脉根部脓肿修复的标准选择。针对根部脓肿，同种主动脉瓣有较多优点：首先，其具有组织柔韧性，与因感染和清创而受损的主动脉根部组织有良好的契合性；其次，保留的二尖瓣前叶还可用于心内修复，如室间隔缺损和（或）瘘管的修补；最后，移植物的生物特性有助于预防早期再感染，并简化后期再感染的处理。

当然，同种瓣也存在以下缺点：首先，同种瓣本身的供应有限，且植入手术技术复杂，因此，这种手术多半都是在具备这一手术能力且有低温保存条件的部分中心进行；其次，同种瓣存在结构衰败的问题，其结果是瓣膜钙化和撕裂，这使得再次手术变得异常困难且充满风险。虽然经导管主动脉瓣置换术（TAVR）是退化的同种主动脉瓣置换方式的一种选择，但部分病例由于同种主动脉瓣管腔的严重钙化和狭窄，导致 TAVR 手术因解剖原因无法实施，以致高风险的开放式再次手术成为唯一选择。

有人将无支架异种瓣与同种主动脉瓣做过比较，没有确凿证据表明无支架瓣优于其他可选材料。然而，无支架主动脉瓣的优势在于可选择性大，尺寸及供应量都不受限制；另外，与同种主动脉瓣相比，具有相似的优异血流动力学性能和长期存活率。缺点与同种瓣类似，无支架瓣也会出现衰败，表现为明显的瓣膜钙化、撕裂以及严重的主动脉瓣关闭不全[14]。

目前，没有确凿证据表明一种瓣膜和（或）带瓣管道优于另一种，因此人工瓣膜选择主要取决于外科医生的偏好。对 IE 这类疾病进行主动脉根部置换术，无论是否进行瓣环重建，都是一项极具挑战性的手术。为安全起见，外科医生应选择自己最擅长的人工瓣膜，将围手术期的存活置于优先位置，而手术长期效果或再次手术的风险则是次要考虑。

补片选择

在主动脉根部脓肿手术过程中经常需要使用补片材料，常规都要准备好生物补片或合成补片。目前，可选用补片材料有多种，包括自体心包、戊二醛固定的马心包、主动脉根部同种血管壁、Dacron、自体腹直肌筋膜和牛心包。

我们倾向于使用戊二醛固定的牛心包来重建受感染的组织。这种方法可减少放置在感染区内的假体材料数量，且易于处理和修正，可用于不同情形和部位的重建。David 等认为这种方法具有良好的中长期效果[15]。然而，一些研究者对这种材料的长期耐久性表示担忧，其中一些人提到了晚期材料变性和相关的瓣周漏问题。其他研究者则认为 Dacron 是一种合适的材料，可获得良好的长期效果[16]。

与人工瓣膜的选择一样，目前没有确凿证据表明一种补片材料优于另一种，因此，外科医生应该选择自己熟悉的材料，以便于成功修复。

手术方法

单纯主动脉瓣置换术

一些中心已经报道了对主动脉根部脓肿实施单纯主动脉瓣置换术的结果。这些病例都经过严格筛选，脓腔多局限于单个主动脉瓣叶，没有扩展到邻近结构或心腔，瓣环可简单重建。脓肿造成的缺损可通过折叠缝合或使用心包补片修补。鉴于相关报道显示单纯主动脉瓣置换术的效果较差，我们倾向于对脓肿进行根部整体置换[17]。

双补片技术

双补片技术最早由 David 等描述，是一种用于治疗累及主动脉瓣、二尖瓣以及中心纤维三角（IFB）的手术方法[18]。现已被多个中心报道及改良，且给出了多个名称，包括"Commando 手术"和"UFO 手术"。

通常，这种方法采用标准的胸骨正中切口，上、下腔静脉插管，逆灌加冠状动脉开口直接顺行灌注心脏停搏液，同时全身降温至 32℃。心脏停搏后，横断主动脉，探查主动脉瓣，切除主动脉瓣，探查 IFB 是否受累。一旦确定 IFB 受累，则须行全主动脉根部置换。此时将主动脉切口向无冠瓣延伸，切开主动脉瓣瓣环，并将切口延至左心房房顶，除纽扣状保留冠状动脉开口外，彻底切除主动脉根部组织。一般情况下，在冠状动脉口周围保留 2~4 mm 的主动脉壁组织，用于冠状动脉开口再植。充分游离冠状动脉，保证冠脉开口吻合时不存在张力，这一点非常重要。接下来，暴露并切除二尖瓣连同 IFB，将任何肉眼可见感染受累的组织一并切除。IFB 的切除范围因疾病的程度而异，可能是仅限于二尖瓣前叶的中央部分，也可能是累及二尖瓣、IFB 和左心房房顶的整块组织。总之，必须清除所有感染组织和假体材料。

接下来就是二尖瓣人工瓣膜的植入。瓣膜的大小至关重要，因为过大的瓣膜会导致 LVOT 梗阻。如果以前植入过二尖瓣人工瓣膜，谨慎起见，只需植入相同大小的新瓣膜即可。如果以前未曾植入过瓣膜，可能情况下，在切除 IFB 之前做评估相对容易，能较为准确判断瓣膜的大小。理想的放置是，植入瓣膜缝合环的 2/3 缝在二尖瓣后瓣环。此外，还应注意瓣膜的方向，避免瓣柱突出到 LVOT。

然后使用"双舌状"牛心包补片重建 IFB，并将其缝合到新植入的二尖瓣环前 1/3 部。这一位置缝合进针应格外小心，以避免体外循环撤除后的严重出血。因为一旦心脏复跳，这类根部出血就很难显露、止血。然后将双舌后侧补片缝在左心房房顶开放部分，前侧补片固定在 LVOT 和主动脉壁的游离缘，以构建一个新的 IFB。如果只需要进行主动脉瓣置换，则可将部分补片用于缝闭主动脉切口；如果主动脉根部置换，则在主动脉瓣环上方几厘米处分割双舌补片，作为主动脉根部缝合瓣环的固定点。

同种主动脉瓣植入

如果进行主动脉根部置换，一些中心认为主动脉同种瓣是理想的选择，因为它不使用假体材料，保留了原有根部大部分组织，可以利用同种瓣整体结构包括二尖瓣前瓣叶完成 IFB 和二尖瓣的修复。首先是显露、插管和心肌保护，与上述步骤相同。清除所有感染组织后，再确定同种瓣的大小。确定瓣膜大小是一个关键步骤，应避免移植物过小，因为这会导致多种并发症，包括早期和晚期移植物衰败、感染、假性动脉瘤和瓣叶脱垂。测定主动脉瓣环的大小需要在清除所有感染组织后进行。我们一般使用 Hegar 探条来测定主动脉瓣环的内径，然后，选择一个直径与测量的主动脉瓣环大小基本相等的同种瓣。与非感染原发性主动脉瓣疾病的同种瓣植入有所不同，心内膜炎的主动脉瓣环通常无明显扩张，因此不需要进行主动脉瓣的瓣环环缩，可直接选择使用与测量的瓣环直径大致相等的同种瓣。

同种瓣的植入方式多种多样，但在主动脉根部脓肿的情况下，最常用的是主动脉根部整体置换。由于感染导致正常解剖标志丧失，使植入手术变得更为复杂。为了解决这一问题，可将同种瓣二尖瓣前瓣叶与患者的纤维三角和二尖瓣前瓣叶进行对齐定位。

在放置同种瓣之前，我们一般先期修剪 LVOT 边缘肌肉并在该结构周围使用一牛心包条加固。使用 3-0 Prolene 缝合线进行水平连续缝合固定，然后放置同种瓣并予以固定，这一过程中须确保 LVOT 没有受到过度的牵张或扭转。可使用 3-0 Prolene 连续缝合将同种瓣直接植入患者的 LVOT，或采用 3-0 Prolene 线水平间断褥式缝合或单纯间断缝合。然后常规植入冠状动脉纽扣，使用牛心包修复左心房顶缺损。

无支架主动脉瓣植入

虽然无支架主动脉瓣在植入技术上比传统的主动脉瓣置换更具挑战性，但无支架瓣膜，如 Freedom 人工瓣膜（LivaNova；Milan，Italy），在主动脉根部脓肿的修复时具有较多优点。

Freedom 人工瓣膜可以内面外翻地放置在 LVOT 内，这有利于显露及确切缝合瓣膜密封缝合线，并在必要时可植入较深位置。此外，该瓣膜没有人工纤维加固，有可能降低持续感染或再感染的发生率。然而，心内膜炎并发主动脉根部脓肿往往需要进行主动脉根部置换，这就限制了 Freedom 的使用。在这种情况下，可以使用猪的主动脉根部假体，如 Freestyle 瓣膜（Medtronic；Minneapolis，MN）。

常规使用 Hegar 探条确定选用 Freestyle 无支架瓣的大小。探条主要用于测量主动脉瓣瓣环直径，当然这一评估还应将主动脉根部的瘢痕组织和空间大小考虑在内。Freestyle 无支架瓣的优点是适用于狭小的空间，具有良好的血流动力学性能。因此瓣膜选择无须过大，通常选择比主动脉根部 Hegar 测定值大 2～3 mm 的假体即可。另外，Freestyle 测量器也可用于测量。

在瓣膜缝合方法上，一般使用 2-0 Ethibond 缝线进行单纯间断缝合以固定 Freestyle 瓣膜（图 18.4）。在瓣膜放置方向上，将 Freestyle 一个冠状动脉口直接对准患者的冠状动脉左主干。然后将瓣膜"落座"对位，在瓣膜缝合线之间放置一小条毛毡，形成主动脉根部缝合线的毛毡加固垫圈（图 18.5）。而后打结固定瓣膜，使用 4-0 或 5-0 Prolene 缝线连续缝合植入左冠状动脉纽扣开口。如果假体上的第二个冠状动脉开口与患者的右冠状动脉对位不佳，可用 3-0 Prolene 加固缝合无法使用的冠状动脉开口，并在假体适当位置使用 15 号手术刀做一新的圆孔，按照标准方式植入右冠状动脉纽扣开口。在冠脉处理过程中，必须充分游离两个冠状动脉开口，以便吻合后不存在牵拉张力，植入位置应适当，避免扭结，以防心脏复跳时影响舒张期冠状动脉的灌注。许多外科医生建议在右冠状动脉再植之前完成主动脉远端吻合，以便使心脏充盈、主动脉膨胀，以此选择一个适当的右冠状动脉植入位置。但这种方法的一个潜在缺点是，在做冠脉吻合口时难以观察猪瓣膜叶，有误伤瓣叶的可能，因此在操作过程中须格外小心。为防止这一并发症，可在进行主动脉吻合之前，在无支架瓣的外表面标记右冠瓣-无冠瓣交界的位置，这是右冠状动脉植入手术打孔时应避开的位置。

定制带瓣管道植入

主动脉根部置换中经常会用到个性化定制的生物瓣或机械瓣带瓣管道，多项

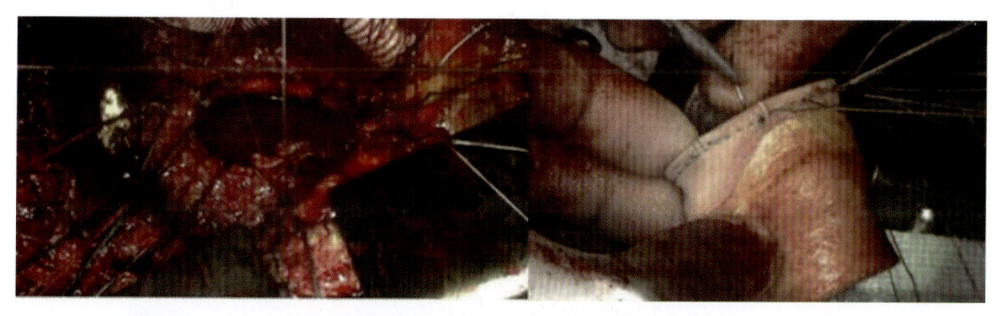

图 18.4 使用单纯间断的 2-0 Ethibond 缝合线植入 Freestyle 无支架瓣

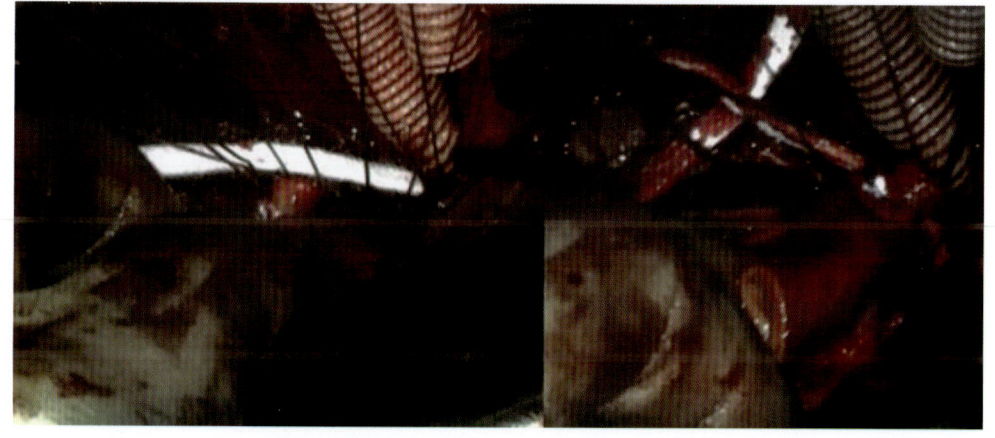

图 18.5 毛毡条放置在瓣膜缝合线之间，为主动脉根部缝合起到垫圈加固作用

研究已经证明这些带瓣管道适用于伴有主动脉根部脓肿的心内膜炎手术。值得注意的是，这些研究多是单中心经验，样本量较小。最近，一种叫"ready-made"的带瓣管道已经上市，由 Edwards Konect Resilia 生物瓣带瓣管道结合 Inspiris 瓣膜和带 Valsalva 窦的 Dacron 血管制作而成，它具有宽大的人工缝合环，这有助于植入和止血。有关这种带瓣管道长期效果的进一步研究还在进行中。

如果主动脉瓣环在清创后仍然完整，则可采用标准的根部置换技术处理带瓣管道近端的缝合。如果主动脉瓣环或 IFB 受到严重破坏，带瓣管道的尺寸可比 LVOT 大 2~3 mm，可缝合固定于室间隔、二尖瓣人工瓣的缝合环或重建 IFB 的补片材料上（见上文）。这种技术的优点是易于确定带瓣管道的尺寸，植入技术是标准主动脉根部置换的常用技术，外科医生对这种技术比较熟悉。缺点是：由于瓣膜位于环上位置，因此需要对冠状动脉纽扣进行广泛游离，同时带瓣管道的植入导致感染区存在假体材料。

网膜覆盖

如果出现严重感染、大量出血和（或）曾用人工材料进行主动脉瓣置换，首先要计划好再次手术，术中用抗生素溶液冲洗纵隔，然后用网膜覆盖手术区。这种情况下，胸骨切口向下延伸到上腹部，并进入腹腔。采集带血管蒂网膜后，将其转移到主动脉根部术区，然后围绕网膜蒂关闭腹部，并以标准方式关胸。虽然有几个中心已经报道了这种手术的良好结果，但长期的再感染率还有待确定。

结　果

由于患者的人口统计学特征、疾病严重程度、手术的紧迫性以及主动脉瓣心内膜炎伴主动脉根部脓肿的手术方式存在很大差异，各方报道的死亡率也存在很大差异。随着时间的推移，报道的死亡率始终保持在 6.7%~32%。更有甚者，有报道称 1 年的死亡率高达 52%，且再感染发生率相对较高[19-22]。

分析结果，死亡率的增加与合并肾衰竭和需要同时进行冠状动脉旁路移植有关。长期死亡率与双瓣膜（主动脉瓣和二尖瓣）置换术、肾衰竭和年龄有关。虽然早期和晚期死亡率都很高，但考虑到主动脉瓣心内膜炎伴主动脉根部脓肿的病情较重，这一死亡率也是合理的[19-22]。

总　结

主动脉瓣心内膜炎伴主动脉根部脓肿的手术是一项极具挑战性的复杂手术，其并发症发生率和死亡率都很高。瓣膜和补片有多样化的选择，但所选择的人工瓣膜及选择的术式并没有显示出各自的明确优势。因此，针对相关病例，我们建议彻底清创，使用外科医生最熟知的瓣膜和补片材料进行重建。

参考文献

[1] Hoen B, Beguinot I, Rabaid C, et al. The Duke criteria for diagnosing infective endocarditis are specific: analysis of 100 patients with acute fever or fever of unknown origin. Clin Infect Dis, 1996, 23: 298–302.

[2] David TE, Komeda M, Brofman PR. Surgical treatment of aortic root abscess. Circulation, 1989, 80: 1269–1274.

[3] Rohmann S, Erbel R, Mohr-Kahaly S, et al. Use of transesophageal echocardiography in the diagnosis of abscess in infective endocarditis. Eur Heart J, 1995, 16: S54–S62.

[4] Slipczuk L, Codolosa JN, Davial CD, et al. Infective endocarditis epidemiology over five decades: a systematic review. PloS One, 2014, 9: e111564.

[5] Gould FK, Denning DW, Elliott TS, et al. Guidelines for diagnosis and treatment of endocarditis in adults: a working party of British Society for Antimicrobial Chemotherapy. J Antimicrob Chemother, 2012, 67: 269–289.

[6] Shapiro SM, Young E, De Guzman S, et al. Transesophageal echocardiography in diagnosis of infective endocarditis. Chest, 1994, 105: 377–382.

[7] David TE. Surgical treatment of aortic valve endocarditis//Cohn LH. Cardiac surgery in the adult. 4thed. New York, NY: McGraw-Hill, 2012: 767–73.

[8] Nishimura RA, Otto CM, Bonow RO, et al. 2014 AHA/ACC guideline for the management of patients with valvular heart disease: a report of the American College of Cardiology/American Heart Association task force on practice guidelines. J Am Coll Cardiol, 2014, 63: e57–e185.

[9] Prendergast BD, Tornos P. Surgery for infective endocarditis: who and when? Circulation, 2010, 121: 1141–1152.

[10] Moon MR, Dc M, Moore KC, et al. Treatment of endocarditis with valve replacement: the question of tissue versus mechanical prosthesis. Ann Thorac Surg, 2001, 71: 1164–1171.

[11] Lytle BW, Priest BP, Taylor PC, et al. Surgical treatment of prosthetic valve endocarditis. J Thorac Cardiovasc Surg, 1996, 111: 198–210.

[12] Jassar AS, Bavaria JE, Szeto WY, et al. Graft selection for aortic root replacement in complex active endocarditis: does it matter? Ann Thorac Surg, 2012; 93: 480–487.

[13] Avierinos JF, Thuny F, Chalvignac V, et al. Surgical treatment of active aortic endocarditis: homografts are not the cornerstone of outcome. Ann Thorac Surg, 2001, 71: 1164–1171.

[14] Borger MA, Prasongsukarn K, Armstrong S, et al. Stentless aortic valve reoperations: a surgical challenge. Ann Thorac Surg, 2007, 84: 737–743.

[15] David TE, Kuo J, Armstrong S. Aortic and mitral valve replacement with reconstruction of the intervalvular fibrous body. J Thorac Cardiovasc Surg, 1997, 114: 766–772.

[16] D'Udekem Y, David TE, Feindel CM, et al. Long term results of operation for paravalvular abscess. Ann Thorac Surg, 1996, 62: 48–53.

[17] Ting M, Wang CH, Chi NH, et al. Outcome for surgical treatment of infective endocarditis with periannular abscess. J Formos Med Assoc January, 2020, 119(1 Pt 1): 113–124.

[18] David TE, Kuo J, Armstrong S. Aortic and mitral valve replacement with reconstruction of intervalvular fibrous body. J Thorac Cardiovasc Surg, 1997, 114: 766–771.

[19] Leontyev S, Davierwala PM, Krögh G, et al. Early and late outcomes of complex aortic root surgery in patients with aortic root abscesses. Eur J Cardio Thorac Surg, 2016, 49: 447–454.

[20] Forteza A, Centeno J, Ospina V, et al. Outcomes in aortic and mitral valve replacement with intervalvular fibrous body reconstruction. Ann Thorac Surg, 2015, 99: 838–845.

[21] Stamou SC, Murphy MC, Kouchoukos NT. Left ventricular outflow tract reconstruction and translocation of the aortic valve for annular erosion: early and midterm outcomes. J Thorac Cardiovasc Surg, 2011, 142: 292–297.

[22] John RJM, Treaure T, Sturridge MF, et al. Aortic root complications of infective endocarditis: influence on surgical outcomes. Eur Heart J, 1991, 12: 241–248.

第19章
感染性心内膜炎的复杂多瓣膜手术

Corbin E. Goerlich, Hamza Aziz, Ahmet Kilic
The Johns Hopkins Hospital, Baltimore, MD, United States

引 言

随着时间的推移,虽然感染性心内膜炎(IE)的发病率维持相对稳定,但IE类型及手术干预频率却已变化。目前老年患者越来越多,风湿病变已不常见,因有创心脏手术植入装置而患病的人数不断增加,静脉吸毒导致的IE人数也在增多,以上因素进而导致手术复杂性的增加[1-2]。有40%~45%的IE病例最终需要手术干预,自2007年发布IE抗生素预防指南以来,这一比例已趋于稳定[3-4]。尽管如此,仍有相当比例的IE患者需手术治疗,随之而来的即是对更复杂、多瓣膜受累病变进行手术的需求[5]。手术治疗IE的指征包括瓣膜功能障碍导致心力衰竭、新发心律失常、持续性脓毒性肺栓塞或全身性栓塞、赘生物持续存在并>1 cm,或高毒力致病菌感染(如金黄色葡萄球菌、真菌或多重耐药菌)在完成全程抗生素治疗后仍持续存在左侧心内膜炎[6]。

术中,所有IE受累组织都必须彻底清除。多瓣膜受累,无论是否需要行中心纤维体(IFB)及心房的重建,本身就是手术治疗的明确指征。在IE病例中,双瓣叶手术最为常见,但也有3~4个瓣叶置换的报道[7-9]。本章重点介绍主动脉瓣和二尖瓣的双瓣叶置换和修复手术的相关临床表现和手术处理,双瓣叶受累心内膜炎的治疗原则也可用于其他更复杂的病情。而单瓣叶心内膜炎则在其他章节阐述。

流行病学

IE多瓣膜受累的研究数据有限。在一项单中心研究中,共纳入1571例接受手术治疗的患者,其中46%接受了主动脉瓣置换(AVR),31%接受了二尖瓣置换(MVR),14%接受了AVR和MVR联合术(其中11%的病例IFB受累)。IFB受累的所有患者均进行了AVR和MVR,另有16%的患者进行了三尖瓣修复,其他同期进行的手术包括主动脉根部置换(60%)、升主动脉或部分主动脉弓置换(20%)以及冠状动脉旁路移植术(32%)[10]。在另一项单中心研究中,有72名主动脉瓣合并二尖瓣受累的IE病例,其中瓣环受累者达12.5%[11]。由此可见,多瓣膜受累的 IE 除需要广泛彻底清除感染组织外还须进行大范围的修复重建，手术大、风险高。据报道，无论感染是否累及 IFB，双瓣叶受累的心内膜炎院内死亡率为 18%，5 年生存率介于 25%～94%[10-11]。对 37 例侵袭性主动脉瓣 IE 合并二尖瓣前瓣病变及 IFB 受累的患者进行的中长期随访发现：院内死亡率为 8%，出院后死亡率为 5%，1 年和 3 年存活率分别为 91% 和 82%[12]。

术前评估

临床最常见的多瓣叶受累 IE 是主动脉瓣心内膜炎向下单纯累及二尖瓣前叶，而侵蚀性脓肿蔓延累及 IFB 则较为少见。术前经胸超声心动图（TTE）辅以术中经食管超声心动图（TEE）有助于确定手术方式。对于那些怀疑有冠状动脉疾病的病例，必须进行心导管检查，但冠状动脉 CT 造影（CTA）可用于不同情形的冠脉评估，尤其是主动脉瓣受累的病例。值得一提的是，如果出现化脓性心包炎，则强烈提示 IFB 受累[13]。所有患者在接受心脏手术治疗前都应进行口腔检查，评估与脓肿的关系，除非患者血流动力学不稳定需要紧急行手术。同样，在手术前，对于存在腹腔感染者，肠道微生物的培养有助于判断病原菌。如有可能（即可以不在急性 IE 活动期进行手术），建议尽可能在手术治疗前清除菌血症。

手术方法

常规采用胸骨正中切口，上、下腔静脉插管，这样便于同时对左、右心进行全方位修复，包括复杂的主动脉根部或 IFB 重建手术[13]。临手术前行 TEE 检查以详尽评估心脏受累情况，确保 IE 未累及更多瓣膜，且没有血栓发生，或赘生物前期特征无变化。此外，操作过程中尽量避免搬动或激惹心脏，以防赘生物脱落发生脓毒性栓塞。即便术前预测只有主动脉瓣或二尖瓣单瓣膜受累，术中也应对其他瓣膜受累情况进行检查。手术方式方面，如有条件，尽量选择瓣膜修复而非置换，这样有助于预防后续的人工瓣膜心内膜炎。但由于瓣膜成形较为复杂，术中手术方式的选择需要视瓣叶损毁程度而审慎决定（见单瓣膜修复章节）。如果发现脓肿，则应对病变周围组织进行彻底清创，并予以充分引流。如果是广泛环状脓肿甚至累及 IFB，则可能需要使用 Dacron 或心包补片进行重建。若出现房室分离，可使用人工补片修复连接[10-11,14]。

"Hemicommando" 和 "Commando" 手术主要应用于主动脉瓣和二尖瓣双瓣叶伴 IFB 受累的 IE 病例[15-16]。"Commando" 手术包括双瓣膜置换和 IFB 重建。首先横断主动脉根部，纽扣状游离冠状动脉开口（图 19.1A）。充分暴露并切除主动脉瓣瓣叶，至周围健康组织清晰可见，暴露二尖瓣及瓣下结构（图 19.1B）。切开无冠瓣瓣环及 IFB，根据需要切除二尖瓣瓣叶及瓣环（图 19.1C）。完全切除二尖瓣（此处描绘的是人工二尖瓣）和主动脉瓣后，可以看到一个单一的房室腔（图

19.2）。接下来植入新的二尖瓣，缝合从后瓣环开始，向前缝合，最前端的二尖瓣瓣环与 IFB 和主动脉瓣环的无冠瓣部分相接，也就是靠近左冠瓣和无冠瓣的交界处（图 19.1D）。在此位置，IFB 可以用自体或上次已有过手术的主动脉瓣和二尖瓣的周围组织或心包补片加固（图 19.1E）。在完成修复新的 IFB 和主动脉根部之上，再缝合植入同种异体主动脉瓣（图 19.1F）。有时为了改善二尖瓣的手术视野，可以切开左房顶，此时则使用适当大小的心包补片将其缝合关闭（图 19.1G）[14,17]。

目前，人工瓣膜、同种瓣和自体瓣膜（Ross 手术）均已被用于 IE 的手术治疗，但它们的长期疗效无明显差别，因此临床应根据患者的需要及相关风险因素进行选择[18-21]。同种瓣因其感染复发率低和血流动力学好而深受欢迎，缺点是供不应

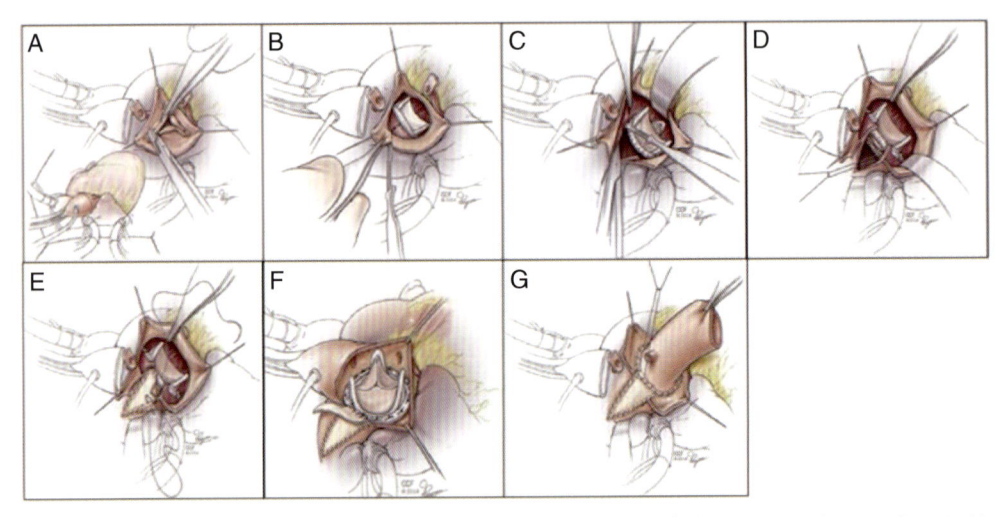

图 19.1 感染性心内膜炎 Commando 手术，可见主动脉瓣感染、人工二尖瓣和中心纤维体（IFB）受累。引自：G.B. Pettersson, S.T. Hussain, R.M. Ramankutty, et al. Reconstruction of fibrous skeleton: technique, pitfalls and results. Multimed Man Cardiothorac. Surg(MMCTS), 2014, mmu004.

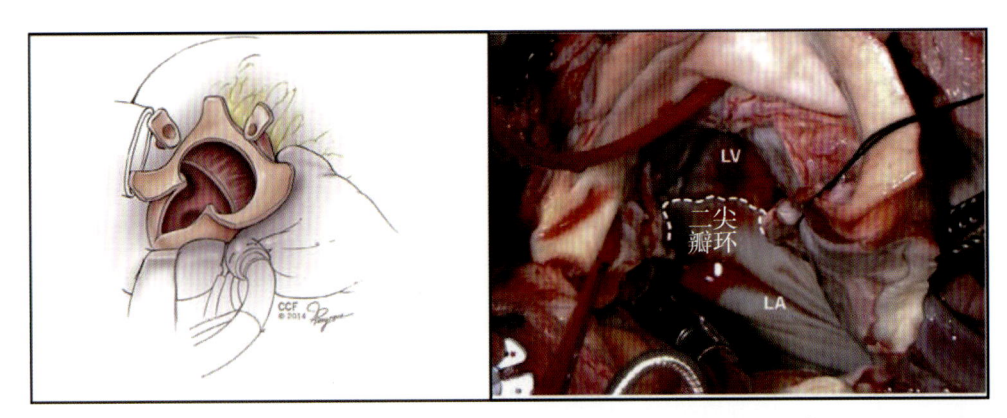

图 19.2 在横断中心纤维体（IFB）、切除人工二尖瓣和主动脉瓣后的单腔视图。主动脉瓣环和二尖瓣环呈直角。LV：左心室；LA：左心房。引自：G.B. Pettersson, S.T. Hussain, R.M. Ramankutty, et al. Blackstone. Reconstruction of fibrous skeleton: technique, pitfalls and results. Multimed Man Cardiothorac. Surg(MMCTS), 2014, mmu004.

求且耐久性差，需要更换时，再手术非常困难。Ross 手术被认为是年轻患者的有效选择，自体肺动脉瓣可抵抗复发性感染、避免抗凝，并具有生长能力，缺点是需要更换一个健康、未感染的瓣膜。在所有选择中，机械瓣的耐用性最好，但需要终生抗凝，还存在不可忽视的感染风险。

病例学习

一例男性患者，76 岁，有高血压病史，最近到印度旅行后出现全身无力、不适、食欲下降、体重减轻和贫血。怀疑尿路感染（UTI），自行开始服用环丙沙星。血培养提示缓症链球菌阳性，遂静脉给予广谱抗生素。入院时白细胞计数为 12.6×10^9/L[3]。无发热及急性呼吸窘迫。肌钙蛋白水平升高至 0.46 ng/mL（μg/L），肌酐为 1.26 mg/dL（111.38 μmol/L），B 型钠尿肽为 572 ng/L。胸部 X 线片仅显示右半膈升高。胸部 CT 显示肺门血管突出，考虑与肺动脉高压有关。脾轻度肿大，肝脏有一小囊肿。TTE 显示左心室大小和功能正常，射血分数为 57%。在主动脉瓣的无冠瓣上发现一个小到中等大小的活动性赘生物，伴有中度主动脉瓣反流（图 19.3）。二尖瓣上也发现了一个小的活动性赘生物，伴轻度二尖瓣反流（图 19.4）。由于血培养中发现了口腔菌群，且牙齿状况不佳，为此进行了颌面部 CT 检查，未发现脓肿。入院接受 IE 治疗 2 d 后，患者出现急性呼吸窘迫和突发性肺水肿，使用无创正压通气治疗。通过积极的利尿治疗避免了气管插管。然而，尽管进行了适当的药物治疗，患者仍出现进行性心功能障碍；因此，在获得患者本人同意后，医生对其进行了手术治疗。

术中 TEE 证实左心室和右心室功能正常，此外，还发现二尖瓣前叶有一大的赘生物伴瓣膜穿孔，主动脉瓣也有一赘生物，两个瓣膜均伴有严重反流。采用胸骨正中切开，建立体外循环，心脏停搏满意后，横断主动脉。

术中可见主动脉瓣为三叶瓣，左冠瓣和无冠瓣都有一个大的赘生物。切除主动脉瓣三个瓣叶，切开左心房探查二尖瓣。二尖瓣上有一约 2.5 cm 大的赘生物，巨大赘生物包绕 A1/A2 以及前瓣叶下方（图 19.5），瓣叶穿孔损毁严重，修复不可行。故切除前瓣叶，保留其瓣环，后瓣叶未受感染累及，使用 27 mm Medtronic

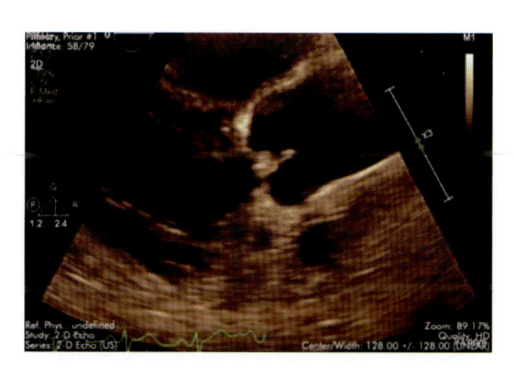

图 19.3　经胸超声心动图胸骨旁长轴切面可见无冠瓣上的赘生物

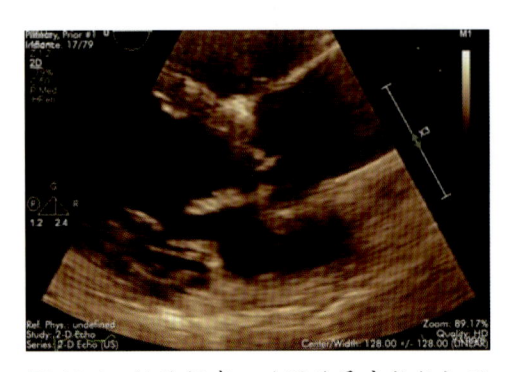

图 19.4　经胸超声心动图胸骨旁长轴切面可见二尖瓣前叶赘生物

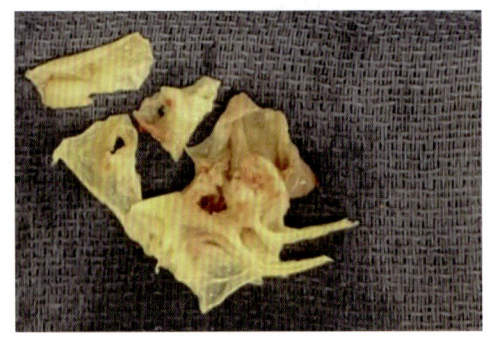

图 19.5　手术大体标本，左冠瓣和无冠瓣赘生物并侵蚀穿孔（左），二尖瓣前瓣叶上巨大赘生物（右）

Mosaic 瓣行保留后瓣的二尖瓣置换术。术中经主动脉切口、左心室流出道探查，二尖瓣人工瓣膜放置位置良好。随后，使用 23 mm St. Jude Trifecta Glide Technology 瓣行主动脉瓣置换。大量冲洗术区后，关闭了主动脉切口和左心房切口。复温并开放主动脉，患者立即恢复了正常的窦性心律。两个生物瓣均功能正常，无瓣周漏，手术效果良好。在极少量正性肌力药物条件下脱离了体外循环，术后恢复满意。

总　结

随着带植入物的侵入性外科手术的复杂性增加，需要外科干预的多瓣膜 IE 手术可能会继续存在。适用于单瓣膜 IE 的外科手术原则，同样适用于多瓣膜 IE。对所有感染受累组织进行大范围彻底清创的同时，如有可能，尽量挽救自身有活性瓣膜组织，以减少在感染区使用外源性材料。IFB 清创术技术要求很高，但对于疾病进展和邻近组织受到侵蚀的病变仍有其存在的必要性。多瓣膜受累 IE 具有很高的并发症发生率和死亡率，在对其进行任何外科干预之前，应多学科协同诊治，以降低疾病风险。

参考文献

[1] Tleyjeh IM, et al. A systematic review of population-based studies of infective endocarditis. Chest, 2007, 132: 1025-1035.

[2] Hoen B, et al. Changing profile of infective endocarditis: results of a 1-year survey in France. J Am Med Assoc, 2002, 288: 75-81.

[3] Pant S, et al. Trends in infective endocarditis incidence, microbiology, and valve replacement in the United States from 2000 to 2011. J Am Coll Cardiol, 2015, 65: 2070-2076.

[4] McDonald JR. Acute infective endocarditis. Infect Dis Clin, 2009, 23: 643-664.

[5] Delahaye F, et al. In-hospital mortality of infective endocarditis: prognostic factors and evolution over an 8-year period. Scand J Infect Dis, 2007, 39: 849-857.

[6] Pettersson GB, Hussain ST. Current AATS guidelines on surgical treatment of infective endocarditis. Ann Cardiothorac Surg, 2019, 8: 630-644.

[7] Seeburger J, et al. Quadruple valve replacement for acute endocarditis. J Thorac Cardiovasc Surg, 2009, 137: 1564-1565.

[8] Kim TY, Kim KH. Simultaneous triple valve replacement for triple valve infective endocarditis with intact cardiac skeleton. J Card Surg, 2020, 35: 260–263.

[9] Alsoufi B, et al. Short- and long-term results of triple valve surgery in the modern era. Ann Thorac Surg, 2006, 81: 2172–2178.

[10] Davierwala PM, et al. Double valve replacement and reconstruction of the intervalvular fibrous body in patients with active infective endocarditis. Eur. J. CardioThorac. Surg, 2014, 45: 146–152.

[11] Tas S, et al. Surgical treatment of double valve endocarditis. Heart Surg Forum, 2014, 17: 28.

[12] Elgharably H, et al. The incorporated aortomitral homograft for double-valve endocarditis: the 'hemi-Commando' procedure. Early and mid-term outcomes. Eur. J. Cardio-Thorac. Surg, 2018, 53: 1055–1061.

[13] Kirklin JW, Kouchoukos NT. Kirklin/Barrat-Boyes cardiac surgery morphology, diagnostic criteria, natural history, techniques, results, and indications. Philadelphia: Elsevier/Saunders, 2013.

[14] David TE, Kuo J, Armstrong S. Aortic and mitral valve replacement with reconstruction of the intervalvular fibrous body. J Thorac Cardiovasc Surg, 1997, 114: 766–772.

[15] Tedoriya T, Hirota M, Ishikawa N, et al. Reconstruction of aorto-mitral continuity with a handmade aortomitral bioprosthetic valve for extensive bivalvular endocarditis. Interact Cardiovasc Thorac Surg, 2013, 16: 405–407.

[16] Obadia JF, et al. Monobloc aorto-mitral homograft or mechanical valve replacement: a new surgical option for extensive bivalvular endocarditis. J Thorac Cardiovasc Surg, 2006, 131: 243–245.

[17] Pettersson GB, Hussain ST, Ramankutty RM, et al. Reconstruction of fibrous skeleton: technique, pitfalls and results. Multimed Man Cardiothorac Surg, 2014, 2014:mmu004.

[18] Kim JY, et al. Long-term outcomes of homografts in the aortic valve and root position: a 20-year experience. Korean J. Thorac. Cardiovasc. Surg, 2016, 49: 258–263.

[19] Ratschiller T, et al. Long-term evaluation of the Ross procedure in acute infective endocarditis. Semin Thorac Cardiovasc Surg, 2017, 29: 494–501.

[20] Flynn CD, et al. Systematic review and meta-analysis of surgical outcomes comparing mechanical valve replacement and bioprosthetic valve replacement in infective endocarditis. Ann Cardiothorac Surg, 2019, 8: 587–599.

[21] Bechtel JFM, et al. The Ross operation: two decades of clinical experience//MD CAY, MD YW, MD RH. Aortic root surgery. NEW YORK: Springer, 2010: 74–85.

第20章
感染性心内膜炎并发急性卒中的手术时机

Lise Tchouta[1], *Shinichi Fukuhara*[2]

[1]Columbia University Medical Center, New York City, NY, United States;
[2]University of Michigan Health Systems, Ann Arbor, MI, United States

引 言

神经系统并发症是感染性心内膜炎（IE）最常见、最具破坏性的并发症之一，发生率为10%~75%[1-3]，死亡率为20%~58%[4-7]。从数据上看，出现神经系统并发症比无这一并发症者死亡率明显增高[8-9]，因此对并发脑损伤的IE病例的处理应及时、慎重。IE的神经系统并发症主要包括缺血性脑卒中（70%）和脑出血（10%）。另外，蛛网膜下腔出血、脑膜脑炎和脑脓肿等较少见的并发症约各占5%。目前针对IE的手术指征主要包括：使用抗生素后脓毒症仍无法控制者（如主动脉根部脓肿、抗生素使用期间持续发热、反复发生栓塞事件），严重瓣膜反流导致心力衰竭者[10-11]。根据以上指征，约50%的IE病例在抗生素治疗的同时接受了心脏手术[12-16]。然而，对于并发脑卒中的IE病例，病情的处理就显得更复杂，术前需要对其手术风险和获益做出详细的评估。

手术的决策需要权衡以下两方面：一方面，有心脏手术适应证的病例其手术的紧迫性；另一方面，脑出血可能加剧神经损伤的风险（出血源于出血性卒中或缺血性卒中的出血转化），另外，体外循环引起的低血压、栓塞事件也可加重神经损害。目前鲜有大型前瞻性研究就IE卒中后手术干预的最佳时机提供指导。本章将就IE出现神经系统并发症时进行心脏手术的数据结果加以概括分析，以期为此类病症提供处理意见，并对目前各学会相关指南推荐加以讨论。

缺血性卒中与手术时机

缺血性卒中是IE最常见的神经系统并发症。值得注意的是，早期研究显示，在缺血性卒中急性期进行心脏手术死亡率将明显升高。一项日本的多中心回顾性研究共纳入181名IE相关脑卒中患者，结果显示推迟心脏手术时间可降低神经系统恶化的发生率，具体如下：心脏手术在卒中发生后24 h内进行，这一发生率为45.5%；在1周内进行，为43.8%；在初次发病后1~2周内进行，为16.7%；在缺血性卒中4周后进行，为2.3%[17]。他们的结论是，心脏手术可在初次脑梗死后4周左右安全进行。Garcia-Cabrera等的报道也指出进一步脑损伤的风险与手术干预的时间成反比：手术在<2周、2~3周和>3周进行，颅内出血的风险分别为50%、33%和20%[18]。Angstwurm等也有类似的结论，他们发现：在发病后3 d内进行手术，神经功能恶化的风险为20%；如果在4~14 d进行手术，为20%~50%；如果手术延迟至14 d后，则为<10%；如果手术时间推迟至初始栓塞事件4周后，风险可降到<1%[19]。

然而，近期数据与早期研究明显矛盾。最近的报道显示，脑卒中后早期手术并未出现不良后果，从而导致手术时间的前移，推荐早期手术，而临床关注的重点转向颅内出血的病例。2015年，Sorabella等发现，在一组≤14 d接受早期手术的病例中，无论既往有无栓塞性脑卒中病史，其术后新发卒中率没有差异（9.3% vs.7.1%，P=0.57）[20]。

死亡率

IE的手术死亡率已大幅降低。最近的数据表明，无论患者是否出现神经系统并发症，早期手术，即便是在感染急性期，均可提高生存率。在一篇包含21项研究的meta分析中，Yanagawa等发现早期手术（手术时间<7 d）在倾向性评分匹配前（OR=0.61，95% CI=0.50~0.74；P<0.001）和匹配后（OR=0.41，95%CI=0.31~0.54；P<0.001）均有生存获益。在一项具有类似结论的前瞻性随机试验中，Kang等发现发病48 h内手术可降低全因死亡率（HR=0.10，95%CI=0.01~0.82；P=0.03）。研究认为，对于大多数没有极高手术风险因素的病例来说，延期手术几乎没有获益。然而，IE出现神经系统并发症的研究数据间还存在细微差异，应细化分析。

约40%的IE病例存在脑损伤的临床证据（缺血性损害、脑出血、感染性动脉瘤、脑脓肿或脑膜炎），这在IE患者群体中占相当大的比例，因此对并发神经系统损伤的患者进行死亡风险专项评估就十分必要。在一项日本的队列研究中，Okita等发现：与颅内出血7 d内接受手术的患者相比，在8~21 d和22 d以后接受手术的院内死亡率较低（OR=0.79，P=0.843 vs. OR=0.12，P=0.200）[21]。这些结果与脑梗死病例形成鲜明对照：他们在15~28 d和29 d后接受手术的院内死亡率则更高（OR=5.90，P=0.107 vs. OR=4.92，P=0.137）。尽管统计学上无显著性差异，但鉴于以上结果，作者建议在发生IE相关颅内出血的7 d内应避免手术。Piper等也得出类似结论，在对108例IE并发血栓栓塞性卒中患者进行的前瞻性研究中发现：发病72 h内手术的患者存活率较高（40个月时为76%，P<0.000 1）[22]。

以上基于不同手术时机带来的结果差异（无论是死亡还是进一步的神经损伤），其原因尚不十分清楚，但可以用不同研究的选择偏倚和观察者偏倚来解释。许多IE并发卒中的患者，尤其是那些之前还患有其他内科疾病或既往接受过多次心脏手术者，其手术风险过高，通常不会选择瓣膜置换术，这就造成了选择偏倚。同理，尽管接受了最佳的药物治疗，但神经系统仍受到严重破坏的患者往往因临床病情恶化也不会接受手术治疗。相反，在接受药物治疗的同时，神经功能逐渐恢复或没有明显恶化的患者会被考虑手术治疗，并获得更好的治疗效果。他们的存活可能不能完全归因于推迟手术时间，而是他们有较好的功能储备，术前内科治疗功能恢复良好，或总体病情较轻。目前还不清楚在不同的评估队列中，上面提到的其他情况较为健康或手术风险较低的患者是如何积极接受手术治疗的，这可能会带来观察者偏倚。本文报告的研究数据并未阐明患者选择手术的决策过程，这是回顾性研究固有的局限性。

当前指南

包括欧洲心脏病学会（ESC）在内的现行心脏学会指南均推荐在发生神经系统事件后进行手术，并建议必须权衡好围手术期风险与术后获益[23]。ESC 的推荐可归纳如下：

– 无症状脑栓塞或短暂性脑缺血（TIA），如有手术指征，可立即进行手术（Ⅰ类，证据级别 B 级）[8]。

– 缺血性卒中并非心脏手术禁忌，除非神经系统预后极差[9]。

– 卒中与心脏手术之间的最佳时间间隔存在争议，但最近的研究倾向于早期手术[24-25]。

– 对于颅内出血患者，手术应推迟至少 1 个月（Ⅱa 类，证据级别 B 级）[17,26-27]。

– 如果头颅 CT 或 MRI 已排除脑出血，且患者神经系统未受到严重损伤（即昏迷），手术适用于心力衰竭、感染未控制、脓肿和持续性栓塞，手术无须延迟且神经系统风险较低（3%～6%）（Ⅱa 类，证据级别 B 级）[9,24]。

2016 年美国胸外科学会（AATS）关于 IE 并发卒中后手术时机的共识指南指出，对于近期颅内出血（Ⅱa 类）者，手术延迟 3 周或更长时间是合理的[10]。AATS 对 IE 并发卒中推荐的最佳手术时机与 ESC 基本一致，可归纳如下：

– 如果已确诊为真菌性脑动脉瘤，患者的治疗和随访应与神经内科和神经外科专家密切协作（Ⅰ类，证据级别 C 级）。

– 对于近期发生颅内出血的患者，推迟 3 周或更长时间手术是合理的（Ⅱa 类，证据级别 B 级）。

– 对于非出血性卒中且有强烈的心脏手术指征，需要紧急手术的，早期手术是合理的（Ⅱa 类，证据级别 B 级）。

– 大面积和多发性脑卒中以及有严重神经系统症状的患者在接受手术前应由神经科医生进行全面评估（Ⅰ类，证据级别 B 级）。

– 对于出现神经系统症状及明显颅内出血的 IE 患者，应考虑进行血管造影检查以排除真菌性脑动脉瘤（Ⅱa 类，证据级别 B 级）。

作者的临床实践与 ESC 和 AATS 指南推荐一致，倾向于早期手术，除非患者出现颅内出血或大面积致残性卒中，且出血转化风险很高。急性期进行手术的好处是可以最大限度地减少 IE 对瓣膜结构的破坏。

准确预测 IE 并发症的风险有助于手术计划的制定。然而，目前能可靠预测栓塞风险或药物治疗失败的工具很少。法国一个多中心队列研究根据 1000 多名 IE 患者的资料开发了一种栓塞风险（ER）计算工具[28]。在单变量分析中，年龄、糖尿病、心房颤动、既往栓塞、赘生物长度和金黄色葡萄球菌感染被确定为栓塞事件的风险因素，并在验证模型中得到证实，该模型可预测 6 个月内的栓塞风险（图20.1）。该计算工具的预测准确性是通过评估预测的和观察到的栓塞事件之间的一致性来获得的，结果非常好。该模型中包含的这些特征先前已表明与较高的栓塞风险有关[29-31]，但由于回顾性研究只调查了患者入院时常规测量的变量，存在检测偏倚，因此应谨慎使用此类风险计算工具。正如计算模型的作者所强调的，

法国栓塞风险计算器		
感染性心内膜炎（IE）6 个月时的栓塞风险计算		
IE 患者入院时采集如下临床、超声心动图和微生物学信息。随后，不同时间点的栓塞风险预测值将自动生成。		
入院时数据		
临床数据	年龄（岁）	75
	糖尿病（0：无；1：有）	1
	栓塞史（0：无；1：有）	0
	房颤（0：无；1：有）	1
超声心动图	赘生物 ≤ 10 mm（0：否；1：是）	0
	赘生物 > 10 mm（0：否；1：是）	1
微生物	金黄色葡萄球菌（0：否；1：是）	1
预测的栓塞风险计算		
时间(d)	预测的栓塞风险	
1	6%	
2	7%	
3	12%	
4	15%	
5	16%	
6	18%	
7	18%	
10	20%	
11	21%	
12	23%	
13	26%	
14	27%	
18	28%	
19	29%	
23	30%	
28	31%	
35	31%	
47	32%	
48	33%	
180	33%	

图 20.1　栓塞风险计算器[28]。一名 75 岁患者的栓塞风险计算图示，该患者有糖尿病和心房颤动病史，既往无栓塞史，超声心动图显示赘生物（> 10 mm）且金黄色葡萄球菌培养阳性

该模型并未测量或评估可能增加栓塞风险的凝血障碍或血栓前状态等变量。作者也没有在模型中评估自体瓣膜与人工瓣膜，或二尖瓣与主动脉瓣的作用。尽管存在上述局限性，但包括日本和菲律宾队列在内的多项研究已对该栓塞风险计算工具进行了外部验证[32-33]。

围手术期的辅助治疗

IE 并发脑卒中的心脏手术治疗必须仔细规划手术时机，以减少上述所讨论的并发症。作为手术评估的一部分，许多患者都要接受冠状动脉导管检查，以便在开放性心脏手术前进行风险分层，并可能同时进行冠状动脉旁路移植术（CABG）。在讨论最佳手术时机时，了解这一介入检查措施的必要性及其对预后的影响至关重要；因为进行非必要的冠状动脉导管检查可能会导致不必要的手术时间延迟，这不利于有神经系统并发症的患者尽早接受手术，以挽救生命。

我们的回顾性研究显示，72% 的 IE 手术患者接受过常规冠状动脉导管检查。有趣的是，尽管 35.4% 的患者有冠状动脉疾病（CAD）（30.8% 为单支血管病变，33.3% 为两支血管病变，35.9% 为三支血管病变），但只有少数患者（9.1%）接受了 CABG。因为在无冠状动脉症状的 IE 患者中，这些冠状动脉病变并不严重，手术干预往往无关紧要。从冠状动脉造影到手术（CABG 和瓣膜置换术）的中位时间为 15.5 d，只有 16.7% 的患者在接受导管检查后 48 h 内接受手术。即使是那些被分类为需要限期手术的患者，从血管造影到瓣膜置换术的中位时间也有不容忽视的延长（6 d）[34]。有趣的是，与术前未接受血管造影的患者相比，两组患者的 30 d 死亡率没有差异（2.6% *vs.* 2.4%；P=0.89）[34]。

虽然医务人员可能会倾向于筛查 CAD，以避免在瓣膜置换术后再次开胸手术，但常规进行冠状动脉造影可能会因推迟 IE 的外科干预时间而造成更大的伤害。我们建议谨慎地有选择性地针对有 CAD 风险因素（包括吸烟、糖尿病、高血压和高脂血症）的病例进行冠状动脉造影。在多变量分析中，Dalati 等人发现只有高血压是 IE 患者进行 CABG 的预测因素[34]。如果 IE 患者之前有心绞痛症状、CAD 风险因素、既往心肌缺血病史或冠状动脉血运重建史，那么在瓣膜手术前考虑进行冠状动脉造影是合理的。作为冠状动脉造影的替代方法，冠状动脉 CT 侵袭性小，易于实施，具有很好的 CAD 诊断灵敏度（91%）和特异性（92%），可加快检查过程[35]。以上对于 CAD 理想筛查方式的决定，或瓣膜手术前介入指征的判断，均须依赖多学科会诊，这就完美地诠释了多学科管理 IE 的重要性。

多学科的手术评估

对伴有或不伴脑卒中的 IE 病例的治疗需要一个由心脏内科、心脏外科、神经科和感染科等多个专科医生组成的多学科团队。如前所述，手术与否的决定是基于抗感染治疗的有效性、神经功能恢复的可能性和心功能恶化的风险等因素做出的。为此，强烈推荐多学科团队协作，以获得最佳疗效。这种获益不仅存在于理论上，有数据表明：实施团队管理后，1年死亡率降低，抗感染治疗依从性更好，栓塞相关死亡率下降，继发性器官损伤减少[36]。

多学科团队治疗IE也会影响资源分配，从而实现高效护理。西班牙安达卢西亚的一家三级医院组建了一个专门针对IE的团队，与团队之外接受相关治疗的人群相比，团队方式可使更多患者手术时间提前（48.6% vs. 23.3%；$P<0.001$），脓毒性休克的发生率下降（9.7% vs. 24.5%；$P=0.009$），神经系统并发症减少（19.4% vs. 29.0%；$P=0.25$）[37]。虽然早期手术尚未明确证明能改善预后，但多学科团队能提高手术团队对患者的早期认识，并在必要时防止手术干预的延误。

总　结

一般而言，IE的手术指征包括：经适当的抗菌治疗感染未能得到控制，瓣膜反流导致心力衰竭，复发性栓塞。理想的手术干预时机应基于当前的指南推荐和相关数据分析，一般倾向于早期手术，但颅内出血除外，手术应推迟3~4周。最终，是否手术应取决于保守治疗可能出现的并发症风险、神经系统损伤的严重程度、患者的意愿及手术风险预测。

参考文献

[1] Hoen B, Duval X. Infective endocarditis. N Engl J Med, 2013, 369(8): 785. https://doi.org/10.1056/NEJMc1307282.

[2] Hess A, Klein I, Iung B, et al. Brain MRI findings in neurologically asymptomatic patients with infective endocarditis. AJNR Am J Neuroradiol, 2013, 34(8): 1579–1584. https://doi.org/10.3174/ajnr.A3582.

[3] Snygg-Martin U, Gustafsson L, Rosengren L, et al. Cerebrovascular complications in patients with left-sided infective endocarditis are common: a prospective study using magnetic resonance imaging and neurochemical brain damage markers. Clin Infect Dis, 2008, 47(1): 23–30. https://doi.org/10.1086/588663.

[4] Barsic B, Dickerman S, Krajinovic V, et al. Influence of the timing of cardiac surgery on the outcome of patients with infective endocarditis and stroke. Clin Infect Dis, 2013, 56(2): 209–217. https://doi.org/10.1093/cid/cis878.

[5] Heiro M, Nikoskelainen J, Engblom E, et al. Neurologic manifestations of infective endocarditis: a 17-year experience in a teaching hospital in Finland. Arch Intern Med, 2000, 160(18): 2781–2787. https://doi.org/10.1001/archinte.160.18.2781.

[6] Pruitt AA, Rubin RH, Karchmer AW, et al. Neurologic complications of bacterial endocarditis. Medicine, 1978, 57(4): 329–343. https://doi.org/10.1097/00005792-197807000-00004.

[7] Salgado AV, Furlan AJ, Keys TF, et al. Neurologic complications of endocarditis: a 12-year experience. Neurology, 1989, 39(2 Pt 1): 173–178. https://doi.org/10.1212/wnl.39.2.173.

[8] Thuny F, Avierinos J-F, Tribouilloy C, et al. Impact of cerebrovascular complications on mortality and neurologic outcome during infective endocarditis: a prospective multicentre study. Eur Heart J, 2007, 28(9): 1155–1161. https://doi.org/10.1093/eurheartj/ehm005.

[9] Ruttmann E, Willeit J, Ulmer H, et al. Neurological outcome of septic cardioembolic stroke after infective

[10] AATS Surgical Treatment of Infective Endocarditis Consensus Guidelines Writing Committee Chairs, Pettersson GB, Coselli JS, et al. 2016 the American Association for Thoracic Surgery (AATS) consensus guidelines: surgical treatment of infective endocarditis: executive summary. J Thorac Cardiovasc Surg, 2017, 153(6): 1241–1258.e29. https//doi.org/10.1016/j.jtcvs.2016.09.093.

[11] Pettersson GB, Hussain ST. Current AATS guidelines on surgical treatment of infective endocarditis. Ann Cardiothorac Surg, 2019, 8(6): 630–644. https://doi.org/10.21037/acs.2019.10.05.

[12] Murdoch DR, Corey GR, Hoen B, et al. Clinical presentation, etiology, and outcome of infective endocarditis in the 21st century: the International Collaboration on Endocarditis-Prospective Cohort Study. Arch Intern Med, 2009, 169(5): 463–473. https://doi.org/10.1001/archinternmed.2008.603.

[13] Wang A, Athan E, Pappas PA, et al. Contemporary clinical profile and outcome of prosthetic valve endocarditis. J Am Med Assoc, 2007, 297(12): 1354–13561. https://doi.org/10.1001/jama.297.12.1354.

[14] Tornos P, Iung B, Permanyer-Miralda G, et al. Infective endocarditis in Europe: lessons from the Euro heart survey. Heart, 2005, 91(5): 571–575. https://doi.org/10.1136/hrt.2003.032128.

[15] Castillo JC, Anguita MP, Ramírez A, et al. Long term outcome of infective endocarditis in patients who were not drug addicts: a 10 year study. Heart, 2000, 83(5): 525–530. https://doi.org/10.1136/heart.83.5.525.

[16] Selton-Suty C, Célard M, Le Moing V, et al. Preeminence of Staphylococcus aureus in infective endocarditis: a 1-year population-based survey. Clin Infect Dis, 2012, 54(9): 1230–1239. https://doi.org/10.1093/cid/cis199.

[17] Eishi K, Kawazoe K, Kuriyama Y, et al. Surgical management of infective endocarditis associated with cerebral complications. Multi-center retrospective study in Japan. J Thorac Cardiovasc Surg, 1995, 110(6): 1745–1755. https://doi.org/10.1016/S0022-5223(95)70038-2.

[18] García-Cabrera E, Fernández-Hidalgo N, Almirante B, et al. Neurological complications of infective endocarditis: risk factors, outcome, and impact of cardiac surgery: a multicenter observational study. Circulation, 2013, 127(23): 2272–2284. https://doi.org/10.1161/CIRCULATIONAHA.112.000813.

[19] Angstwurm K, Borges AC, Halle E, et al. Timing the valve replacement in infective endocarditis involving the brain. J Neurol, 2004, 251(10): 1220–1226. https://doi.org/10.1007/s00415-004-0517-x.

[20] Sorabella RA, Han SM, Grbic M, et al. Early operation for endocarditis complicated by preoperative cerebral emboli is not associated with worsened outcomes. Ann Thorac Surg, 2015, 100(2): 501–508. https://doi.org/10.1016/j.athoracsur.2015.03.078.

[21] Okita Y, Minakata K, Yasuno S, et al. Optimal timing of surgery for active infective endocarditis with cerebral complications: a Japanese multicentre study. Eur J Cardio Thorac Surg, 2016, 50(2): 374–382. https://doi.org/10.1093/ejcts/ezw035.

[22] Piper C, Wiemer M, Schulte HD, et al. Stroke is not a contraindication for urgent valve replacement in acute infective endocarditis. J Heart Valve Dis, 2001, 10(6): 703–711.

[23] Habib G, Lancellotti P, Antunes MJ, et al. 2015 ESC guidelines for the management of infective endocarditis The task force for the management of infective endocarditis of the European society of cardiology (ESC)endorsed by: European association for cardio-thoracic surgery (EACTS), the European association of nuclear medicine (EANM). Eur Heart J, 2015, 36(44): 3075–3128. https://doi.org/10.1093/eurheartj/ehv319.

[24] Kang D-H, Kim Y-J, Kim S-H, et al. Early surgery versus conventional treatment for infective endocarditis. N Engl J Med, 2012, 366(26): 2466–2473. https://doi.org/10.1056/NEJMoa1112843.

[25] Thuny F, Beurtheret S, Mancini J, et al. The timing of surgery influences mortality and morbidity in adults with severe complicated infective endocarditis: a propensity analysis. Eur Heart J, 2011, 32(16): 2027–2033. https://doi.org/10.1093/eurheartj/ehp089.

[26] Yoshioka D, Sakaguchi T, Yamauchi T, et al. Impact of early surgical treatment on postoperative neurologic outcome for active infective endocarditis complicated by cerebral infarction. Ann Thorac Surg, 2012, 94(2): 489–495. https://doi.org/10.1016/j.athoracsur.2012.04.027. discussion 496.

[27] Wilbring M, Irmscher L, Alexiou K, et al. The impact of preoperative neurological events in patients suffering from native infective valve endocarditis. Interact Cardiovasc Thorac Surg, 2014, 18(6): 740–747. https://doi.org/10.1093/icvts/ivu039.

[28] Hubert S, Thuny F, Resseguier N, et al. Prediction of symptomatic embolism in infective endocarditis: construction and validation of a risk calculator in a multicenter cohort. J Am Coll Cardiol, 2013, 62(15): 1384–1392. https://doi.org/10.1016/j.jacc.2013.07.029.

[29] Vilacosta I, Graupner C, San Román JA, et al. Risk of embolization after institution of antibiotic therapy for infective endocarditis. J Am Coll Cardiol, 2002, 39(9): 1489–1495. https://doi.org/10.1016/s0735-1097(02)01790-4.

[30] Steckelberg JM, Murphy JG, Ballard D, et al. Emboli in infective endocarditis: the prognostic value of echocardiography. Ann Intern Med, 1991, 114(8): 635–640. https://doi.org/10.7326/0003-4819-114-8-635.

[31] Erbel R, Rohmann S, Drexler M, et al. Improved diagnostic value of echocardiography in patients with infective endocarditis by transoesophageal approach. A prospective study. Eur Heart J, 1988, 9(1): 43–53. https://doi.org/10.1093/ehj/9.1.43.

[32] Takahashi Y, Izumi C, Miyake M, et al. Diagnostic accuracy of the Embolic Risk French Calculator for symptomatic embolism with infective endocarditis among Japanese population. J Cardiol, 2017, 70(6): 607–614. https://doi.org/10.1016/j.jjcc.2017.04.003.

[33] Aherrera JAM, Abola MTB, Balabagno MMO, et al. Prediction of symptomatic embolism in Filipinos with infective endocarditis using the embolic risk French calculator. Cardiol Res, 2016, 7(4): 130–139. https://doi.org/10.14740/cr490w.

[34] El-Dalati S, Shea M, Fukuhara S, et al. The role of coronary catheterization with angiography in surgically managed infectious endocarditis. Am J Med January, 2020, 133(9): 1101–1104. https://doi.org/10.1016/j.amjmed.2019.12.019.

[35] Danilo N, Daniele R, Chiara C, et al. Detection of significant coronary artery disease by noninvasive anatomical and functional imaging. Circulation: Cardiovascular Imaging, 2015, 8(3): e002179. https://doi.org/10.1161/CIRCIMAGING.114.002179.

[36] Botelho-Nevers E, Thuny F, Casalta JP, et al. Dramatic reduction in infective endocarditis-related mortality with a management-based approach. Arch Intern Med, 2009, 169(14): 1290–1298. https://doi.org/10.1001/archinternmed. 2009.192.

[37] Carrasco-Chinchilla F, Sánchez-Espín G, Ruiz-Morales J, et al. Influence of a multidisciplinary alert strategy on mortality due to left-sided infective endocarditis. Rev Esp Cardiol, 2014, 67(5): 380–386. https://doi.org/10.1016/j.rec.2013.09.010.

第21章
静脉吸毒者心内膜炎的医疗伦理

Lloyd M. Felmly [1,2], *Robert M. Sade* [1,2]

[1] Medical University of South Carolina, Charleston, SC, United States;
[2] Division of Cardiothoracic Surgery, Department of Surgery, Medical University of South Carolina, Charleston, SC, United States

引 言

感染性心内膜炎（IE）是一种由细菌或真菌引起的心脏瓣膜和内膜的感染，Jean François Fernel 早在 1554 年首次提到了这种疾病，至今已近 500 年。其后，William Osler 在 1885 年的一系列演讲中详细描述了该病[1]。近几十年来，心内膜炎的临床情况发生了快速而显著的变化。随着新技术的进步和社会环境的改变，IE 相关的微生物学和风险因素也在不断变化，其中一个重要的风险因素就是静脉违禁药物的使用，如海洛因和可卡因。而这种疾病演变的核心正是所谓"阿片类药物泛滥"，目前，这一趋势正影响着美国和其他一些国家[2]。

临床特征和结局

IE 是一种罕见疾病，但近年来其发病率迅速蹿升。近期数据显示，截至 21 世纪初，全球每年 IE 的发病率为（3~10）/10 万[2]，但 IE 的发病率一直在上升，虽然存在地区差异，但美国的 IE 发病率居全球之首——达到 15/10 万[3]。

IE 的主要致病菌已从口腔链球菌转变为葡萄球菌，其中原因很多，包括有效抗生素的研发、假体植入物使用的增加、侵入性静脉导管的使用、免疫抑制剂，以及本章要讨论的核心问题——静脉吸毒（IVDU）[4]。心内膜炎的诊断需要结合病史、体格检查和超声心动图检查。抗生素是其治疗首选，但由于流行病学和疾病急性程度的变化，心内膜炎已逐渐成为一种外科疾病[5]。心内膜炎的治疗效果仍不理想：据报道，院内死亡率可高达 20%[6]。

IE 的手术结果差异很大，这一差别主要取决于受累的瓣膜、疾病的侵袭性和共病。围手术期总体死亡率低于 10%[7]。局限于瓣叶的孤立性自体主动脉瓣和二尖瓣感染的围手术期死亡率差别不大，分别为 7% 和 6%；但侵袭性（感染范围超出瓣叶，累及邻近结构）和多瓣膜受累 IE 的治疗效果较差。IE 的 5 年总体存活率为 66%，其中，非侵袭性主动脉瓣心内膜炎的存活率较高，而二尖瓣、多瓣膜受累和侵袭性 IE 的存活率较低。IVDU 是影响长期生存的一个重要因素，复吸和再感染可导致较差的长期预后[8]。

阿片类药物滥用

过去几十年，处方镇痛药的使用在美国急剧增加，估计有430万人在非医疗情况下使用了处方镇痛药。他们当中IVDU的可能性是普通人的40倍[9]，约80%的新发海洛因使用者以前曾滥用过处方镇痛药[10]。

在2002—2016年的15年间，美国静脉吸毒相关感染性心内膜炎（IVDU-IE）的发病率翻了1倍[11]，仅2010—2015年，IVDU-IE在所有IE病例中的占比从15.3%增至29.1%[12]。虽然IVDU-IE患者的短期存活率高于非IVDU患者，这可能与他们较为年轻有关，但他们再入院率和毒品使用率更高[12]。他们的中期预后并不乐观，在3~4个月时，IVDU-IE患者发生死亡或再次手术的风险是非IVDU-IE的10倍以上[13]。此外，与非IVDU-IE相比，IVDU-IE的长期预后更差：5年和10年存活率分别为46.7%和41.1%，而前者分别为71.1%和52.0%[8]。

主要伦理问题

在治疗IVDU-IE的过程中，伦理困境很常见，并可能严重影响治疗和结局。常见的问题往往源于对IVDU者的偏见，例如质疑对有明显自残行为的患者进行治疗的意义，在现代医疗体系中面对高昂的治疗成本如何分配有限的资源，以及对患者可能会因持续吸毒而造成长期治疗结局不佳的疑虑。在某些病例中，可能会出现一些不常见的问题，但仍可能造成严重的两难困境，例如，在活胎妊娠的情况下对IVDU-IE的治疗。

对自残患者的医疗

对IVDU-IE患者的医疗在多个层面上具有挑战性，但许多困难不是来自"如何治疗"，而是来自"我们是否应该治疗"。临床医生在工作中获得的成就感来自在正确的时间为正确的患者提供正确的治疗，患者的病情会得到很好的控制。相反，如果临床判断告诉医生，无论他们做什么，患者的情况都会很糟糕，成就感就会减弱。有些人可能会认为，无论为IVDU者提供什么治疗，患者在出院后不久就会重新开始吸毒，因而存在较高的IE复发风险。此外，IVDU者通常会受到诋毁；尽管阿片类药物使用障碍（OUD）是一种公认的诊断和疾病过程，但吸毒成瘾往往被视为"道德败坏"[14]。许多研究表明，对IVDU者的负面态度和看法十分普遍[14-16]。对IVDU的污名化可对相关治疗产生很大影响，常会引起医患双方相互的不满，并可能损害治疗效果。

- **基于患者生活方式或行为的有限或可变通的医疗**

"自残"行为的存在及其对疾病的危害，影响着许多医护工作者的态度。大多数外科医生会为第一次患心内膜炎的IVDU者进行手术。但许多外科医生可能会就此划清界限，施行"一次出局"的原则对待这类瓣膜置换术，也就是只做这一次手术，再次出现问题则不予过问。显然，IVDU 是患者的个人行为，但成瘾过程是复杂的，许多外部因素会影响成瘾行为。那种认为患者对自己的健康不负责的说法貌似有理，其实反而是弱化了自主性原则的基础，因为其他因素在这一过程中可能起着重要作用。例如，阿片类药物成瘾通常源于处方镇痛药，缺乏适当的成瘾治疗可能会减缓或阻碍康复，加上社会问题或心理问题可能会使戒毒更加困难。OUD 与其他精神障碍高度相关，需要同时进行治疗才能达到最佳效果[17]。如果医生仅仅因为患者存在未得到充分治疗的吸毒行为而简单地拒绝治疗复发性 IE 是不负责任的，会剥夺患者所需的治疗[18]。OUD 被认为是一种医学疾病，现有证据表明，对 OUD 相关的 IE 和其他 IVDU 相关感染的治疗普遍不足[19]。

IVDU-IE 并不是唯一一种明显由自我伤害引起的疾病。但心胸外科医生在同一问题上的立场表现却截然不同：他们会拒绝为复发性 IVDU-IE 患者做手术，但对因吸烟而复发的肺癌或对肥胖、已放置冠脉支架且血糖未得到控制的糖尿病患者，需要做冠状动脉旁路移植手术时，却毅然决然，立即手术。

Baldassarri 等做过一个有趣的比较——将 IVDU-IE 与其他被更正面看待的危险生活方式引起的伤害或疾病进行对比[20]。他们列举了狂热徒步旅行者的例子，其中有些人因在户外接触蜱虫而反复患蜱传播疾病；还有自行车骑手或摩托车骑手因骑行时发生意外而反复骨折。这些疾病都是由于参加了被社会视为积极生活方式的活动而引起的。尽管患者知道参加这些活动的风险，而且以前发生过不良事件，仍继续参加这些活动，但没有医生会拒绝治疗他们。作者断言，IVDU 者的神经生化在病理上受到化学依赖性的影响，与徒步旅行者或骑自行车者相比，对于出现并发症，他们的责任相比还要小一些。一般人可以对参加各种活动的相对风险存在质疑，但如果医生也对这些危险行为持有如此不一致的观点，其观察结果发人深省。

根据患者的生活方式为其改变治疗方案，一个具体的例子就是为年轻的 IVDU-IE 患者选择瓣膜类型。据我们所知，目前还没有针对这一问题的正式研究，但一般经验是，IVDU-IE 年轻患者接受生物瓣膜治疗的情况比较普遍。仅从年龄来看，他们使用机械瓣膜可能会获得更好的长期效果，但这类患者通常被认为在抗凝药物的依从性方面"不可靠"。如果这种假设是正确的，患者就可能免于瓣膜血栓形成、卒中和早期死亡。但这一处理方式对那些能够坚持长期抗凝治疗的患者则很不幸，这些患者需要承受瓣膜衰败的后果，并可能在未来某个时间需要再次手术。

一项关于心内膜炎手术结果的单中心研究指出：尽管队列中 IVDU-IE 患者的平均年龄为 43 岁，但 95% 以上的患者接受了生物瓣置换；相比之下，平均年龄为 48 岁的非 IVDU-IE 患者中只有 73.7% 接受了生物瓣置换[8]。尽管 IVDU-IE 患者年龄较小，但术后中位生存期仅为 3 年，且这些患者再次手术的风险并没有增加。

作者的结论是，对于 IVDU-IE 患者，无论年龄大小，使用生物瓣膜都是合理的。值得注意的是，在少数接受机械瓣置换的 IVDU-IE 患者中，没有一例出现与瓣膜相关的并发症。

• 药物使用合同有效吗？

Merriam-Webster Dictionary 将合同定义为"两人或两人以上或多方之间具有约束力的协议，尤其是具有法律约束力的协议"[21]。阿片类药物合同或镇痛合同是处方开出者与患者之间的正式书面协议，概述了适当使用阿片类药物的基本规则，旨在阻止阿片类药物滥用。但与传统合同不同，它们不具有约束力或法律强制力。鉴于此，抑或由于对"合同"一词感到不适，一些医生开始使用阿片类药物或镇痛"协议"一词。然而，协议是由"更具话语权"的医生起草的，因此这种不对等使得医患之间合作的表象和达到的共识失去了实际意义[22]。阿片类药物合同包含规范阿片类药物处方、配药和使用的规则和条款，以及违反这些规则的后果，但很少或根本没有涉及应达到的医疗目标。阿片类药物合同的执行表明医护对患者缺乏信任度。虽然医生对患者缺乏信任可能是合理的，但当患者发现这种缺乏信任的情况时可能会破坏医患关系。

阿片类药物合同取得成功的案例已见诸报道。一项针对内科签订了长期阿片类药物合同患者的回顾性研究发现，63% 的患者在研究期间始终遵守合同条款。在 37% 未遵守合同条款的患者中，20% 为自愿停止治疗，17% 因"违约"而被医生解除合同[23]。该研究纳入的患者包括以前未服用阿片类镇痛药的慢性疼痛患者。研究未报告吸毒史，也未报告研究参与者中是否之前曾有过 IVDU。遗憾的是，这一策略能否防止患者从长期口服阿片类药物发展为静脉注射阿片类药物尚不明确。在这一人群中，预计随机尿检会出现阿片类药物阳性反应。鉴于这些原因，这项研究的结果可能无法推广到 IVDU-IE 人群中。

阿片类药物使用合同也适用于外科治疗。瓣膜置换术后使用阿片类药物合同对预防复吸的有效性尚未确定。在前面提到的无药物成瘾史的慢性疼痛患者群体中，有近 20% 的患者被发现违反了阿片类药物合同[23]。可以预见，在 IVDU 群体，这种违约率还会高得多。正如 Wurcel 等在社论中所说："药物/物质使用障碍具有复杂的病理生理学，在很大程度上受到合并精神疾病和社会经济因素的影响……在这一极端特殊的医疗背景下，指望在一张纸上签字就能避免患者再次吸毒是不现实的"[24]。对这篇社论的回应认为，如果不接受治疗，OUD 就是一种致命疾病，外科医生坚持要求患者"同意在手术后认真努力地遵循治疗计划"并非不合理[25]。OUD 是 IVDU-IE 的一个重要共病，必须进行治疗，以尽可能达到最佳的长期效果。如果患者能够充分理解 IVDU 是导致其发生危及生命的瓣膜感染的原因，那么从逻辑上讲，他们就想停止使用毒品，此时，安排适当的戒毒治疗似乎比签订戒毒合同更有可能奏效。

为术后成瘾治疗制定书面协议似乎本质上并无害处或是不道德，但如果要签署这样一份协议，文件的目的应该是明确患者和医生的共同目标，并关注可预见的问题和可用资源。协议无须罗列吸毒时所采取的惩罚性措施，因为这可能会降低患者在复吸时寻求帮助的可能性。此外，医生应该有一种清晰的认识，即他们与患者之间签订的任何药物使用或成瘾治疗协议都不具有法律约束力，以此文件拒绝为患者提供治疗，无论在道德上还是法律上都是站不住脚的。正如 DiMaio 等提醒我们的那样，医生的义务是为患者做出医疗决定，而不是对其进行道德绑架[18]。

· **照护"第二个生命"——在涉及怀孕案例中的产妇权利与胎儿权利**

妊娠期心内膜炎非常罕见，每 8000 例妊娠中仅有 1 例[26]。但由于母体和胎儿的需求之间可能存在冲突，处理起来会相当复杂。心脏手术后的胎儿死亡率为 16.7%～30%[26-27]，妊娠早期（前 3 个月）的胎儿死亡率更高[27]。相比之下，孕产妇死亡率为 2%～3%。胎儿器官形成在妊娠的前 3 个月，这表明手术应推迟到妊娠中期（中间 3 个月）[26]。也有人建议等到第 28 周再进行手术[27]，但妊娠晚期进行手术同样有增加早产的风险[26]。

IVDU 者妊娠期间发生 IE，在医疗上，母体和胎儿处理优先权方面就存在显著的冲突。首先，准妈妈吸毒会给胎儿带来风险，因此必须极力劝阻患者不要再吸毒，并安排最佳的戒毒治疗。其次，对孕妇有益的不一定对胎儿有益。如果在怀孕期间患上 IE，手术最好推迟到分娩后进行。孕期限期手术会给胎儿带来巨大风险。在妊娠早期和妊娠中期前段分娩的胎儿无法存活，推迟限期手术很可能会导致孕妇和胎儿死亡。因此如要手术，则应清楚一点：在这种情况下终止妊娠的风险很高。妊娠晚期进行手术胎儿死亡风险较低，尽管早产儿有相当大的死亡风险或远期的神经系统问题，但剖宫产仍不失为一个合理的选择[26]。综上，手术的决定必须根据胎儿的胎龄和孕妇疾病的严重程度个性化处理。

孕妇可能会不顾医疗团队的劝阻，拒绝接受剖宫产等有指征的手术。幸运的是，准妈妈们几乎总是以胎儿的利益为重[26]，但当她们不考虑胎儿的利益时，她们自身的利益就会与胎儿的利益产生冲突。除非患者因精神疾病而缺乏做决定的能力，否则她有权自主决定对其身体采取何种处理。然而，胎儿的权利就不那么明确了，这就取决于当地的文化。在美国，妇女的权利高于胎儿的权利[28]；而且共识表明，为了胎儿的利益而强迫孕妇进行手术是不正当的[29]。在孕产妇和胎儿利益不一致的情况下，最好的办法可能是将胎儿的存活和健康作为所有相关方的共同目标[26]。

· **安装心律失常治疗装置患者的特殊注意事项**

起搏器和植入式心律转复除颤器（ICD）是可以挽救生命的医疗装置，但也是容易受到感染的血管内异物，尤其是在 IVDU 相关菌血症的情况下。对于如何处理 IVDU 者的起搏器和 ICD 感染的伦理问题，相关文献很少。一项报道提到了相关问题，但只得出了一个结论：在讨论知情同意时，IVDU 患者应被告知静脉注射会增加设备感染的风险[30]。报道特别提到，处理被感染的起搏器或 ICD 比处理被感染的人工瓣膜更为直截了当，因为移除起搏器电极导线或 ICD 比再次手术置换瓣膜更简单。而决定是否重新植入起搏电极则显得更加困难。依赖起搏器或有心源性猝死病史的患者当然必须接受再植入手术，这时如果植入心外膜或皮下电极，在 IVDU 者，感染的可能性就会降低。对于植入起搏器适应证不明确的患者，例如既往因症状性心动过缓而植入起搏器但目前不再需要起搏治疗的患者，不重新植入起搏器是合理的，对此类患者可进行密切监测并转而接受成瘾治疗。

"难治性"患者的伦理考量

在 IE 患者中，IVDU 患者是最难治疗的。正如 Buchman 和 Lynch 所说，"医院环境对吸毒者往往并不友好"[31]。医护人员通常对 IVDU 者持消极态度，合并精神障碍可能引发患者与医护人员之间的冲突。此外，使用静脉注射抗生素治疗 IE 通常需要长时间住院，让医患的沮丧情绪进一步强化。在 IE 人群中，IVDU 者违背医嘱（AMA）离院的可能性明显高于非吸毒者[32]。IVDU-IE 的成功彻底治疗需要具备管理患者和医护人员两个方面的措施。

·医护人员的注意事项

医护人员普遍对 IVDU 者持消极态度[14-16]。一项关于患者拒绝接受所需治疗的报道指出："在某些情况下，被视为'不受欢迎'的患者被允许拒绝接受治疗，医护人员希望他们能因此尽快出院"[33]。对许多医生、护士和辅助人员来说，IVDU-IE 患者属于"不受欢迎"的一类，他们可能宁愿看到患者提前出院，也不愿继续照护他们。这种情绪可能源于患者与医护人员之间不愉快的互动，也可能源于他们认为 IVDU-IE 是一种"自作自受"的疾病。对于这类患者的负面情绪，医护人员可能会做出如下反应：视而不见、延迟使用镇痛药物、禁止接触想要的物品或设备（如电视）以及迅速减少美沙酮用量[32]。适当的员工干预措施包括支持性地倾听受挫医护人员的意见，定期召开医护人员会议，特别邀请心理咨询师参与会议，他们可以帮助医护人员理解患者的行为，改善与患者的沟通。

·对于拒绝治疗患者的处理

IVDU 者在治疗 IE 期间出现 AMA 离院的风险很高。一项对所有心内膜炎患者性格倾向的研究显示：6 年内，9 名 IVDU-IE 患者中有 8 人因 AMA 离院，而 17 名不吸毒的患者中无一人离院[32]。有些患者可能仅仅为了自己或他人的利益而非自愿入院治疗。民事收治条律（civil commitments）由美国各州法律管辖，其中包括允许的收治期限。一般来说，如果患者对自己或他人构成威胁，或患上了精神疾病、学习障碍，或因药物导致对现实的认知产生扭曲，就可非自愿收治[34]。

对于 IVDU-IE 患者来说，留在医院继续接受治疗对他们最有利。这类人群中的 AMA 出院率较高，这可能是由于医院中的冲突或他们自身想要复吸造成的。然而，如果 IVDU 者选择 AMA 离院，就会出现受益原则和自主原则之间的伦理学冲突：对这类患者最好的办法是让他们继续住院，但这样做又侵犯了他们自主决策的权利。

由于民事收治过程侵犯了个人自由，医生必须考虑收治患者的法律后果。IVDU 者有很高的精神疾病共病率，但规范民事收治的法律仅支持根据上述标准对患者实施非自愿收治[34]。仅有 OUD 本身而收治是不够的，甚至于如果 IVDU-IE 患者心智健全，他们如果选择 AMA 离院，医务人员都无权阻止，这一状况可能会令人沮丧。尽管如此，医生仍应与患者详细讨论 AMA 离院的后果，并应询问患者，给他们提供某些未满足但可补救的需求，或帮助解决潜在的问题，以期说服其留院完成治疗。一项单中心研究发现，美沙酮、丁丙诺啡和纳曲酮等药物与 AMA 离院率的降低有关，但这项低效能研究的结果差异并无统计学意义[35]。

特殊情况下可允许仅因吸毒而被收治。在美国 23 个州，怀孕期间吸毒被视为虐待儿童；在明尼苏达州、南达科他州和威斯康星州则被视为民事收治的依据[36]。因此，在特定情况下，孕妇可能会被非自愿收治，以确保她们不再继续吸毒，因为这种行为会危及胎儿和她自身的生命安全。

医生在医疗成本评估和资源分配中的作用

当前各家医疗机构都很重视成本控制，医生在分配稀缺或昂贵资源方面扮演什么角色？社会的需求和患者的需求往往背道而驰，医生可能会被夹在中间。此外，医疗机构可能会出于财务原因向医生施压，要求他们基于经济因素而非医疗因素进行医疗决策。IVDU 者往往没有保险，医院也无法从中获利；对其社会价值的先入之见使人们对他们未来的生产力充满疑虑，也使他们无法获得昂贵的医疗服务和接受手术治疗。医疗决策中的成本控制有时很容易，比如更换缝合材料的品牌，但在决定谁应该接受挽救生命的手术时却充满了伦理学难题。

·因资源有限而拒绝为 IVDU 者进行手术是否符合伦理？

IE 的治疗费用高昂。IVDU-IE 患者通常被认为是"不受欢迎的人"，这既是因为在社会层面上他们为吸毒者，也因为他们可能没有保险。美国疾病控制与预防中心最近报道称，IVDU-IE 患者的平均住院费用约为 5 万美元，其中 42% 的患者没有保险或是通过医疗补助计划（Medicaid）获得保险[9]。这一较大比例的无保险或需要公费医疗的患者将治疗 IE 的经济负担转嫁给了纳税人和当地医疗系统。仅在 5 年间，IVDU-IE 的住院人数就增加了 12 倍，而住院费用增加了 18 倍。根据 2011 年的报道，美国每年因违禁药品造成的经济损失为 1930 亿美元，而现在这个数字肯定还要高得多[37]。这一数字包括医疗花费、犯罪活动引起的直接和间接浪费以及生产力丧失所带来的损失。据最近估计，每年因吸食或注射海洛因造成的社会损失高达 512 亿美元，其中约 20% 来自生产力损失[38]。

鉴于这些事实，IVDU 者是否应该接受昂贵的医疗，如心脏手术？自体瓣膜 IE 且符合手术条件的 IVDU 者几乎都会接受瓣膜置换术，争议主要围绕在如果继续吸毒，是否还要再次进行瓣膜手术这一问题上。

对于 IVDU-IE 再手术问题，基于社会和经济利益考量，也可能是出于某些人的个人偏见，可能会做出不再进行手术的决定。IVDU-IE 的治疗费用昂贵，但从美国使用合法药物的经济成本来看，这一经济成本不足以成为不为 IVDU-IE 患者提供手术的理由。美国每年因过度饮酒造成的经济损失高达 2490 亿美元[39]。吸烟的成本也同样高昂，每年造成的损失超过 3200 亿美元，其中 1700 亿美元用于医疗[40]，1500 亿美元是生产力损失[41]。这两种行为也都属于自我伤害，是可以避免的。尽管成本高昂，但没有人反对治疗酗酒和吸烟的并发症。我们很难泾渭分明地区分出"可接受"和"不可接受"的自残行为[42]，同样，要量化多大程度上是基于社会价值偏见，多大程度上是基于对保险覆盖面和支付医疗费用能力的考量而做出相应的医疗决策也一样困难。

从历史的角度来看待治疗 IE 的经济学问题很有启发性[43]。在 1965 年建立医疗保险（Medicare）和医疗补助计划（Medicaid）之前，贫困患者在公立和私立医院接受慈善治疗。1965 年后，因患者无力支付医疗费用而拒绝为其提供所需的医疗服务被认为是不道德的。法律上也有先例，在面对昂贵的医疗服务时，医生应从患者疾病治疗的角度出发去做决策，医生是患者的代理人，而不是社会的代理人[43]。

为 IVDU 者成功实施 IE 手术后，他们会重返社区。他们可能会重新开始吸毒，在返回医院时又会出现新的并发症，并产生更多相关费用。如果患者因得不到治疗而死亡，虽然避免了未来的医疗费用，但也导致了未来生产力的损失。有关资源分配的决策必须在社会政策层面做出，而不是医生在病床边做出[44]。医生不应将自己的社会责任视为必须剔除负担沉重的患者以节省公共资金。相反，在治疗急性心脏病之后，医生应努力帮助这些患者治疗他们的第二种疾病——毒瘾。这样，他们就能为患者提供最好的治疗，这更符合医疗职业道德的要求，并将一个有可能恢复正常劳动力的人交还给社会。

无效性评估

成功治疗 IVDU-IE 的一个重要阻碍是先入为主地认为治疗是徒劳的。在这种疾病的治疗中，"无效"可以有两种解释。医学上的无效是指在医学上不可能达到任何目标，因此停止治疗在伦理学上是可以接受的。将医疗无效的概念应用于 IVDU-IE 中较为复杂，可能要面临多样的情形，面对不同的结果。总体而言，对 IVDU-IE 进行干预可能被认为最终是无效的，因为患者的长期存活率很低。但眼前的现实是，抗生素和瓣膜置换是治疗感染性瓣膜病变非常有效的疗法，且短期疗效通常较好。"社会心理无效"已被应用于成瘾和不良适应行为，这些行为极有可能导致再次吸毒，并因此导致 IE 复发、寿命缩短[20]。心脏外科医生会常规评估手术风险，可以对手术短期和长期并发症及死亡的发生风险做出比较直接明确的分析。困难的是，如何评估有关治疗在社会心理学层面的无效性，因为 IVDU 患者可能已经过了能够克服毒瘾的阶段。

• IVDU-IE 患者的长期存活率如何？

IVDU-IE 患者的短期疗效往往优于非 IVDU-IE 患者，因为他们的年龄轻，合发症少[13]。但长期疗效却因复吸的高再感染率而受到影响，再感染是这一人群的主要死因[45]。然而，再感染并不是吸毒的唯一致死并发症，因为吸毒者也可能死于暴力或吸毒过量[3]。

一项单中心系列研究发现：IVDU 者在心内膜炎手术后的中期死亡率（6 个月至 5 年）明显高于非吸毒者，分别为 53% 和 31%，尽管非 IVDU-IE 患者的年龄明显更大（平均年龄 60 岁 vs.38 岁）[46]。另一项单中心研究发现：IVDU-IE 患者的中位生存期为术后 3 年，术后 5 年和 10 年的存活率均明显低于非 IVDU-IE 患者（46.7% vs. 71.1%；41.1% vs. 52%）[8]。一项多中心研究发现，IVDU-IE 和非 IVDU-IE 患者的长期预后相似：5 年存活率为 78.9% vs.76.1%，10 年存活率为 69.5% vs. 68.7%[47]。与之前的单中心研究相比，该研究的组间年龄差异更大（分别为 23 岁和 5 岁），这可能是长期存活率结果不同的原因。以上 3 项研究均发现 IVDU 增加了再感染的风险，但只有多中心研究发现 IVDU 与再手术率增加有关。这或许表明各医疗单位对再次手术的态度不同，这可能会影响患者的长期生存。Straw 等发现 IVDU-IE 患者的 5 年存活率低于 50%[48]，Shrestha 等发现 5 年存活率为 50%~60%[13]。一项包括 19 项研究的 meta 分析也发现：与非 IVDU-IE 相比，IVDU-IE 的长期存活率更低，5 年存活率为 70% vs. 62%，10 年存活率为 63% vs.56%[49]。

对接受过瓣膜手术的 IVDU 者的长期存活率研究发现，尽管这些患者年龄较轻，但存活率并不高，5 年存活率较高的为 78%[47]，大多数是 40%~60%[8,13,48]。存活率如此之低，难道 IVDU-IE 患者的手术治疗是徒劳吗？我们可以同时考虑一下心肺衰竭的手术治疗效果。左心室辅助装置（LVAD）治疗和肺移植的 5 年存活率均为 54%，但这两种疗法既不被认为是徒劳的干预措施，也不被认为是浪费资源[50-51]。与内科治疗相比，肺移植和 LVAD 治疗均能提高患者的存活率；但关于瓣膜置换手术是否能改善 IVDU-IE 的长期预后，目前还没有高质量的数据。据报道，接受手术治疗的 IVDU-IE 患者的死亡率高于接受药物治疗的患者，但这些都是回顾性数据，可能是因为手术组患者的病情更重[48]。一项研究报道了因再感染而再手术的情况，显示再手术率最高的患者群具有最好的长期疗效[47]，这表明如果对复发性 IE 的再手术采取更积极的态度，患者的长期存活率可能会提高。

• 判断患者可戒毒的难度

治疗 IVDU-IE 最具挑战性的问题可能是预测患者是否会停止继续吸毒。对药物辅助疗法（MAT）的研究显示，与其他疗法相比，MAT 的复吸率明显降低，消除了人们对于这一疗法的疑虑[52-54]。不过，目前对外科患者使用阿片类替代药物或阿片类药物拮抗剂似乎尚未得到广泛采纳。虽然自 20 世纪 60 年代以来，美沙酮一直用于治疗海洛因成瘾，疗效良好，但相关数据可能并不广为人知[55]。更有甚者，围绕 OUD 的污名化以致大家都不愿开具这些药物；另外，获得专业的成瘾治疗指导的途径又非常有限，导致这一疗法尚未得到推广。尽管如此，复吸仍是导致再感染和死亡的最重要因素，而 IE 与 OUD 密切相关，并非独立过程。因此，为了确保良好的长期疗效，必须将心内膜炎的手术治疗与戒毒相关的药物治疗和精神治疗相结合。

双重疾病的治疗——瓣膜疾病和成瘾

越来越多的人认识到，需要对 IVDU-IE 患者进行双重疾病的治疗。2016 年美国胸外科协会 IE 外科治疗共识指南将这一治疗方案作为 I 类方案予以推荐，即"有 IVDU 史的患者应接受成瘾治疗"[56]。现在，OUD 被认为是一种医学疾病，因此相关外科医生应将成瘾视为一种共病而非性格缺陷。这一推荐的重要性就像心脏外科医生使用冠状动脉旁路移植术治疗冠心病的同时还需要治疗其共病高脂血症和糖尿病一样。在治疗 IVDU-IE 患者的心脏疾病时，还需提供目前治疗 OUD 的最佳方法——MAT，以优化长期疗效。

· 成瘾治疗转诊率

遗憾的是，对 IVDU-IE 群体中的成瘾治疗远远不足。住院接受成瘾治疗是一种强有力的措施，住院 MAT 的启动可提高门诊 MAT 的依从性，降低非法阿片类药物的使用率[57]。然而，在一家医疗中心收治的 IVDU-IE 患者中，只有 24% 的患者接受了住院成瘾治疗或精神科咨询；更糟糕的是，只有 7.8% 的患者在出院时制定了 MAT 计划，没有一人在出院时服用治疗成瘾的药物[19]。

· 单纯戒断与药物辅助治疗的比较

目前的戒毒疗法包括一系列药物和精神疗法。许多药物已被证明能有效抑制吸毒者对毒品的需求，并有助于防止复吸。此外，认知行为疗法和其他精神治疗方法可以帮助患者合理用药并培养应对技能。

MAT 是指使用阿片类替代药物或阿片类药物拮抗剂，如美沙酮、丁丙诺啡和纳曲酮，治疗 IVDU 以防复吸高风险。这与"单纯戒断"形成鲜明对比，后者不使用任何药物治疗，希望患者依靠自身意志力停止吸毒，或采用认知行为疗法等精神治疗方法。在美国，"单纯戒断"尽管不能充分解决作为一种医学疾病的 OUD 问题，但仍然是一种普遍使用的方法。另外，与 MAT 相比，这种方法的 OUD 复发率较高。

MAT 源于 Dole 和 Nyswander1965 年的一项具有里程碑意义的研究，他们报道使用美沙酮成功治疗了 22 名海洛因成瘾者[55]。所有患者都说用药后"麻醉药物渴望感"（narcotic hunger）有所减轻，并能避免继续吸毒，恢复工作和生活。其他一些替代药物的研究也显示很有疗效。在一项关于丁丙诺啡与安慰剂的随机对照试验中，两组患者都接受了认知行为疗法和每周一次的心理咨询，1 年后的结果差异令人惊叹：75% 接受丁丙诺啡治疗的患者仍在接受治疗，而安慰剂组则无一人仍在接受治疗[52]。在另一项试验中，缓释纳曲酮（XR-NTX）与安慰剂相比显示：XR-NTX组的阿片类药物使用明显减少（纳曲酮组99%的天数不使用阿片类药物，而安慰剂组仅为60%），且保留在组内继续治疗的时间也更长（平均168 d *vs.* 96 d）[53]。还有一项专门针对美国刑事罪犯的XR-NTX研究发现，服用XR-NTX者复吸率较低（43% *vs.* 64%），过量吸毒发生率也较低（0% *vs.* 4.5%）[54]。

在治疗OUD方面，MAT明显优于单纯戒断。然而，MAT并未被广泛用于治疗成瘾：只有34%的患者接受了MAT治疗OUD[58]。MAT推广应用的障碍存在于个人认知、基础设施和政策层面。人们普遍将吸毒视为耻辱，许多个体医疗服务提供者认为MAT只是用一种毒瘾替代另一种毒瘾。另外，患者和医疗服务提供者通常都对OUD和MAT缺乏足够的了解[59]。再者，缺乏合格的成瘾问题专家可能会限制这些药物的使用，因为全科医生可能不熟悉这些药物的使用，而较少开出。一项旨在广泛调查MAT应用阻碍的研究发现，美国各州MAT实施情况差异很大[60]。拥有良好基础设施的州，特别是拥有适当规模的戒毒专家队伍和充足资金的州，采用MAT的比例较高。而那些对12步戒毒计划和其他"社会戒毒"计划投入巨大的州则对MAT的采用抱强烈的抵触情绪，其中许多州不允许对OUD门诊患者使用美沙酮。此外，政策制定者和立法者可能对MAT持有偏见，这严重阻碍了MAT的采用。

- **减少危害策略**

减少危害是一种旨在减少吸毒负面影响的策略，目的是使吸毒更安全，而不是预防或阻止吸毒[61]。当前的措施包括针头交换计划（NEP）和安全注射教育。尽管许多人认为以任何方式持续使用毒品都是令人厌恶的，但这种对吸毒者不带偏见的态度反而可能有助于他们逐步戒除毒瘾。患者应被纳入医疗保健系统，并建立治疗关系。相反，如果在患者没有思想准备之前就强迫他们参加戒毒或MAT计划，则有可能失去患者的信任，甚至失去联系，直到吸毒造成灾难性后果。许多研究数据表明，减少危害策略是有效的。从技术上讲，MAT也是减少危害的一种形式。但在本节，我们将重点讨论注射卫生教育、安全注射点（也称监督注射点）和针头交换计划。

一项针对针头卫生和安全注射方法的随机对照干预研究发现：接受干预后，吸毒者的不安全注射行为大幅减少，细菌性皮肤感染风险降低[62]。针头交换计划允许吸毒者退还用过的针头以换取新针头。理论上讲，这可以降低感染并发症的发生，如人类免疫缺陷病毒（HIV）、丙型肝炎病毒（HCV）感染和心内膜炎及其他细菌感染。安全注射点允许患者在专业医务人员在场的情况下安全、卫生地进行注射，而不是在公共场所或其他吸毒场所进行注射，因为这两种场所都会增加感染风险[63]。多项研究证明了针头交换计划和安全注射点的安全性和有效性，并记录到了过量用药、重复使用和共用针头以及在公共场合使用或丢弃针头等情况的减少[61]。

针头交换计划在美国备受争议，但已变得越来越普遍。截至 2018 年，已有 39 个州加上华盛顿特区和波多黎各通过了相关法律，允许实施针头或注射器交换计划[64]。要想取得成功，针头交换的概念必须得到普遍接受，还须执法部门予以配合。如果执法人员盯住针头交换点，将其作为轻易逮捕吸毒者的机会，那么针头交换计划就无法达到预期目的。安全注射点与针头交换计划有本质区别，因为它们不仅提供设备，而且实际上提供了非法吸毒的场所。安全注射点已在欧洲和加拿大成功施行多年，但目前在美国还是非法的[65]。

从伦理上讲，减少危害计划符合自主和非恶意原则。吸毒者选择继续吸毒的权利得到尊重，危害的风险也会降低。而从继续吸毒是一种自我伤害行为的意义上讲，减少危害计划的实施会违背受益原则，或者相反，减少危害计划可能会促使吸毒者参与 MAT 或戒毒治疗，这将带来显著获益。总的来说，减少危害计划似乎大多是有益的。从法律上讲，纵容和帮助吸毒有违正义：在许多司法管辖区，吸毒者仍然受到追捕和起诉。此外，减少危害计划可以使吸毒者保持与医疗专业人员的接触，并建立融洽的关系，这可能会促进戒毒。从伦理上讲，这些项目符合正义原则，因为它们的存在不是为了吸毒，而是为了吸毒者的安全，吸毒者与所有寻求改善健康状况的人一样应受到尊重。显然，减少危害计划并无有悖伦理。

- **经外周中心静脉置管在减少危害中的作用**

对 IVDU 者在门诊使用经外周中心静脉置管（PICC 管路）的问题存在争议。PICC 管路是治疗严重细菌感染的标准工具，依此，患者可在门诊接受静脉注射抗生素治疗，从而腾出住院病床和资源，并可降低住院治疗的相关风险。为 IVDU 者置入 PICC 管路的一个主要顾虑是这种管路为注射毒品提供了便利，为此，目前的普遍做法是，不允许 IVDU-IE 患者带着 PICC 置管出院，以进行院外长期静脉注射抗生素治疗。一项针对 PICC 管路的高危吸毒者的研究显示，即使他们没有出院回家，在医院或疗养院期间，重新开始 IVDU 的比例高达 40%，这凸显了他们毒瘾的严重性[66]。在门诊 IVDU 者中使用防"篡改"PICC 后，96% 的患者成功完成了门诊抗生素治疗，且没有证据表明 PICC 被"篡改"用于吸毒[67]。这项研究的纳入标准相对严格，包括对"篡改"PICC 的"零容忍"政策。

门诊 PICC 可作为一种减少危害的策略，这种管路有助于促进出院，从而节省宝贵的医疗资源[31]。但戒毒被认为是一条"崎岖不平的道路"，患者可能会在一段时间内遵从医嘱，也可能会复吸，所以有必要向患者讲授安全的注射方法，这样即便因复吸而出现并发症，其危险性也相对较小。

复发性心内膜炎与再手术

在 IVDU-IE 患者的治疗过程中，最有争议也是被讨论最多的话题可能是，是否应该为接受过瓣膜置换、却因再次 IVDU 发生人工瓣膜感染的患者提供再次瓣膜手术。限定瓣膜置换的次数是一种相对常见的做法[14]，即外科医生提供一次瓣膜置换术，如果患者再次 IVDU 并出现瓣膜感染，则拒绝为其提供再次治疗。而有些外科医生会以手术可行性为前提，尽可能地为这类患者提供多次手术机会。但多数外科医生则会根据实际情况，采用更为细致、稳妥的处理方法。面对这些问题，正确的处理包括以下方面：

- 有目标的进行客观的评估和决策；
- 避免情绪波动和道德评判的影响；
- 同时考虑 OUD 和 IE 这两种既相互独立又相互关联的疾病的各自治疗需要；
- 结合患者的价值观和个人意愿。

Yeo 等认为，对于不遵从医嘱、反复出现 IVDU-IE 的持续吸毒者，不存在再次手术的道德义务[68]。他们首先援引了自主权的论点，声称患者最终要对自己的行为和健康负责；其次援引了正义的论点，指出患者之前有机会改善自己的健康状况，其他人也有权获得有限的资源。他们关注的是群体健康，而不是个人健康。他们认为，对屡教不改的吸毒者的治疗与优化人口健康背道而驰，因为这些患者不会为自己的健康负责，他们过度使用稀缺资源，增加了犯罪率，而且由于他们往往没有经济基础，会造成资源的进一步流失。虽然 Yeo 等承认医疗决定不能以一个人的社会价值为基础，但他们断言这些患者的行为已经违背了已有"社会契约"。他们支持在国家和社会层面进行医疗资源配给，但不鼓励医生个人进行床边配给，认为"医生必须始终是患者的代言人"。

Kirkpatrick 指出，医疗服务的主要支付方要么是政府机构，要么是保险公司，但两者都未能根据患者行为或生活方式为医疗服务配给做出决策[69]。与 Yeo 等一样，他也认为医生没有资格代表政府或保险公司做出决定，医生的职责只是治疗疾病。

Buchman 和 Lynch 认为，如果复吸者表示愿意停止吸毒，就应该给予其第二次瓣膜置换的机会[31]。他们从减少危害的角度出发，将吸毒成瘾描述为一种以复吸为特征的慢性疾病，认为期望 IVDU 者无限期戒毒是不现实的，并建议将讲授安全注射方法作为减少危害策略的一部分。

Hull 和 Jadbabaie 则选择中间道路，试图平衡医生对患者和社会的责任[70]。他们指出，医生不应根据患者的社会价值或道德缺陷来做出医疗决定，同时要成为医疗资源的"好管家"，以免限制了患者获得医疗服务的路径。医生决策的关键在于个性化评估手术和戒毒治疗成功或失败的可能性。与其他医生意见一致，他们也认同必须为术后的成瘾康复做出安排和建议。最终，与"一次性出局"相比，他们提出了"三次出局"的解决方案，给了患者更多的治疗机会，但仍然设定了一个限制，即假定一名患者经历了两次瓣膜手术后仍旧吸毒并引发了下一次的感染，那说明患者已经无法戒掉这种习惯，他们也就不再进行下一次手术了。然而，即便是选择这种方法也需要投入大量资源，以确保这些患者得到最佳的戒毒治疗。

Miljeteig 等则提出了一项有趣的伦理学分析，为 IVDU 复吸者提供了一种系统而公正的分析方法，包括评估患者的知识基础、涉事相关各方意见、已有的法规和建议、可获益状况、各方利益冲突以及所涉及的伦理原则[71]。他们对数据的回顾发现：如果术后继续吸毒，针对复发性 IVDU-IE 的重复瓣膜手术平均可延长患者 1~2 年的寿命；如果停止吸毒，则可能会延长更多。据此，他们认为，医生既然愿意为其他预计可获得 1~2 年存活时间的疾病进行手术，就应为复吸者提供瓣膜手术治疗。当然，他们也承认，如果存在阻碍治疗产生获益的因素，拒绝治疗也是符合伦理的。虽然以前的生活方式不应成为妨碍或改变治疗选择的因素，但可预见的未来生活方式的确可能会影响治疗的选择。虽然作者再次进行瓣膜手术态度积极，但他们对此也有清楚的认识，有些吸毒成瘾病例可能非常严重，即便手术也无疗效。

DiMaio 和 Salerno 之间的争论[18]全面反映了支持和反对二次手术的各种观点。DiMaio 认为外科医生可以拒绝第二次手术，理由包括吸毒者的高死亡率、手术团队受到感染的风险、资源分配问题以及外科医生的职责，即不进行他们认为徒劳无益的治疗。Salerno 则根据其他专业（包括精神科医生和律师）的观点提出了相反的看法。精神病学的观点强调了对 OUD 诊断的医学意义，并强调了成瘾治疗和多学科方法的必要性。从法律角度来看，治疗合同虽不具有法律强制力，但也不是拒绝治疗的正当理由。Salerno 坚持，外科医生的职责是治疗疾病，而不是做道德评判。

·再次手术的决策

复吸者 IE 面临着临床和伦理两方面的挑战。首先，这类患者病情都很严重，已到晚期，需要限期手术，术中还要做广泛的重建，手术难度大。另一方面，在 IVDU-IE 首次瓣膜置换术后，他们都被要求停止吸毒，但却未能做到。此外，他们可能在情绪上非常不稳定，会与医护人员发生冲突。

外科医生在决定是否对这些患者进行再次手术时，首要的问题就是反省自身的认识问题，即自己的个人偏见在决策中起了多大作用。虽然与第一次手术相比，再次手术的风险更高、技术更复杂，如果他们没有吸毒，大多数外科医生都会毫不犹豫地进行手术；但即使继续吸毒，考虑到他们当中许多人都很年轻，或许还有多年的预期寿命，手术还应该是治疗选项。患者以前的行为不应作为现在选择治疗的判定依据，尤其是如果患者愿意接受戒毒治疗。即便是之前签订过不使用毒品的治疗协议，但那既无法律约束力，也不应被视为拒绝治疗的理由，因为这些在伦理和法律上都不能成立。这个外科医生不能做的 IVDU-IE 手术，可能另外一个外科医生能为他做，那么，遇到这种情况，不能因为自己不能做而简单地将患者拒之门外，而应该主动将这类患者转诊给其他能做的外科医生，让后者去考虑手术问题。

吸毒有其神经化学机制模式，认识并接受这一点可以减轻医务人员在治疗吸毒成瘾过程中所遇到的挫败感。这一人群存在问题，但问题终究需要解决，他们来找医生，其实也就是来寻求帮助。医生必须抛开个人偏见，把 OUD 作为临床治疗的一部分，甚至对患者上次 IVDU-IE 治疗时是否忽视 OUD 这一部分进行评估。医生的首要职责是治疗他们面前的病患，而不是从保险公司或政府机构层面去评估相关的支出。人工瓣膜价格昂贵，但并不像移植器官供体那样到了资源有限的地步。有些复发性 IVDU-IE 病例，患者拒绝成瘾治疗、内科治疗无效或外科手术禁忌，临床对此无计可施。这种情况下，医生不予治疗在伦理上无可争议。但对有手术存活可能性，并有 OUD 治疗意愿的，无论患者过去行为如何，医生都应责无旁贷地为其进行手术。

总　结

　　IVDU-IE 的治疗充满了伦理难题，主要有三大原因：IVDU 者成瘾的自毁性、社会和专业人员对 IVDU 者的偏见、成瘾相关的精神问题。

　　IVDU-IE 并不是唯一一种由自我伤害行为引起的疾病，但 IVDU 的并发症非常严重。IVDU 者的预期寿命大大低于正常人，尽管如此，长期存活还是有可能的。导致早期死亡的主要原因是复吸，但要确定哪些患者可能复吸或不再复吸极其困难，这也导致了治疗选择的挑战性。

　　医生对 IVDU 的态度往往是负面的，许多医生认为很难治疗 IVDU-IE 患者。此外，这一人群中还合并有很多精神问题，这使他们的治疗更加令人沮丧，而相关的精神疾病往往未得到充分治疗。由于复吸的愿望、精神因素或与医护人员的冲突，IVDU-IE 患者 AMA 离院的风险很高。虽然强制性住院治疗可能符合某些患者的最佳利益，但在美国大多数司法管辖区，只有当患者患有精神病、谵妄、有自杀或杀人倾向时，才能采取这种极端措施。

　　除了医疗和手术问题，IE 的经济和法律问题也非常重要且复杂。在人们普遍认为 IE 患者的社会价值较低的背景下，IE 的高昂治疗费用和资源分配的合理性往往成为人们考虑的重点。医生发现自己被夹在患者和社会之间的两难境地——既要承受控制成本的外部压力，又要承担自己作为医生治病救人的首要职责。在我们看来，医生最符合伦理要求的立场是继续为患者代言，而把成本因素留给其他人解决。因为医生的可信度以及患者对医生和医疗行业的信任度对疗愈本已受损的医患关系至关重要。

　　从法律角度来看，使用治疗合同并不可取，因为这种合同有损医患关系的融洽，且非强制性，还不能在法律或道德上成为拒绝为患者提供适当治疗的理由。

　　对 IVDU-IE 患者的整体医护最好从 OUD 的角度来看待。医生也是人，既然是人，就会有内在的或外在的偏见。但无论医生如何看待各种不同的生活方式，他们优先要考虑的以及他们的职责都是治病救人。从起初将毒瘾视为道德缺陷，到将 OUD 作为一种复杂的内科疾病，这一过程消除吸毒的污名，使医生能更加客观地看待这些患者及问题。IVDU-IE 是吸毒的后果，仅仅对感染的瓣膜进行手术，而忽视或未对 OUD 给予充分治疗，将是一个巨大的错误。IVDU-IE 的治疗必须是针对这两种不同但又相关的疾病同步进行积极的治疗。事实证明，对于期望戒毒者，MAT能有效减少毒品使用，而对于尚未准备戒毒的，减少危害的策略有助于减少吸毒的并发症，降低由此产生的医疗费用。

即便是首次瓣膜术后IVDU-IE复发的患者也并非不需要帮助。这些患者的成瘾治疗转诊率很低，许多患者在首次瓣膜置换术后并没有接受过适当的成瘾治疗。对这些患者进行评估时应重点考虑其预期寿命以及是否愿意接受成瘾治疗。而对于这种复发性IVDU-IE再次手术的主要依据是手术的技术可行性和治疗的预期效果，而不是过去或现在的吸毒情况。尤其是对那些过去没有接受过适当戒毒治疗的患者，他们在接受高质量的随访和多学科治疗后有可能会取得很好的疗效。

越来越多的人已接受OUD是一种医学疾病，并对其精神并发症有了认识。以此为基础，我们希望IVDU不再被污名化。但目前在为IVDU-IE患者提供最佳治疗方面存在巨大障碍，其中许多是文化障碍。只要具备足够敏锐的洞察力和强大的理解力，相信我们能够克服这些障碍。

参考文献

[1] Millar BC, Moore JE. Emerging issues in infective endocarditis. Emerg Infect Dis, 2004, 10(6): 1110–1116.
[2] Cahill TJ, Prendergast BD. Infective endocarditis. Lancet, 2016, 387(10021): 882–893.
[3] Jamil M, Sultan I, Gleason TG, et al. Infective endocarditis: trends, surgical outcomes, and controversies. J Thorac Dis, 2019, 11(11): 4875–4885.
[4] Cahill TJ, Baddour LM, Habib G, et al. Challenges in infective endocarditis. J Am Coll Cardiol, 2017, 69(3): 325–344.
[5] Pettersson GB, Hussain ST. Surgical treatment of aortic valve endocarditis//Cohn LH, Adams DH. Cardiac Surgery in the Adult, 5e. New York, NY: McGraw-Hill, 2020. Accessed:http://accesssurgery.mhmedical.com.ezproxyv.musc.edu/content.aspx?bookid=2157&sectioned=164303289. [Accessed 4 May 2020].
[6] Murdoch DR, Corey GR, Hoen B, et al. Clinical presentation, etiology, and outcome of infective endocarditis in the 21st century: the international collaboration on endocarditis e prospective cohort study. Arch Intern Med, 2009, 169(5): 463–473.
[7] Hussain ST, Shrestha NK, Gordon SM, et al. Residual patient, anatomic, and surgical obstacles in treating active left-sided infective endocarditis. J Thorac Cardiovasc Surg, 2014, 148(3): 981–988.e4.
[8] Rabkin DG, Mokadam NA, Miller DW, et al. Long-term outcome for the surgical treatment of infective endocarditis with a focus on intravenous drug users. Ann Thorac Surg, 2012, 93(1): 51–57.
[9] Fleischauer AT, Ruhl L, Rhea S, et al. Hospitalizations for endocarditis and associated health care costs among persons with diagnosed drug dependence - North Carolina, 2010—2015. Morb Mortal Wkly Rep, 2017, 66(22): 569–573.
[10] Gostin LO, Hodge Jr JG, Noe SA. Reframing the opioid epidemic as a national emergency. J Am Med Assoc, 2017, 318(16): 1539–1540.
[11] Kadri AN, Wilner B, Hernandez AV, et al. Geographic trends, patient characteristics, and outcomes of infective endocarditis associated with drug abuse in the United States from 2002 to 2016. J Am Heart Assoc, 2019, 8(19): e012969.
[12] Rudasill SE, Sanaiha Y, Mardock AL, et al. Clinical outcomes of infective endocarditis in injection drug users. J Am Coll Cardiol, 2019, 73(5): 559–570.
[13] Shrestha NK, Jue J, Hussain ST, et al. Injection drug use and outcomes after surgical intervention

[14] Hayden M, Moore A. Attitudes and approaches towards repeat valve surgery in recurrent injection drug use-associated infective endocarditis: a qualitative study. J Addiction Med, 2019 [Epub ahead of print].

[15] McLaughlin D, Long A. An extended literature review of health professionals' perceptions of illicit drugs and their clients who use them. J Psychiatr Ment Health Nurs, 1996, 3(5): 283–288.

[16] Lloyd C. Sinning and sinned against: the stigmatisation of problem drug users. UK drug policy commission. (2010-09-29) [2020-05-05]. http://www.ukdpc.org.uk/reports.shtml.

[17] Elbatarny M, Bahji A, Bisleri G, et al. Management of endocarditis among persons who inject drugs: a narrative review of surgical and psychiatric approaches and controversies. Gen Hosp Psychiatr, 2019, 57: 44–49.

[18] DiMaio JM, Salerno TA, Bernstein R, et al. Ethical obligation of surgeons to noncompliant patients: can a surgeon refuse to operate on an intravenous drug-abusing patient with recurrent aortic valve prosthesis infection? Ann Thorac Surg, 2009, 88(1): 1–8.

[19] Rosenthal ES, Karchmer AW, Theisen-Toupal J, et al. Suboptimal addiction interventions for patients hospitalized with injection drug use-associated infective endocarditis. Am J Med, 2016, 129(5): 481–485.

[20] Baldassarri SR, Lee I, Latham SR, et al. Debating medical utility, not futility: ethical dilemmas in treating critically ill people who use injection drugs. J Law Med Ethics, 2018, 46(2): 241–251.

[21] Merriam-Webster Inc. Merriam-Webster's collegiate dictionary. 11th ed. (2003) [2020-05-05]. https://merriam-webster.com.

[22] Buchman DZ, Ho A. What's trust got to do with it? Revisiting opioid contracts. J Med Ethics October, 2014, 40: 673–677.

[23] Hariharan J, Lamb GC, Neuner JM. Long-term opioid contract use for chronic pain management in primary care practice. A five year experience. J Gen Intern Med April, 2007, 22(4): 485–490.

[24] Wurcel AG, Yu S, Pacheco M, et al. Contracts with people who inject drugs following valve surgery: unrealistic and misguided expectations. J Thorac Cardiovasc Surg December, 2017, 154(6): 2002.

[25] Hussain ST, Gordon SM, Streem DW, et al. Contract with the patient with injection drug use and infective endocarditis: surgeons perspective. J Thorac Cardiovasc Surg, 2017, 154(6): 2002–2003.

[26] Paulus DA, Layon AJ, Mayfield WR, et al. Intrauterine pregnancy and aortic valve replacement. J Clin Anesth, 1995, 7(4): 338–346.

[27] Yuan SM. Infective endocarditis during pregnancy. J Coll Physicians Surg Pak, 2015, 25(2): 134–139.

[28] Wade Roe v. 410 U.S. 113. 1973.

[29] Committee on Ethics, American College of Obstetricians and Gynecologists. Patient choice: maternal-fetal conflict. Washington, D.C.: American College of Obstetricians and Gynecologists, 1987.

[30] Sridhara S, Mayer PA. Medical and ethical concerns regarding pacemaker implantation in a patient with substance use disorder. Cureus, 2018, 10(7): e3027.

[31] Buchman DZ, Lynch MJ. An ethical bone to PICC: considering a harm reduction approach for a second valve replacement for a person who uses drugs. Am J Bioeth, 2018, 18(1): 79–81.

[32] Schindler BA, Blum D, Malone R. Noncompliance in the treatment of endocarditis. The medical staff as co-conspirators. Gen Hosp Psychiatr, 1988, 10(3): 197–201.

[33] Appelbaum PS, Roth LH. Patients who refuse treatment in medical hospitals. J Am Med Assoc, 1983, 250(10): 1296–1301.

[34] Testa M, West SG. Civil commitment in the United States. Psychiatry, 2010, 7(10): 30–40.

[35] Suzuki J, Robinson D, Mosquera M, et al. Impact of medications for opioid use disorder on discharge against medical advice among people who inject drugs hospitalized for infective endocarditis. Am J Addict, 2020, 29(2): 155–159.

[36] Substance Use During Pregnancy. Guttmacher Institute. [2020-04-20]. https://www.guttmacher.org/state-policy/explore/substance-use-during-pregnancy#.

[37] National Drug Intelligence Center. The economic impact of illicit drug use on American society.

Washington D.C.: United States Department of Justice, 2011. 2011-Q0317-002.

[38] Jiang R, Lee I, Lee TA, et al. The societal cost of heroin use disorder in the United States. PloS One, 2017, 12(5): e0177323.

[39] Sacks JJ, Gonzales KR, Bouchery EE, et al. 2010 National and state costs of excessive alcohol consumption. Am J Prev Med, 2015, 49(5): e73–e79.

[40] Xu X, Bishop EE, Kennedy SM, et al. Annual healthcare spending attributable to cigarette smoking: an update. Am J Prev Med, 2015, 48(3): 326–333.

[41] National Center for Chronic Disease Prevention and Health Promotion (US). Smoking-Attributable Morbidity, Mortality, and Economic Costs. Office on smoking and health. The health consequences of smoking-50 Years of progress: a report of the surgeon general, vol. 12. Atlanta (GA): Centers for Disease Control and Prevention (US), 2014.

[42] Stimmel B. Unlimited entitlement to healthcare: the dilemma of narcotic dependency. Mt Sinai J Med, 1988, 56(3): 176–179.

[43] La Puma J, Cassel CK, Humphrey H. Ethics, economics, and endocarditis. The physician's role in resource allocation. Arch Intern Med, 1988, 148(8): 1809–1811.

[44] McCarthy P, Lamm R, Sade RM. Medical ethics collides with public policy: LVAD for a patient with leukemia. Ann Thorac Surg, 2005, 80(3): 793–798.

[45] Nguemeni Tiako MJ, Mori M, Bin Mahmood SU, et al. Recidivism is the leading cause of death among intravenous drug users who underwent cardiac surgery for infective endocarditis. Semin Thorac Cardiovasc Surg, 2019, 31(1): 40–45. Spring.

[46] Wurcel AG, Boll G, Burke D, et al. Impact of substance use disorder on midterm mortality after valve surgery for endocarditis. Ann Thorac Surg, 2020, 109(5): 1426–1432.

[47] Kim JB, Ejiofor JI, Yammine M, et al. Surgical outcomes of infective endocarditis among intravenous drug users. J Thorac Cardiovasc Surg, 2016, 152(3): 832–841.e1.

[48] Straw S, Baig MW, Gillott R, et al. Long-term outcomes are poor in intravenous drug users following infective endocarditis, even after surgery. Clin Infect Dis, 2019, 71(3): 564–571. pii: ciz869.

[49] Goodman-Meza D, Weiss RE, Gamboa S, et al. Long term surgical outcomes for infective endocarditis in people who inject drugs: a systematic review and meta-analysis. BMC Infect Dis, 2019, 19(1): 918.

[50] Hanke JS, Rojas SV, Mahr C, et al. Five-year results of patients supported by HeartMate II: outcomes and adverse events. Eur J Cardio Thorac Surg, 2018, 53(2): 422–427.

[51] Yusen RD, Edwards LB, Dipchand AI, et al. The registry of the international society for heart and lung transplantation: thirty-third adult lung and heart-lung transplant report-2016; focus theme: primary diagnostic indications for transplant. J Heart Lung Transplant, 2016, 35(10): 1170–1184.

[52] Kakko J, Svanborg KD, Kreek MJ, et al. 1-year retention and social function after buprenorphine-assisted relapse prevention treatment for heroin dependence in Sweden: a randomised, placebo-controlled trial. Lancet, 2003, 361(9358): 662–668.

[53] Krupitsky E, Nunes EV, Ling W, et al. Injectable extended-release naltrexone for opioid dependence: a double-blind, placebo-controlled, multicentre randomised trial. Lancet, 2011, 377(9776): 1506–1513.

[54] Lee JD, Friedmann PD, Kinlock TW, et al. Extended-release naltrexone to prevent opioid relapse in criminal justice offenders. N Engl J Med, 2016, 374(13): 1232–1242.

[55] Dole VP, Nyswander M. A medical treatment for diacetylmorphine (heroin) addiction. A clinical trial with methadone hydrochloride. J Am Med Assoc, 1965, 193: 646–650.

[56] Pettersson GB, Coselli JS, Hussain ST, et al. 2016 The American Association for Thoracic Surgery (AAT) consensus guidelines: surgical treatment of infective endocarditis: executive summar. J Thorac Cardiovasc Surg, 2017, 153(6): 1241–1258.e29.

[57] Sharma M, Lamba W, Cauderella A, et al. Harm reduction in hospitals. Harm Reduct J, 2017, 14(1): 32.

[58] Knudsen HK, Abraham AJ, Roman PM. Adoption and implementation of medications in addiction treatment programs. J Addiction Med, 2011; 5(1): 21–27.

[59] Oliva EM, Maisel NC, Gordon AJ, et al. Barriers to use of pharmacotherapy for addiction disorders and how to overcome them. Curr Psychiatr Rep, 2011, 13(5): 374–381.

[60] Rieckmann T, Kovas AE, Rutkowski BA. Adoption of medications in substance abuse treatment: priorities and strategies of single state authorities. J Psychoact Drugs, 2010;(Suppl. 6): 227–238.

[61] Logan DE, Marlatt GA. Harm reduction therapy: a practice-friendly review of research. J Clin Psychol, 2010, 66(2): 201–214.

[62] Phillips KT, Stein MD, Anderson BJ, et al. Skin and needle hygiene intervention for injection drug users: results from a randomized, controlled Stage I pilot trial. J Subst Abuse Treat, 2012, 43(3): 313–321.

[63] Beletsky L, Davis CS, Anderson E, et al. The law (and politics) of safe injection facilities in the United States. Am J Publ Health, 2008, 98(2): 231–237.

[64] Kaiser Family Foundation. State health facts: sterile syringe exchange programs. [2020–06–09]. https://www.kff.org/hivaids/state-indicator/syringe-exchange-programs.

[65] Controlled Substances Act. 21 USC, x856. 1971.

[66] Camsari UM, Libertin CR. Small-town America's despair: infected substance users needing outpatient parenteral therapy and risk stratification. Cureus, 2017, 9(8): e1579.

[67] Ho J, Archuleta S, Sulaiman Z, et al. Safe and successful treatment of intravenous drug users with a peripherally inserted central catheter in an outpatient parenteral antibiotic treatment service. J Antimicrob Chemother, 2010, 65(12): 2641–2644.

[68] Yeo KK, Chang WJ, Lau JM, et al. Valve replacement in endocarditis: setting limits in noncompliant intravenous drug abusers. Hawaii Med J, 2006, 65(6): 170–171. 168.

[69] Kirkpatrick JN. Infective endocarditis in the intravenous drug user. Virtual Mentor, 2010, 12(10): 778–781.

[70] Hull SC, Jadbabaie F. When is enough enough? The dilemma of valve replacement in a recidivist intravenous drug user. Ann Thorac Surg, 2014, 97(5): 1486–1487.

[71] Miljeteig I, Skrede S, Langørgen J, et al. Should patients who use illicit drugs be offered a second heart-valve replacement? Tidsskr Nor Laegeforen, 2013, 133(9): 977–980.

第 22 章

感染性心内膜炎的多学科服务

Hariharan Regunath, Stevan P. Whitt
University of Missouri, Columbia, MO, United States

引 言

感染性心内膜炎（IE）是一种会出现多种并发症的疾病，需要在发病早期进行细致的临床评估和风险分层[1-3]。其预后受多种因素影响：患者特征、感染微生物的毒力、发病时的病情严重程度（包括有无心力衰竭、栓塞表现、心源性休克或脓毒性休克）、就诊、诊断和治疗时机是否延误、手术指征和手术时机等。30 d内的死亡率为 10%～50%，且许多患者需要手术治疗[4]。Duke 标准最初是为科学研究而设计，结果发现可为自体瓣膜心内膜炎（NVE）提供诊断指导。但也并非所有确诊的 IE 都符合这一标准[5-7]。另外，对于人工瓣膜心内膜炎（PVE），该标准敏感性较低。近年来，除超声心动图外，新型心脏影像检查手段发挥了越来越重要的临床作用，弥补了这方面的不足[7]。

IE 在社区的总体患病率较低，并非所有医疗机构都具有处理 IE 患者的专业能力。患者可能同时患有心脏、神经、风湿、感染和代谢紊乱等多系统疾病，在缺乏专科医生会诊的情况下，个体医生可能无法对患者进行治疗[2]。目前的指南推荐采用多学科团队（MDT）方案来加强 IE 的临床诊疗[1-3]。虽然这些建议提供了指导决策的一般性原则，但临床实际却往往更为复杂，需要对个体患者进行仔细和持续的评估[8]。此外，不同学会指南之间专家意见的差异以及这些指南引用证据的质量也受到质疑 [例如，美国感染病学会认可的美国心脏协会（AHA）IE 指南中超过 50% 的证据级别为 C 级]，因此需要根据临床情况进行个体化处理，而不是简单教条地遵守指南[1,8-10]。

MDT 方法能促进医务工作者更好地遵守 IE 指南中的一般性原则，减少实践中医务人员之间的处理差异，避免治疗延误，同时允许进行适当的个体化治疗[8,11]。本章中，我们将讨论 IE 管理中的多学科服务问题，并对那些专门描述 MDT 组成和功能的文献进行综述，并总结我们所在中心 IE 团队发展和实践的经验。

心内膜炎团队——欧洲的经验和教训

心脏瓣膜团队管理的早期成功经验已自然而然地被用于 IE 的管理中[12]。欧洲的多项研究表明，专门的心内膜炎 MDT 可改善患者的预后、降低死亡率[11,13-21]。表 22.1 总结了相关主要出版物中所描述的 MDT 组成及其对预后的影响，这些内容已被纳入 IE 的指南。

在 MDT 构架内，成员必须是相关专业高水平的专业人员，这样才能起到改善治疗效果的作用，其中心脏内科、心胸外科和感染科专家是不可缺少的人员[2,22]。MDT 的组成和功能应根据医疗机构的规模、亚专科服务的设置、其他相关资源、有效的沟通策略以及领导层的支持来决定[2,16,23]。如果该医疗机构没有相应的亚专科，则必须将 IE 患者转诊至可提供 IE 多学科治疗的中心，并建立完整的转诊制度，以便在起病的急性期将患者转诊给相应的医疗中心进行诊治。Mestres CA 等在他们的社论中全面概述了西班牙近 30 年来为 IE 患者提供多学科服务的经验，并给出了他们的转诊标准（表 22.2）[15]。住院医生 / 内科医生的作用不容忽视，因为他们通常承担着诊治 IE 患者的主要责任。口腔颌面外科、放射科、神经内科、行为治疗科、骨科 / 脊柱外科等科室的辅助服务在心内膜炎患者的管理中也发挥着重要作用。圆桌讨论（图 22.1）可很好激发团队活力，明确角色定位、互动和统一的参与方式，使团队成员之间可在定期会议中无缝沟通，这对取得成功至关重要[14,17,19-20]。在这些讨论中，应定期核查预先确定的质量控制措施，以改善诊疗服务（表 22.3）。

表 22.1　欧洲关于感染性心内膜炎（IE）多学科团队的研究

作者，国家	方法，瓣膜	MDT 的发展、组成和功能	具有统计学意义的结果
Botelho Nevers 等，法国[14]	· 观察性前 – 后对照研究）（1991—2001，N=173）–（2002—2006，N=160） · 瓣膜类型：NVE 和 PVE · Duke 标准：确诊的 IE	标准化的诊治方案： 1. 1994 年：采用诊断工具（对切除的瓣膜进行系统的血清学检测、血培养、微生物学和组织学分析） 2. 2002 年：全面推行 MDT，制定了相关方案和内 – 外科指南，以多学科方式做出最终决策	1. 死亡率从 18.5% 降至 8.2% 2. 提高了抗感染治疗的依从性 3. 栓塞事件、肾衰竭、多器官衰竭综合征减少
Chirillo 等，意大利[14]	· 观察性前 – 后对照研究）（1996—2002，N=102）–（2003—2009，N=190） · 瓣膜类型：NVE · Duke 标准：确诊的 IE	标准化的诊治方案： 1. 2003 年：强制转诊至 MDT（由心脏内科、感染科、微生物学、心脏外科专家组成） 2. 特别关注血培养和超声心动图的标准化	1. 总死亡率从 28% 降至 13%（手术死亡率为 47%~13%，3 年死亡率为 34%~16%） 2. 血培养阴性 IE 减少 3. 并发肾衰竭患者减少

表 22.1（续）

作者，国家	方法，瓣膜	MDT 的发展、组成和功能	具有统计学意义的结果
Carraschinchilla F 等，西班牙[17]	· 前瞻性队列（2008—2011，N=72）与历史队列对比（1996—2007，N=155） · 瓣膜类型：NVE 和 PVE，但仅限于左心系统 · Duke 标准：确诊或疑似的 IE	自 2008 年起，实施 IE 多学科预警策略（AMULTEI） MDT 组成： · 临床——内科、感染科 · 微生物学 · 超声心动图 · 如果符合 Duke 标准，则纳入心脏外科	1. 早期手术比例上升 2. 住院期间休克发生率明显降低 3. 住院期间和随访第 1 个月内的死亡率降低
Camou 等，法国[8]	· 回顾性观察 – 描述性研究：其团队实施 MDT 4.5 年（2013—2017）的成果 · 瓣膜类型：NVE 和 PVE · Duke 标准：确诊或疑似的 IE	自 2010 年起，每周召开一次区域性心内膜炎多学科会议，旨在对患者进行确诊、制定治疗策略和前瞻性随访 MDT 组成： · 心脏内科专家 · 感染病专家 · 心脏外科专家 · 微生物学家 · 影像学专家 · 重症监护专家	1. 未对 MDT 实施前进行评估，因此无法得出结论 2. 社区获得性和医院获得性 IE 的死亡率无显著差异（9% vs. 14%）
Ruch 等，法国[10]	· 观察性研究（回顾性），MDT 实施前（2012 年 1 月至 2016 年 12 月）与实施后（2017 年 1 月至 12 月） · 瓣膜类型：NVE 和 PVE · Duke 标准：确诊的 IE	自 2012 年起，名为"感染性心内膜炎登记处"的中央数据库收集了所有确诊为 IE 患者的医疗、辅助医疗和治疗决定 MDT 组成： · 感染病专家 · 心脏内科专家 · 心脏外科专家 · 超声专家	院内死亡率无明显下降（实施 MDT 前后分别为 20.3% vs. 14.7%），但以下指标在 MDT 实施后明显下降： 1. 确诊至实施手术时间（16.4 d vs. 10.3 d） 2. 抗生素使用天数（55.2 d vs. 47.2 d） 3. 住院天数（40.6 d vs. 31.9 d） 4. 多变量分析：实施 MDT 后的时间与存活率呈正相关
Issa N 等，法国[21]	· 前瞻性观察研究（2013 年 1 月至 2016 年 3 月，N=357） · 瓣膜类型：NVE 和 PVE · Duke 标准：确诊或疑似的 IE	自 2010 年起，每周举行 MDT 会议	

表 22.1（续）

作者，国家	方法，瓣膜	MDT 的发展、组成和功能	具有统计学意义的结果
Kaura 等，英国[16]	·观察性前-后对照研究，MDT 实施前（2009 年 8 月至 2012 年 6 月）与实施后（2012 年 7 月至 2015 年 4 月）	自 2012 年起实施 MDT。由心脏内科专家对疑似患者进行初步评估，然后进行 TTE/TEE，如高度怀疑，则转至 MDT MDT 组成： ·2 名心脏内科专家 ·1 名微生物学家 ·1 名心脏影像学专家 ·1 名心脏外科专家 ·护士协调员	1. IE 特异性抗生素治疗时间 [(4±4) d vs. (2.5±3.5) d] 和确诊至手术时间 [(7.8±7.3) d vs. (5.3±4.2) d] 缩短 2. 存活率从 42.9% 提高到 66.7%
Mestres 等，西班牙[12]	·一篇社论描述了 30 年来（1985—2014）MDT 的视角和经验	自 1979 年，创建 IE 数据库工作小组、心血管组织库，与感染科、心脏内科和心脏外科合作 1. 自 1993 年起，储存致病菌株，创建实验性心内膜炎实验室 2. 自 1994 年起，每周召开 IE 会议 MDT 组成： ·感染病专家 ·微生物学家 ·心脏瓣膜病和心脏影像学专家 ·心脏外科专家 ·病理学家 ·OPAT 专家	未报告结果数据

NVE：自体瓣膜心内膜炎；PVE：人工瓣膜心内膜炎；MDT：多学科团队；TTE：经胸超声心动图；TEE：经食管超声心动图；OPAT：门诊患者肠外抗菌治疗

表 22.2　无心血管手术条件医院的转院标准

1. 血流动力学不稳定（需正性肌力药物支持、机械通气）
2. 严重瓣膜反流（满足临床和超声心动图标准）
3. 人工心内膜炎
4. 心内装置相关心内膜炎（起搏器、除颤器、再同步化设备）
5. 瓣周并发症（脓肿、瘘管）
6. 持续性脓毒症（血培养阳性＞7 d）
7. 卒中
8. 反复栓塞
9. 残留的较大赘生物（＞10 mm）
10. 侵袭性或难治性微生物（如金黄色葡萄球菌、革兰氏阴性杆菌、真菌、血培养阴性心内膜炎）

经许可引自：Mestres CA, Paré JC, Miró JM. Organization and functioning of a multidisciplinary team for the diagnosis and treatment of infective endocarditis: a 30-year perspective (1985-2014). Rev Esp Cardiol, 2015, 68(5): 363–368.

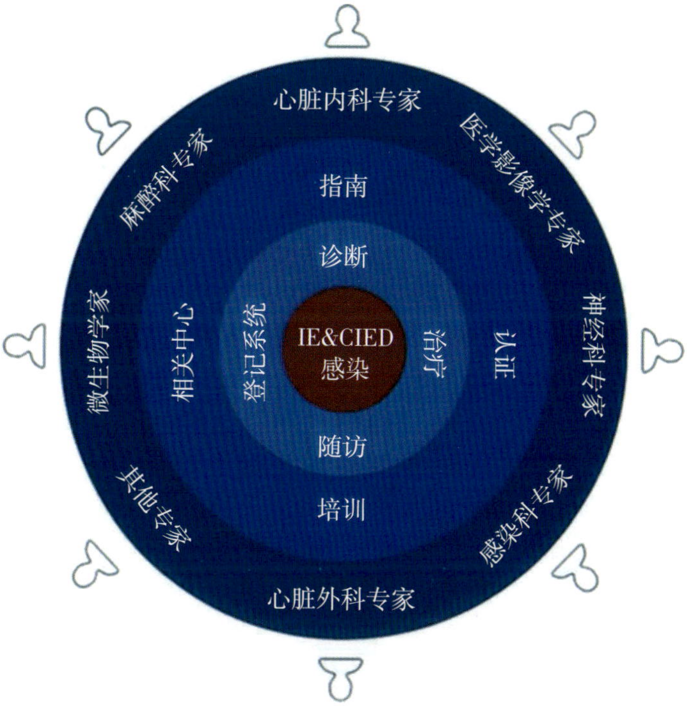

图 22.1 感染性心内膜炎（IE）和心脏植入式电子设备（CIED）感染的圆桌讨论。经许可引自：Kaura A, Byrne J, Fife A, et al. Inception of the 'endocarditis team' is associated with improved survival in patients with infective endocarditis who are managed medically: findings from a before-and-after study. Open Heart, 2017, 4(2): e000699.

表 22.3 感染性心内膜炎（IE）多学科团队的质量控制

组织方面

1. 在 24 h 内回复来自其他中心的咨询，包括通过电话或互联网提出的转院请求
2. 在专门数据库中前瞻性地收集超声心动图、微生物学、外科手术和临床病程等数据
3. 小组所有成员每周开会
4. 预防院内医源性心内膜炎：提供信息和教育，减少导管相关菌血症和植入式心脏设备感染

临床方面

1. 对疑似 IE 病例必须在 48 h 内进行超声心动图检查
2. 72 h 内进行栓塞相关检查，尤其对感染真菌和葡萄球菌（金黄色葡萄球菌、路邓葡萄球菌）的 IE 病例
3. 定期检查经验性和特异性抗感染方案的适用性、用药时间和毒性

微生物方面

1. 对疑似 IE 病例，在不同静脉、至少两次且非同一时间抽血进行血培养。第 3 天和第 7 天对照血培养结果
2. 如果血培养结果显示 IE 典型病原体生长（< 24 h），团队内部的微生物学专家应与感染科专家进行实时沟通
3. 对疑似 IE 病例，所取出的瓣膜赘生物、栓塞物质和心内装置都应进行组织染色、培养和分子生物学检测（16S 和 18S）

表 22.3（续）

手术方面

1. 在 24 h 内与外科医生讨论患者的手术指征
2. 遵守指南中对急诊手术和紧急手术建议的时限
3. 清除所有受感染的心内装置，并对未移除心内装置的患者进行复查和讨论

科学学术问题

1. MDT 内外的继续教育
2. 与地方、国家和国际研究小组合作
3. 进行大会发言，在科学杂志上发表文章，参与制定地方、国家和国际临床指南

通用措施

1. 对 50% 以上的住院死亡病例进行尸检
2. 对所有病例进行至少 1 年的临床、微生物学和超声心动图随访

经许可引自：Mestres CA, Paré JC, Miró JM. Organization and functioning of a multidisciplinary team for the diagnosis and treatment of infective endocarditis: a 30-year perspective (1985-2014). Rev Esp Cardiol, 2015, 68(5): 363–368.

心脏手术

了解患者的病情进展对 IE 的临床治疗至关重要[3,24]。左心系统 IE 比右心系统更常出现严重并发症，其中约有半数患者需要手术干预[25-26]。与常规等待内科治疗清除脓毒症或菌血症后手术相比，早期手术往往能改善左心系统心内膜炎患者的预后[27-28]。表 22.4 列出了 AHA 和欧洲指南中的手术适应证[29]。2016 年美国胸外科医师协会（STS）关于 IE 手术治疗的共识指南就诊断、适应证、手术时机、治疗方案、围手术期管理提出了建议，并提倡心脏外科医生尽早干预[30]。

手术时机：AHA 和欧洲指南对早期手术的定义不同。AHA 指南将早期手术定义为在同次/首次住院期间及抗菌治疗结束前进行的手术，而欧洲指南则分为急诊手术（＜24 h）、限期手术（几天内）和择期手术（抗生素治疗 1 ~ 2 周后）[1-2]。大多数心内膜炎病例可能没有明确或明显的手术指征，病情也是处于稳定与不稳定之间，这时就需要心脏外科医生进行细致评估。正因为如此，由外科医生主导的 MDT 可能是比较合理的安排，同时也需要其他专科的高水平专家参与[10]。在外科医生时间有限的情况下，则以心脏外科、内科、感染科和心脏内科为基础的团队应发挥团队主导或共同领导作用，协助加快术前评估并完善术前准备。

术前风险评估与手术禁忌：根据心内膜炎国际合作–PLUS 前瞻性队列数据，无法进行手术的最常见原因包括预后不良、血流动力学不稳定、术前死亡、卒中和严重脓毒症[31]。这就要求 MDT 应努力加快术前准备，尽早识别即将出现病情恶化的风险，赶在病情出现恶化之前完成手术，以降低死亡率。经典评分系统如 STS 评分和欧洲心脏手术风险评估系统（EuroSCORE），可用于评估心脏手术死亡风险[32-33]。此外，还有不少专门针对 IE 的评分系统：STS-IE 评分，风险–心内膜炎评分（RISK-E），PALSUSE 评分（项目包括：假体、年龄 ≥ 70 岁、大的

表 22.4 美国心脏协会（AHA）和欧洲心脏病学会（ESC）指南中的手术指征

	2015 年 AHA 指南	类别，证据水平	2015 年 ESC 指南	类别，证据水平	时机[b]
心力衰竭	如果 IE 患者出现瓣膜功能障碍，导致心力衰竭的症状或体征，应尽早[a]进行手术治疗	I，B	主动脉瓣或二尖瓣 NVE，或 PVE 出现严重的急性反流、梗阻或瘘管，导致难治性肺水肿或心源性休克	I，B	急诊手术
	对于因人工瓣瓣环裂开、心内瘘或严重人工瓣膜功能障碍而出现心力衰竭症状或体征的 PVE 病例，应尽早[a]进行手术治疗	I，B	主动脉瓣或二尖瓣 NVE，或 PVE 出现严重反流或梗阻，导致心力衰竭症状，或超声心动图显示血流动力学耐受性差	I，B	限期手术
感染难以控制	当 IE 并发心脏传导阻滞、瓣环或主动脉瓣脓肿，或损毁性穿透病变时，患者应尽早[a]进行手术治疗	I，B	无法控制的局部感染（脓肿、假性动脉瘤、瘘、赘生物变大）	I，B	限期手术
	对复发的 PVE 患者而言，早期手术[a]是合理的	IIa，C	真菌或多重耐药菌引起的感染	I，C	限期/择期手术
	应考虑尽早[a]手术，尤其是由真菌或高度耐药菌（如 VRE、多重耐药革兰氏阴性杆菌）引起的 IE	I，B	尽管采用了适当的抗生素治疗并充分控制了脓毒性转移灶，但血培养仍持续呈阳性	IIa，B	限期手术
	在开始适当的抗菌治疗后，如果有持续感染的证据（表现为持续菌血症或持续发热 > 5~7 d，且已排除其他部位的感染），应尽早[a]手术治疗	I，B	由葡萄球菌或非 HACEK 革兰氏阴性菌引起的 PVE	IIa，C	限期/择期手术
预防栓塞	对于那些尽管接受了适当的抗生素治疗，但栓塞仍反复发生、赘生物持续存在或增大的患者，应尽早[a]进行手术	IIa，B	主动脉瓣或二尖瓣 NVE；或 PVE 发生 ≥ 1 次栓塞，尽管接受了适当的抗生素治疗，仍存在 > 10 mm 的赘生物	I，B	限期手术
	对存在瓣膜严重反流、活动性且 > 10 mm 的赘生物，应尽早[a]手术	IIa，B	主动脉瓣或二尖瓣 NVE 伴赘生物 > 10 mm，伴有严重的瓣膜狭窄或反流，手术风险较低	IIa，B	限期手术

表 22.4（续）

2015 年 AHA 指南	类别，证据水平	2015 年 ESC 指南	类别，证据水平	时机[b]
对于活动性赘生物 > 10 mm 的患者，尤其是二尖瓣前叶赘生物并伴有其他相关手术指征的患者，可考虑尽早[a]手术	Ⅱb, C	主动脉瓣或二尖瓣 NVE，或 PVE，伴有孤立的超大赘生物（> 30 mm）	Ⅱa, B	限期手术
		主动脉瓣或二尖瓣 NVE，或 PVE，伴有孤立的大赘生物（> 15 mm），但无其他手术指征	Ⅱb, C	限期手术

[a] 定义为"首次住院期间和完成全疗程抗生素之前"。[b] 定义为：急诊手术 = 在 24 h 内进行手术；限期手术 = 在几天内进行手术；择期手术 = 在至少完成 1～2 周抗生素治疗后进行手术。IE：感染性心内膜炎；HACEK：嗜血杆菌属、凝聚杆菌属、心杆菌属、侵蚀艾肯菌、金氏杆菌属；NVE：自体瓣膜心内膜炎；PVE：人工瓣膜心内膜炎；VRE：万古霉素耐药肠球菌。经许可引自：Cahill TJ, Baddour LM, Habib G, et al. Challenges in infective endocarditis. J Am Coll Cardiol, 2017, 69(3): 325–344.

心内结构破坏、葡萄球菌感染、限期手术、女性）、De Feo-Cotrufo 评分和 Costa 评分[2,34-37]。一项研究显示，STS-IE 评分与其他所有评分（RISK-E 除外）相比，对死亡的预测能力最高；而在另一项研究中，RISK-E 评分优于 STS-IE 评分、EuroSCORE 评分和 PALSUSE 评分[35,38]。

口腔卫生和卒中的评估：口腔卫生不良或龋齿容易导致链球菌性 IE。在未拔除龋齿的情况下安装人工瓣膜，为后续发生人工瓣膜 IE 留下了隐患。因此，在抗生素治疗期间，即应慎重对住院 IE 患者的口腔疾病进行评估和治疗[1]。同样，未确诊的（有 IE 栓塞表现）或近期发生的缺血性或出血性卒中都有可能因持续肝素化抗凝的心脏手术而进一步恶化。如果神经功能损害不明显，通常需要进行脑部 MRI 检查，以完成术前神经系统风险评估；如果有卒中表现，手术时机则根据疾病严重程度（临床和放射学）、年龄和类型来确定。发现颅内出血不一定是早期手术的禁忌证，但如果是高风险病情，心脏手术前则需要进一步的影像学检查或干预，图 22.2 提供了一个用于指导手术时机的流程图[39]。

多学科团队的形成——我们的模式

2016 年，通过持续的绩效改进工作，我们确定了改善 IE 患者临床管理的模式。当时，很少有关于美国医疗系统内发展 MDT 的文章。我们利用质量改进工具发展了 MDT[40]。我们按顺序完成了以下步骤，完整的细节已在其他地方发表[23,41]。

1. Tuckman 团队发展模式（图 22.3）是建立心内膜炎工作组的框架，该工作组由医院内科、感染科、心脏科（包括超声心动图和心力衰竭方面的专家）和心

感染性心内膜炎的多学科服务 第 22 章

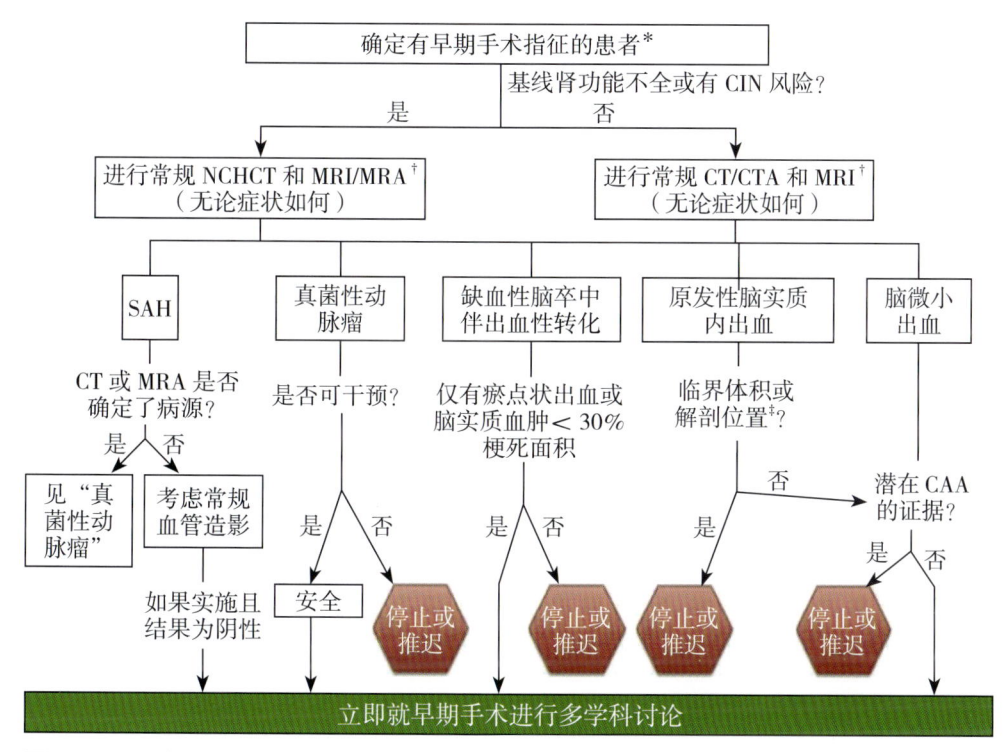

图 22.2 术前评估和处理流程图。CAA：脑淀粉样血管病；CIN：造影剂诱导性肾病；CTA：CT 血管造影；IE：感染性心内膜炎；MRA：磁共振血管造影；MRI：磁共振成像；NCHCT：无增强头部 CT；SAH：蛛网膜下腔出血。*继发于瓣膜功能障碍的心力衰竭，有证据表明心脏组织结构受损（即瓣环或主动脉瓣脓肿、心脏传导阻滞、损毁性病变），需要控制病源 [如使用抗生素 5～7 d 后仍持续感染和（或）反复发生栓塞事件]，由真菌或高度耐药菌引起的感染以及赘生物 >10 mm。†NCHCT 是评估 SAH 和亚急性较大脑梗死的有效检查。如果没有禁忌证，建议使用 CTA 而不是 MRA，因为 CTA 检测小动脉瘤（<5 mm）和真菌性动脉瘤的灵敏度略高于 MRA。常规 MRI 可进一步识别微出血以及早期/急性或小梗死病灶。‡虽然非 IE 卒中文献表明出血量 <30 mL 的患者风险较低，但这一观点尚未在 IE 患者的研究中得到验证，研究仅表明 10 mL 以下病变的手术效果可以接受。高风险部位包括脑室内、脑干下或靠近语言功能区等重要功能区。经许可引自：Venn RA, Ning M, Vlahakes GJ, et al. Surgical timing in infective endocarditis complicated by intracranial hemorrhage. Am Heart J., 2019, 216: 102–112.

胸外科专家组成[23,42]。

2. 制定了鱼骨图，以确定导致医疗服务和质量差异的原因（图 22.4）。

3. 我们回顾了 2016 年 1～12 月所有确诊 IE 患者（经改良 Duke 标准确诊）的临床数据，评估了 2016 年的临床绩效。这些数据是使用特定 IE 诊断代码从电子记录生成的列表中筛选出来的，包括人口统计学、微生物学、死亡率、手术延迟或拒绝手术的原因。

4. 确定"杠杆点"。"杠杆点"是指复杂系统中的可操作点，在此点上实施变革能产生巨大影响（如改善预后）[43]。根据数据，我们注意到改善延迟手术的情况可能是提高疗效的"杠杆点"[23]。

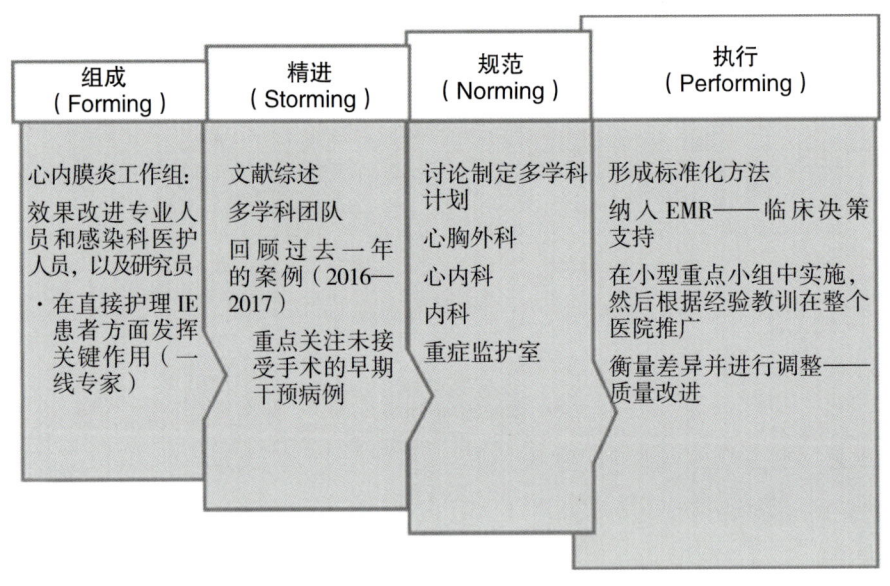

图 22.3 利用 Tuckman 模式建立心内膜炎工作组。EMR：电子病历。经许可引自：Regunath H, Vasudevan A, Vyas K, et al. A quality improvement initiative: developing a multi-disciplinary team for infective endocarditis. Mo Med, 2019, 116(4): 291–296.

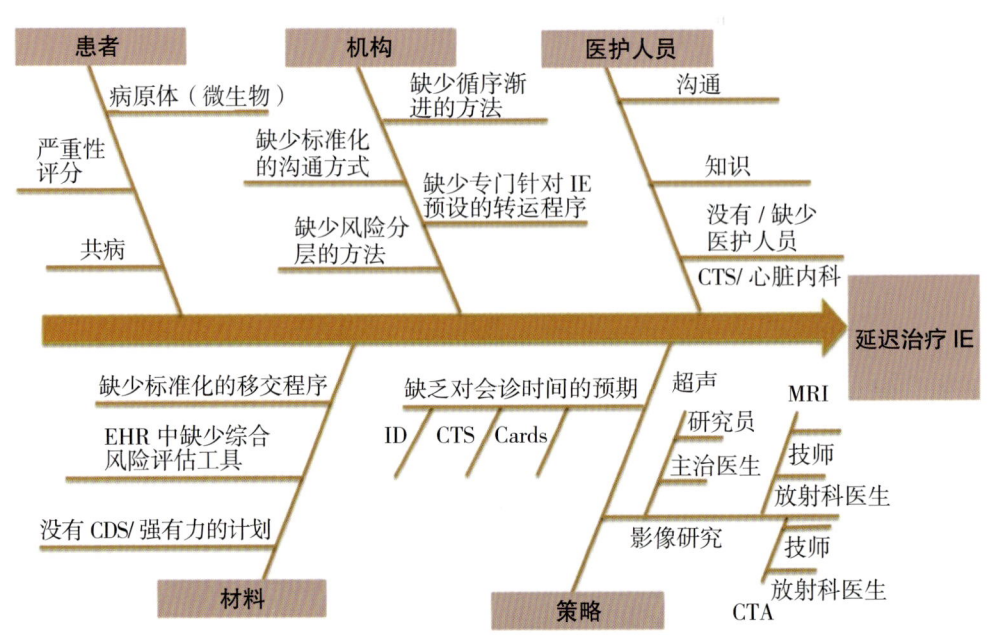

图 22.4 鱼骨图：造成感染性心内膜炎治疗效果差异的可能原因。Cards：心脏病学咨询服务；CDS：临床决策支持；CTA：CT 血管造影；CTS：心胸外科；EHR：电子健康档案；ID：感染科；IE：感染性心内膜炎；MRI：磁共振成像。经许可引自：Regunath H, Vasudevan A, Vyas K, et al. A quality improvement initiative: developing a multi-disciplinary team for infective endocarditis. Mo Med, 2019, 116(4): 291–296.

5. 制定任务说明和目标。

   a. 任务说明：通过制定工作流程图和组建 MDT，使 IE 患者的医疗和护理标准化，从而持续提高诊疗质量；

   b. 目标：通过以下步骤，对 IE 患者实施标准化处理。

      i. 第 1 步：发展由内科、心脏内科和心胸外科医生组成的 MDT；

      ii. 第 2 步：结合 MDT 的工作流程开发临床决策支持工具，并将其纳入电子病历。

临床路径

在随后的 6 个月中，感染科、心脏内科、心脏外科、内科、绩效改进科和信息科的代表每月召开一次会议。我们构建了一个纳入指南建议的标准化流程，并在团队成员之间进行审核，然后将其整合到我们的电子病历系统中。该临床决策支持工具以电子诊疗途径的形式提供分步临床决策支持。

及早识别有心脏、脓毒症或栓塞并发症风险的 IE 病例是我们流程的核心（分诊），并与确保高危人群早期手术的"杠杆点"相一致。我们的路径顺序总结如下（图 22.5）。

1. 触发因素：临床疑似 IE，包括以下高危标志（见下文）。为了避免过于烦琐和低效的工作，我们没有详尽列出导致心内膜炎的心脏、临床、合并疾病和流行病学因素。

   a. 不明原因的发热；

   b. 已知有结构、瓣膜病变及存在心内分流的先天性心脏病；

   c. 接受血液透析的终末期肾病；

   d. 静脉吸毒／滥用药物；

   e. 金黄色葡萄球菌菌血症；

   f. 近期进行过侵入性口腔／内镜操作。

2. 任务：应用改良 Duke 标准将患者分为确诊 IE 和疑似 IE。

3. 分诊：评估是否存在危及生命的情况或并发症。

   a. 心脏：急性瓣膜功能障碍、穿孔、破坏引起的急性心力衰竭、急性肺水肿；

   b. 全身：严重脓毒症或脓毒性休克。

4. 路径。

   a. 快速通道：如果有上述风险因素或病情危重，则安排感染科和心脏内科进行紧急会诊（最好在 6 h 内），然后将患者转至心脏重症监护室，因为那里有胸心外科团队随时待命。

   b. 非紧急通道：如果风险极小或没有风险，则要求感染科和心脏内科进行常规会诊（24 h 内），然后根据指南建议进行心脏外科会诊。

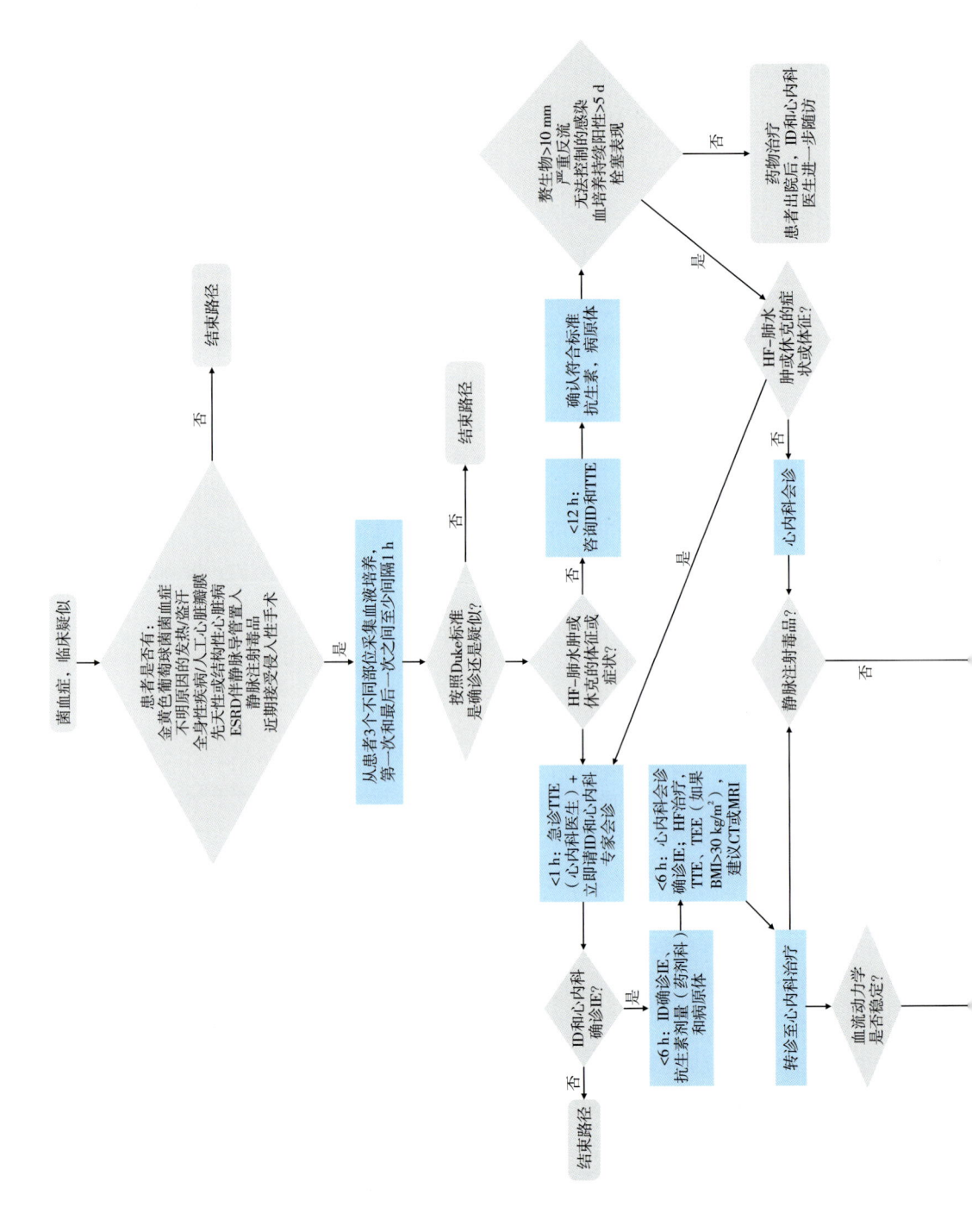

感染性心内膜炎多学科诊疗 *Infective Endocarditis A Multidisciplinary Approach*

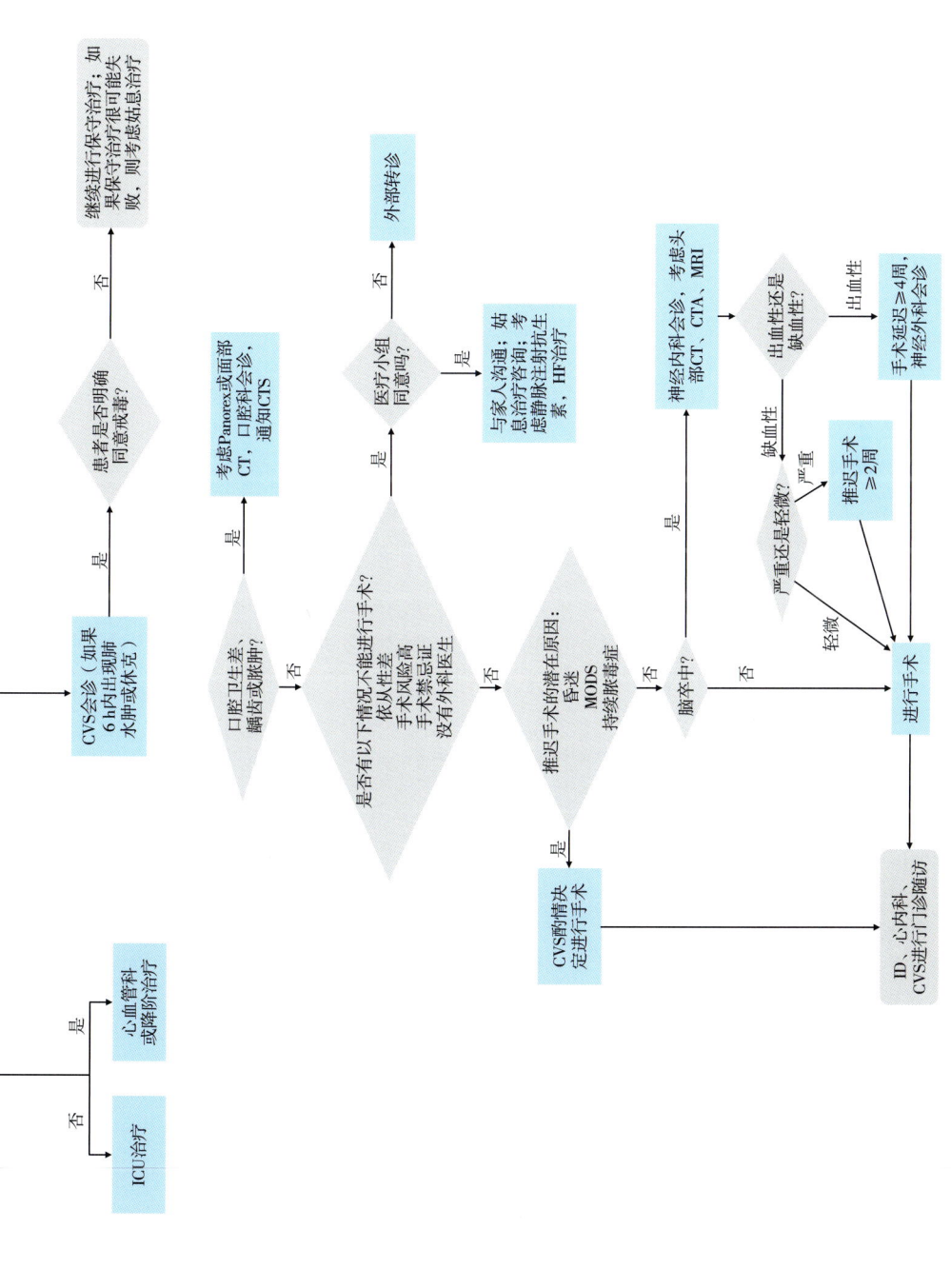

图22.5 美国密苏里大学的临床决策支持流程。BMI：体重指数；CTA：CT血管造影；CTS：心胸外科；CVS：心血管外科；ESRD：终末期肾病；ICU：重症监护室；ID：感染科；IE：感染性心内膜炎；HF：心力衰竭；TEE：经食管超声心动图；TTE：经胸超声心动图；MODS：多器官功能障碍综合征；MRI：磁共振成像

确诊 IE

病理学标准：通过对赘生物、赘生物栓子或心内脓肿标本进行培养或组织学检查发现微生物，或有病理性病变；通过组织学检查证实赘生物或心内脓肿为活动性心内膜炎。

临床标准：2 项主要标准、1 项主要标准和 3 项次要标准，或 5 项次要标准。

疑似 IE

1 项主要标准和 1 项次要标准，或 3 项次要标准。

排除 IE

有解释 IE 证据的确诊的其他诊断；或经抗生素治疗≤ 4 d 后 IE 缓解；或经抗生素治疗≤ 4 d 后，手术或尸检无 IE 病理证据；或不符合上述疑似 IE 的标准。

主要标准

- IE 血培养阳性

1. 两次独立的血培养中检出符合 IE 的典型微生物：草绿色链球菌、牛链球菌、HACEK 菌属、金黄色葡萄球菌；或无原发病灶的社区获得性肠球菌；或符合以下定义的持续血培养阳性的 IE 致病菌：两次抽血间隔至少 >12 h 的血样本培养阳性，或所有 3 次血培养均阳性，或≥ 4 次的血培养中多数为阳性（第一次与最后一次抽血的间隔≥ 1 h）。

2. 贝氏柯克斯体单次血培养阳性或其 IgG 抗体滴度 > 1∶800。

- 心内膜受累的证据

超声心动图检查提示 IE 阳性 [建议对人工瓣膜患者、根据临床标准至少评定为疑似 IE 或复杂 IE（瓣周脓肿）进行 TEE 检查，其他患者首先进行 TTE 检查]，定义如下：瓣膜或支持结构上、反流喷射路径上或植入材料上有活动性心内团块，且无其他解剖学解释；脓肿；或人工瓣膜新出现的部分瓣环撕脱或新的瓣膜反流（杂音强度加重、音调改变或之前杂音不足以说明问题）。

次要标准

1. 易患因素：心脏本身存在易患因素，或静脉吸毒；
2. 发热：体温 >38℃；
3. 血管征象：大动脉栓塞、感染性肺梗死、真菌性动脉瘤、颅内出血、结膜出血以及 Janeway 病变；
4. 免疫学表现：肾小球肾炎、Osler 结节、Roth 斑和类风湿因子；
5. 微生物学证据：血培养阳性，但不符合上述主要标准（不包括凝固酶阴性葡萄球菌和不引起心内膜炎的微生物的单次阳性培养），或与 IE 相符的微生物活动性感染的血清学证据；
6. 超声心动图不符合主要标准。

改良的 Duke 标准经许可改编自：Baddour LM, Wilson WR, Bayer AS, Fet al. Infective endocarditis in adults: diagnosis, antimicrobial therapy, and management of complications. Circulation, 2015, 132(15): 1435–1486.

5. 检查。

  a. 经食管超声心动图、脑影像学检查、反复血培养直至阴性、口腔及其他影像学检查等。

6. 转诊。

  a. 如果心脏外科医生和医疗团队认为手术风险可以接受（使用评分工具或

主观评分），则准备进行手术，并根据所实施的外科手术向术后护理过渡；

b. 如果手术风险被认为很高，或者内科团队和外科团队的意见有冲突，则由主要团队决定进一步的治疗方案。例如，与患者/家属一起做出明智的决定，转到其他中心或姑息治疗。

随后，我们的工作组通过讲座和大查房向住院医生、进修医生以及医院内科、心脏内科、心脏外科和感染科的主治医生提供教育。我们发现，在诊断延迟、亚专科咨询服务和术前检查方面还存在可改进空间。目前的模式要求感染科、心脏内科（心力衰竭和超声心动图专家）、心脏外科医生和基层团队对每一例 IE 进行直接讨论。内科团队加速评估并确定是否存在手术指征。如果有，则与心脏外科会诊，同时根据路径完成手术要求。我们根据计划–执行–研究–行动（PDSA）循环绩效改进框架，随访多项指标，包括心脏评估时间、发病至手术时间、住院时长和获得临床治愈的时间，每年追踪两次。

多学科团队在美洲的进展

2015 年 10 月，加拿大多伦多桑尼布鲁克健康科学中心（Sunnybrook Health Sciences Center）实施了一项病例会议方案，其中包括一个由感染科、心脏内科、心脏外科、重症监护和神经科临床医生组成的工作小组[44]。他们的病例会议由一名工作组成员担任讨论组长。只要有手术指征，这些会议就要求进行线下面对面的病例讨论。如果没有手术指征，则通过电子邮件与所有成员通信，只有在未达成共识时才召开病例会议。对干预前（2013 年 10 月至 2015 年 10 月）与干预后（2015 年 10 月至 2017 年 10 月）的数据进行比较后发现：心脏评估（63.9%～81.3%，$P=0.01$）和手术数量（21.7%～44.6%，$P=0.007$）均显著增加，并具有统计学差异；在并发症发生和死亡率方面没有发现差异，其原因可能是研究效能较低，大多数接受手术的患者病情危重，干预后并未能加快手术实施[44]。

2017 年，华盛顿大学医疗系统成立了一个 MDT，包括 3 家参与的学术型医院和多家诊所[45]。他们的方法与我们类似。此外，由于很大一部分病例与静脉吸毒有关，他们还成立了一个多学科成瘾医学小组，以协助筛查、干预和转诊成瘾治疗[45]。目前还没有关于 MDT 对其结果影响的纵向数据。

2018 年 5～6 月，美国密歇根大学安娜堡分校成立了 IE MDT[46]。2018 年 6 月至 2019 年 6 月期间，在 56 例至少有一个手术指征的确诊 IE 患者中，MDT 的方法使患者的全因死亡率从 29.4%（2014—2015）降至 7.1%，并且 84% 的患者改变了诊疗计划（63% 的患者改变了抗生素方案，21% 的患者改变了手术方案）。此外，经食管超声心动图、神经影像学以及其他诊断和感染相关检查的数量也有所增加[46]。在对内科、感染科、心脏内科和心脏外科医生的后续调查中，98% 的人认为 MDT 促进了沟通，85% 的人认为 MDT 增加了手术机会、改变了临床决策、最大限度地减少了错误并降低了死亡率[47]。

总结与展望

MDT 诊治护理 IE 患者的方法可改善临床诊疗、降低死亡率。最重要的优势是可以识别出能从早期手术中获益的患者，并加快他们的术前准备工作。欧洲的医疗中心拥有最强大的 MDT，可以作为有效的诊疗模式。美国和加拿大越来越多的高质量医疗系统也对 IE 实施了 MDT 管理。IE 患者的临床和流行病学特征，以及医疗保健系统的结构和资源可以指导制定和实施 IE MDT 所需的适当策略。正规的开展和质量改进工具及流程有助于确定 MDT 在一段时间内的表现及其对 IE 死亡率的最终影响。

参考文献

[1] Baddour LM, Wilson WR, Bayer AS, et al. Infective endocarditis in adults: diagnosis, antimicrobial therapy, and management of complications. Circulation, 2015, 132(15): 1435–1486.

[2] Habib G, Lancellotti P, Antunes MJ, et al. 2015 ESC guidelines for the management of infective endocarditis: the task force for the management of infective endocarditis of the European society of cardiology (ESC) endorsed by: European association for cardio-thoracic surgery (EACTS), the European association of nuclear medicine (EANM). Eur Heart J, 2015, 36(44): 3075–3128.

[3] Pettersson GB, Hussain ST. Current AATS guidelines on surgical treatment of infective endocarditis. Ann Cardiothorac Surg, 2019, 8(6): 630–644.

[4] Mistiaen WP. What are the main predictors of in-hospital mortality in patients with infective endocarditis: a review. Scand Cardiovasc J, 2018, 52(2): 58–68.

[5] Habib G, Derumeaux G, Avierinos JF, et al. Value and limitations of the Duke criteria for the diagnosis of infective endocarditis. J Am Coll Cardiol, 1999, 33(7): 2023–2029.

[6] Li JS, Sexton DJ, Mick N, et al. Proposed modifications to the Duke criteria for the diagnosis of infective endocarditis. Clin Infect Dis, 2000, 30(4): 633–638.

[7] Millar BC, Habib G, Moore JE. New diagnostic approaches in infective endocarditis. Heart, 2016, 102(10): 796–807.

[8] Huang G, Gupta S, Davis KA, et al. Infective endocarditis guidelines: the challenges of adherence-a survey of infectious diseases clinicians. Open Forum Infect Dis, 2020, 7(9).

[9] Fanaroff AC, Califf RM, Windecker S, et al. Levels of evidence supporting American college of cardiology/American heart association and European society of cardiology guidelines, 2008—2018. J Am Med Assoc, 2019, 321(11): 1069–1080.

[10] Vlahakes GJ. "Consensus guidelines for the surgical treatment of infective endocarditis": the surgeon must lead the team. J Thorac Cardiovasc Surg, 2017, 153(6): 1259–1260.

[11] Camou F, Dijos M, Barandon L, et al. Management of infective endocarditis and multidisciplinary approach. Med Maladies Infect, 2019, 49(1): 17–22.

[12] Lancellotti P, Rosenhek R, Pibarot P, et al. ESC working group on valvular heart disease position paper-heart valve clinics: organization, structure, and experiences. Eur Heart J, 2013, 34(21): 1597–1606.

[13] Ruch Y, Mazzucotelli J-P, Lefebvre F, et al. Impact of setting up an "endocarditis team" on the management of infective endocarditis. Open Forum Infect Dis, 2019, 6(9).

[14] Botelho-Nevers E, Thuny F, Casalta JP, et al. Dramatic reduction in infective endocarditis-related mortality with a management-based approach. Arch Intern Med, 2009, 169(14): 1290–1298.

[15] Mestres CA, Paré JC, Miró JM. Organization and functioning of a multidisciplinary team for the diagnosis and treatment of infective endocarditis: a 30-year perspective (1985—2014). Rev Esp Cardiol, 2015, 68(5): 363–368.

[16] Kaura A, Byrne J, Fife A, et al. Inception of the 'endocarditis team' is associated with improved survival in patients with infective endocarditis who are managed medically: findings from a before-and-after study. Open Heart, 2017, 4(2): e000699.
[17] Chirillo F, Scotton P, Rocco F, et al. Impact of a multidisciplinary management strategy on the outcome of patients with native valve infective endocarditis. Am J Cardiol, 2013, 112(8): 1171–1176.
[18] Anguita Sánchez M, Torres Calvo F, Castillo Domínguez JC, et al. Short-and long-term prognosis of infective endocarditis in non-injection drug users: improved results over 15 years (1987—2001). Rev Esp Cardiol, 2005, 58(10): 1188–1196.
[19] Erba PA, Habib G, Glaudemans AWJM, et al. The round table approach in infective endocarditis & cardiovascular implantable electronic devices infections: make your e-Team come true. Eur J Nucl Med Mol Imag, 2017, 44(7): 1107–1108.
[20] Carrasco-Chinchilla F, Sánchez-Espín G, Ruiz-Morales J, et al. Influence of a multidisciplinary alert strategy on mortality due to left-sided infective endocarditis. Rev Esp Cardiol, 2014, 67(5): 380–386.
[21] Issa N, Dijos M, Greib C, et al. Impact of an endocarditis team in the management of 357 infective endocarditis. Open Forum Infect Dis, 2016, 3(Suppl.1): 1122.
[22] Chambers J, Sandoe J, Ray S, et al. The infective endocarditis team: recommendations from an international working group. Heart, 2014, 100(7): 524–527.
[23] Regunath H, Vasudevan A, Vyas K, et al. A quality improvement initiative: developing a multi-disciplinary team for infective endocarditis. Mo Med, 2019, 116(4): 291–296.
[24] Pettersson GB, Hussain ST, Shrestha NK, et al. Infective endocarditis: an atlas of disease progression for describing, staging, coding, and understanding the pathology. J Thorac Cardiovasc Surg, 2014, 147(4): 1142–1149.e2.
[25] Murdoch DR, Corey GR, Hoen B, et al. Clinical presentation, etiology, and outcome of infective endocarditis in the 21st century: the international collaboration on endocarditis-prospective cohort study. Arch Intern Med, 2009, 169(5): 463–473.
[26] Kiefer T, Park L, Tribouilloy C, et al. Association between valvular surgery and mortality among patients with infective endocarditis complicated by heart failure. J Am Med Assoc, 2011, 306(20): 2239–2247.
[27] Anantha Narayanan M, Mahfood Haddad T, Kalil AC, et al. Early versus late surgical intervention or medical management for infective endocarditis: a systematic review and meta-analysis. Heart, 2016, 102(12): 950–957.
[28] Liang F, Song B, Liu R, et al. Optimal timing for early surgery in infective endocarditis: a meta-analysis. Interact Cardiovasc Thorac Surg, 2016, 22(3): 336–345.
[29] Cahill TJ, Baddour LM, Habib G, et al. Challenges in infective endocarditis. J Am Coll Cardiol, 2017, 69(3): 325–344.
[30] Pettersson GB, Coselli JS, Hussain ST, et al. 2016 The American Association for Thoracic Surgery (AATS) consensus guidelines: surgical treatment of infective endocarditis: executive summary. J Thorac Cardiovasc Surg, 2017, 153(6): 1241–1258.e29.
[31] Chu VH, Park LP, Athan E, et al. Association between surgical indications, operative risk, and clinical outcome in infective endocarditis. Circulation, 2015, 131(2): 131–140.
[32] Gaca JG, Sheng S, Daneshmand MA, et al. Outcomes for endocarditis surgery in North America: a simplified risk scoring system. J Thorac Cardiovasc Surg, 2011, 141(1): 98–106.e2.
[33] Nashef SA, Roques F, Michel P, et al. European system for cardiac operative risk evaluation (EuroSCORE). Eur J Cardio Thorac Surg, 1999, 16(1): 9–13.
[34] De Feo M, Cotrufo M, Carozza A, et al. The need for a specific risk prediction system in native valve infective endocarditis surgery. Scientific WorldJournal, 2012, 2012: 307571.
[35] Olmos C, Vilacosta I, Habib G, et al. Risk score for cardiac surgery in active left-sided infective endocarditis. Heart, 2017, 103(18): 1435–1442.
[36] Martínez-Sellés M, Muñoz P, Arnáiz A, et al. Valve surgery in active infective endocarditis: a

simple score to predict in-hospital prognosis. Int J Cardiol, 2014, 175(1): 133–137.
[37] Costa MA, Wollmann Jr DR, Campos AC, et al. Risk index for death by infective endocarditis: a multivariate logistic model. Rev Bras Cir Cardiovasc, 2007, 22(2): 192–200.
[38] Varela L, López-Menéndez J, Redondo A, et al. Mortality risk prediction in infective endocarditis surgery: reliability analysis of specific scoresy. Eur J Cardio Thorac Surg, 2017, 53(5): 1049–1054.
[39] Venn RA, Ning M, Vlahakes GJ, et al. Surgical timing in infective endocarditis complicated by intracranial hemorrhage. Am Heart J, 2019, 216: 102–112.
[40] Vasudevan A, Vyas K, Chen L-C, et al. 1910. Developing a multi-disciplinary team for infective endocarditis: a quality improvement project. Open Forum Infectious Diseases, 2018, 5(Suppl. 1). S549–S.
[41] Regunath H, Cochran K, Cornell K, et al. Is it painful to manage chronic pain? A cross-sectional study of physicians in-training in a university program. Mo Med, 2016, 113(1): 72–78.
[42] Tuckman BW. Developmental sequence IN small groups. Psychol Bull, 1965, 63: 384–399.
[43] Meadows D. Places to intervene in a system. Whole Earth, 1997, 91(1): 78–84.
[44] Tan C, Hansen MS, Cohen G, et al. Case conferences for infective endocarditis: a quality improvement initiative. PloS One, 2018, 13(10): e0205528– .
[45] Gibbons EF, Huang G, Aldea G, et al. A multidisciplinary pathway for the diagnosis and treatment of infectious endocarditis. Crit Pathw Cardiol, 2020, 19(4): 187–194.
[46] El-Dalati S, Cronin D, IV JR, et al. 713. The clinical impact of implementation of a multidisciplinary endocarditis team. Open Forum Infect Dis, 2020, 7(Suppl. 1):S407–8.
[47] El-Dalati S, Khurana I, Soper N, et al. Physician perceptions of a multidisciplinary endocarditis team. Eur J Clin Microbiol Infect Dis, 2020, 39(4): 735–739.

第23章
感染性心内膜炎的未来研究方向

Lauren V. Huckaby[1], *Arman Kilic*[2]

[1]University of Pittsburgh Medical Center, Pittsburgh, PA, United States;
[2]John M. Kratz Endowed Chair in Cardiac Surgery, Medical University of South Carolina and Surgical Director of the Heart Failure and Heart Transplant Program, Charleston, SA, United States

引 言

医学文献中首次出现对心内膜炎的描述是在17世纪,当时人们对心脏的解剖和生理特征并不完全了解[1]。随着时间推移,医学取得巨大的进步,包括影像技术、抗生素治疗和外科手术干预的发展,从而开启了感染性心内膜炎(IE)治疗的新纪元。这种疾病曾经让Giovanni Morgagni(译者注:意大利解剖学家)和Rudolf Virchow(译者注:德国病理学家)等众多享誉医学史的著名教授都感到十分困惑,然而即使在今天,它仍然是临床医生面临的一大挑战。当然,现今IE的治疗结果无疑已显著改善[1-2]。本章中,我们将探讨IE目前的发展趋势,以应对这一疾病未来在诊断和治疗方面所面临的机遇和挑战;此外,我们还要加强那些传统研究领域的工作,以便更好地理解这一疾病复杂的病理过程。

静脉吸毒的趋势

近年来,阿片类药物的滥用以一种令人担忧的趋势发展,已被视为美国的全国性公共卫生危机[3-4]。在过去10年中,处方阿片类药物滥用的问题日益凸显,海洛因和芬太尼的使用量也出现了令人不安的增长趋势[5]。1999—2017年间,仅与海洛因相关的吸毒过量死亡发生率已从0.7/10万增至4.9/10万,虽然近期这一增长率似乎趋于平稳[5]。正如预期的那样,与静脉吸毒(IVDU)相关的IE发病率也同步上升,从而改变了IE的流行病学特征[6-7]。与IVDU相关的IE更有可能为右侧IE,感染的病菌毒力更强,而且由于持续使用毒品,此类患者的长期临床病程可能更加复杂[8]。共用针头、舔舐针头、注射前未进行皮肤消毒以及药物混合物中的污染物,这些都可能导致菌血症,并增加罹患IE的风险。因此,旨在遏制传染病传播的措施,如针头交换计划和阿片类受体激动剂治疗等,可能会对降低IE的风险产生积极影响[9]。

然而，IVDU的发展趋势很难预测，未来它对IE的影响也不明确。但可以肯定的是，这一公共卫生危机不会消失。自2013年以来，合成阿片类药物（如芬太尼）的使用量急剧上升，滥用处方阿片类药物（如羟考酮）的患者转而吸食海洛因的可能性增加了19倍[10-11]。对此，美国已采取了多层面的应对措施，主要集中在戒毒和其治疗服务以及相关领域的研究，以更好地量化疾病负担，并制定戒毒治疗和无阿片类药物疼痛管理的创新策略。这些公共卫生措施旨在解决目前存在的IVDU人群以及处方阿片类药物的分发问题，因为这是使用处方阿片类药物人群可能发展为静脉注射毒品的关键因素，效果如何仍有待观察。但可以确定，这两方面的措施将共同决定未来IE患者的整体状况。

上述趋势也显示出成瘾治疗在IVDU相关IE患者长期管理中的重要作用。由于持续IVDU，这类患者的再入院率和IE复发率都很高，这就不难解释为何复吸是IVDU相关IE患者的主要死因[8,12]。此外，与首次IE手术相比，再次瓣膜手术也可导致30 d死亡率显著增加[13]。目前，遏制持续IVDU的努力尚未取得成效，作为IE长期管理的重要组成部分，同时也能降低医疗成本[14]，成瘾医学专家参与到这类患者的治疗中已显示出有助于降低他们的再入院率[15]。当然，要确保这类患者戒除IVDU，降低IE复发的风险，多学科参与必不可少，同时还应将IVDU相关IE患者首次住院后的门诊随访纳入一同管理。

危险分层

IE仅发生在少数植入人工瓣膜或有易感因素的患者中，因此预测IE高风险患者人群对于制定有效的预防性治疗和指导检查流程至关重要。研究人员建立了各种模型，不仅可以估算IE风险，还可以预测患者最终是否需要手术，以及内科或外科治疗后的长期结局。通过大规模的队列研究，这些工具可以帮助医生更好地理解疾病的发展趋势，并为患者提供个性化的治疗策略。

首先，许多研究都特别关注接受高风险手术的人工瓣膜患者发生IE的风险，以便为他们提供适当的抗生素预防指导。美国心脏协会（AHA）最新的IE预防指南可追溯到2007年，其中明确规定了高危患者人群和基于不同手术类型的预防建议[16]。但作者也承认，由于IE的总体发病率较低，很难获得充分的数据来支持他们的建议，因此他们呼吁进行更多的抗生素与安慰剂对照的随机试验，以明确不同人群的相对风险和获益情况[16]。虽然牙科手术可能会引起短暂性菌血症，但这与IE之间的关系仍不明确。由于缺乏充分的证据，不同国家和地区制定了与AHA完全不同的指南：AHA建议仅对高危人群使用抗生素预防，而英国则不建议常规使用抗生素预防[17]。为此，开展大规模的人群研究，进行长期的随访调查，收集有关侵入性手术类型、预防性抗生素使用剂量和时机的详细数据就显得十分必要。另外，从成本-效益的角度来看，有研究表明抗生素预防可能仅对高风险病例是有益的；因此，未来指南的推荐应将成本-效益和临床结局相结合进行综合分析后予以发布[18]。

其次，相关研究还集中在评估修复术后患者的死亡率，以预判手术效果，与 IE 死亡相关的因素包括老龄、人工瓣膜相关感染、致病菌和整体病情严重程度[19-21]。这些研究中就包括 EndoSCORE，它是专门为预测术后死亡率而开发的评分系统，预测因素包括年龄、性别、共病、是否存在瓣周脓肿、术前心肾功能和感染病原体种类[22]。但这些研究大多来自对现有数据库的回顾性分析，其中许多数据库并不包含 IE 治疗的具体数据，如致病微生物和一些复杂手术的具体细节，而在瓣周受累的病例中可能需要这些数据，这限制了使用美国胸外科医师学会（STS）数据库等资源进行复杂病例的分析预测。可见，如果需要提高对不同治疗方案下患者预后评估的准确性，未来的研究则应结合前瞻性数据进行更为复杂的分析，以期达到对 IE 的风险做出分层。此外，使用经过验证的风险评分系统对 IE 患者进行前瞻性风险分层，结合多种不良预后的风险因素，可为如何对这些患者进行最佳治疗提供客观的指导。

预防 IE 装置的研制

人工瓣膜已成为 IE 负担的重要因素，与这些外源性假体相关的感染风险增加了人们对设备工程的兴趣，并以此为机遇试图开发具有较低感染风险的假体。许多研究都试图对人工瓣膜的设计进行改进，以减少细菌定植和生物膜的形成。体外研究对有抗生素涂层的人工瓣膜上的细菌数量进行了检测，结果显示细菌数量有所减少，这表明此类瓣膜在预防早期 IE 方面可能具有临床效果[23-24]，但尚未应用于临床。人工瓣膜心内膜炎减少试验（Artificial Valve Endocarditis Reduction Trial）是一项旨在评估一种采用镀银人工瓣环的机械瓣设计（Silzone, St. Jude Medical；St. Paul，Minnesota）与传统缝合瓣环相比，可否降低主动脉瓣或二尖瓣人工瓣膜置换后心内膜炎发生率的临床研究[25]。该试验于 1998 年启动，2000 年终止，原因是接受 Silzone 瓣膜后瓣周漏发生率增加，导致患者需要再次手术[26-27]。目前，研究人员正在探索将新材料（如脱细胞组织）整合到人工瓣膜设计中，以期阻止生物膜的形成。然而，这些新设计瓣膜的临床表现和长期耐用性仍需进一步研究[28]。

虽然装置相关性 IE 预防的重点是人工瓣膜，但对于 IE 风险相对较小的心脏植入式电子设备（如起搏器和除颤器）也做了相应的研究。随着老年患者人数的增加，这些设备的使用率在未来还会增加[29]。全球随机抗生素封套感染预防（Worldwide Randomized Antibiotic Envelope Infection Prevention）试验发现，使用可吸收抗生素洗脱封套可以显著减少植入心脏起搏器和（或）除颤器后的主要感染，包括伤口和深部手术部位感染[30]。然而，考虑到抗生素封套组和对照组的菌血症和心内膜炎发生率均 < 1%，因此，使用封套并没有观察到显著的 IE 减少[30]。而随后的一项荟萃分析则表明使用抗生素封套对减少局部并发症有一定的效果，但

研究并未专门检视其对 IE 发生率的影响[31]。据此推测，心内膜炎的预防通过装置电极的工程学改进或许更为有效，这样才可增强抗生物膜形成的能力，而不是单纯使用封套解决囊袋的感染问题。

登记方案的发展

鉴于心内膜炎患者管理的复杂性和精细化要求，我们迫切需要收集大量不同类型患者的数据，以确定最佳的临床实践方法。欧洲感染性心内膜炎登记处作为一个前瞻性的多中心队列，收集了接受内科或外科治疗的、疑似或确诊 IE 的成年患者的信息[32-33]。这一协作组织提供了全面的关于心内膜炎患者病因、治疗方法及疗效的概况，反映了当前临床模式[32]。瑞典与意大利的 IE 患者登记处，连同其他国家设立的类似机构，均已开始运作并收集关于心内膜炎管理与预后的详细数据[34-35]。值得一提的是，意大利登记处从 1979 年开始登记患者，可以对 IE 的关键信息（如影像学检查和培养结果）进行纵向评估，从而揭示 IE 临床治疗方法的趋势及病因的变化，如 IVDU 的增加。

尽管 STS 数据库收集了大量信息，但基于注册的 IE 数据大多来自欧洲。STS 数据库收集了许多接受手术治疗的 IE 患者，但其局限性在于只包括了最终接受手术治疗的患者，因此可能会遗漏那些成功接受药物治疗的患者，或有手术指征但未接受手术治疗的患者。此外，STS 数据库并未纳入非典型病例或未全面纳入手术难度较高的复杂病例。诚然，对美国的 IE 患者进行药物治疗和手术治疗的前瞻性研究任务艰巨，但这一研究将对临床管理做出重大贡献，尤其是在伴随着 IVDU 增加和病原学演变的背景下。

大数据应用

无论是前瞻性还是回顾性收集的 IE 患者数据，都凸显出我们需要新的数据分析和解读方法来为临床实践提供依据。尽管 STS 的数据集包含了大量的变量和相当大规模的样本量，但 IE 病理生理学、诊断和处理的精细化要求不仅需要一个相当大的样本量，而且还需要详尽的细节，以阐明这类患者医疗的复杂性。同时，需采用先进的统计和计算方法准确解读和分析相关数据，为临床实践提供依据。

机器学习利用其强大的计算能力，以已知信息为基础构建特定主题的模型，并将这些信息进行前瞻性应用。这种方法克服了传统统计方法的局限性，并有可能厘清以前无法确定的因素，从而提高模型的效能。机器学习最近被应用于 IE，探索生物标志物，对死亡风险进行分层。研究人员利用分类树发现，C-反应蛋白、C-C 基序趋化因子配体和白细胞介素 -15 的升高与院内死亡显著相关[36]。对这些血清标记物的进一步研究，再结合已知的导致 IE 的风险因素，有望进一步改善内科和外科治疗的预后。

机器学习还可用于影像学数据的解读。一项早期研究利用机器学习来对常规超声心动图中的限制性心包炎和缩窄性心包炎进行鉴别诊断[37]。还有研究利用机器学习来分辨超声心动图上的心室组织特性[38]，并将所测指标与射血分数结合预测死亡率[39]。类似方法还可用于经胸超声心动图（TTE）对二尖瓣病变的诊断，通过机器学习可提高我们的诊断能力，从而减少侵入性经食管超声心动图（TEE）的使用。同样，机器学习可以帮助我们利用现有的成像模式，提升对手术修复的复杂性和范围的预测能力，从而能更加准确地判断术后结局。

很少有研究专门将机器学习用于 IE，但这种方法可以提高对患者进行个性化处理的能力，并根据患者的独特表现和病理生理学设定期望值。此外，这些人工智能模式的应用有可能克服现有影像和生化检测方法的局限性，指导我们对某些患者的手术决策。然而，将机器学习融入临床实践需要大量数据集的验证，并且可能只适用于特定的患者群体。这同时是一个迭代过程，机器学习需要根据每一次新的临床进展（如新成像方法的引入）进行重新评估，尽管如此，与现有的统计方法相比，这种利用所有可用数据的学习能力已经在一些研究中显示出了较高的预测准确性，表现出了较好的应用前景[39]。

诊断和治疗展望

IE 的临床诊断依赖于改良 Duke 标准，该标准包括影像学、实验室、体格检查和病史等多方面信息。尽管如此，一些患者的 IE 诊断仍然难以确定，许多患者需要通过侵入性影像学检查（如 TEE）来确诊、评估更复杂的疾病及监测病情的改善。因此，新的研究重点在于如何提高 IE 的诊断能力或更好地描述 IE 的特征。除了诊断方面的改进外，内外科治疗的进步也将有助于降低该病的死亡率，减轻对医疗系统的影响。

影像学手段作为改良 Duke 标准用于进行临床诊断的一部分，经常用于检查是否存在瓣膜赘生物、评估心内膜炎病变的血流动力学状态以及监测感染的清除情况。在许多情况下，对瓣膜结构（尤其是二尖瓣）的准确评估依赖于 TEE；因此，最近的研究聚焦于对这一疾病负担采用非侵入性放射学评估。例如，近期一项荟萃分析探讨了 ^{18}F- 氟脱氧葡萄糖（^{18}F–FDG）PET/CT 对自体瓣膜和人工瓣膜心内膜炎的诊断准确性[40]。研究发现，与单独使用改良 Duke 标准相比，PET/CT 提高了心脏植入式电子设备或植入人工瓣膜患者的诊断准确性[41]。尽管这种成像技术并未广泛普及，但在其他疾病中的应用正逐渐增多，可能也会增加其在 IE 诊断中的可用性。

其他各种技术也被用于提高 IE 的诊断率，特别是对培养阴性的心内膜炎病例致病微生物的鉴定，这是指导抗生素治疗的关键因素。常规血培养是鉴定微生物的标准方法，但之前使用过抗生素可能会干扰培养的结果，导致部分微生物在常规培养中不会增殖，出现培养阴性结果。利用聚合酶链反应（PCR）从切除的心脏组织中鉴定微生物有望改进微生物学诊断[42]。荧光原位杂交技术也可提高诊断能力，同时还能区分活跃的生物膜和降解的细菌[43]，并可观察抗生素治疗后细菌的持续增殖，有助于指导抗生素的选择和疗程规划。

静脉注射抗生素（通常为 6 周）一直是 IE 治疗的重要部分，然而，近期研究表明，通过肠道途径给予抗生素可能同样有效。一篇关于口服抗生素降级疗法的综述指出，在菌血症消除后使用生物利用度高的口服抗生素可能并不劣于静脉注射抗菌药物[44]。虽然这一概念需要通过大型随机对照试验来验证，而且可能只适用于某些致病菌和病情稳定的患者，但这在避免长期静脉注射带来的并发症和降低相关费用方面可能会减轻 IE 对医疗系统造成的负担。对于有 IVDU 史的患者而言，这一变化尤为重要，因为这类患者往往需要在出院后到护理机构接受长时间的肠外抗生素治疗。新型抗菌药物的出现有望在保持疗效的同时减轻治疗负担。奥利万星（oritavancin）是一种针对革兰氏阳性菌的新型静脉用抗生素，其半衰期超过 2 周，每周仅需给药一次，已用于治疗耐万古霉素肠球菌引起的人工瓣膜心内膜炎[45]。这种治疗方法可能为 IE 患者提供一种更便捷的门诊抗生素治疗方案。

除了诊断和药物治疗的进步，伴随时间的推移及其他心脏手术的进展，IE 的外科治疗方法也在不断改善，疗效也得到了显著提升。IVDU 相关 IE 的发病率越来越高，此类病例通常涉及侵袭性更强的微生物，结果是瓣周脓肿和瘘管等并发症的发病率增加，导致手术的复杂性增加。然而，IVDU 患者普遍较年轻、共病较少，因此在治疗策略上倾向于采取更为积极的手术干预是合理的。随着 IVDU 的发展趋势，这些更复杂的手术可能会成为 IE 手术中的常见手术；而随着经验的增加，特别是在大型中心，这些手术的死亡率和术后效果无疑会得到改善。微创技术的不断成熟为 IE 治疗提供了新的可行性，其在特定病例中的应用逐渐被视为一种可行的治疗手段[16-17]。此外，通过真空抽吸系统经皮清除赘生物的方法也得到了研究，这可能是一种重要的辅助治疗方法，尤其适用于因各种原因不适合手术的病例[48]。手术时机是一个争论不休的话题，急需进一步明确，尤其是对心脏以外其他脏器受累的病例[49-50]。由于难以获得前瞻性数据以及患者群体的异质性，使得许多相关研究的临床应用受到了限制。在大型中心进行 IE 区域化治疗可能有助于开展以手术适应证和手术实施为重点的研究工作，以改善患者的医疗质量。

此外，针对 IE 手术时的全身炎症反应的前期研究工作已初步展开。REMOVE 研究是一项随机对照试验，旨在评估放置在体外循环回路中的非选择性细胞因子吸附柱 CytoSorb（CytoSorbents，Monmouth Junction；New Jersey）对 IE 手术后多器官功能障碍的影响[51]。虽然与接受非感染性瓣膜病手术的患者相比，IE 患者的循环细胞因子水平更高，但之前的一项前导研究显示，心脏手术使用 CytoSorb 和未使用血液吸附技术的结果之间并无显著差异[51-52]。因此，这种使用术中尝试性免疫调节对炎症标志物的客观水平和临床结局所产生的影响仍有待观察。

多学科协作

"心脏团队"在复杂病例心脏手术指征决策时所取得的临床成功经验，引起了学界对于建立专门的多学科团队来管理 IE 患者的浓厚兴趣。考虑到已知的高复吸风险，特别是对于 IVDU 相关的 IE 患者，这一举措尤为重要。正如欧洲心脏病学会 IE 指南所强调的，心内膜炎团队应通过与来自多个专科的医疗人员合作来应对 IE 病理生理学中的细微变化，以优化这些患者的治疗效果[53]。AHA 在其瓣膜性心脏病指南中也建议对 IE 采取团队合作的方法，尤其是在讨论手术干预时机时[54]。多学科团队的影响会覆盖病程的所有阶段，包括诊断、治疗、随访和长期预后。除心脏内科、感染科和心脏外科医生外，神经内科、神经外科和风湿病学领域的医疗人员也可为这些复杂患者的优化处理提供宝贵意见[55]。IVDU 相关 IE 患者还可受益于社会工作者、精神科医生和成瘾医学专家的早期参与，以确保戒毒，从而避免 IE 复发。

多学科团队的实践得到了广泛认同，这可能有助于推进质量改进和研究实施[55-56]。即使在 IE 发生率相对较低的中心，同样应该采用多学科方法，必要时可请收治量较高的三级医疗中心的团队参与会诊，以达到遵循业内指南推荐，确保循证管理的目的。相关工作人员定期会面不仅有助于正确分诊和确立初步诊断后的管理目标，还有助于与门诊工作人员进行协调，讨论停止抗生素治疗的相关问题，并确定长期随访、治疗或延迟手术（如有必要）计划。心脏团队取得的成功和对其价值的普遍认可会促进许多已经建立了多学科管理基础设施的医疗机构成立专门的心内膜炎小组。尽管心内膜炎小组并不是一个新概念，但它是全面应对和整合 IE 患者医疗的未来发展关键。

总　结

自几个世纪前首次发现 IE 以来，其诊断和治疗一直是临床一大挑战。对 IE 的治疗在很大程度上依赖于实验室检测、影像学和手术方法的共同进步。然而，医护人员越来越清楚地认识到，IE 的复杂性和异质性要求聚焦于相关研究，以降低与其病理生理学相关的高死亡率。加强对高危患者的实践认知将有助于制定预防策略。对大量数据的准确解读和临床应用有望弥补成像技术的局限性。IE 未来进展的一个关键环节就是 IVDU 相关的 IE 负担，这一类型极大地改变了该疾病的流行病学特征，严重影响了 IE 患者的治疗效果和长期预后。在这方面，临床经验和多学科团队的参与成为战胜这一疾病的最大希望，同时，所有这些领域的进步都将对目前 IE 的高并发症发生率和死亡率产生重要影响。

参考文献

[1] Major RH. Notes ON the history OF endocarditis. Bull Hist Med, 1945, 17(4): 351–359.
[2] Contrepois A. Towards a history of infective endocarditis. Med Hist, 1996, 40: 25–54.

[3] Murthy VH. Ending the opioid epidemic—A call to action. N Engl J Med, 2016, 375: 2413–2415.

[4] Schwetz TA, Calder T, Rosenthal E, et al. Opioids and infectious diseases: a converging public health crisis. J Infect Dis, 2019, 220(3): 346–349. https://doi.org/10.1093/infdis/jiz133.

[5] Hedegaard H, Miniño AM, Warner M. Drug overdose deaths in the United States, 1999—2018. NCHS Data Brief, 2020, (356): 1–8.

[6] Schranz AJ, Fleischauer A, Chu VH, et al. Trends in drug use-associated infective endocarditis and heart valve surgery, 2007 to 2017: a study of statewide discharge data. Ann Intern Med, 2019, 170(1): 31–40. https://doi.org/10.7326/M18-2124.

[7] Kadri AN, Wilner B, Hernandez AV, et al. Geographic trends, patient characteristics, and outcomes of infective endocarditis associated with drug abuse in the United States from 2002 to 2016. J Am Heart Assoc, 2019, 8(19): 1–10. https://doi.org/10.1161/JAHA.119.012969.

[8] Nguemeni Tiako MJ, Mori M, Mahmood SU B, et al. Recidivism is the leading cause of death among intravenous drug users who underwent cardiac surgery for infective endocarditis. Semin Thorac Cardiovasc Surg, 2019, 31(1): 40–45. https://doi.org/10.1053/j.semtcvs.2018.07.016.

[9] Macneil J, Pauly B. Needle exchange as a safe haven in an unsafe world. Drug Alcohol Rev, 2011, 30(1): 26–32. https://doi.org/10.1111/j.1465-3362.2010.00188.x.

[10] Compton WM, Jones CM, Baldwin GT. Relationship between nonmedical prescription-opioid use and heroin use. N Engl J Med, 2016, 374(2): 154–163. https://doi.org/10.1056/NEJMra1508490.

[11] Daniulaityte R, Juhascik MP, Strayer KE, et al. Trends in fentanyl and fentanyl analogue-related overdose deaths—montgomery County, Ohio, 2015-2017. Drug Alcohol Depend, 2019, 198(March): 116–120. https://doi.org/10.1016/j.drugalcdep.2019.01.045.

[12] Rosenthal ES, Karchmer AW, Theisen-Toupal J, et al. Suboptimal addiction interventions for patients hospitalized with injection drug use-associated infective endocarditis. Am J Med, 2016, 129(5): 481–485. https://doi.org/10.1016/j.amjmed.2015.09.024.

[13] Mori M, Mahmood SU B, Schranz AJ, et al. Risk of reoperative valve surgery for endocarditis associated with drug use. J Thorac Cardiovasc Surg, 2020, 159(4): 1262–1268.e2. https://doi.org/10.1016/j.jtcvs.2019.06.055.

[14] Tookes H, Diaz C, Li H, et al. A cost analysis of hospitalizations for infections related to injection drug use at a county safety-net hospital in Miami, Florida. PloS One, 2015, 10(6): 1–11. https://doi.org/10.1371/journal.pone.0129360.

[15] Marks LR, Munigala S, Warren DK, et al. Addiction medicine consultations reduce readmission rates for patients with serious infections from opioid use disorder. Clin Infect Dis, 2019, 68(11): 1935–1937. https://doi.org/10.1093/cid/ciy924.

[16] Wilson W, Taubert KA, Gewitz M, et al. Prevention of infective endocarditis: guidelines from the American heart association. Circulation, 2007, 116(15): 1736–1754. https://doi.org/10.1161/CIRCULATIONAHA.106.183095.

[17] Cahill TJ, Harrison JL, Jewell P, et al. Antibiotic prophylaxis for infective endocarditis: a systematic review and meta-analysis. Heart, 2017, 103(12): 937–944. https://doi.org/10.1136/heartjnl-2015-309102.

[18] Franklin M, Wailoo A, Dayer MJ, et al. The cost-effectiveness of antibiotic prophylaxis for patients at risk of infective endocarditis. Circulation, 2016, 134(20): 1568–15678. https://doi.org/10.1161/CIRCULATIONAHA.116.022047.

[19] Olmos C, Vilacosta I, Habib G, et al. Risk score for cardiac surgery in active left-sided infective endocarditis. Heart, 2017, 103(18): 1435–1442. https://doi.org/10.1136/heartjnl-2016-311093.

[20] Park LP, Chu VH, Peterson G, et al. Validated risk score for predicting 6-month mortality in infective endocarditis. J Am Heart Assoc, 2016, 5(4): 1–13. https://doi.org/10.1161/JAHA.115.003016.

[21] Gaca JG, Sheng S, Daneshmand MA, et al. Outcomes for endocarditis surgery in North America: a simplified risk scoring system. J Thorac Cardiovasc Surg, 2011, 141(1): 98–106.e2. https://doi.org/10.1016/j.jtcvs.2010.09.016.

[22] Di Mauro M, Dato GMA, Barili F, et al. A predictive model for early mortality after surgical

treatment of heart valve or prosthesis infective endocarditis. The EndoSCORE. Int J Cardiol, 2017, 241: 97–102. https://doi.org/10.1016/j.ijcard.2017.03.148.

[23] Darouiche RO, Fowler VG, Adal K, et al. Antimicrobial activity of prosthetic heart valve sewing cuffs coated with minocycline and rifampin. Antimicrob Agents Chemother, 2002, 46(2): 543–545. https://doi.org/10.1128/AAC.46.2.543-545.2002.

[24] Mashaqi B, Marsch G, Shrestha M, et al. Antibiotic pretreatment of heart valve prostheses to prevent early prosthetic valve endocarditis. J Heart Valve Dis, 2011, 20(5): 582–586.

[25] Schaff HV, Carrel TP, Steckelberg JM, et al. Artifical valve endocarditis reduction trial (AVERT): protocol of a multicenter randomized trial. J Heart Valve Dis, 1999, 8(2): 131–139.

[26] Schaff HV, Carrel TP, Jamieson WRE, et al. Paravalvular leak and other events in silzone-coated mechanical heart valves: a report from AVERT. Ann Thorac Surg, 2002, 73(3): 785–792. https://doi.org/10.1016/S0003-4975(01)03442-7.

[27] Jamieson WRE, Fradet GJ, Abel JG, et al. Seven-year results with the St Jude medical silzone mechanical prosthesis. J Thorac Cardiovasc Surg, 2009, 137(5): 1109–1115.e2. https://doi.org/10.1016/j.jtcvs.2008.07.070.

[28] Horke A, Tudorache I, Laufer G, et al. Early results from a prospective, single-arm European trial on decellularized allografts for aortic valve replacement: the ARISE study and ARISE Registry data. Eur J Cardio Thorac Surg, 2020, 58(5): 1045–1053. https://doi.org/10.1093/ejcts/ezaa100.

[29] Bradshaw PJ, Stobie P, Knuiman MW, et al. Trends in the incidence and prevalence of cardiac pacemaker insertions in an ageing population. Open Hear, 2014, 1(1): 1–6. https://doi.org/10.1136/openhrt-2014-000177.

[30] Tarakji KG, Mittal S, Kennergren C, et al. Antibacterial envelope to prevent cardiac implantable device infection. N Engl J Med, 2019, 380(20): 1895–1905. https://doi.org/10.1056/NEJMoa1901111.

[31] Koerber SM, Turagam MK, Winterfield J, et al. Use of antibiotic envelopes to prevent cardiac implantable electronic device infections: a meta-analysis. J Cardiovasc Electrophysiol, 2018, 29(4): 609–615. https://doi.org/10.1111/jce.13436.

[32] Habib G, Erba PA, Iung B, et al. Clinical presentation, aetiology and outcome of infective endocarditis. Results of the ESC-EORP EURO-ENDO (European infective endocarditis) registry: a prospective cohort study. Eur Heart J, 2019, 40(39): 3222–3232B. https://doi.org/10.1093/eurheartj/ehz620.

[33] Habib G, Lancellotti P, Erba PA, et al. The ESC-EORP EURO-ENDO (European infective endocarditis) registry. Eur Hear J - Qual Care Clin Outcomes, 2019, 5(3): 202–207. https://doi.org/10.1093/ehjqcco/qcz018.

[34] Van Vlasselaer A, Rasmussen M, Nilsson J, et al. Native aortic versus mitral valve infective endocarditis: a nationwide registry study. Open Hear, 2019, 6(1). https://doi.org/10.1136/openhrt-2018-000926.

[35] Di Mauro M, Foschi M, Dato GMA, et al. Surgical treatment of isolated tricuspid valve infective endocarditis: 25-year results from a multicenter registry. Int J Cardiol, 2019, 292: 62–67. https://doi.org/10.1016/j.ijcard.2019.05.020.

[36] Ris T, Teixeira-Carvalho A, Coelho RMP, et al. Inflammatory biomarkers in infective endocarditis: machine learning to predict mortality. Clin Exp Immunol, 2019, 196(3): 374–382. https://doi.org/10.1111/cei.13266.

[37] Sengupta PP, Huang YM, Bansal M, et al. Cognitive machine-learning algorithm for cardiac imaging; A pilot study for differentiating constrictive pericarditis from restrictive cardiomyopathy. Circ Cardiovasc Imaging, 2016, 9(6): 1–10. https://doi.org/10.1161/CIRCIMAGING.115.004330.

[38] Narula S, Shameer K, Salem Omar AM, et al. Machine-learning algorithms to automate morphological and functional assessments in 2D echocardiography. J Am Coll Cardiol, 2016, 68(21): 2287–2295. https://doi.org/10.1016/j.jacc.2016.08.062.

[39] Samad MD, Ulloa A, Wehner GJ, et al. Predicting survival from large echocardiography and electronic health record datasets: optimization with machine learning. JACC Cardiovasc Imaging, 2019, 12(4): 681–689. https://doi.org/10.1016/j.jcmg.2018.04.026.

[40] Mahmood M, Kendi AT, Ajmal S, et al. Meta-analysis of 18F-FDG PET/CT in the diagnosis of infective endocarditis. J Nucl Cardiol, 2019, 26(3): 922–935. https://doi.org/10.1007/s12350-017-1092-8.

[41] Pizzi MN, Roque A, Fernández-Hidalgo N, et al. Improving the diagnosis of infective endocarditis in prosthetic valves and intracardiac devices with ^{18}F-fluordeoxyglucose Positron emission tomography/computed Tomography angiography: initial results at an infective endocarditis referral center. Circulation, 2015, 132(12): 1113–1126. https://doi.org/10.1161/CIRCULATIONAHA.115.015316.

[42] Liesman RM, Pritt BS, Maleszewski JJ, et al. Laboratory diagnosis of infective endocarditis. J Clin Microbiol, 2017, 55(9): 2599–2608.

[43] Eichinger S, Kikhney J, Moter A, et al. Fluorescence in situ hybridization for identification and visualization of microorganisms in infected heart valve tissue as addition to standard diagnostic tests improves diagnosis of endocarditis. Interact Cardiovasc Thorac Surg, 2019, 29(5): 678–684. https://doi.org/10.1093/icvts/ivz159.

[44] Spellberg B, Chambers HF, Musher DM, et al. Evaluation of a paradigm shift from intravenous antibiotics to oral step-down therapy for the treatment of infective endocarditis: a narrative review. JAMA Intern Med, 2020, 180(5): 769–777. https://doi.org/10.1001/jamainternmed.2020.0555.

[45] Johnson JA, Feeney ER, Kubiak DW, et al. Prolonged use of oritavancin for vancomycin-resistant Enterococcus faecium prosthetic valve endocarditis. Open Forum Infect Dis, 2015, 1(4): 1–5. https://doi.org/10.1093/ofid/ofv156.

[46] Van Praet KM, Kofler M, Sündermann SH, et al. Minimally invasive approach for infective mitral valve endocarditis. Ann Cardiothorac Surg, 2019, 8(6): 702–704. https://doi.org/10.21037/acs.2019.07.01.

[47] Zhigalov K, Khokhlunov M, Szczechowicz M, et al. Right anterior minithoracotomy for endocarditis after transcatheter aortic valve replacement. Ann Thorac Surg, 2020, 109(1): e17–e19. https://doi.org/10.1016/j.athoracsur.2019.04.104.

[48] Starck CT, Dreizler T, Falk V. The AngioVac system as a bail-out option in infective valve endocarditis. Ann Cardiothorac Surg, 2019, 8(6): 675–677. https://doi.org/10.21037/acs.2019.11.04.

[49] Wang A, Chu VH, Athan E, et al. Association between the timing of surgery for complicated, left-sided infective endocarditis and survival. Am Heart J, 2019, 210: 108–116. https://doi.org/10.1016/j.ahj.2019.01.004.

[50] Venn RA, Ning MM, Vlahakes GJ, et al. Surgical timing in infective endocarditis complicated by intracranial hemorrhage. Am Heart J, 2019, 216: 102–112. https://doi.org/10.1016/j.ahj.2019.07.011.

[51] Diab M, Platzer S, Guenther A, et al. Assessing efficacy of CytoSorb haemoadsorber for prevention of organ dysfunction in cardiac surgery patients with infective endocarditis: REMOVE-protocol for randomized controlled trial. BMJ Open, 2020, 10(3): 1–8. https://doi.org/10.1136/bmjopen-2019-031912.

[52] Poli EC, Alberio L, Bauer-Doerries A, et al. Cytokine clearance with CytoSorb during cardiac surgery: a pilot randomized controlled trial. Crit Care, 2019, 23(1): 1–12. https://doi.org/10.1186/s13054-019-2399-4.

[53] Habib G, Lancellotti P, Antunes MJ, et al. 2015 ESC guidelines for the management of infective endocarditis. Eur Heart J, 2015, 36(44): 3075–3128. https://doi.org/10.1093/eurheartj/ehv319.

[54] Nishimura RA, Otto CM, Bonow RO, et al. 2017 AHA/ACC focused update of the 2014 AHA/ACC guideline for the management of patients with valvular heart disease: a report of the American college of Cardiology/American heart association task force on clinical practice guidelines. J Am Coll Cardiol, 2017, 70(2): 252–289. https://doi.org/10.1016/j.jacc.2017.03.011.

[55] Davierwala PM, Marin-Cuartas M, Misfeld M, et al. The value of an "endocarditis team. Ann Cardiothorac Surg, 2019, 8(6): 621–629. https://doi.org/10.21037/acs.2019.09.03.

[56] El-Dalati S, Khurana I, Soper N, et al. Physician perceptions of a multidisciplinary endocarditis team. Eur J Clin Microbiol Infect Dis, 2020, 39(4): 735–739. https://doi.org/10.1007/s10096-019-03776-9.